Orthopaedic Surgery in Infancy and Childhood

Fourth edition

Orthopaedic Surgery in Infancy and Childhood

Fourth edition

ALBERT BARNETT FERGUSON, JR., B.A., M.D.

Silver Professor of Orthopaedic
Surgery and Chairman, Department of Orthopaedic Surgery, University of Pittsburgh

Chief of Orthopaedic Service, University
of Pittsburgh Medical Center

Senior Staff—Children's
Hospital, Presbyterian—University Hospital, Pittsburgh

Active Staff—Allegheny General
Hospital, Pittsburgh

Chief Consultant—Veteran's Hospital (Oakland), Pittsburgh

Consultant—Mercy Hospital,
St. Francis Hospital, St. Margaret's Hospital, Montefiore Hospital, Pittsburgh

Williams and Wilkins Company, Baltimore

Made in the United States of America

Library of Congress Cataloging in Publication Data

Ferguson, Albert Barnett, 1919—
Orthopaedic surgery in infancy and childhood.

   1. Pediatric orthopedia. I. Title. [DNLM: 1. Orthopedics. 2. In infancy and childhood. WS270 F3520 1975]
RJ480.F47 1974   617'.3   74—5311
ISBN 0—683—03166—X

Composed and printed at the Waverly Press, Inc., Mt. Royal and Guilford Aves. Baltimore, Md. 21202, U.S.A.

Contributors

Mary Williams Clark, B.A., M.D.

Assistant Professor of Orthopaedic Surgery, University of Pittsburgh. Director of Physical Medicine Services, Children's Hospital of Pittsburgh. Assistant Chief, Rehabilitation Medicine, Health Center Hospital of Pittsburgh. Associate Staff, Children's Hospital, Presbyterian-University Hospital, Pittsburgh

William Fielding Donaldson, B.A., M.D., F.A.C.S.

Clinical Professor of Orthopaedic Surgery, University of Pittsburgh. Senior Staff—Children's Hospital Presbyterian-University Hospital, St. Francis Hospital, Shadyside Hospital, Pittsburgh. Attending Staff, Veteran's Hospital, (Oakland) Pittsburgh. Consultant, St. Margaret's Hospital, Home for Crippled Children, Pittsburgh.

William Thomas Green, Jr. B.A., M.D., F.A.C.S.

Assistant Professor, Department of Orthopaedic Surgery, University of Pittsburgh. Associate Staff, Children's Hospital, Presbyterian-University Hospital, Pittsburgh. Consultant, Veteran's Hospital (Oakland), John J. Kane Hospital, Pittsburgh

Ronald Carl Hillegass, B.A., M.D.

(Formerly) Assistant Professor of Orthopaedic Surgery, University of Pittsburgh. Attending Staff, Roger Williams Hospital, Rhode Island Hospital, Providence Rhode Island

James Henry McMaster, B.A., M.D.

Assistant Professor of Orthopaedic Surgery, University of Pittsburgh. Associate Staff, Children's Hospital, Presbyterian-University Hospital, Pittsburgh. Consultant, Veteran's Hospital, (Oakland) Pittsburgh. Director of Orthopaedic Research Laboratory, University of Pittsburgh

John A. Ogden, B.A., M.D.

Assistant Professor of Orthopaedic Surgery, Yale University Medical School. Director, Orthopaedic Section Human Growth and Development Unit, Yale University. Attending Staff, Yale-New Haven Hospital, Newington Children's Hospital, Connecticut. Consultant, Veteran's Hospital, West Haven, Connecticut

Frank H. Stelling III, M.D., F.A.C.S.

Chief Surgeon, Shriners Hospital for Crippled Children, Greenville Unit, Greenville, South Carolina. Associate Clinical Professor of Orthopaedic Surgery, Medical University of South Carolina. Assistant Clinical Professor of Orthopaedic Surgery, Duke University School of Medicine. Chairman, Education, Orthopedic Department, Greenville Hospital System

Charles S. Stone, B.S., M.D.

Clinical Instructor of Orthopaedic Surgery, University of Pittsburgh. Associate Staff, Children's Hospital, Presbyterian-University Hospital, St. Francis Hospital, St. Margaret's Hospital, West Penn Hospital, Shadyside Hospital, Pittsburgh

Harold Edward Swensen, B.S., M.D.

Clinical Assistant Professor of Orthopaedic Surgery, University of Pittsburgh. Associate Staff, Children's Hospital, Presbyterian-University Hospital, West Penn Hospital, Pittsburgh. Consultant, Magee-Womens Hospital, Western Psychiatric Hospital, Pittsburgh

H. Andrew Wissinger, B.S., M.D., F.A.C.S.

Clinical Associate Professor of Orthopaedic Surgery, University of Pittsburgh. Senior Staff, Children's Hospital, Presbyterian-University Hospital, St. Francis Hospital, St. Margaret's Hospital, Pittsburgh. Associate Director, Child Amputee Clinic of Pittsburgh. Consultant, State Crippled Children's Program of Pennsylvania. Consultant, Western State School and Hospital of Canonsburg, Pennsylvania

Preface to the first edition

This volume is the outgrowth of that period in life when the subject matter of orthopaedic surgery was laboriously amassed by running from text to text and article to article. Excellent though so many volumes are, none of them appeared to have gathered under one cover details regarding the many odd syndromes encountered in the practice of orthopaedic surgery dealing with infants and children. Pediatricians and residents have often indicated by their questions that they were undergoing a similar experience.

No syndrome, photograph or roentgenogram is presented which was not personally seen by the author. No feature of disease is reiterated which has not been a feature in our own experience.

Obviously no text arises without roots in the past, and the excellent volumes of Colonna, Howorth, Mercer, Platt, Wiles, Fairbank, Shands, Campbell, Luck, Smillie and DePalma have also served as references. This text does not include a consideration of fractures, for the subject is adequately covered in Walter Blount's recent book, *Fractures in Children*.

If clarity in visualizing these syndromes has been achieved, it is a reflection of the teaching of Joseph Barr, William T. Green and Albert B. Ferguson, Sr. They are not responsible for what others may deem as errors, however.

Certain areas in the book have been done by others. Frank Stelling has contributed his knowledge of reconstruction of the hand to the section on the upper extremity. Scoliosis is the work of William Donaldson of Pittsburgh. John Donaldson of Pittsburgh has added the chapter on the neck. Robert Klein encompasses rickets and scruvy from the metabolic point of view. Albert Ferguson, Sr., writes of defective formation of bone from cartilage. All these authors are deserving of my humble thanks in enabling a sound production of a book on orthopaedic surgery in the infant and childhood years.

The Children's Hospital of Pittsburgh is blessed with men of selfless spirit whose help has been invaluable. This is particularly true of Bertram Girdany, George Fetterman and Thomas Brower; although no one failed to respond when called upon. The pleasant and productive atmosphere of this hospital is a reflection of its guiding spirit and medical director, Edmund McCluskey.

The manuscript has been typed, retyped and retyped again by my secretary already overloaded with budgets, bills, and records. This type of dedication is typical of Mary Cosgrove.

My children and my wife, Louise, have taken night work, which deprived them of companionship, with good spirit. My wife's patient understanding is not found often in this world—without it such an arduous task could not be completed.

The drawings are the result of the talents of Margaret Croup except for those accompanying the section on the upper extremity. The photographs and roentgenogram reproductions were done by Albert Levine and James Stark. The patient cooperation exhibited by these worthy individuals has been a source of pleasure and has eased the task immeasurably.

The publishers and particularly Dick Hoover have been patient and have exhibited the skills of their profession with consummate ease.

Great care and effort have been used to duly credit thoughts, drawings and photographs whose origin might in any way be elsewhere. Should any omission have arisen, it is entirely inadvertent and not by conscious design.

The regional arrangement of the text will, we hope, make reference easy and invite a return visit.

A. B. F., Jr.

Preface to the fourth edition

There have been a number of objectives for this fourth edition. The illustrations, particularly those relating to surgical technique, have been increased in number, improved in quality, and made more informative. Information relating to any particular syndrome has been enlarged, with new information developed in greater depth and heavily referenced. Completeness has been a goal and all areas and types of disease and the relevant therapy increased in its coverage.

In addition, specific new material has been added, especially important here are "Developmental Anatomy" by John Ogden, specific scoliosis subjects by Charles Stone and William T. Green, Jr., the "Lower Extremity in Myelodysplasia" by Andrew Wissinger, "Hemophilia" by Ronald Hillegass, and "Amputations" by Mary Williams Clark.

Areas of recent interest and development such as congenital dislocation of the hip have been largely rewritten. New operations developed and followed by the author such as the treatment of plantar-flexed talus, dislocated hips and many others are included.

The fundamental approach to children's orthopaedics in a growing, maturing child is emphasized throughout.

The drawings, which are beautifully executed, are the work of Ron Filer, who very clearly grasps the principle being protrayed. Ann Eakins has taken great care with the photography, assuring that each illustration would clearly tell the message involved.

Mary Cosgrove has organized, typed and retyped and researched for material and is an indispensable part of the book's development.

With the help of many people this book is maturing into a valuable reference and text and is aimed to satisfy both the beginner and the highly trained orthopaedic surgeon. It it hoped that those who read it find it valuable.

PRECAUTION

I never dared be radical when young

For fear it would make me conservative when old.

Robert Frost

Table of contents

CONTENTS

CHAPTER 1

Orthopaedic Treatment of Childhood Disability

The child is a growing, maturing individual, a fact that must be kept in mind in the treatment phases of orthopaedic disability.

Braces must be used to enlarge, not limit, a child's horizon. All aspects of the child's development must be given attention at a time when the tendency is to rivet the attention on the single aspect of a deformity or loss of function under treatment. If treatment is always thought of in terms of total function of the child, these things can be brought into proper perspective. Surgical decisions are accurately made when the contribution of the surgical procedure to the total function of the child is ascertained. Decisions for long term hospitalization or physiotherapy must be made only after being weighed against the removal of the child from an area where emotional and intellectual development can be served. The rapid improvement in function occasionally possible with surgery is a point in its favor if it returns the child to a growth environment with greater opportunity to take part in it.

Many procedures fail because of a poor concept of what is necessary to make them work and increase the child's function. The procedure includes the postoperative period and the type of cast, traction, or physical therapy, the return home with adequate instruction for the parents and child, and the follow-up in the years following so that maximum function is achieved.

Factors which tend to make a deformity recur, such as growth, must be considered in on-going care. Unbalanced muscle pull and diseased tissue must be corrected or the limb braced until they can be corrected. The natural vigor of the child's tissues aids in regeneration of tissues if protection of the area is continued sufficiently long. During this period the hobbling effect of the treatment must be minimized so that the child can still take part in learning activities of all types.

GROWTH AFFECTING SKELETON

Many orthopaedic diseases may represent the development of a congenital abnormality. The variation usually appears in the specific age group in which the particular portion of the skeleton normally is differentiated. Growth may affect the degree of development of an abnormality such as scoliosis. The effect of growth on the development of deformity in the presence of unbalanced musculature of the limb is a very important underlying consideration in orthopaedics. The growing child with one muscle group dominating another, as in poliomyelitis, must be braced; but the unbraced adult with the same clinical picture does not necessarily develop a deformity.

Some understanding of human skeletal growth and its effects is essential to an understanding of orthopaedic disease.

Skeletal Growth

In order to appreciate growth at a given age, two types of studies may be done. Cross sectional studies, to be significant, require a large number of children, but they are more commonly carried out than longitudinal studies because of the time involved in studying one child throughout his growth period. From cross sectional studies, the mean measurement of any particular skeletal attribute is obtained. From longitudinal studies, the rate of change can be determined. Longitudinal studies are quite readily available to the orthopaedist because he usually follows up a patient throughout the growth period when a particular abnormality is present.

There is an exponential fall in the rate of mean gain in standing height for the human being except for two periods. The first delay in this fall is noted between 5½ and 7 years and is called the midgrowth spurt. The second delay is the adolescent growth spurt between 13 and 15 years (Fig. 1.1).

The growth rates in boys and girls are essentially the same except for the following variations. Boys may be slightly longer at birth, and they may grow slightly faster in the first year. Girls begin their adolescent growth spurt 2 years earlier than boys (at 11 instead of 13 years). During this spurt, they grow faster and larger than boys, but, slowing quickly, they are finally smaller than boys in all dimensions except pelvic width. The boys, commencing their adolescent growth spurt 2 years later, go on to grow for a longer period and to larger dimensions.

Because their growth period is longer, the boys have longer legs. Hormonal influences give the boys wider shoulders and the girls a wider pelvis. In boys there is also a relative increase in the amount of growth of the trunk (sitting height) to that of the legs (Fig 1.2). The

tremendous variation in this pattern in any one individual, racial group, or body type is readily evident.

Factors Affecting Growth

Prenatal

The influence of inherited factors is accepted. Such orthopaedic conditions as achondroplasia, spina bifida, dislocation of the hip, and osteogenesis imperfecta in genetic studies have been shown to result from a single gene mutation. The state of health of the mother also obviously affects the developing fetal skeleton.

Postnatal

Environmental and sociologic factors may influence the onset of puberty. Genetic factors

Fig. 1.1. Note the declination in height per year as growth progresses. The two periods during which this rate of decline levels off are known as the midgrowth spurt and the adolescent growth spurt. (This chart and the following one (Fig. 1.2) are reprinted with the permission of J. B. Lippincott Co., from R. Duthie: The significance of growth in orthopaedic surgery, *Clinical Orthopaedics, 14:* 7, 1959. They were prepared from data that originally appeared in K. Simmons: *The British Foundation Study of Child Growth and Development, II. Physical Growth and Development,* Monograph, Society for Research in Child Development, Vol. 9, No. 1, Serial 37, 1944.)

Fig. 1.2 Gain in millimeters per year in sitting height and leg length is contrasted in boys and girls. The later increase in leg length and sitting height of boys is evident.

are also still of importance. The state of health of the individual can result in skeletal dwarfism. Dietary factors are important.

Relation of Growth to Orthopaedic Conditions

The so-called osteochondritides are distinguished by their preference for a specific age group and often for a specific sex. If all cases were considered to occur at a physiologic rather than a chronologic age, their relationship to a specific age might be still more remarkable. Girls, because of their earlier skeletal maturation, would be expected to experience an earlier onset of these diseases, and, in osteochondritis involving the spine and Osgood-Schlatter disease, they do in fact (Fig. 1.3).

Tumors such as osteogenic sarcoma, neuroblastoma, and Ewing's chondrosarcoma and giant cell sarcoma are distinguished by their occurrence in specific age groups.

Scoliosis is a noteworthy anomaly in terms of relating growth to skeletal disease. That the curve in idiopathic scoliosis ceases to progress when spine growth is complete is documented (Fig. 1.4). Paralytic curvatures that have been doing well often develop into severe deformity during the adolescent growth spurt.

Temporary deformities that normally occur during development, such as genu valgus, which appears between the ages of 2 and 4 years and gradually improves thereafter, internal tibial torsion, and anteversion of the hip, are evidence of the influence of growth on the skeleton. The examples are many, for the influence of growth can be seen in most skeletal changes—normal and abnormal—of childhood.

References

1. Crompton, C. W.: Physiological age, a fundamental principle, *Child Develop., 15:* 1, 1944.
2. Duthie, R. B.: The significance of growth in orthopedic surgery, *Clin. Orthop., 14:* 7, 1959.
3. Price, C. H. S.: Osteogenic sarcoma; an analysis of the sex and age incidence, *Brit. J. Cancer, 9:* 558, 1955.
4. Simmons, K., and Todd, T. W.: Growth of well children: analysis of stature and weight, 3 months to 13 years, *Growth, 2:* 93, 1938.

Osteochondritis of:	Usual Age at Diagnosis	Range of Age Incidence	Sex Incidence	Year of Appearance of Epiphysis MALE FEMALE	
Upper Femoral Epiphysis (Legg-Calve-Perthes' Disease)	5 - 9	$3\frac{1}{2}$ - 15	M > F	1	$\frac{1}{4}$
Tuberosity of Tibia (Osgood-Schlatter's Disease)	12 - 15	10 - 23	M > F	11	11
Navicular Bone (Kohler's Disease)	3 - 8	$2\frac{1}{2}$ - 10	M > F	2 - 4	2 - 4
Calcanean Tubercles (Haglund's Disease)	$8\frac{1}{2}$ - 15	8 - 22	M > F	10	8
Head of Second Metatarsal Bone (Freiberg's Disease)	10 - 18	10 - 45	F > M	3	2
Upper and Lower Epiphyses of Vertebrae (Scheuermann's Disease)	10 - 21	.	M > F	10	10

Fig. 1.3. Relationship of some orthopaedic conditions in childhood to specific age groups. Growth and its effects may be a prime underlying factor in delineating these age groups. (Reproduced with the permission of J. B. Lippincott Co., from R. Duthie: The significance of growth in orthopaedic surgery, *Clinical Orthopaedics, 14:* 7, 1959.)

GROWTH OF EPIPHYSIS

There is a startling ability of the epiphysis to recover from injury. This is substantiated by animal experiments. On the other hand, trauma (the effects of which are virtually undiscernible on the roentgenogram) may result in real growth inhibition and subsequent deformity in the human (Fig. 1.5).

Selye[4] removed the entire epiphysis in rats and found that a complete new functional epiphysis developed in 12-15-day-old rats. This potential was confined to very young animals and did not occur in mature rats. Ford and Key[1] found that drilling the central portion of the epiphyseal plate produced no deformity in rabbits, whereas peripheral damage caused extensive changes. Langenskiold and Edgren[2] produced small central areas of destruction with x-ray and found that there was ingrowth of cartilage cells from the surrounding undamaged areas and no deformity resulted with growth. Friedenberg[2] found after partial resection of the epiphysis in rabbits that the shortening and deformity that occurred was related to the remaining length of the undamaged epiphyseal line and the extent of reactive bone bridging the epiphyseal line. There was no evidence of cartilage regeneration. Normal growth in the remnants of the epiphyseal line occurred in some specimens where there was obvious bridging.

References

1. Ford, L. T., and Key, J. A.: A study of experimental trauma to the distal femoral epiphysis in rabbits, *J. Bone Joint Surg., 38A:* 84, 1956.
2. Friedenberg, L. A.: Reaction to partial surgical resection of the epiphysis, *J. Bone Joint Surg., 39A:* 332, 1957.
3. Langenskiold, A., and Edgren, W.: Imitation of chondrodysplasia by localized reontgen ray; an experimental study of bone growth, *Acta Chir. Scand., 99:* 352, 1949.
4. Selye, H.: On the mechanism controlling growth in long bones, *J. Anat., 68:* 289, 1934.

DEVELOPMENT OF EPIPHYSIS AND GROWTH PLATE

An understanding of the dynamic development of the growth plate is implicit to comprehension of the multiple problems of pediatric orthopaedics. This structure is responsible for the enlargement of immature bone, by elaboration of both cellular constituents and intercellular matrices. The most important aspect of the growth plates is that they provide for a controlled, rapid expansion of preformed cartilage models.

A discrete structure that can be classified as a growth plate appears relatively late in the development of long bones, and even later in the development of epiphyses, apophyses, and the small bones of the wrist and ankle. Initially the axial skeleton and, shortly thereafter, the

Fig. 1.4. Relation of increase in curvature in children with infantile scoliosis to the gain in millimeters per year in sitting height.

limb buds form mesenchymal condensations that begin conversion to cartilage by the fifth to sixth weeks. These small cartilagenous anlagen then enlarge by interstitial and appositional expansion of cells throughout their length, and particularly at the ends. The cartilage cells in the center of the anlage then begin to hypertrophy (Fig. 1.6a). A periosteal cuff forms around the center of the anlage by the end of the sixth week. The hypertrophic central cartilage continues to mature and calcify, and subsequently begins ossification concomitant with the penetration of the irruption artery. The central shaft converst to bone and leaves cartilage at each end. This junction between bone and cartilage is initially not a discrete structure (Fig. 1.6b). By the third month these junctional cartilage cells have assumed a typical columniated appearance (Fig. 1.6c). From this point of differential develop-

Fig. 1.5. *(A)* This 14-year-old boy has shortening and angulation of the tibia secondary to epiphyseal injury. *(B)* The growth arrest occurred medially at the proximal tibial epiphysis. The continued growth of a major portion of the lateral segment produced the severe deformity.

ment, further specialization of the growth plate is contingent upon the type of bone and varies considerably.

There are two basic types of growth plate, discoid and spherical. Most primary growth plates of the long bones are discoid—a relatively planar area of rapidly differentiating and maturing cartilage between the epiphysis and metaphysis. These contribute to longitudinal as well as circumferential increase in bone size. These discoid growth plates are also found between apophyses and shafts. There are several anatomic variations. In shorter, tubular bones, such as the metacarpals, metatarsals, and phalanges, two discoid growth plates are initially present, but, with further skeletal growth and maturation, only one end of the bone forms a true epiphysis. The growth plate at the opposite end becomes juxtaposed to the developing articular cartilage and more closely resembles a spherical, rather than discoid, growth plate (Fig. 1.7). The growth plate of the calcaneal apophysis, although discoid, curves around the posteroinferior body of the calcaneus. A spherical growth plate is found in the small bones of the wrist and ankle, as well as in early development of the secondary ossification centers of the epiphyses and apophyses. The

growth plate surrounds an evolving ossific nucleus that is analogous to the metaphysis. In the small bones of the wrist and ankle, as well as the apophyses, this spherical growth plate gradually assumes the contour of the bone. In the epiphyses the spherical growth plate and ossification centers enlarge and lead to juxtaposition of the spherical secondary center growth plate and discoid primary growth plate (Fig. 1.8), temporarily creating a bipolar growth zone between the epiphyseal ossification center and the metaphysis. The spherical secondary center growth plate is eventually replaced by a subchondral bone plate where it is apposed to the primary discoid growth plate. However, the spherical growth plate does remain along the epiphyseal borders and under the articular surface to allow expansion of the epiphysis commensurate with diametric growth of the shaft. The vertebral body initially has a spherical growth plate (Fig. 1.9), which disappears by gradual expansion of the ossification center and becomes two parallel discoid growth plates on the upper and lower surfaces of the vertebral body. However, no true vertebral epiphyses develop (in essence, the intervertebral disc occupies the analogous anatomical position of the epiphysis). The bipolar growth plate of

Fig. 1.6. Stages in the early development of the growth plate. Readings refer to crown-rump length of the embryo or fetus. At 20 mm *(a)*, a midshaft periosteal cuff is beginning to form. No growth plate is present. At 12 cm *(b)*, the primary ossification center has extended along the shaft. There is a distinct margin between cartilage and bone. But the characteristic columniation is not yet present. By 15 cm (*c*), about 4½ months, the growth plate has assumed its characteristic appearance. Also, the chondroepiphysis is now beginning to develop a circulatory (cartilage canal) system.

Fig. 1.7. First phalanx of the foot in a full-term fetus. Note the contour differences between the proximal (discoid) growth plate and the distal (spherical) growth plate. Also note that the ends of the phalanges and metatarsal that will form true epiphyses have a cartilage canal system, while the distal end of the proximal phalanx, which does not form bony epiphysis, has no cartilage canal system.

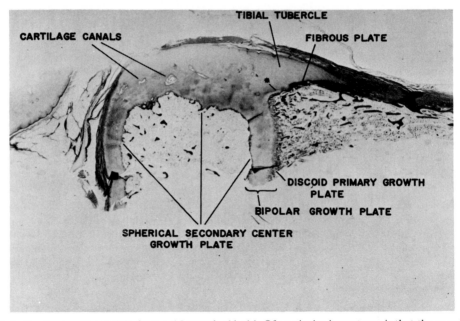

Fig. 1.8. Proximal, anterior tibia from a 15-month-old girl. Of particular importance is that the growth plate stops at the beginning of the tibial tubercle (*), and does not extend down the posterior aspect of the tubercle, as is usually described. This area is instead comprised of fibrous tissue.

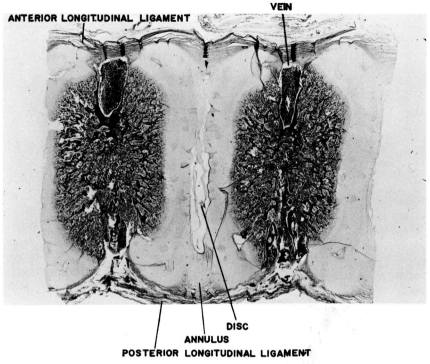

ANTERIOR LONGITUDINAL LIGAMENT

VEIN

DISC
ANNULUS
POSTERIOR LONGITUDINAL LIGAMENT

Fig. 1.9. Lumbar vertebrae from a 2-month-old neonate. Both the anterior and posterior longitudinal ligaments are well developed. The disc (nucleus pulposus) occupies a much larger area than in the adult.

the triradiate (acetabular) cartilage develops by the juxtaposition of spherical growth plates of the various pelvic ossification centers.

The growth plate has a characteristic and virtually unchanging architectural pattern from early fetal life to skeletal maturation. The structure can be arbitrarily broken down into different zones using either histologic or functional criteria—the zone of growth, the zone of cartilage maturation, and zone of transformation (Fig. 1.10).

The zone of growth is concerned with longitudinal and diametric expansion of the bone. It is the only area where cell addition and multiplication occurs (the other regions are concerned with matrix elaboration and transformation to bone). The resting cells are intimately associated with the blood vessels that cover the zone of growth (E-vessels). These vessels may be instrumental in providing undifferentiated cells that will become the resting chondrocytes. Additional resting cells are also elaborated peripherally through the perichondrial ring (zone of Ranvier). The next stage in the zone of growth is cell division. This occurs

in transverse and longitudinal directions and leads to the formation of the cell columns characteristic of the growth plate. These cell columns constitute about one-half of the overall height of the growth plate. The randomly dispersed collagen of the resting/dividing regions becomes longitudinally oriented along these cell columns.

The next area is the zone of cartilage transformation. In this zone the intercellular matrix undergoes the significant biochemical changes necessary for eventual ossification. The matrix becomes metachromatic and calcifies. The chondrocytes become hypertrophic, a reflection of their increased metabolic activity. The fate of these chondrocytes at the end of the zone of cartilage transformation is controversial—some feel that the cells degenerate, while others feel the cells modulate to become osteoblasts. It is quite likely that both processes occur.

The last zone is that of cartilage transformation. The cartilage matrix is replaced by bone. Most characteristic of the region is vascular invasion (M-vessels). Electron micros-

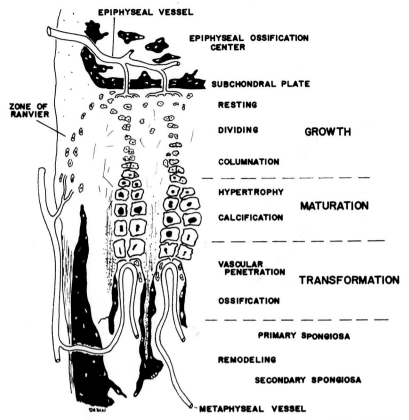

Fig. 1.10. Schematic depiction of the architecture of a discoid growth plate. The spherical growth plate is similar, but there is no subchondral plate and the cell columns are quite short.

copy has confirmed that these capillary loops are a closed circulation. They undoubtedly are a source of cells necessary to the formation of bone. Osteoblasts elaborate osteoid on the performed calcified cartilage, transforming it to bone. This bone surrounding cartilage is the primary spongiosa. By remodeling, this bone is replaced by a more mature secondary spongiosa. In the neonatal skeleton this zone of very active bone formation and remodeling is the weakest structurally, and fractures during birth or infancy occur in this region of the metaphysis, rather than through the growth plate itself, as in the classical Salter I or II injury of the older child.

The growth plate derives blood supply from three major regions, the epiphyseal circulation (E-vessels), the metaphyseal circulation (M-vessels), and the perichondrial circulation.

The epiphyseal circulation varies considerably, depending upon whether the epiphysis is principally cartilage or bone. The vessels enter in regions characteristic for each epiphysis, usually in the regions of capsular and perichondrial attachment. In the apophyses there is extensive vascular penetration along the tendinous insertions.

Vessels enter the chondroepiphyses in cartilage canals (Fig. 1.11). These canals course throughout the cartilage, supplying discrete regions, with minimum anastomosis between major canal systems. These canal systems send branches down to the resting cell region of the growth plate. Occasionally these vessels communicate across the growth plate, anastomosing with the metaphyseal circulation (Fig. 1.12). The vessels that cross the growth plate tend to be found in the larger epiphyses (proximal and distal femur, proximal humerus) for several months, but become less frequent as the secondary ossification center forms and enlarges. By the time the subchondral plate is formed, no vessels cross the growth plate.

The cartilage canals have several important

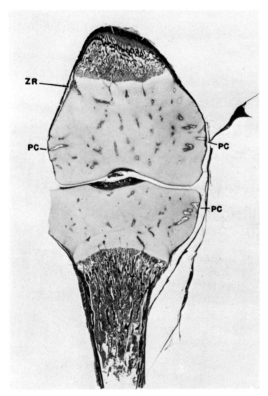

Fig. 1.11. Sagittal section of the knee of a 7-month-old fetus showing the extensive cartilage canal system. (*RZ,* zone of Ranvier; *PC,* perichondrium.)

characteristics. First, and most important, they supply discrete regions within the epiphysis, with virtually no anastomosis between canalicular systems of adjacent regions. Second, the canals enter the epiphysis at fairly regular intervals along the growth plate periphery, but much more irregularly in other regions of the epiphysis. Third, the canals probably serve as a source of chondroblasts for interstitial enlargement of the epiphysis. Fourth, the canals are surrounded by a more dense area of cartilage and intercellular matrix that probably renders an internal support system to the chondroepiphysis and protects the canals from collapse during load-bearing stress (Fig. 1.13). And fifth, the canals play an integral role in the development of the secondary ossification center (Fig. 1.14).

Once the ossification center begins to form and enlarge, the epiphyseal circulatory pattern changes. Several cartilage canal systems send vessels into the ossification center, creating significant anastomoses between canal systems that previously were virtually endarterial. Enlargement of the ossification center leads to the formation of a subchondral bone plate adjacent to the growth plate. Small branches cross this bone plate and form vascular expansions that supply regions containing several cell columns (Fig. 1.15). The proximity of vessels and resting cells suggests that the resting cells may originate from vascular endothelium or privascular tissue. These arborizing vessels never penetrate between cell columns. There do not appear to be any anastomoses between these perforating arteries after they cross the subchondral plate. However, before crossing the bony plate there are extensive anastomoses.

If a portion of the epiphyseal circulation is compromised, the zones of growth and transformation associated with the affected vessels cannot undergo appropriate cell division and maturation. The unaffected surrounding growth plate continues to grow longitudinally, resulting in the affected portion being "pulled" toward the metaphysis (Fig. 1.17). The rate of growth of the cells adjacent to the infarcted area would be more compromised (by tethering effect) than the rate of growth of cells much further away. If the involved area is peripherally situated, this results in tilting of the epiphysis relative to the metaphysis. If the circulatory compromise occurs while the epiphysis is still primarily cartilaginous, the infarcted area may continue to grow, but at a significantly decreased rate compared to adjacent growth plate. But in the older child with an ossification center, the damaged segment of the growth plate may be "pulled" far enough into the metaphysis to allow a bony bridge to replace the damaged cartilage, connecting the metaphysis and epiphyseal ossification center. If a large enough segment of the growth plate is replaced by a bone bridge, an epiphyseodesis may result. If the subchondral plate is damaged during the injury to the epiphyseal circulation, significant epiphyseodesis invariably results.

The metaphyseal circulation is derived primarily from the nutrient artery. However, small branches from the perichondrial circulation also enter the periphery of the metaphysis (Fig. 1.16). The terminal portions of both arterial systems form a series of parallel loops that

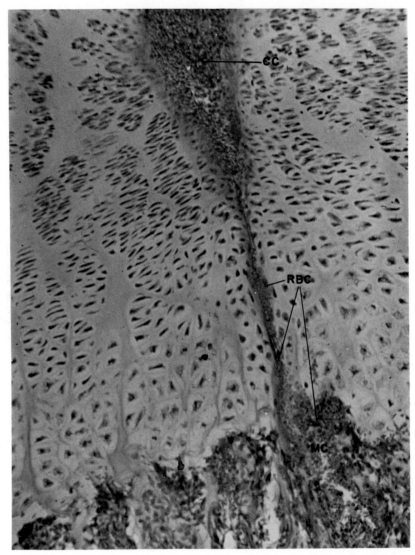

Fig. 1.12. A blood vessel crossing the growth plate of the proximal femur in a full-term fetus. (*CC*, cartilage (epiphyseal) canal; *RBC*, red blood cells in the communicating canal; *MC*, metaphyseal circulation.)

Fig. 1.13. Representative cartilage canal in a 2-month-old neonate, showing the artery *(A)*, vein *(V)*, undifferentiated mesenchymal tissue *(M)*, the densely stained matrix surrounding the canal *(DM)*, and the differentiating and maturing hyaline cartilage *(HyC)*.

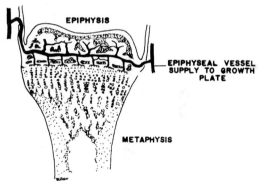

Fig. 1.15. Epiphyseal circulation, with vessels penetrating the subchondral bone plate to supply the growth plate.

penetrate between the trabeculae of the primary spongiosa to reach the end of the hypertrophic region. These vessels do not form an open communication with the "empty" lacunae. The venule side of the loops terminate

Fig. 1.14. Cartilage canal glomerular ending *(CCG)* in the middle of a group of hypertrophic hyaline cartilage cells *(HC)*, from the early ossification center of the proximal humerus of a 2-month-old neonate.

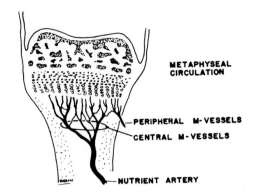

Fig. 1.16. Metaphyseal circulation, with contributions from the perichondral and nutrient circulations.

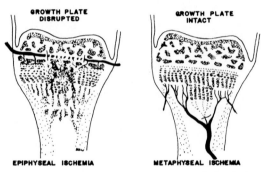

Fig. 1.17. Disruption of the epiphyseal circulation usually leads to damage to the structural integrity of the growth plate, whereas metaphyseal ischemia results in widening of the growth plate, but leaves the basic structure intact.

as large sinusoids. These capillary loops and venous sinusoids are not associated with any reticuloendothelial system, which, along with the rheologic changes in this type of network, may explain the predisposition to infection localization adjacent to the growth plate.

Interruption of the metaphyseal circulation has no effect on chondrogenesis and maturation of the growth plate, but transformation to bone is blocked. This causes significant widening of the affected portion as more cartilage is added in the resting/maturation regions, while no cartilage is replaced by bone in the transformation region (Fig. 1.17). When the metaphyseal circulation is reestablished (which occurs quickly, since the metaphyseal circulation has significant anastomoses near the terminal loops), the broad, already calcified region is rapidly penetrated and ossified, returning the growth plate to normal width.

The perichondral circulation, besides providing branches to the metaphyseal circulation peripherally, also supplies the peripheral regions of the growth plate in a region called the zone of Ranvier. This region is necessary to the appositional enlargement of the growth plate. Compromise of the vessels probably causes decreased diametric expansion of the growth plate.

Characteristically growth of long bones is considered a *longitudinal* phenomenon. However, the growth plates may expand in two other significant ways. The discoid growth plate must also grow in a diametric, or latitudinal, direction. This occurs by cell division and matrix expansion within the plate (interstitial expansion) or by cell addition at the peripheral zone of Ranvier (appositional expansion). The spherical growth plate expands primarily by rapid interstitial expansion, with radially directed "longitudinal" growth that corresponds to the longitudinal metaphyseal erosion of the discoid growth plate (Fig. 1.18). Such interstitial expansion of the epiphyseal growth plate occurs throughout the existence of the ossification center, even after it has assumed the general contour of the epiphysis. Interstitial growth in the discoid growth plate is probably directly related to the epiphyseal ossification center. When there is a chondroepiphysis, or even when a small epiphyseal ossification center is present, the pliable hyaline epiphyseal cartilage continuous with the growth plate probably does not present a mechanical barrier to interstitial expansion. But with increasing development of the epiphyseal ossification center, a discrete subchondral bone plate forms, to which the underlying portions of the discoid growth plate become "attached." Further in-

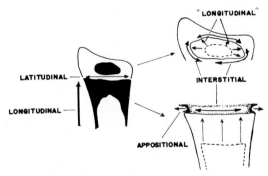

Fig. 1.18. Types of growth in the discoid and spherical growth plates.

terstitial, latitudinal expansion of the discoid growth plate is precluded in the areas under this subchondral plate (Fig. 1.19). When the secondary ossification center approximates the diametric size of the juxtaposed metaphysis, latitudinal expansion of the discoid growth plate is possible only at the periphery (appositional growth).

Two regions of the developing skeleton show growth variations that can be explained by the presence or absence of this mechanical limitation to interstitial expansion. The distal humerus of the neonate has a capitulum and trochlea of approximately equal cross sectional areas. The ossification center of the capitulum develops during the third to fifth months, and thus presents an early limitation to interstitial expansion of that portion of the distal humeral growth plate associated with the capitulum. In contrast, the ossification center of the trochlea does not appear until 7-8 years of age, allowing both interstitial as well as appositional expansion of the distal humeral growth plate associated with the trochlea. The mature trochlea is considerably larger than the mature capitulum. Eventually these two ossification centers coalesce, and permit continued expansion of the distal humerus in fully integrated fashion. The proximal femur similarly shows the appearance of two separate ossification centers (capital femur and greater trochanter) at different times. However, the central region, which will eventually become the intertrochanteric groove, never has a limiting bony plate and continues interstitial expansion, contributing to the length of the femoral neck (Fig. 1.20).

In the epiphysis the articular cartilage and nonarticular contours do not present as rigid a limiting structure to interstitial expansion of the spherical growth plate of the epiphyseal ossification center.

The effects of force on growth cartilage and epiphyseal cartilage are incompletely understood. Physiologic stress appears necessary for continued, orderly development of both discoid and spherical growth plates. These stresses may result from compression or tension forces. All growth plates must be able to initially respond to both compression and tension induced stress. However, as each growth plate develops, it may become primarily responsive to either compression (epiphyseal growth plates) or tension (apophyseal growth plates). Since a growth

Fig. 1.19. Maturation of the ossification center precludes further interstitial enlargement of the growth plate and limits latitudinal expansion to appositional growth.

plate, such as the proximal femur, may develop into one section that responds to tension (under the greater trochanter), it is reasonable to assume that there is a biologic range of compression-tension response for each growth plate. Within this physiologic range, increasing tension or compression probably accelerates growth, whereas decreasing tension or compression decelerates growth. Beyond the physiologic limits of compression, growth may be significantly decreased. The response (i.e., rate of growth) is probably greater to compression than tension (e.g., the differential rates of growth of the capital femoral and greater trochanteric sections of the proximal femoral growth plate).

The discoid growth plate is never completely planar, but rather is variably convoluted, because each growth plate tends to align its various regions to be perpendicular to the absorbed forces in each region. This minimizes shear stresses within the discoid growth plate. Similarly, the spherical growth plates of the epiphyses, carpus, and tarsus respond to compression and tension forces *within* the chondroepiphysis, and form characteristic shapes that best respond to the stress patterns (e.g., the nonspherical shape of the early proximal tibial ossification center).

When the hyaline cartilage of the chondroepiphysis first forms, there is no significant difference histochemically between the cartilage at the joint surface and the cartilage within the epiphysis. But during the last month of intrauterine development and particularly during the first year of life, significant changes occur such that the articular cartilage becomes histochemically different from the underlying hyaline cartilage. Further, this articular cartilage will not calcify or ossify. If a piece of articular cartilage is embedded in the hyaline

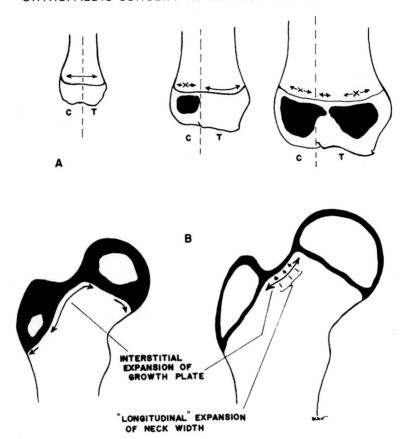

Fig. 1.20. *(A)* Sequential development of the distal humerus. Development of the ossification center of the capitulum (*C*) first limits interstitial expansion on the lateral half of the distal humeral growth plate. Eventual development of the trochlear (*T*) ossification center then limits interstitial enlargement of the medial half of the distal humeral growth plate. These two ossification centers then fuse, completely stopping interstitial expansion. *(B)* Sequential development of the proximal femur. Unlike the distal humerus, the two initially separate ossification centers do not fuse, allowing continued interstitial expansion to form the length of the femoral neck. In addition, this portion of the growth plate also grows "longitudinally," contributing to overall neck diameter. Disruption of this region can lead to shortening and narrowing of the femoral neck.

cartilage, the epiphyseal ossification center will develop all around it, but the cartilage will remain unchanged. As skeletal maturity is reached a tidemark develops that delineates articular cartilage from underlying mature epiphyseal cartilage and subchondral bone.

BY JOHN OGDEN, M.D.

DISTINGUISHING GROWTH LINES FROM FRACTURE LINES*

Distinguishing the growth line from the fracture line can be a very troublesome medico-

legal problem. A knowledge of their characteristics and features in their occurrence is at times helpful.

This is illustrated in spondylolisthesis where the defect in the neural arch may be pointed out following trauma as due to the injury. The clue to the correct diagnosis is furnished by the sacrum. Ordinarily its superior border is the same width as the inferior border of the fifth lumbar vertebra. With forward slip of the vertebra, however, the sacrum builds up an anterior prominence resulting in the widening of its superior border, which would not be present if the injury were a fracture.

---

* This section, "Distinguishing Growth Lines from Fracture Lines," is reprinted from A. B. Ferguson, Jr.:

Growth lines versus fracture lines, *Journal of the Medical Association of Georgia, 46:* 55, 1957.

X-ray Characteristics

A fracture line varies in width and has sharp angles and edges. A growth line is the same width all the way across with rounded edges (Fig. 1.22).

The suture lines of a skull are growth lines. Here the line has maintained its width throughout or, if narrowing, does so in a symmetrical artistic manner, one edge of the line undulating with the other. Inspection reveals apparently sharp angles to actually be rounded or blunted.

The problem of distinguishing growth lines from fracture lines is not always easy. The pull off fracture at the base of the fifth metatarsal is a good example. The shell of bone forming a

Fig. 1.21. An accessory center of ossification, when it is combined with the parent bone, forms a bone that is larger than the normal size of the particular bone. Diagram of the normal *(A)* is compared with an accessory ossification center *(B)* at the medial malleolus; the combined size of the ossification center and the medial malleolus is larger than normal.

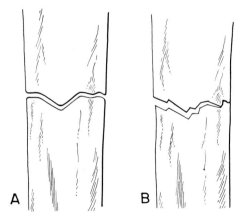

Fig. 1.22. The growth line *(A)* is of equal width throughout and has rounded points rather than sharp angles. The fracture line *(B)* is of uneven width and has sharp angles.

separate growth center in this area can easily be mistaken for fracture unless the fundamental characteristics of the fracture line are borne in mind (Fig. 1.21).

The accessory growth center at the medial or lateral malleolus about the ankle joint is similarly difficult and leads us to several additional characteristics which may be helpful. Soft-tissue swelling in the area of injury helps lead the eye to the injured area, but may be stimulated by ankle sprain. More important is the fact that the accessory center in combination with the parent bony area is always larger than the expected size of the part with a single growth center. In cases where for one reason or another the growth line is difficult to see, this point may assume great importance.

Some areas where separate growth centers occur normally include the lower pole of the patella where the characteristic growth line can be seen separating the apophysis from the parent bone (Fig. 1.23).

Fracture Lines That Cannot Be Seen

Where the fracture line is invisible to ordinary roentgen technique, other signs must be relied upon.

The epiphyseal line fracture when little or no displacement of the epiphysis has occurred is one of these. It must be recognized that the epiphyseal line fracture occurs on the metaphyseal side of the line and always takes with it a triangle of metaphyseal bone, however small.

Where the epiphyseal line appears intact, a search for this triangle of metaphyseal bone will frequently lead to the diagnosis which otherwise might be missed. Where epiphyseal displacement is marked, there is no diagnostic problem—in these cases the triangular area of metaphyseal bone can be seen. Common areas for this type of fracture are the distal radius and the lateral condyle of the humerus. In either case the soft-tissue swelling and slight elevation of the metaphyseal cortex may be the only leads.

In infants where the growth center for the epiphysis has not yet been seen, the diagnostic problem becomes even more difficult. Epiphyseal line fractures at this time of life are frequently called dislocations if seen early before a calcifying callus is seen, or bone tumors when seen late with a massive and

Fig. 1.23. Apophysis ossifiying at the lower pole of the patella. A growth line, not a fracture line, divides it from the parent bone. Note the rounded edges and constant width of the line.

apparently wild growth of bone engulfing the metaphyseal area.

The reason for the appearance of dislocation is obvious. The metaphysis and diaphysis of the involved bone no longer have the expected anatomical relationship to the joint. The epiphysis, however, remains in the joint, the fracture allowing the remainder of the bone to displace away from it. The small triangle of metaphyseal bone will be present, however, still attached to the epiphysis. Knowledge of the weakness of this area as compared to the possibility of dislocation helps and will prevent useless manipulation to reduce the joint. Such fractures surround themselves with such exuberant callus that rapid remodeling in the presence of good general limb alignment tends to obliterate all evidence of the fracture. The displacement into varus or valgus at either side of the knee

joint may be troublesome, however, and require several years to recover normal alignment.

The two most common situations in which this injury is mistaken for dislocation include the elbow and hip.

MULTIPLE TRAUMA

The chief complaint when infants and children subject to multiple trauma are seen is unexplained inability to use a limb. Some patients, however, arrive with multiple contusions and occasionally with obvious severe injuries and poor systemic conditions verging on shock. Investigation of the circumstances of an obvious severe injury leads in the usual course of events, to an uncovering of the family situation that is responsible for the injury.

Diagnosis of the more isolated, but recurring, disability requires more subtlety. These children come to orthopaedic attention as diagnostic problems from the roentgenographic point of view. Confusion with metabolic bone disease may arise.

Clinical Picture

In addition to soft-tissue contusions, swelling at the distal end of one or more of the long bones is often seen. The general health on examination is usually found to be good, although malnutrition of the infant or child may be present. The initial history of the injury is vague because the person bringing the child attempts to conceal the true nature of events from the examiner.

Roentgen Picture

The usual injury is an epiphyseal fracture without marked displacement. Such fractures are recognized by the triangular area of metaphysis which is fractured off in the process of even a minimal displacement (Figs. 1.24-1.26). They take place on the metaphyseal side of the epiphyseal line but are always accompanied by the metaphyseal fragment as well.

BIRTH FRACTURE

EPIPHYSEAL FRACTURE

Fig. 1.24 *(Left)*. The typical birth fracture at the ends of long bones is an epiphyseal fracture. When the epiphysis has not ossified, the fracture may be mistaken for dislocation due to displacement of the shaft in relation to the joint. In the diagram, the femoral head is stippled to indicate its location, but all that is seen by roentgenogram is the small triangle of metaphysis carried with it. Epiphyseal fractue is much more likely than dislocation secondary to birth trauma.

Fig. 125 *(Right)*. Epiphyseal fracture is recognized by the small triangular fragment of the metaphysis that is carried with the epiphysis even when displacement is minimal.

Suspicion of the diagnosis is aroused by evidences of other trauma. These may consist of fractures of a minimal nature so far as displacement is concerned and in various stages of healing. Rib fractures or old healed malunions may be noted. Confusion sometimes arises because of thickening of the diaphysis caused by repeated subperiosteal hemorrhages. These result in bizarre-appearing bones without evidence of normal remodeling (Fig. 1.27).

Treatment

The individual fractures are usually without marked displacement and require the usual plaster immobilization. Of far more importance is the attempt to save these children from further injury. A close interrogation of the person bringing the child to medical attention in most cases brings the reason for the child's dilemma to light.

Possible causes include psychiatric disturbance in the mother or father, alcoholism in the family, or brutality from other children. The physician who makes the diagnosis is responsible for following through with a social investigation of the family background and for procuring the help of whatever agencies may be available to seek a solution to the situation.

References
1. Caffey, J.: Multiple fractures in long bones of infants suffering from chronic subdural hematoma, *Am. J. Roentgenol., 56:* 163, 1946.
2. Friedman, M. S.: Traumatic periotitis in infants and children, *J.A.M.A., 166:* 1840, 1958.
3. Miller, D. S.: Fractures among children. I. Parental assault as causative agent, *Minn. Med., 42:* 1209, 1959.
4. Silverman, F. N.: Roentgen manifestations of unrecognized skeletal trauma in infants, *Am. J. Roentgenol., 69:* 413, 1953.

UNEQUAL LEG LENGTH

Unequal length of the upper extremities is virtually unnoticeable except in extreme cases. On the other hand, a difference in length of more than ½-inch in the lower extremities constitutes a definite disability.

The limp produced is marked and necessitates application of a noticeable raise to the shoe, and the psychic distress and motor disability justify corrective measures.

Fig. 1.26. Anteroposterior view *(top)* of the distal tibial epiphyseal line bilaterally is not very remarkable. The lateral view *(bottom)* shows the slight displacement of the epiphysis and the small triangle of metaphysis carried with it posteriorly.

Etiology

Overgrowth

Overgrowth stems from one of two main causes. It is a result either of a congenital disability or of some local cause of excessive blood supply to an epiphyseal area. Entities such as hemihypertrophy fall in the first group. The second class contains chronic synovitis of the knee, vascular tumors, and arteriovenous shunts. Neurofibroma with elephantiasis of an extremity and chronic osteomyelitis associated with long-standing hyperemia, but not with destruction of the epiphyseal line, also result in increased growth. Fractures of the midshaft, particularly when the reduction is not anatomic, are likely causes of abnormal gain in length.

Delayed Growth

Again, congenital abnormalities may give rise to severe discrepancies. These include hemiatrophy, congenital short femur (Fig. 1.31), chondrodysplasia, and congenital absence of

Fig. 1.27. In a child with multiple trauma, fractures in various stages of healing can be seen. Here, the two rib fractures, one almost healed, are evident, and ossification at the distal end of the humerus due to old epiphyseal fracture is seen. Note also the widening of the medullary canal of the distal humerus due to repeated subperiosteal hemorrhages and the remodeling that is not quite sufficient to withstand repeated episodes of trauma.

the tibia or fibula. Disorders caused locally include the atrophy of poliomyelitis and denervation with undergrowth of the affected extremity. Loss of soft tissues due to trauma, actual destruction of the epiphyses due either to trauma or to infection may affect leg length. Radiation trauma may be especially significant in infants. Trauma to the epiphyseal plate of a crushing nature may affect the plate to varying degrees, or growth may occur asymmetrically with resultant deformity. Epiphyses have been noted to undergo premature closure, which is often associated with prolonged disability, for example, in conjunction with bone and joint tuberculosis.

Clinical Picture

The patient often first complains chiefly of limp. Prominence of one hip may be noted (Figs. 1.28 and 1.29).

When the child stands, the pelvic crests, posterosuperior spines of the sacrum, and knee

creases are not symmetric. An appropriate raise applied under the heel of the short leg balances the pelvic crests and spines and gives an estimate of the discrepancy. The so-called "real" measurement of the leg is taken from the anterosuperior spine of the ilium to the medial malleolus. This is still not an accurate bone measurement, but it is a good clinical guide. The relationship of the hip to the pelvis may affect the functional length of the leg. Adducting the hip results in elevation of the pelvis and consequent shortening. Abducting the hip gives rise to relative lengthening. These effects are taken into account by measuring from the umbilicus to the medial malleolus bilaterally.

Other factors that affect leg length include fixed pelvic obliquity, and the ability of the pelvis to change position freely in relation to the lumbar spine must be demonstrated.

The underlying etiology of the leg length discrepancy must be sought if the future course of the inequality is to be foreseen. Some growth disturbances, such as hemihypertrophy, formidable undertakings, fraught with complications that require expert care. In clinics in which a special interest has been taken in these procedures, complications have been kept to a minimum.

Fig. 1.28. Shortening due to poliomyelitis with apparent atrophy of the right lower extremity. The effect of the posture is apparent.

add an increment each year; others, such as poliomyelitis, may be erratic and difficult to predict.

The height, body build, and race of each of the parents should be known.

Treatment

Femoral and tibial shortening and lengthening procedures have been developed. These are

Fig. 1.29. Shortening due to congenitally short femur.

Tibial Lengthening

In the field of bone lengthening the fact that the tibia can be lengthened without important complications or undue morbidity has been emphasized by M. V. Anderson of Edinburgh and, following his principles, by Sherman Coleman of Salt Lake City.

Coleman and Noonan[1] have clarified the technique and indications for tibial lengthening. The group of youngsters who are ideal candidates for this procedure according to Coleman are between 8 and 12 years of age. Since this is a major procedure the limb should not·be essentially normal but should face the need for either a prosthetic device or amputation as an alternative to the lengthening procedure. The more simple procedure of epiphyseal arrest of the appropriate tibia should not be possible or desirable. This usually means a predictable shortening of at least 4 cm.

The procedure consists of accomplishing a carefully directed osteoclasis which maintains a closed space for a fracture hematoma. This area is then distracted by proximal and distal tibial pins affixed to an appropriate apparatus.

The foot may be drawn into valgus by this procedure. In order to avoid this complication and to ensure uniform lengthening of both the tibia and fibula, a preliminary synostosis of the distal tibia and fibula is performed. The ankle mortise is thereby preserved.

Nonunion of the tibia is a complication of this procedure. It has been found responsive to secondary grafting, however.

Femoral Lengthening

Lengthening of the femur has additional complications such as sciatic nerve palsy. In this procedure it is important that the proximal fragment be fixed so that the hip is not drawn out of the acetabulum. A periosteal tube is constructed so that the bone fragments can slide within it. A transverse cut in the bone is made, an intramedullary nail is inserted, and the distal fragment drawn along it by traction on both the distal femur and proximal tibia. Westin has procured lengthening of 1½-2 inches by this method over a period of 3-4 weeks with further immobilization needed thereafter for the new bone forming in the periosteal tube to reach maturity. Desperation to increase the functional range of the child results in the occasional necessity for these procedures, but they must be carefully overseen.

Growth Stimulation

This is a particularly desirable approach to a short leg in childhood since it would not shorten the total height as does epiphyseal arrest, but it is not yet a clinically sure-footed procedure. Growth stimulation is based on division of the intramedullary artery. In order to further increase the magnitude of the periosteal vascular response the periosteum is usually elevated up and down the diaphysis and into the metaphysis if possible. A circular section of the diaphyseal bone is removed at the level of the junction of the diaphysis and metaphysis. A curette is used to divide the medullary contents transversely, and the circular piece of cortical bone that had been removed is placed transversely to try and prevent rapid reconstitution of the medullary artery.

Although occasional femoral fractures with considerable displacement are found to have produced 1 inch of growth stimulation, this magnitude of stimulation has not been observed in the planned procedure. Occasional cases are believed to have resulted in a ½ inch increase, the effect of the stimulation lasting but 1 year.

Epiphyseal Arrest

Epiphyseal arrest of the long extremity in those children whose ultimate height is sufficient to tolerate some loss has proved to have predictable results in equalizing leg lengths. Green and Anderson have devised a chart based on enough data that an accurate prediction of the effect of epiphyseal arrest at the distal femur or proximal tibia can be determined.

Epiphyseal arrest, as devised by Phemister,[2] involves the removal of a block of bone traversed at the juncture of its mid and distal, or mid and proximal, thirds by the epiphyseal line. The line is then curetted, and the bone block is rotated 180° so that the epiphyseal end of the block lies well down the metaphysis. A similar approach is made from the other side of the bone.

Epiphyseal arrest is also accomplished by placing a sufficient number of staples (usually three on each side) across an epiphyseal line (Blount). There appears to be a delay in the effectiveness of this type of arrest, as compared to that of the Phemister type, although it is not sufficient to rule out the effective clinical application of the method. Stapling is also done at a time when the result of the growth arrest is predictable. Haphazard application and removal of staples cannot be undertaken with the expectation that normal growth will resume.

The appropriate time of arrest is based on skeletal age rather than chronologic age (Fig. 1.30). Skeletal age is determined by the skeletal development of the hand and wrist; the Todd or the Greenlich-Pyle atlas should be used as a standard.

An accurate roentgen method of measuring the skeleton is essential.

The patient should be observed several times before a time for arrest is chosen. The increment of change, as well as the absolute difference due to growth, can thus be estimated. It is obvious that if the discrepancy between the leg lengths is decreasing at a rate sufficient to equalize them, no growth arrest is necessary.

References
1. Coleman, S. S., and Noonan, T. D.: Anderson's method of tibial lengthening by percutaneous

osteotomy and gradual distraction, *J. Bone Joint Surg., 49A:* 263, 1967.
2. Phemister, D. B.: Operative arrest of longitudinal growth of bone, *J. Bone Joint. Surg., 15:* 1, 1933.

MOTOR DEVELOPMENT

Some standard pattern of motor development must be borne in mind by the physician examining children. It is well to remember, for instance, that to prefer to use one upper extremity rather than the other before the age of 1 year is abnormal. Before the age of 18 months, such a preference raises the suspicion of the examiner and suggests the possibility of underlying neural damage, such as might exist with hemiplegia in cerebral palsy.

A normal sequence of motor events is roughly as follows (Fig. 1.32). In the first 2 weeks, the infant exhibits mass activity of the limbs, and the eyes focus on light and on the face of the observer. Crying occurs with discomfort. At 1 month, the chin and chest are up and the eyes follow a moving object. At 3 or 4 months, the infant laughs and brings the hand to the mouth. The feet push and the reach for a rattle occurs. In the 6-8-month range, the infant learns to sit alone, to transfer a toy from one hand to the other, and to pull the hair of an observer. By 8 or 9 months, the youngster

Fig. 1.30. Useful tables in choosing the appropriate time to perform an epiphyseal arrest on the long leg. If an epiphyseal arrest is to accomplish its purpose, the short leg must still have growth potential so that it will catch up after the rate of growth in the long leg is slowed. Various factors, such as the height of the parents and the relative maturity of the child, are helpful in judging the appropriate time for epiphyseal arrest. The centimeter scale in this chart relates to the number of centimeters of discrepancy to be gained if the growth rate of both the long and short leg are known. (Reprinted with permission of W. T. Green, M.D.)

Fig. 1.31. In this case of congenitally short femur, the discrepancy is slight enough that epiphyseal arrest will be of great aid. For a girl this deformity is a major obstacle to a full life and major procedures could be justified to obtain knees at the same level.

Fig. 1.32. A general guide to the development of motor skills in a child. There is wide normal variation.

stands with support. By 11 or 12 months, he can pull himself up to stand; and at 12 or 14 months he can walk, repeat words, recognize sounds, and name a few objects. Running starts at 16-18 months. By 24 months, the child climbs on furniture and jumps off, obeys simple commands, and investigates objects of interest. He opens cupboards and drawers and begins to use simple sentences.

All such indications of timing are rough approximations and guides, not absolute rules.

Secondary Effects of Immobilization

Immobilization removes a child from an opportunity for learning experience. In addition, immobilization results in an adjustment of the muscles of the limb or trunk to a new fixed position.

This adjustment is termed "myostatic" contracture. It may be defined as the adaptation of an innervated muscle to a new functional length. Such a process cannot occur in a flail muscle without tone. It cannot occur in joint capsule or synovia which is in a normal state, except over a very prolonged period of time when the collagen fibers could become reoriented to new stresses. The principal cause for joint stiffness when a plaster cast is removed is the development of a myostatic contracture in the muscles.

There are no joint adhesions in the normal joint although they may exist in the inflamed or diseased joint. Trauma and the development of edema inflammation and fibrin deposits in tendon sheaths, torn muscle bellies, and around joint capsules may aid this process.

The treatment of myostatic contracture is active exercise controlled by the patient. Passive stretching may tear tissues and compound the process. The treatment of limited motion at the elbow resulting in flexion contracture, for instance, is active flexion and extension of the elbow—not carrying a pail of water. This latter type of passive stretching results in a painful, still further limited elbow with muscle spasm.

Immobilization atrophy is not a loss of water in the muscle, but a total loss of muscle tissue, the relative percentage of water remaining the same.

Immobilization of the total patient results in a negative nitrogen balance, with loss of protein

and mineral from the skeleton. Where the process is rapid there may be secondary complications in areas such as the genitourinary tract.

JOINT STABILITY MAINTAINED BY ATMOSPHERIC PRESSURE*

There are a number of factors involved in the support of a human joint: ligaments, the architectural shape of the joint, muscle pull, and atmospheric pressure. How great is the role of atmospheric pressure? We carried out a number of experiments in an attempt to accurately calculate this force in its role of aiding joint stability.

Human metacarpophalangeal joints and knees were subject to distraction to the point at which vaporization occurred in the joint and the effect of atmospheric pressure was neutralized. Determination of the force necessary to do this combined with the surface area of the joint made it possible to calculate the force of atmospheric pressure supporting the joint. It was shown that this force in an intact congruous joint is much larger than that necessary to stretch the joint ligaments.

Fluid Behavior

The syringe experimental model offers an opportunity to test the behavior of various types of fluids in both atmospheric pressure and partial vaccum without the complicating factors present in the joint. Synovial fluid has some of the physical properties of an aqueous solution such as surface tension. In order to show that the plunger in the syringe is not held by surface tension alone, the following experiment was performed. The distraction force necessary to pull the plunger from the syringe creating a vapor phase was determined at atmospheric pressure for water, glycerin, liquid petrolatum, isopropyl alcohol, normal saline solution, and synovial fluid obtained from human knees where the effusion was due either to traumatic causes or degenerative arthritis. The same experiment was carried out in a

---

* This section, "Joint Stability Maintained by Atmospheric Pressure," is reprinted in part from K. Semlak and A. B. Ferguson, Jr.: Joint stability maintained by atmospheric pressure; an experimental study, *Clinical Orthopaedics, 68:* 294, 1970.

Fig. 1.33. Distraction curve of the third and fifth metacarpophalangeal joints. Note the continuous distraction of the fifth metacarpophalangeal joint. The third metacarpophalangeal joint shows negligible distraction until the appearance of a vapor phase. Insertion of a needle into the metacarpophalangeal joint of the third finger gives a distraction curve illustrated by the *triangle*. With a vapor phase constantly in the joint, the soft tissues are the only resisting force to distraction.

vacuum jar and the level of vaccum required to permit the plunger to fall from the syringe was determined for the above fluids. A fixed weight of 143 g/cm^2 was attached to the plunger. The results, shown in Table 1.1, indicate that in its ability to initiate vaporization, synovial fluid most closely resembles pure water. Synovial fluid as an aqueous dialysate of plasma contains 2.5 g of plasma protein per 100 ml (about one-third as much as plasma), of which 60-75% is albumin, and about 0.36 g of hyaluronate per 100 ml. The forces needed to cause formation of a gas bubble inside the syringe when synovial fluid is used lie between the amount needed for an aqueous solution and that needed for an organic solution.

Organic fluids with a lower heat of vaporization would be expected to distract with lower forces than required by water. However, the increased viscosity of these organic fluids and their decreased heat conductivity does affect the kinetics and reduces the rate of nucleation and growth of a gas bubble, thus leading to an expectation that the forces required would be quite similar to an aqueous solution.

It is apparent that atmospheric pressure forms an almost solid bar to distraction of the joint until it is overcome. Either considerable laxity of the walls or incongruity of the joint so

that a seal cannot be obtained, the rapid appearance of increasing volumes of fluid, or communication with the atmosphere negates this affect. The failure of a vapor phase to appear in the synovial fluid marks this situation and progressive distraction resisted solely by the soft tissues occurs.

The amount of nitrogen, oxygen, and carbon dioxide dissolved in synovial fluid was calculated as 3.80 ml/100 ml from the partial pressures determined on 5 fluid samples. The small amounts of synovial fluid present in normal joints would not be sufficient to produce a gas bubble of 1-2 ml seen in these experiments. The vapor phase produced in the joint by distraction disappeared quickly. Contrast air injected into a joint for arthrography usually remained for several days.

The initial nucleation apparently comes from gas in solution in synovial fluid. It must be augmented by the vapor phase of the fluid, however, to produce a bubble of the size seen.

Both the knee and metacarpophalangeal joint experiments detailed here reveal that if the joint is not effectively sealed against atmospheric pressure either by damage to its intact structure or by excess joint fluid, the distracting force is immediately thrown on the ligaments. The difference in the force necessary to distract the joint between a knee with an effusion and one without, points out the considerable role that atmospheric pressure may play. In the experiment, a 5-kg force was all that was necessary to stretch the ligaments of a knee with a surface area of 50 cm^2 when it contained an effusion. This contrasts with a calculated value of a 60-kg force necessary to distract the intact joint.

Thus, a patient with a joint effusion has a greater risk of stretching his knee ligaments than a patient with a normal joint who has atmospheric pressure as a real force aiding stability. This may explain the development of ligamentous laxity in a joint with a chronic effusion.

Excess fluid or a readily available reservoir of fluid will negate the effect of atmospheric pressure by supplying additional fluid to eliminate the pressure on it and prevent vaporization. The vaporization is taken as a mark of the reality of force being exerted on the fluid rather than in itself a form of resistance. Women retaining fluid thus have available a

Fig. 1.34. *(A)* The third and fifth metacarpophalangeal joints are under an 8-lb distraction force and the fifth distracts to 3.2 mm; the third is unaffected. *(B)* Increasing the force to 11 lb. on the third metacarpophalangeal joint causes distraction to 2.8 mm with the formation of a gas bubble in the joint. *(C)* Inserting an open needle to the atmosphere and to the joint negates the effect.

Fig. 1.34*B*

Fig. 1.34C

Table 1.1. Pressure Effects on Fluids

Substance	Pressure of Distraction Force at 20 C and 750 mm Hg	Vacuum Required to Cause Distraction at Weight of 143 g/cm² and 20 C*
	g/cm²	mm Hg
H₂O	984	100
Glycerin	1010.5	92
Liquid petrolatum	948	103
Isopropyl alcohol.....	940	118
Normal saline solution (0.9%)	1010	102
Synovial fluid .	965	96†
	955	92‡

* All vacuum measurements are the averages from 3 experiments.

† Obtained from degenerative arthritis.

‡ Obtained from traumatic effusion.

reservoir to negate this effect. The effect is more evident in very congruous joints than in those with eccentric anatomic formation.

These experiments suggest that atmospheric pressure is an important force aiding joint stability and protecting ligaments from being overstretched.

References

1. Evans, W. A., Jr.: The roentgenological demonstration of the true articular space, *Am. J. Roentgenol., 43:* 860, 1940.
2. Fick, R.: *Anatomie and Mechanid der Gelenke.* Jena: G. Fischer, 1911.
3. Fuiks, D. M., and Grayson, C. H.: Vacuum pneumoarthrography and spontaneous occurrence of the gas in the joint spaces, *J. Bone Joint Surg., 32A:* 933, 1950.
4. Gerschow, C., I.: Internal derangement of the knee joint; the diagnostic scope of soft tissue roentgenogram examination and the vacuum technique demonstration of the meniscus, *Am. J. Roentgenol., 54:* 338, 1945.

CHILDHOOD AMPUTEES

In discussing childhood amputees, one includes not only those children with traumatic loss of a limb or a segment of it, but those with congenital conditions which either primarily or secondarily require a prosthetic appliance and training for maximal function. There has been a great increase in the amount of function that can be achieved for children with an amputation through improved equipment, increased knowledge, and better training.

The child is a unit in a family situation, and the orthopaedist must recognize that rehabilitation can be achieved for the child only if the family supports and desires it. Unless the family wants prosthetic restoration of a limb and increased function for the child, the program will fail. So much depends on guidance by the family that if it is lacking the child will not use the prosthetic device and will fail to develop skill in its use. The family must be educated along with the child.

The amputee clinic for the child includes among its personnel the orthopaedic surgeon, the physical therapist, the occupational therapist, the prosthetist, and the medical social worker. Following up treated patients and finding untreated ones depends on the skill of the social worker, without whose work the program must fall short of its objectives.

Children grow as adults do not, and the level of proficiency achieved varies among the different age groups. In setting goals the physical therapist, occupational therapist, and surgeon must bear in mind the child's age, future problems, and development.

JUVENILE AMPUTATIONS AND CONGENITAL LIMB DEFICIENCIES

Juvenile amputees include children with congenital limb deficiencies and those with acquired amputations for trauma, tumor, or other disease. They need long-term care and concern, and their problems fall properly in the orthopaedic field. Fortunately, knowledge, equipment, and techniques are constantly improving and provide increasingly better function for these patients. All orthopaedists should be familiar with current principles of good treatment and stay aware of the new developments in this changing area.

How many juvenile amputees are there in the United States? We have some statistics available from the 31 participating clinics in the National Research Council's Cooperative Child Amputee

Research Program. During 1972 the clinics saw 644 new patients, an average of 20 per year for each clinic.[12] Of these, 66% had congenital problems. Several years ago two large clinics saw congenital problems reflect increased local care of children with uncomplicated acquired amputations outside of regional clinics; this means that the absolute number of new amputees per year is probably even greater than that shown by clinic statistics.

Acquired Amputations

About 35-45% of all juvenile amputations are acquired.[5] Trauma causes approximately 70% of these, and power tools (including farm machines), vehicular accidents, and gunshots or explosions are almost equally responsible.

The most common nontraumatic cause of amputation in children is tumor; the most common childhood malignant tumor of the extremities is osteogenic sarcoma. Vascular and neurogenic disease or malformation are the most common of other diseases which can require amputation. About 70% of all acquired amputations are of the lower extremity, and most of these are below the knee.

Surgical Principles

The severity and extent of trauma usually dictates the amputation level that it causes, but there are some general principles which can apply to both traumatic and surgical amputations in children.

A. Save all length possible, whether lower or upper extremity. The greater the length, the greater the proprioception and the longer the lever arm for control of the prosthesis.

Use skin grafts if necessary to preserve length. Today's prosthetic fabrication techniques for plastic total contact sockets allow comfortable weight bearing with some relief of grafted skin and few breakdown problems.

Open amputations for markedly contaminated wounds or very short stumps are feasible to preserve length and prevent infection. Skin traction and frequent dressing changes in the first postoperative week provide a good granulating surface suitable for grafting.

B. Save epiphysis whenever possible, for two reasons: to preserve length (and assure adequate length after growth), and to prevent the

complication of bony overgrowth which is very common after section of a long bone in children. The contributions of the various epiphyses to growth are shown in Tables 1.2 and 1.3.

C. If section of a long bone is necessary, avoid stripping periosteum of the portion of the bone which will remain; to do so will allow the raised periosteal remnants to produce irregular new bone growth which will be painful under a prosthesis, and may cause a ring sequestrum if circumferential.

D. It is better not to use techniques of myodesis which require drilling near the bone end; the drilled holes may increase the tendency to bony overgrowth.

E. Handle nerves with care and do the least possible amount of trauma to them. Pull them gently distally and cut sharply with one stroke of a fresh scalpel blade allowing them to retract from the scar area. Attempts to reduce neuroma formation by injection, ligation, and bending, have all proved to increase scarring and are no longer felt to be good practice. Vessels on larger nerves such as the sciatic and the tibial may be dissected free and clamped or ligated separately.

Table 1.2. Epiphyseal Growth Contributions

Epiphysis	Contribution	
	Proximal	Distal
	%	%
Humerus	80	20
Radius	20	80
Ulna	25	75
Femur	30	70
Fibula	60	40
Tibia	55	45

Table 1.3. Contribution to Total Lower Extremity Growth by Individual Epiphyses

Epiphysis	Contribution
	%
Proximal femur	10
Distal femur	40
Proximal tibia	30
Distal tibia	20

F. Remember that rigid dressing immediately postoperatively, according to the principles detailed by Burgess[8],[9] can markedly decrease edema formation and speed healing. This dressing is as appropriate in children as in adults. (See further discussion below.)

Surgical Techniques

The details of the operative procedures are covered well in *Campbell's Operative Orthopaedics,*[11] and the July 1972 issue of *Orthopaedics Clinics of North America.*[22] These are as applicable to children as adults, bearing in mind the principles outlined above.

Comprehensive Care Principles

A. Rigid Dressing. Casting in the operating room immediately after amputation (with sterile lambswool distally, then elastic plaster over a spandes stump sock, padded with felt or foam to relieve bony prominences, reinforced with standard plaster, and suspended from a waist or shoulder belt) will prevent the development of edema and has proved far superior to "conventional" elastic wrapping for below knee stumps.[19] It is also applicable to upper extremity amputations. The techniques are more complicated and the results less easy to achieve with above-knee stumps or proximal disarticulations.

A pylon attachment for standing may be added immediately or deferred for 1 or 2 weeks and applied after a cast change reveals the wound to be healing well. Use of semi-rigid unna paste dressings has been recently published;[17] we have no long-term experience with it. It appears promising for such difficult to cast areas as above-elbow and above-knee stumps.

B. Exercise Program and Stump Care. No matter what stump dressing and weight-bearing routine is followed, an exercise program taught and encouraged daily by a physical therapist is essential. The program should be taught preoperatively if possible so that postoperatively it is familiar and will be easier in spite of discomfort. It should include active strengthening exercises to the unaffected extremities and active range of motion exercises to the stump, followed by strengthening as healing allows. Walking should begin in parallel bars and progress to crutches, whether or not partial weight bearing in a pylon cast is allowed.

Flexion contractures occur easily at the hip, shoulder, and knee and interfere with the fitting and use of a prosthesis. Once present they are difficult to get rid of; it is far better to prevent them instead. Postoperative elevation of the bed in Trendelenberg position is better than using pillows to decrease edema. Pillows under below-knee stumps can allow the knee to flex and should be discouraged. Wheelchairs for below-knee amputees should have an extension board under the affected limb to keep the knee straight. All lower extremity amputees should spend several half-hours each day lying prone to prevent hip flexion contractures. Active range of motion exercises for the involved shoulder should be begun early for the upper extremity amputee. External rotation and abduction of the stump should be discouraged in above-knee amputees.

Stump wrapping with elastic bandages is an important part of an amputee's self-care and must be taught to the child or his parents. Even those patients dressed initially with a rigid cast must begin stump wrapping when the cast is discontinued. Wrapping is an art which must be practiced so that the compression is always greatest distally and gradually decreases proximally with no proximal constriction. This means that below-knee stump wrapping must be carried above the knee, because suspension of a wrap that ends below the knee depends on tightness proximally, producing constriction. An above-knee stump wrapping must be carried around the waist in a spica for the same reasons. Few individuals can wrap a stump well, but those involved with amputee care should learn. A new stump must always be wrapped when the prosthesis is not on, and rewrapped when the bandages slide or curl at the edges (several times a day, at least). After 6 months to 1 year, the stump will no longer swell when out of the prosthesis and wrapping may be discontinued.

C. Skin Care. The skin on the stump needs to be kept clean and dry. Sometimes patients and family have a disturbing tendency to treat the wrapped limb as something apart from the patient, to be surprised that it needs to be washed, and to be shocked that they will be expected to wrap it themselves. Occasionally nurses also suffer the same misconceptions, but on a well organized orthopaedic floor with good communication among doctors, nurses, and patients this should not remain a problem for long.

Both stump and prosthetic socket should be washed daily with soap and water and dried thoroughly. Dry skin is the best defense against bacterial invasion. Skin softeners are not necessary and may predispose to maceration and superficial infection. Occasionally an area of skin subject to pressure is slow to develop the thickened keratin layer it needs, and some patients have found that patting the area with wet tea bags and allowing it to dry is helpful. It may be the tannic acid in the tea that produces the desired effects; it is at least not harmful.

Specific Skin Problems. (1) *Reactive hyperemia.* Reddening of the skin, particularly in the areas of pressure, subsides with time as the skin adapts; both the keratin layer and the living skin layers increase in thickness. (2) *Stump edema syndrome.* Later development of reactive hyperemia (beyond the initial prosthetic training period) may progress to a serous ooze with some capillary rupture. Treatment: stop wearing prosthesis, wrap with elastic bandages, and elevate. (3) *Contact dermatitis.* This may be a primary irritation or an allergy. The first is due to a substance which is itself an irritant (soap, turpentine). Some patients use such substances in an effort to toughen the skin or clean it. Allergic reactions are due to a substance to which the patient has been exposed and become allergic. Common allergens for amputees are nickel, chrome, polyester resins, lacquer, dyes, and antoxidants used in foam rubber. In all these cases the dermatitis is limited to the area of contact, which helps in the identification of the offending agent. (4) *Epidermoid cysts.* Usually occurring at or near the brim of the socket, they appear at points of rolling friction, pushing keratin fragments into the dermis; they rarely occur if the prosthesis is well fitted and well aligned. Treatment: stop wearing the prosthesis, incise and drain or excise the cyst; realign and fit the prosthesis. (5) *Pyogenic infections.* (*a*) Folliculitis: superficial; usually occurs early with wearing of a new prosthesis. Treatment: an antibiotic ointment or lotion. (*b*) Furuncles: treat as elsewhere with incision and drainage. (*c*) Hidradenitis: infection in the apocrine sweat glands, in the axilla and groin; these glands empty into the hair follicles, secrete slowly and with thick secretion; infections of them are deep seated

and difficult to treat, sometimes requiring wide excision and skin grafting. (6) *Fungal infections.* These infections usually occur in the groin, and more often in fat people, whose skin is less dry than that of thin people. As amputees have loss of heat-radiating surface, they begin to sweat at lower temperatures, and wet intertriginous areas predispose to these infections. They are characteristically patches of red scaly dermatitis which enlarge and clear in the center. Treatment: Griseofulvin orally. *Candida albicans* infection typically produces red, moist, oozing skin, with small pimples at the periphery with canida yeast spores present in the pus. This occurs frequently in diabetics and obese patients. Treatment: topical Nystatin. (7) *Tumors.* Warts, keratoses, etc., under a prosthesis can produce painful pressure points and should be removed if they do. All suspicious nodules should of course be biopsied.

Teaching the parents the details of stump care and exercise programs, and allowing them to help the therapist before discharge of the patient will help ensure success of the program at home.

D. Psychologic Support. Children having to undergo amputation have a great deal of adjustment to make before they can come eventually to acceptance. Most go through a denial-anger depression-bargaining-acceptance cycle similar to that described in dying or grieving people,[16] though the phases or the cycle are not always equally evident or in the same order. Some patients have to accept both the fact of an amputation and that of having a malignancy and an uncertain future. They need help with this; someone must be able to listen, to offer answers to the many questions, and to understand when the anger comes out in words and actions. Fear is worse when it is of things unknown, and knowing in advance some details of the dressing, the exercising, and the fitting of the prosthesis can help a patient make the fear manageable. Experienced nurses can be very helpful in this area; we have at times been lucky enough to have available a nurse clinical specialist who has more time available than the floor nurses or the doctors, and spends it with these patients and their families, to the benefit of all. The details of management can be frightening to the patient if given too soon or at a time when he is worrying about something else, and all of those who care (in all senses) for these patients must be alert for the signs that show when they need to talk and about what. Reviewing current material on dying and grief reactions[16] is worthwhile.

Prosthetic Fitting

A. Timing. If long-term follow-up is not to be done by the primary surgeon, early consultation with an appropriate physician is necessary. If immediate postoperative ambulation with the cast-pylon technique is planned, the prosthetist or a physician experienced with the technique should be present at the time of the amputation to apply the cast.

If there is any doubt about the potential healing of the stump (e.g., if the amputation was done for ischemia) it may be best to delay weight bearing.[19] A rigid dressing is still useful, and the wound may be checked at 1 week or 10 days. If the wound is healing well a second cast can be applied with a weightbearing pylon attached, or a mold for an intermediate prosthesis taken by the prosthetist. The intermediate ("temporary") limb has a plastic total-contact socket with a modular adjustable pylon attached; it may be covered with cosmetic foam. It can usually be made in less than 1 week, and in the interim the stump may be recast (and will remain the same size) or elastic wrapping may be begun (with the advantage of continued stump shrinkage and usually perfect fit with a stump sock).

The permanent prosthesis can be made when the stump is no longer shrinking noticeably and there are no areas of palpable edema. The further, slower shrinkage of the stump which occurs over 6-8 months can be accomodated for by adding 3- or 5-ply wool stump socks as necessary. A child requires a new prosthesis because of growth or wear every 18 months on the average, but in the first year after amputation the time may be closer to every 6 or 8 months. Upper extremity prostheses need replacement less frequently because length requirements are less precise than for lower extremities.

Some physicians delay prosthetic fitting of patients with malignant tumors for an arbitrary number of months following amputation, or omit it altogether if a metastasis is present. Statistics show that patients with metastases use a prosthesis for an average of 1 year, and many longer.[5] Now that fitting and fabrication

techniques take only 1 or 2 weeks and inpatient gait training another week, denying a prosthesis and the independence it allows to any patient seems totally unjustified.

B. Prosthetic Prescription. Prescription is legally and traditionally the sole responsibility of the physician, but the advice of experienced prosthetists and therapists can be invaluable. Each case of acquired amputation is individual and had its own particular considerations. Current laminated sockets, fabricated over a mold of the stump, allow total contact which distributes pressure evenly. These are more comfortable and more efficient than the previously used open ended sockets. A list of the most frequently used prostheses for each level of amputation and some of the options follows.

Lower Extremity

1. Hemipelvectomy: Plastic total contact socket with Canadian hip joint, single-axis knee, and SACH (solid-ankle-cushion-heel) foot.
2. Hip disarticulation (Fig. 1.35): Same as above.
3. Above knee (Fig. 1.36): Quadrilateral total contact socket; may be suction; may be used with hip joint and pelvic belt, or a Silesian belt. May use single axis, constant friction knee joint or hydraulic knee unit; SACH foot.
4. Through knee: Knee-disarticulartion type plastic total contact socket, with entrance panel for molded suspension, or the new silastic air-pocket "diaphragm" suspension: SACH foot.
5. Below-knee (Fig. 1.37): Patellar-tendon bearing (PTB) total contact socket with either cuff or wedge suspension; SACH foot. Occasionally knee joint side hinges and thigh lacer may be necessary, but the thigh lacer has the disadvantage of usually producing quadriceps atrophy.
6. Symes (Fig. 1.38) socket with front, side, or back entrance panel: Of the new and promising (and more cosmetic) silastic air panel suspension.
7. Partial foot: Shoe fillers, some attached to molded heel and ankle sockets.

Upper Extremity

1. Shoulder disarticulation and forequarter amputation: Molded shoulder cap and extension over opposite shoulder; or a chest-strap harness; shoulder hinge with

Hip Joint (CANADIAN)

Hip Flexion Control
and Kick Strap

Left Side Lateral Detail

CANADIAN HIP DISARTICULATION PROSTHESIS
TYPE: Hip disarticulation
BUCKET: Plastic
THIGH: Wood or plastic
SHANK: Wood or plastic
KNEE: Single pivot constant friction
FOOT: Prescription choice

Fig. 1.35. Hip disarticulation prosthesis, Canadian type.

motion in two planes to allow for dressing, abducting over chair arm, etc.; mechanical or motorized aids can improve operation of elbow flexion or elbow lock. (Terminal devices will be discussed separately below.)

2. Above-elbow (Fig. 1.39): Total contact plastic socket with figure-of-eight harness, positive locking elbow (with 11 locking positions, and turntable to allow internal and external rotation—without the humeral condyles, shoulder rotation cannot be transferred to the prosthesis).

3. Elbow disarticulation: Same as for above-elbow, but the currently available outside locking hinges have only 7 locking positions available, as opposed to the 11 of the more bulky "inside" positive locking elbows, and are not as durable.

4. Below-elbow (Fig. 1.40): Total contact double-wall plastic socket, with figure-8 or single loop (figure-9) harness, triceps cuff, single pivot hinges, and constant friction wrist unit. Polycentric hinges allow more

antecubital space, multiple-action or step-up hinges allow more flexion for a very short stump, when used with a split socket; it is more common to use a pre-flexed socket to achieve full flexion with a very short stump. A triceps *pad* (smaller than cuff) and flexible hinges allow pronation and supination if the stump is long enough; 50% of available rotation of a forearm stump is lost in the harnessing, therefore only long below-elbow stumps will have enough useful rotation to take advantage of flexible hinges.

5. "Muenster" below-elbow socket: A molded supracondylar fit with olecranon-notch molding (Fig. 1.41); for very short below-elbow stumps; eliminates separate suspension and only harnessing necessary if for cable control of the terminal device. Does limit flexion to about $90°$

6. Wrist disarticulartion: Fitted as for a long below-elbow stump; an oval constant friction wrist is available which can be

Fig. 1.36. *(A)* Above knee prosthesis, quadrilateral suction socket; SACH foot is now preferred. *(B)* The toddler's harness for the early walker.

laminated into the socket more easily and takes slightly less room than the standard below-elbow constant friction wrist unit.

7. Partial hand: There are no really useful partial hand prostheses at present; surgical reconstruction of pinch and grasp is necessary.

8. Harnessing: As described above, a cable is anchored to the harness and the prosthesis so that the body motions of shoulder flexion (and scapular abduction when necessary will exert tension on the cable and open the terminal device; the first part of these motions will cause a second cable to flex the elbow and lock it for an above-elbow amputee. Voluntary opening terminal devices close by rubber bands about the bases of the fingers of the device, exerting about 1 lb of pressure per rubber band.

9. Other wrist units. *Flexion:* Necessary only with bilateral upper extremity amputations to bring one terminal device close to the body. *Quick-change:* Useful for those who wear both a hook terminal device and a cosmetic hand; allows easy one-handed change.

10. Terminal devices: All available for children

Fig. 1.37. Below knee prosthesis, patellar tendon-bearing type (PTB), with cuff suspension and SACH foot.

Fig. 1.38. Symes prosthesis, with removable entrance panel.

are voluntary-opening. Voluntary-closing devices are available for adolescents and adults and are useful for those activities requiring more precise regulation of pinch force.

11. Standard adult terminal devices, suitable for adolescents:

Dorrance 5: Stainless steel; weight, 7 oz.

Dorrance 5X (Fig. 1.42): Same, with Neoprene lining of fingers for better prehension.

Dorrance 5XA: Same as 5X in aluminum; weight, 3 oz.

Dorrance 7 (Fig. 1.43): "Farmer's hook" stainless steel; weight, 8 oz. Adapted for nail, knife, and tool holding.

12. Smaller devices, suitable for children:

Dorrance 8: Weight is 5-3/4 oz., otherwise equivalent to Dorrance 5.

Dorrance 8X: Weight is 5-3/4 oz., equivalent to Dorrance 5X.

Dorrance 88X: Aluminum; weight 2-1/3 oz., equivalent to 5XA: 4-3/8-inch long; suitable for ages 10-14 years.

Dorrance 99X (Fig. 1.44): Aluminum; weight, 2 oz., 3-3/8 inches long; suitable for 3-6 years.

Dorrance 10P: Plastisol covered fingers; 3½ inches long; weight, 3 oz.; for 3-6 years.

Dorrance 12P: Plastisol covered fingers; 2¾ inches long; weight, 2 oz.; steel; for 1-4 years.

Plastic mitt: 2-1/4 inches long; weight 2 oz.; useful for 6 months to 1 year.

Myoelectric prostheses are now in the experimental stages, and will probably become the most useful prostheses in the near future when they are perfected. They operate by utilizing days is best because the patient's early efforts can be supervised and awkward body movements changed before they become bad habits. The limb should be delivered to the training facility after final fitting for check out by the physician or therapist according to a protocol. If training is to be outpatient, the limb should not go home with the patient until both he and his parents are familiar with the correct gait pattern.

Ambulation begins in parallel bars and progresses usually to crutches, then to one or two canes, and then to independence. Training should include steps (with and without railings), ramps, rough ground, and falling and getting up again while wearing the prosthesis.

It is helpful to keep in mind the normal progression of gait in childhood, from toddling at about 1 year to an adult heel-toe pattern at about age 5 years. The gait sought with an artificial limb should be kept appropriate to the child's age. Children can usually be taught to

Fig. 1.39. Above elbow prosthesis, with figure-8 harness, standard positive locking elbow, and hook terminal device.

action potentials of the remaining muscles of the stump to activate a controller switch which allows a battery to supply power to the prosthesis.

Training

A. Lower Extremity. Gait training should be begun by an experienced physical therapist on a daily schedule. Inpatient training for several

Fig. 140. Below elbow prosthesis standard, with triceps cuff, single-pivot hinges, and hook terminal device.

Fig. 1.41. Below elbow prosthesis, Muenster type, with figure-9 harness for cable control of terminal device.

use crutches at about age 3; younger children can toddle independently, in a sling walker or around furniture.

B. Upper Extremity. This training should also be done daily, by an experienced physical therapist or occupational therapist; it can be accomplished within about a week for unilateral amputee old enough to cooperate well. Training periods for children are limited by their attention span, which has been estimated at *1 min* for each year of age. At the present time initial training with a hook type of terminal device is highly recommended, and is actually a rule in some clinics, even for patients who are sure (or whose parents are sure) they will only accept a cosmetic hand. Functional hand prosthesis are currently far from satisfactory—their action is less precise, and they are far less durable. Even appearance-conscious adolescents usually use a hook at school and work, and a hand only for social events, if at all (Fig. 1.44.1).

Training is mainly work on the body-control motions necessary to activate the terminal device (below-elbow) and the elbow flexion and lock (above-elbow). Patients with shoulder disarticulations or forequarter amputations need work on breathing exercises as well to increase chest expansion and decrease the energy expenditure necessary for operation of the limb.

Both child and parents should learn how to watch for impending skin and fit problems. Some children show a distressing tendency to gain weight rapidly after amputation; the parents must understand that rapid changes in weight will affect prosthetic fit and atention to careful diet may be necessary.

Long-term Follow-up

Children with amputations should be followed every 3 or 4 months at a minimum until growth is complete. The average time between

Fig. 1.42. Dorrance 5X terminal device.

new prostheses is 18 months but during growth spurts may be much less. Limb lengthening without fabrication of a whole new prosthesis is necessary an average of every 6 months.

Overgrowth is a common complication after transverse section of a growing long bone, occurring in 16% of Dr. Aitken's cases.[1] It is appositional new bone laid down distally and epiphyseodesis will not prevent or halt it. The only treatment is stump revision when the prosthesis is no longer comfortable, and this may have to be repeated several times. Although overgrowth is not epiphyseal, once skeletal maturity is reached, overgrowth stops. It occurs most frequently in humerus, fibula, and tibia in that order.

Follow-up is best done in a children's amputee clinic, staffed by a physician (orthopaedist, physiatrist, or pediatrician), certified prosthetist(s), physical therapists, occupational therapists, and social worker; frequently the staff includes a nurse-specialist, and a psychologist or psychiatrist.[17] The presence of all these people together allows easy exchange of information and evaluation of the patient from the various points of view. Another advantage is the chance children and parents have to see and know others with similar problems.

Congenital Limb Deficiencies

About 60% of all juvenile amputees are the result of congenital limb deficiencies; about 70% of these are upper extremity problems. About one-third of congenital limb deficient patients have more than one limb involved, and 10% are quadrimembral (Fig. 1.45).[5]

The term "congenital amputee" is an inac-

Fig. 1.43. Dorrance 7 (Farmer's) hook terminal device.

curate but shorter way to speak of children with congenital limb anomalies. True congenital amputations usually due to a constricting band with a developed but gangrenous or separated limb present, are very rare. However, failure of the limbs to develop occurs in many various ways, most of which can be best treated prosthetically and managed as amputees whether or not they have in fact had an amputation.

Classification

The variety of forms of developmental limb anomalies makes classification necessary for better communication (Table 1.4). At this time there are several classification systems in use, but none is universally accepted. The one most frequently used in most child amputee centers in this country is that of Frautz and O'Rahilly[13] or Burtch's revision of it.[10]

These classify limb defects as *terminal* (everything distal to a certain point missing) or *intercalary* (a portion missing with more distal parts present), and *transverse* (defect similar in both bones of forearm or leg) or *longitudinal* (one or a portion of one bone of the two-bone segments present and the other missing). The basic defects are amelia (absent limb) or meromelia (partial limb). (The older term "hermimelia" has been changed to meromelia in newer classifications to avoid the implication of "half-limb" rather than "partial.") The missing segment of a longitudinal defect is named, thus absence of the tibia becomes "tibial meromelia" and may be partial or

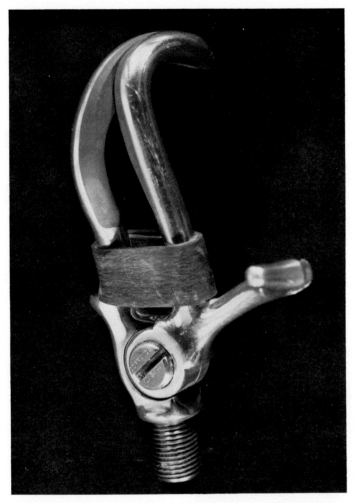

Fig. 1.44. Dorrance 99X terminal device; note scale compared to Figure 1.42 wrist-connect threaded units are the same size.

complete, and terminal (tibia and medical tarsals and digits missing) or intercalary (tibia only missing).

In practical conversation an absent tibia is still referred to as just that and not "a complete intercalary tibial meromelia," but for accurate record keeping, documentation of incidence, and better care, a good understanding and consistent use of a classification system is a necessity.

Treatment Principles

Aitken[5] emphasizes that the major problems which may be presented by upper extremity anomalies are (1) loss of prehension, (2) lack of promimal power and stability, (3) difficulty with hand placement due to limitation of proximal joint motion, (4) malrotation, and (5) severe length inequalities. Problems of lower extremity anomalies are (1) severe length inequalities, (2) instability impairing weight bearing, and (3) malalignment.

These problems will be present in varying degrees in individual cases but must be evaluated and accommodated for in some way. Current plastic fabricating techniques allow the fitting of nonstandard prostheses; these are most successful when the *most distal stable* joint in the limb is identified and everything distal to it is treated as stump for purposes of fitting. This identification of the joint with the

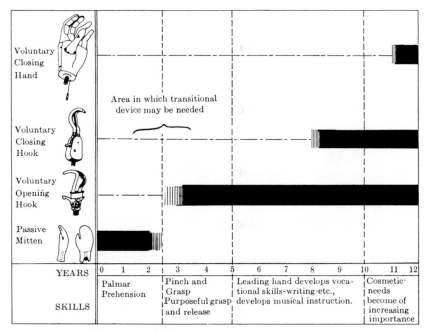

	YEARS	0	1	2	3	4	5	6	7	8	9	10	11	12
		Palmar Prehension			Pinch and Grasp Purposeful grasp and release			Leading hand develops vocational skills-writing-etc., develops musical instruction.				Cosmetic needs become of increasing importance		

Area in which transitional device may be needed

Fig. 1.44.1. This chart showing the development of prehension by age helps in the fitting of terminal devices for upper extremity prostheses. (From G. T. Aiken and C. F. Frantz: Management of the child amputee, *Instructional Course Lecturer; American Academy of Orthopaedic Surgeons, 1960.*)

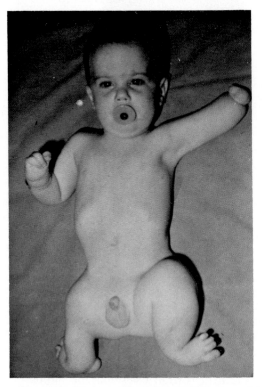

Fig. 1.45. Many problems for rehabilitation exist

most useful range of motion and adequate motor power allows prescription as for an amputation above or below the knee, or elbow; the anomalous limb becomes an amputation homologue.

Timing of prosthetic fitting should be based on consideration of normal developmental patterns; as far as possible a child should progress through his motor and social skills at appropriate ages and if he needs a prosthesis to do so, that is the best indication for fitting.

At 6 months of age, the average child begins to creep and sit; he also begins to use palmar grasp for objects. At 8 or 9 months he is pulling up to stand, and is using a "3-jaw-chuck" finger grasp. At 1 year he can stand unsupported and has mastered release of objects held in his hand. Exploring his world by crawling, standing, and reaching is necessary for his mental and social development. A child with a severe leg length inequality needs a prosthesis when he begins to stand. If he has a lower extremity amelia severe enouth to impair his sitting balance, he needs to be fitted with a plastic "bracket" to sit in, at 6

for a child with multiple anomalies of the upper and lower extremities.

Table 1.4. Nomenclature for Congenital Skeletal Limb Deficiencies*

Terms	
Amelia	COMPLETE absence of a free limb (exclusive of girdle).
Meromelia	PARTIAL absence of a free limb (exclusive of girdle).
Terminal deficiency	Absence of all skeletal elements distal to the proximal limit of the deficiency, along the designated axis (longitudinal or transverse).
Intercalary deficiency	Absence of middle part(s) lying between a proximal-distal series of limb components; elements proximal to and distal to the absent part(s) are present.
Transverse	Absence extending across the width of the limb.
Longitudinal	Absence extending parallel with the long axis of the limb, (forearm and/or hand, or leg and/or foot), either pre-axial, postaxial, or (as in the hand or foot) central in nature.
Pre-axial	Absence of the portion of the forearm and/or hand, or leg and/or foot on the thumb or the great toe side of the limb (radial or tibial portion).
Postaxial	Absence of the portion of the forearm and/or hand, or leg and/or foot on the side of the limb opposite the thumb or the great toe (ulnar or fibular portion).
Central	Absence of one or more of the intermediate digital rays (for example, Ray III).
Rudimentary	A remnant of an osseous element. If the remnant is identifiable (for example, the humerus), the term "rudimentary humerus" would be applicable. If the remnant cannot be identified, the symbol "X" (unknown) would be cited (for example, "rudimentary X").
Ray	A digit.

Symbols		
I = Intercalary	?	= Questionable identity of element cited (for example, radius ?).
T = Terminal		
— = Transverse	X	= Unknown (unidentifiable).
Pre- = Pre-axial	:I, II, III, IV, or V =	Digital ray(s) involved, starting
Post = Postaxial		from pre-axial to postaxial side of limb.

* From the Report of the Consultants to the Subcommittee on Child Prosthetics Problems of the Committee on Prosthetics Research and Development.

months or younger. Early fitting of upper extremity prostheses, even with nongrasping "mitten" hands, allows normal crawling patterns, and normal two-handed examination of objects at arm's length. Also, the earlier that children are fitted the sooner they become accustomed to the harnessing, and the artificial limb becomes incorporated in their own body image.

Development of motor power and coordination allows modification of the initial prothesis at an appropriate time, such as a cable-activated terminal device at 12-18 months; an elbow lock control cannot usually be operated before about 3 years of age, and before that time a constant friction passive joint is used. At 2-3 years of age an above knee prosthesis can be articulated at the knee; normally knee-flexion patterns are not present in a child's gait before this age. Timing of these steps must depend on

evaluation of the individual child and his progress in development, as most children are not "average."

Surgical "Conversion"

Amputation of part of an anomalous limb may be thought as "surgical conversion" to a more standard amputation stump. In lower extremity anomalies it may be necessary to allow proper weight-bearing function of the limb and a better gait. In upper extremities it is almost never indicated as all portions of the limb may be useful to the child for tactible sensation and examination of objects without a prosthesis, *and* almost any movable part, however small, can be utilized to push a switch, pull a lock, etc., to conserve energy in the use of a prosthesis. For these reasons primary surgical conversion is not recommended in the upper extremity. In large clinics approximately 50% of anomalous lower extremities require surgical conversion, but in most cases this is not done until after fitting around the original has proved inadequate. There are probably only three congenital lower extremity problems whose usual life history is well enough known that it makes primary surgical conversion an accepted method of treatment. These are proximal femoral focal deficiency, fibular meromelia, and tibial meromelia; they will be discussed in greater detail below.

Specific Congenital Anomalies

A. Proximal Femoral Focal Deficiency (PFFD). In the past 10 years much work has been done to differentially diagnose and classify this problem which is not uncommon. It may be difficult to distinquish at birth from infantile or congenital coxa vera, or "congenital short femur" of another etiology. In 1967, Aitken[4] presented a classification which allows consideration of the natural history of each type, and treatments appropriate for each.

The classification is based on radiologic findings. Clinically the patients all present with a shortened, flexed, and externally rotated thigh; in some instances the shortening is such that the foot on the affected side is at the level of the opposite knee.

In Classes A and B, both an adequate acetabulum and a femoral head are present, with a short femoral segment. Initially there is no connection between the femoral shaft and head, but at maturity in Class A there is bony connection, usually with subtrochanteric varus and occasionally with a pseudarthrosis. In Class B there is never any bony connection between head and shaft, and probably no cartilaginous connection.

In Classes C and D, there is no femoral head and the acetabulum is severely dysplastic or absent. In Class C, an ossified tuft is present at the proximal end of the short femoral shaft; in Class D this is absent.

These classes (and some of the conditions with which PFFD may be confused clinically) may not be clear radiologically until age 6 months or 1 year.

Treatment usually involves a combination of surgery and prosthetic treatment. Initially a platform brace may be fitted to equalize leg lengths, but this is usually an awkward and ugly appliance and a nonstandard prosthesis fitted over the foot with the foot in equinus may be better. A modified Symes amputation (ankle disarticulation with Symes flap) simplifies future fitting and eliminates the unsightly anterior bulge of a prosthesis fitted over the foot.

Arthrodesis of the knee can stabilize the lever arm of the limb and considerably reduce the limp. King has shown that this can be done as early as 3 to 4 years of age; if done carefully, and stabilized with a Küntscher rod, the epiphyses remain open and continue to contribute to needed length.[4,14]

Stabilization or reconstruction about the hip can only be useful in Classes A and B, and is not uniformly successful. Attempts at hip fusion have not been successful.

Rotation osteotomies of the tibia through 180°, to allow the foot to be fitted as a below-knee stump, have been found by Van Nes[25] to yield good results. Their disadvantages are a high incidence of derotation with growth, and the need to use a platform brace to preserve the foot until the patient is large enough to have the operation.

In cases of bilateral PFFD consideration should be given to preserving the feet (without rotation) so that around the house the patient may ambulate without prostheses. Knee arthrodesis in these cases is also felt to interfere with independent (nonprosthetic) ambulation.

B. Fibular Meromelia. This deficiency is one of the most frequent congenital limb deformities, and often occurs with other anomalies (for instance, it is seen in more than 50% of all patients with PFFD). The major problem it presents is leg length discrepancy, which is progressive. Kruger[3] found that this discrepancy was greater unfortunately in those patients who retained a normal foot (intercalary deficiency), and less in those with terminal deficiencies and only a partial foot remaining. Many of these patients have associated shortening of the epsilateral femur; the tibia is also frequently bowed anteriorly at the junction of the middle and distal thirds; both of these problems increase the leg length discrepancy.

Modified Symes amputation (as described above, or fusing the os calcis and attached heel pad to the distal tibia) offers many advantages to these patients, e.g., the avoidance of multiple osteotomies, lengthening procedures, procedures to stabilize the ankle; the better cosmesis of a prosthesis compared to a platform brace (Fig. 1.46).

Keeping the heel pad correctly located after a Symes amputation is a difficult problem in a growing child. The use of a Steinman pin through the pad into the tibia, and a well molded cast for 6 weeks postoperatively is helpful.

C. Tibial Meromelia. This deficiency is less common; it may be partial or complete and may be associated with distal reduplication (the only reduction deformity documented to do this). It is also known to occur in siblings and in

more than one generation of the same family, often with a familial incidence of clawhand deformities as well.

The fibula head lies more proximal than normally and is lateral and posterior at the knee. Clinically the patients present with a flexed knee and varus foot; the foot may be complete (intercalary deficit) or incomplete, and associated tarsal anomalies are common.

As leg length discrepancy in the unilateral cases precludes normal use of the foot, it cannot usually be preserved. Achievement of the useful knee, to be fitted with a below-knee prosthesis can sometimes be accomplished by

Fig. 1.46. A useful termination for the amputation stump in childhood is the heel pad still attached to the os calcis. *(A)* Anteroposterior view shows os calcis firmly united to the hypertrophied distal end of the fibula which had previously been united to the remnant of the proximal tibia. *(B)* Lateral view shows firm adherence of the heel pad to the os calcis. This prevents many of the complications of amputation in childhood. The heel pad stays in place and the bone does not grow through the skin.

Fig. 1.46*B*

centralization of the proximal fibula. Myers[20] in 1905 published one of the first reports of this operation, with a 5-year follow-up, but it was Brown[6,7] who has reintroduced it. Brown emphasizes in his follow-up review[7] attachment of the patellar ligament to the fibula, hamstring releases if necessary, and in obtaining and maintaining full extension. The biggest postoperative difficulty is flexion deformity, and secondary release or other procedures may be necessary and are worthwhile. The earlier this procedure is performed, of course, the better adaptation of proximal fibular cartilage to form a joint with the femur will occur; Brown recommends operating as early as possible, the patient will have a limb suitable for a below-knee prosthesis; knee joints and a thigh lacer must be used because of persistent mediolateral instability. Strengthening exercises for the quadriceps and hamstrings are important postoperatively.

If a portion of the tibia is present prox-imally, the fibula can be transferred centrally into it; this has to be done after a portion of the tibial remnant has ossified, to allow bone-to-bone apposition.

Bilateral cases may cause consideration of ways to preserve the feet, but instability at the ankle is usually extreme, and short stature is marked. These patients are best treated by ankle disarticulation and Brown procedure, or knee disarticulation if these fail.

BY MARY WILLIAMS, M.D.

Elective Revision

Elective revisions of the stump have one fundamental etiology peculiar to children. This is bone overgrowth, which results in stretching of the soft tissues over the stump end, ulceration, trophic changes, and a nonfunctional situation. Painful and functionally limiting neuromas occur in children as they do in adults.

The fibula is a particularly troublesome bone with respect to overgrowth and its secondary sequelae, perhaps because of its narrow cross sectional diameter and poor adherence to the skin over it. Overgrowth does not necessarily follow the growth potential of the proximal epiphysis.

Bursae are a complication particularly in childhood. It is not unusual to find them in anyone who plays basketball or football, not in a wheelchair, but as one of the active participants. This kind of activity, seldom practiced by the adult, tears at the stump and its tissue, which is not intended for weight bearing. Bursae thus formed usually require surgical excision, but the stump does not necessarily need to be shortened.

References

1. Aitken, G. T.: Amputation as a treatment for certain lower extremity congenital abnormalities, *J. Bone Joint Surg., 41A:* 1267, 1959.
2. Aitken, G. T. (ed.): *The Child with an Acquired Amputation,* Washington, D. C.: National Academy of Sciences, 1972.
3. Aitken, G. T. (ed.): *Selected Lower Limb Anomalies,* Washington, D.C.: National Academy of Sciences, 1971.
4. Aitken, G. T. (ed.): *P.F.F.D: Congenital Anomalies,* Washington, D. C.: National Academy of Sciences, 1969.
5. Aitken, G. T., and Lambert, C.: The Management of the Juvenile Amputee, Manual and Lectures for Prosthetics 631, Prosthetic-Orthotic Center, Northwestern University Medical School, 1972.
6. Brown, F. W.: Construction of a knee joint in congenital total absence of the tibia; a preliminary report, *J. Bone Joint Surg., 47A:* 695, 1965.
7. Brown, F. W., and Pohnert, W. H.: Construction of a knee joint in meromelia tibia; a 15-year follow-up study, *J. Bone Joint Surg., 54A:* 1333, 1972.
8. Burgess, E. M., and Romano, R. L.: Immediate post-surgical prosthetic fitting, *Bulletin of Prosthetic Research, 10*(4), 1965.
9. Burgess, E. M., Romano, R. L., and Zettl, J. H.: Management of Lower Extremity Amputees, TR 10-5, Veteran's Admnistration, Washington, D. C. 1969.
10. Burtch, R. L.: Nomenclature for congenital skeletal limb deficiencies; a revision, *Artif. Limbs, 10:* 24, 1966.
11. Crenshaw, A. H. (ed.): *Campbell's Operative Orthopedics,* St. Louis: C. V. Mosby Co., 1971.
12. Fishman, S.: Report of NYU Studies, 1972 Clinic Chiefs Meeting, Atlanta, 1972.
13. Frantz, C. H., and O'Rahilly, R.: Congenital skeletal limb deficiencies, *J. Bone Joint Surg., 43A:* 1202, 1961.
14. *Inter-Clinic Information Bulletin,* New York University Postgraduate Medical School, New York; monthly publication.
15. Kay, H. W., and Dolan, C.M.E.: Some guidelines for operation of child amputee clinics, *Inter-Clinic Information Bulletin, 7*(9), 1968.
16. Kübler-Ross, E.: *On Death and Dying,* New York: Macmillan, 1969.
17. LaForest, N. T., and Regon, L. W.: The physical therapy program after an immediate semirigid dressing and temporary below-knee prosthesis, *Phys. Ther., 53:* 497, 1973.
18. Levit, F.: Dermatological Considerations, Lecture for Prosthetics 622, Prosthetic-Orthotic Center, Northwestern University Medical School, 1971.
19. Mooney, V.: Comparison of post-operative stump management, *J. Bone Joint Surg., 53A:* 241, 1971.
20. Myers, T. H.: *Am. J. Orthop. Surg., 3:* 72, 1905.
21. Myers, T. H.: Further report on a case of congenital absence of the tibia, *Am. J. Orthop. Surg., 8:* 398, 1910.
22. *Orthopedic Clinics of North America, 3*(2), July 1972; Amputation Surgery and Prosthetics.
23. Schoenberg, B., Carr, A. C., Peretz, D., and Kutscher, A. H.: *Loss and Grief: Psychological Management in Medical Practice,* New York: Columbia University Press, 1970.
24. Swinyard, C. (ed.): *Limb Development and Deformity,* Springfield, Ill.: Charles C Thomas, 1969.
25. Van Nes, C. P.: Rotation-plasty for congenital defects of the femur, *J. Bone Joint. Surg., 32B:* 12, 1950.

DEVELOPMENTAL ANATOMY

The gross anatomy of the infant or child exhibits marked differences from the adult. This is most manifest in the musculoskeletal system. Since a complete survey of anatomical changes from birth to physeal closure is not feasible, salient areas will be emphasized.

Upper Extremity

The upper limbs are relatively long compared to the rest of the body. Their overall length averages 16.5 cm, which is about the same as the lower limb. Structurally and functionally the upper limb is better developed than the lower limb.

Shoulder

The clavicle is the first bone to form a primary ossification center, about the sixth week of development. It forms an epiphysis and discoid growth plate at the proximal end (sternoclavicular joint), while the distal (acromioclavicular) end has a subarticular spherical growth plate analagous to that in the phalanges (Fig. 1.7). The scapula forms a large, flat ossification center with two significant discoid growth plates, one along the medial edge and one adjacent to the glenoid. Like the acetabulum, the glenoid is entirely composed of hyaline cartilage at birth, with some fibrocartilage along the rim. The proximal humerus develops an ossification center just before or after birth. Figure 1.47A shows the proximal humerus of a neonate. The ossification center is just beginning to form. By 15 months (Fig. 1.47B) the first epiphyseal ossification center

has appeared and the second one has started in the region of the greater tuberosity. The proximal humeral growth plate contributes 40% of the length of the upper extremity and 80% of the length of the humerus.

Elbow

Development of the distal humerus has been alluded to in a previous section. No ossification centers are present at birth, but during the first year the ossification center appears in the capitellar portion of the distal humeral epiphysis. The ossification center of the trochlear portion of the epiphysis does not appear until

Fig. 1.47. *(A)* Neonatal humerus. The epiphysis is entirely cartilaginous. The epiphyseal ossification center *(EOC)* is just beginning to form. This area is shown in more detail in Figure 1.8. *(B)* Proximal humerus from a 15-month-old infant, showing two well developed ossification centers. The *arrow* indicates a blood vessel connecting the two centers. Cartilage transformation is occurring around this vessel.

Fig. 1.47*B*

approximately 7 years. The distal humerus contributes 10% of the length of the upper extremity and 20% of the length of the humerus. The proximal radius has no ossification center until 3 years of age, whereas the proximal ulnar ossification center appears at 7-8 years. The proximal ulna shows considerable variation in the structure of the growth plate (Fig. 1.48). The most proximal portion is a normally structured plate, engaged in longitudinal growth. But the segment under the elbow joint has narrower, shorter cell columns (a reflection of the lessening role in longitudinal development of this area of the proximal ulna). The proximal radial and ulnar growth plates contribute 11% of the overall length of the upper extremity, and, respectively, 25% and 20% of radial and ulnar length. Only 21% of overall arm length occurs at the elbow.

Wrist

The distal radius and ulna are relatively underdeveloped (Fig. 1.49). The radial growth plate is slightly more proximal than the ulnar growth plate. Both epiphyses are of similar volume, a relationship that will change very rapidly over the next 2-3 years. The distal radial and ulnar growth plates contribute 39% of overall length of the upper extremity, and, respectively, 75% and 80% of radial and ulnar length. The carpal bones do not begin to ossify until the end of the first year of life. The pisiform does not develop until just before puberty.

Hand

The newborn hand is functionally very mature, being capable of relatively strong grasp.

Fig. 1.48. Olecranon from a 2-month-old infant. The portion of the growth plate oriented perpendicular to the longitudinal axis has a normal architecture, whereas that part under the joint has much shorter cell columns and is primarily undergoing interstitial rather than longitudinal growth.

The length is about one-quarter that of the upper extremity (about 4-5 cm). The phalanges develop similarly to the toe phalanx shown previously (Fig. 1.7); i.e., a discoid growth plate and epiphysis at one end and a slowly diminishing chondroepiphysis and spherical growth plate at the other end.

Vertebral Column

The average neonatal vertebral column is 19-20 cm from C1 to L5, with the thoracic spine comprising 50% of the length, and the cervical and lumbar regions 25% each. With development, the thoracic portion remains about the same, but the cervical decreases and the lumbar increases. There are *no* fixed curves at birth, unless a structural abnormality is present. The spine is so flexible that the dissected column can be bent into a semicircle. After birth the thoracic spine rapidly develops and stabilizes a fixed curve. The cervical curve develops a few weeks later as the infant begins to lift his head. The lumbar curve does not develop until the child begins to stand and walk. At birth each vertebra (except C1 and C2) has three separate ossification centers (one in the body and two in the posterior elements). The atlas (C1) has only two ossification centers (both in the posterior elements), whereas the axis (C2) has four centers (two posterior, one in the body, and one in the odontoid process). Most of the vertebra is comprised of hyaline cartilage. The necleus pulposus is relatively large in the neonate, with a much smaller anulus (Fig. 1.9).

Lower Extremity

Relative to the upper limbs the legs are poorly developed at birth, both structurally and functionally. They are proportionately much smaller than the upper limbs, when considering final adult size. Intrauterine positioning is much more manifest, causing significant flexion and abduction at the hip, flexion at the knees, and supination at the foot. There is moderate resistance to manipulative correction of these positional "contractures."

Fig. 1.49. Distal radius *(R)* and ulna *(U)* of a neonate. The growth plate of the ulna is more distal than the radius. The radius has a more significant zone of Ranvier (*).

Hip

The neonatal femur is a straight bone that averages 8.5 cm in length. The femoral head is approximately 1 cm in diameter. A femoral neck is virtually nonexistent. The head is incompletely covered by the acetabulum. The ligamentum capitum femoris is relatively long. The musculature is better developed medially than laterally. Since hip disorders are a major problem in infants, the detailed anatomy will be discussed.

The femoral nerve, artery, and vein are relatively large structures that occupy the middle one-third of the proximal lower leg (Fig. 1.50). The adductor muscle group is much better developed than the abductor group. The iliopsoas is separated from the overlying nerve and blood vessels by a fascial sleeve that creates a tunnel from the inguinal ligament to the lesser trochanter (Fig. 1.51). The role of the iliopsoas functionally varies, depending upon the position of the femur relative to the pelvis. When the hip is neutral, the iliopsoas crosses only a small portion of the medial femoral head and acetabulur rim. With flexion the iliopsoas relaxes significantly. But with increasing abduction, the iliopsoas translocates laterally to cover

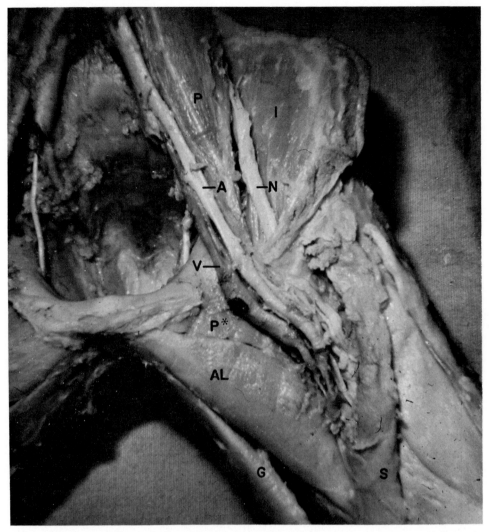

Fig. 1.50. Superficial anatomy of the infant thigh. (*P*, psoas; *I*, iliacus; *A*, femoral artery; *N*, femoral nerve; *V*, femoral vein; *P*,* pectineus; *AL*, adductor longus; *G*, gracilis; *S*, sartorius.)

more of the femoral head and cross the acetabulum rim more laterally and superiorly (Fig. 1.52). As the iliopsoas shifts laterally, its function changes to a significant hip abductor.

The hip capsule is attached to the proximal femur along the groove between femoral head and greater trochanter (intraepiphyseal groove). In the neonate the medial most attachment of the capsule to the proximal femur is adjacent to the growth plate. Therefore, most of the proximal femoral growth plate at this stage is extra-articular. With subsequent development the growth plate eventually becomes an intra-articular structure. The capsular attachments on

the acetabular side are several millimeters beyond the labrum, and not directly at the edge of the labrum (Fig. 1.53). The labrum is then an intra-articular, rather than periarticular structure.

The acetabulum is composed of two significantly different types of cartilage during early development (Fig. 1.54). The most peripheral portion of the labrum is composed of fibrocartilage, while the bulk of the labrum and acetabulum is composed of hyaline cartilage. The limbus forms from hypertrophy of the fibrocartilaginous portion of the acetabulum. The labrum, especially the fibrocartilaginous

Fig. 1.51. Fascial tunnel separating the iliopsoas from the overlying neurovascular structures.

portion, can be easily deformed by manual pressure (Fig. 1.55).

The proximal femur of the neonate has a single epiphysis and a single growth plate (Fig. 1.54). This is transversely oriented, just above the lesser trochanter. However, as the infant grows, differential growth rates cause the central portion of the epiphysis to grow faster both longitudinally as well as interstitially, such that the growth plate becomes "pyramidal." The proximal femoral growth plate contributes 15% of the overall leg length and 30% of femoral length.

The blood supply of the proximal femur stems primarily from the deep (profunda) femoral artery, which gives off two significant branches—the lateral and medial circumflex arteries. The lateral circumflex artery divides into ascending, transverse, and descending branches. The transverse branch goes between the rectus femoris and iliopsoas to reach the anterolateral proximal femur (Fig. 1.56). Several branches ramify over the greater trochanter, and a small branch courses in the intraepiphyseal groove to anastomose with the terminal portion of the medial circumflex artery. The medial circumflex artery goes between the iliopsoas and adductor muscles to reach the medial side of the proximal femur just above the lesser trochanter (Fig. 1.57). Small branches enter the epiphysis just above the growth plate. The medial circumflex artery then continues around to the posterior surface to reach the intraepiphyseal groove. The artery

Fig. 1.52. Lateral translocation of the iliopsoas *(IP)* when the hip is flexed and abducted. *(LT,* lesser trochanter.)

courses along this groove onto the anterior portion to anastomose with the lateral circumflex termination. The major penetrating arteries to the epiphysis and growth plate arise from the medial circumflex artery posteriorly in the intraepiphyseal groove. This artery in the intraepiphyseal groove is subject to compression during positioning.

Positioning significantly affects the relationship between the intraepiphyseal groove and its contained arteries and the acetabulum, and thereby affects the circulation to the proximal femur. When hips are put through various ranges of motion, or held in the commonly used treatment positions, the superior and posterior acetabulum fit tightly into the intraepiphyseal groove, interlocking similar to pieces of a jigsaw puzzle (Fig. 1.58). Not much pressure is necessary to firmly wedge the labrum into the groove, especially with increasing abduction, compromising the space available in the groove for the blood vessels that supply the femoral head. In the Lorenz and "frog-leg" positions, the labrum and groove are maximally compressed together. In less extreme treatment positions, such as the "human position" of Salter, compression in the intraepiphyseal groove is minimized. Thus, one of the major effects of treatment in positions emphasizing marked abduction is to variably occlude the blood supply as it courses along the posterior intraepiphyseal groove.

Circulatory compromise may also occur as the medial circumflex artery courses between the iliopsoas and adductor group. By abducting the hip the medial circumflex artery may be stretched and partially occluded as it courses over the iliopsoas tendon (Fig. 1.59). Internal

Fig. 1.53. Attachment of hip joint capsule several millimeters beyond the acetabular rim, leaving a potential space between the rim and capsule. This area fills with dye in an arthrogram, visualizing the "rose thorn."

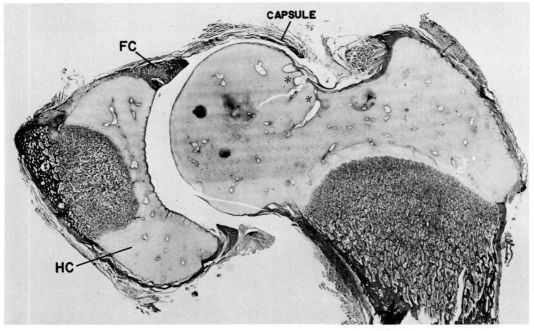

Fig. 1.54. Sagittal section of the proximal femur and acetabulum of a 2-month-old infant. Note the extensive cartilage canal system, with major penetrating canals (*) from the interepiphyseal groove. (*FC*, fibrocartilaginous acetabular rim; *HC*, hyaline cartilage of the acetabulum.) The articular cartilage of the acetabulum is histochemically different (darker staining).

Fig. 1.55. Deformity of the posterior acetabular rim.

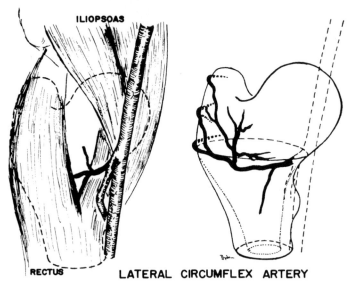

Fig. 1.56. Lateral circumflex arterial circulation. The artery stems from the profunda femoris and crosses the iliopsoas and then goes between the two heads of the rectus femoris to reach the anterior proximal femur, where distribution is primarily to the trochanteric region.

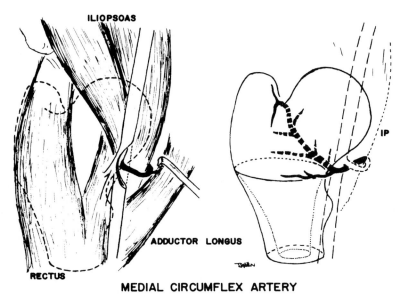

MEDIAL CIRCUMFLEX ARTERY

Fig. 1.57. Medial circumflex arterial circulation. The artery usually stems from the profunda femoris. It crosses the iliopsoas and then wraps around the iliopsoas tendon to reach the medial portion of the proximal femur. It then courses along the posterior intraepiphyseal groove, providing the major blood supply to the chondroepiphysis and central and medial portions of the growth plate.

Fig. 1.58. Abduction and flexion cause impingement between the rim of the acetabulum and the intraepiphyseal groove.

Fig. 1.59. Abduction and flexion stretch the medial circumflex, as it is fixed where it courses between the iliopsoas and the adductor longus.

rotation increases the degree of stretching. There may also be arterial compression deeper, between the iliopsoas tendon and the pectineus/adductor muscles. One of the beneficial effects of adductor tenotomy may be to lessen such arterial compression.

Congenital Hip Dislocation. The pathologic anatomy of congenital hip dislocation will be discussed in detail in the section dealing with hip disease. However, some normal anatomy is pertinent to discuss here. The ligamentum capitum femoris is relatively long. If the capsule is transected, the femoral head can be dislocated over the lateral rim, but it cannot be dislocated into the usual superoposterior position due to limitation imposed by the ligamentum capitum femoris (Fig. 1.60). The intact capsule and its intrinsic supporting ligaments further limit lateral motion of the femoral head.

The adductor/pectineus muscle group is much better developed than the abductors (gluteus medius, minimus) and external rotators, which tends to direct the femoral head into a more uncovered position. The iliopsoas is significantly displaced when the hip is dislocated (Fig. 1.61). The iliopsoas crosses the evacuated acetabulum, creating the characteristic hourglass capsular contraction. The iliopsoas also pulls the dislocated head back against the labrum, deforming it initially, and even invaginating the fibrocartilaginous portion. This inverted fibrocartilaginous rim may hypertrophy to create the pathologic limbus.

Knee

The distal femoral chondroepiphysis characteristically has a secondary ossification center at birth (Fig. 1.62). The distal femoral growth plate makes the most significant contribution to overall leg length (40%), as well as femoral length (70%). The proximal tibia may have a secondary ossification center at birth. This

Fig. 1.60. With the ligamentum capitum femoris intact, the femoral head can be displaced only to the acetabular rim.

Fig. 1.61. When the hip is completely dislocated, the iliopsoas *(IP)* crosses the vacated acetabulum, compressing the capsule into the joint, and causing the "hourglass" constriction.

Fig. 1.62. Distal femoral epiphysis of a newborn, showing the well developed ossification center that is present at birth. The *arrow* indicates a cartilage canal artery entering the vascular system of the ossification center.

rapidly expands because of growth and forces across the knee during the first year of life (Fig. 1.63). The proximal tibia contributes 27% of overall leg length and 55% of tibial length. Thus the knee growth plates contribute 67% of the entire leg length, a significant difference compared to the elbow contribution to arm length. The tibial tubercle does not develop an ossification center until relatively late (8-10 years). This may arise as a separate ossification center, or may extend from the main proximal tibial ossification center. It is classically taught that the growth plate of the proximal tibia turns to extend downward under the tibial tubercle. This does *not* occur. The cellular growth plate is replaced by a fibrous plate between the tibial tubercle cartilage and proximal tibial metaphysis (Fig. 1.64). This fibrous plate is more susceptible to shear stress than the cellular growth plate, and may explain how the tibial tubercle pulls away in a disease such as Osgood-Schlatter's.

Fig. 1.63. Proximal tibial epiphysis of a 15-month-old infant showing the well developed ossification center.

Ankle

The distal tibia and fibula are entirely cartilagenous at birth, while the talus and calcaneus have already commenced ossification. Significant blood vessels enter the lateral side of the tibial epiphysis (Fig. 1.65). This blood supply may be injured in a fracture of Tillaux. The distal tibia (and fibula) contribute 18% of overall leg length and 45% of tibial length.

Foot

By the end of the second fetal month the developing foot is formed, but markedly supinated. Not until the seventh fetal month does the process of gradual pronation commence, although at birth and for the first few weeks of life many children may still have some supination. Pronation occurs because of structural changes in the shape of the talus and calcaneus, and by the rapid growth of the medial side of the foot. At birth the foot is capable of considerable dorsiflexion because of the shape of the articular surface of the body of the talus. In contrast, plantar flexion may be limited, partially because of shortness of the foot extensor tendons. The feet are relatively long and narrow compared to the rest of the lower extremity, with an average length of 6.5 cm (the hip to heel length averages 16-18 cm). The foot appears to have no arches because of a thick, fibrous, plantar fat pad. The longitudinal arch of the neonate is actually relatively higher

Fig. 1.64. Section of the tibial tubercle showing the end of the cellular growth plate *(large arrow)* and the fibrous "growth" plate under the tibial tubercle.

than during later development. Failure of the transition from a supinated to a pronated foot, along with intrauterine positioning, probably play a major role in the evolution of the clubfoot.

Clubfoot. The clubfoot that proves resistant to treatment, or recurs after nonoperative treatment, usually has significant chronic alterations in the anatomy of the ankle, subtalar, and midtarsal articulations. There are major soft tissue contractures. The head and neck of the talus become structurally deformed, even while the body of the talus retains a relatively normal relationship with the mortise.

The most important "joint" is a multiple articulation that includes the talonavicular joint and the anterior and middle talocalcaneal joints. These articulations have a common synovial cavity that is separate from the posterior subtalar articulation. The anterior calcaneus and navicular are maintained as a structural unit by strong ligaments, the most important of which is the inferior calcaneonavicular, or spring ligament. This "joint" can be

considered a ball-and-socket joint, with the head of the talus (ball) articulating in the calcaneonavicular complex (socket).

Normal plantar flexion of the foot includes supination of the forefoot and calcaneovarus. The calcaneovarus occurs by a pivotal motion focused at the middle of the calcaneus: the anterior portion moves downward and medial, while the posterior portion moves upward and lateral. Concomitantly, the navicular, which must move integrally with the anterior calcaneus, also moves medially, but rotates instead of going downward. This exposes a greater portion of the talar head laterally, since the talus is normally unable to significantly abduct and adduct within the ankle mortise.

In the resistant or recurrent clubfoot, pathologic contractures of the soft tissue prevent the reduction of the calcaneonavicular complex on the head of the talus. These posterior, medial, and subtalar soft-tissue contractures are more significant than the structural deformity of the talus. Figures 1.66 and 1.67 show gross and schematic depictions of these contractures. The

Fig. 1.65. Distal tibia, fibula, calcaneus *(C)*, and talus *(T)* of a 2-month-old infant. This sagittal section is posterior to the ossified portions of the talus and calcaneus. The *arrow* indicates a major vessel entering the lateral side of the tibial epiphysis.

posterior contractures involve the posterior capsules of the ankle and subtalar joints, the heel cord, and the posterior tibiofibular and calcaneofibular ligaments. These latter contractures also lead to a more posterior displacement of the fibula. The medial contractures include the deltoid and spring ligaments; the talonavicular joint capsule; the posterior tibial, flexor digitorum longus, and flexor hallucis longus tendons; and the anterior tibial and extensor hallucic longus tendons. Subtalar contractures involve the anterior subtalar interosseous liga-

ment and the bifurcated (Y) ligament.

Since the talus has no musculotendinous connections, its position and shape are mediated by surrounding structures. As the talus is forced into equinus, the posterior calcaneus is displaced upward and lateral. This is due to contractures of the posterior capsule, the heel cord, and the calcaneofibular ligament. Since the calcaneus pivots centrally, the anterior segment is displaced downward, medially, and under the head of the talus. In this position contractures of the deltoid and spring ligaments

Fig. 1.66. Gross and schematic anatomy of a resistant clubfoot (anterior view).

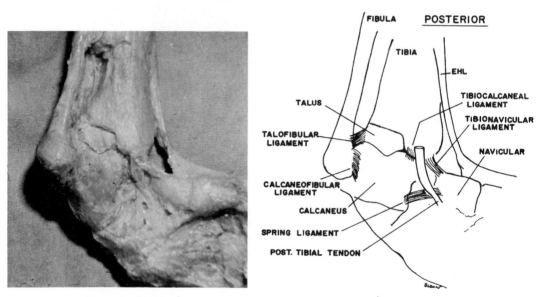

Fig 1.67. Gross and schematic anatomy of a resistant clubfoot (posterior view).

and posterior tibial tendon worsen and accentuate the deformity, and undoubtedly play a role in the deformation of the more cartilaginous head and neck of the talus. The navicular is displaced medial to the head of the talus and may even articulate with the medial malleolus. The severity of the contractures juxtaposes the navicular bone, the sustentaculum tali, and the medial malleolus. The pathologically contracted ligaments form a dense medial mass that obscures the joint lines and neck of the talus anteriorly and posteriorly.

BY JOHN OGDEN, M.D.

HOW TO READ AN ORTHOPAEDIC X-RAY FILM, SELF-TEACHING

INTRODUCTION

This is a program on the fundamentals of x-ray diagnosis of bone and joint lesions. It is arranged as a branching program. It begins with a single major concept or idea. You read this. You are then asked a question and given a number of possible answers from which you select one you think is correct. Only one answer is actually correct. The others are selected because they are typical or plausible mistakes.

The answers are numbered and they have been scrambled in the remainder of this portion of the text. Turn to the numbered answers that you selected.

If you are correct, you will be given additional new material followed by an option for an additional question, and thus will advance through the material.

If you are incorrect, you will be given a short explanation of why and asked to return to the original numbered segment from which you started. You may then select another answer.

Remember, this material is not arranged in consecutive order and you must progress by numbered segments, choosing your next reading on the basis of the options offered you at the end of each portion of new material.

PROGRAM

1

The important attribute that anyone reading orthopaedic x-ray films must have is that of making an observation of the individual roentgen features present on the film. These changes in various combinations lead one to surmise the pathologic process that is taking place. Ultimately, with logical reasoning, and the addition of other facts about the patient, such as age and sex, the observer is led to the diagnosis.

All of this depends on the observation of individual roentgen features. It must be looked at in detail rather than in a total impression. A beginning is made when one can distinguish fluid and muscle density from fat density, bone density, and metallic density.

On an x-ray film there are a number of densities apparent. Air or gas are least dense. Fat as exemplified in subcutaneous tissue is next in density. The third density is that of water, which is exemplified by muscle density in the soft tissues. Bone is obviously more dense than any of these. If one contrasted bone and metal on the x-ray film, he would expect metal to be most dense.

Water density is:

Less dense than fat	32
Less dense than muscle	13
More dense than bone	39
More dense than fat	17

2

YOUR ANSWER: Bone density is the density of medullary contents of the bone.

You are incorrect. Bone density is principally formed by the extremely dense cortex.

Return to number 33 and try again.

3

YOUR ANSWER: A swelling is most likely to be associated with a tumor.

You are incorrect. A swelling is caused by inflammatory edema. This could occur with a tumor but is not likely. Most likely is the x-ray definition of a mass caused by growth of the tumor. It has well defined edges as it displaces normal tissue.

Return to number 6 and try again.

4

YOUR ANSWER: The metaphysis is more likely to be the seat of disease than other areas of the bone because embolic phenomena lodge in the metaphysis due to the formation of endarterial loops in this area.

You are correct. Infection, tumor, and metabolic products all tend to lodge in the metaphysis, carried there by the general circulation.

Blood-borne bacteria lodging in the metaphysis would produce an inflammation. This would first be evident on the x-ray film as a soft-tissue swelling. Nine to 11 days later one might have sufficient destruction of the cortex to distinguish the lesion in the bone.

The swelling associated with osteomyelitis would involve the deep soft tissues next to the bone. Deep soft tissue swelling can be distinguished from superficial soft tissue swelling involving the subcutaneous tissues. Superficial soft tissue swelling is associated with cellulitis rather than osteomyelitis.

An osteomyelitis first is evident on the x-ray film as:

An area of bone destruction in the metaphysis	5
An area of superficial swelling centered about the metaphysis	52
An area of deep soft tissue swelling centered about the metaphysis	61
An area of bone destruction in the diaphysis	25

5

YOUR ANSWER: An osteomyelitis first is evident on the x-ray film as an area of bone destruction in the metaphysis.

You are incorrect. The change of bone destruction is a late change only visible when enough of the cortex has been destroyed. The first change is a deep soft tissue swelling centered about the metaphysis.

Return to number 4 and try again.

6

YOUR ANSWER: A swelling obscures the fat lines running through the muscle density areas because swellings have density comparable to muscle.

You are correct. Swellings have water density comparable to muscle density and therefore eliminate contrast areas within the muscle shadow. In the illustration for frame 6 there is a swelling about the distal femoral metaphysis. It is partly obscured by the wrapping holding the infant to the x-ray cassette, but note that its exact limits are hard to determine.

A swelling enlarges an area of water density. A mass also enlarges an area of water density. A mass has a clear-cut and distinct edge, in contrast to a swelling which has indistinct edges gradually fading into the shadow created by other soft tissues. A mass would be most likely to be associated with a tumor or an infection? If you answered tumor, you were correct.

Between these two which would be most likely to be associated with swelling?

Tumor	3
Infection	56

7

YOUR ANSWER: Tumor bone tends to a pattern which is around rather than in the tumor.

You are incorrect. Tumor bone is formed by the tumor and is the distinguishing feature of osteogenic sarcoma. Bone formed around the tumor is a reaction of the host and formed by normal tissues.

Return to number 59 and try again.

8

YOUR ANSWER: *B* is more dense than *D*.

You are incorrect. *B* is the subcutaneous tissue or fat. It is not as dense as bone.

Return to number 17 and try again.

9

YOUR ANSWER: A bone cyst could be larger than evident on the x-ray film.

You are correct. What is seen is those areas where the cortex has been thinned. Actual cystic involvement could extend beyond this point, involving or replacing the medullary contents as in *A* or *B* in figure for frame 9.

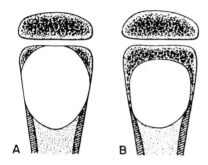

A   B

Ordinarily lines of contrasting density are seen running through the area occupied by muscle. These are created by fat lying in tissue planes. A swelling has vague outlines fading into the water density, but obscures these fat lines, rendering the shadow relatively homogeneous. These lines are obscured because a swelling has water density.

A swelling obscures the fat lines running through the muscle density areas because:

Swellings have fat density.	41
Swellings have air density.	51
Swellings have density comparable to muscle.	6

10

YOUR ANSWER: A tumor that is designated an osteogenic sarcoma always arises from marrow elements.

You are incorrect. Arising from marrow elements is not a characteristic of osteogenic sarcoma.

Return to number 36 and try again.

11

YOUR ANSWER: Total destruction of the bone area occupied is characteristic of metastases from breast carcinoma.

You are incorrect. The roentgen appearance of breast carcinoma may be one of varying

degrees of sclerosis giving rise to alternate areas of density as the host tissues are excited to lay down bone.

Return to number 53 and try again.

12

YOUR ANSWER: The number of visible vessel lines would be expected to increase with a swelling.

This is true. Vascular dilation is associated with inflammation. An inflammation causes a swelling. One can see evidence of this increased vascularity in the subcutaneous tissue where the vessel lines of water density contrast with the fat density of subcutaneous tissue.

An area of active destruction in the metaphysis of a long bone associated with soft tissue swelling would presumably be an infection. An area of active destruction in a bone associated with a mass would presumably be a malignant tumor.

Active destruction is associated with either osteomyelitis or a malignant process.

Osteomyelitis can be distinguished from destruction of bone due to malignancy by:

The nature of destructive line	24
The decision as to whether a mass or a swelling accompanies the destruction	59
The area of bone involved	35

13

YOUR ANSWER: Water density is less dense than muscle.

You are incorrect. Water density and muscle density are synonymous so far as x-ray interpretation is concerned.

Return to number 1 and try again.

14

YOUR ANSWER: The metaphysis is more likely to be the seat of disease than other areas of the bone because it is the most active portion of the bone from the standpoint of metabolism.

You are incorrect. It is true that metabolism is most active in the metaphysis. Bone as an organ mirrors body states in this area, but disease phenomena are transmitted to this area from the rest of the body and the nature of the metaphyseal circulation becomes extremely important.

Return to number 42 and try again.

15

YOUR ANSWER: Numbers 1 and 3 are true; number 2 is false.

You are incorrect. Metastases from the thyroid are totally lytic and prostatic metastases can be both sclerotic and lytic. However leukemia with its cellular infiltrates tends to run between bone trabeculae, giving rise to a lagging type of destruction by roentgenogram.

Return to number 28 and try again.

16

YOUR ANSWER: The diagnosis would be fracture line if soft tissue swelling were present.

You are incorrect. Soft tissue swelling does not differentiate a growth line from a fracture line since this finding could accompany either.

Return to number 46 and try again.

17

YOUR ANSWER: Water density is more dense than fat.

This is correct. Fat does not contain water, and its structure is such that it is not as dense on the roentgen film as water density as exemplified by muscle shadows on the x-ray film.

The illustration is the roentgen picture of an extremity. The various densities are tagged with letters. Select the proper answer below.

B is more dense than *D*.	8
B is less dense than *A*.	21
B is less dense than *C*.	33

18

YOUR ANSWER: The diagnosis would be fracture line if the radiolucent line was of uneven width with sharp angles and irregular edges.

Your are correct. The growth line, by contrast, has even width and rounded edges.

A fracture line is associated with soft-tissue swelling. Would you expect this to be deep soft-tissue swelling or superficial soft-tissue swelling? If you said deep soft-tissue swelling, you were correct, since the onset of the swelling, at least, is due to the developing hematoma about the fracture. Where the injury has been crushing in nature the superficial tissues may be swollen as well.

A fracture line is most likely associated with:

Deep soft-tissue swelling	20
No soft-tissue swelling	63
Superficial soft-tissue swelling	54

19

YOUR ANSWER: Bone density is principally formed by the cortex.

You are correct. A lesion in the bone, if it involved the medullary contents only and not the cortex, might not be visible on the roentgen film.

A, B, and C in the figure illustrate varying degrees of involvement of the cortex in fibrous dysplasia. If the medullary lesion was similar in density to the medullary contents and did not involve cortex it would not be evident on the roentgen film.

A lesion of bone is going to be most evident on the x-ray film if it affects the medullary contents of the bone or the cortex? If you answered cortex, this is true. Here we have a very dense substance by x-ray. It can overlay a considerable medullary lesion and make it impossible to be seen. To be seen by roentgenogram, a lesion must create a contrast.

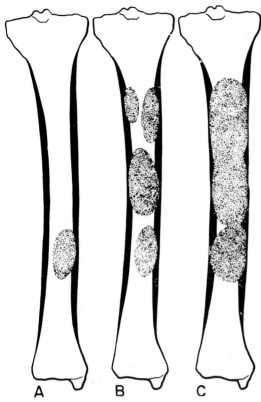

A B C

A bone cyst could be:

Larger than evident on the x-ray film   9
Smaller than evident on the x-ray film   48

20

YOUR ANSWER: A fracture line is most likely associated with deep soft-tissue swelling.

You are correct. The developing hematoma associated with a fracture soon makes deep soft-tissue swelling evident.

A vertebral fracture produces a typical deformity. Soft-tissue swelling cannot be ascertained through the overlying structures. The deformity due to trauma occurs by fracturing the superior cortex. This produces an angulation of the anterior margin as the anterior cortex is broken, and decreases the height of the vertebra anteriorly.

The deformity of a vertebra due to osteoporosis is quite different. Here the intervertebral disc, being of fluid nature and relatively incompressible, maintains its height. The vertebra loses height more anteriorly than posteriorly, but without pushing out the superior,

anterior angle of the vertebra. Both superior and inferior cortices are depressed in rounded fashion by pressure from the intervertebral disc, giving rise to a biconcave vertebra.

In the drawings for frame 20 select the vertebral outline which is due to fracture.

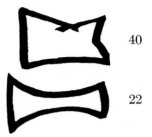

40

22

21

YOUR ANSWER: *B* is less dense than *A*.

A is the background density of the film itself. *B* is subcutaneous tissue of fat density recording a shadow against the background density and consequently more dense.

Return to number 17 and try again.

22

YOUR ANSWER: The vertebral outline in the figure for frame 20 is due to fracture. You are correct.

The compression and fracture of the superior cortex breaks out an anterior beak superiorly as the anterior cortex also fractures. This is a typical vertebral fracture outline.

The density of a bone is a reflection of its metabolic equilibrium with the body. This equilibrium cannot be maintained if the blood supply to a bone or a portion of it is cut off. The bone about this area remains responsive to changes in this equilibrium but the dead bone remains at a static density. Thus, disuse which accompanies the pain associated with this lesion leaves the dead portion at its original density as the bone about it loses density.

The roentgen appearance of avascular bone is such that it is more dense than the surrounding bone.

In order to recognize the avascular state of a segment of a bone by roentgenogram:

More calcium salt must go into the avascular segment.	23
The original density of the bone segment must change.	57
A contrasting change in density is necessary in the bone about it.	47

23

YOUR ANSWER: In order to recognize the avascular state of a segment of bone by roentgenogram more calcium salt must go into the avascular segment.

You are incorrect. Since there is no longer a vascular penetration of this segment it is impossible for additional metabolic products to be deposited.

The density of this segment remains the same. The bone about it becomes less dense, increasing the contrast between the two.

Please return to number 22 and try again.

24

YOUR ANSWER: Osteomyelitis can be distinguished from destruction of bone due to malignancy by the nature of the destructive line.

You are incorrect. In both cases active destruction of bone is present. This is distinguished by a minutely spiculated rather than a smooth edge.

Return to number 12 and try again.

25

YOUR ANSWER: An osteomyelitis first is evident on the x-ray film as an area of bone destruction in the diaphysis.

You are incorrect. Osteomyelitis is blood-borne to the metaphysis, not the diaphysis, and the metaphysis is the characteristic location for it. The diaphysis is a relatively inactive portion of the bone principally used for support.

Return to number 4 and try again.

26

YOUR ANSWER: Numbers 1, 2, and 3 are true.

You are correct. Metastases from the thyroid are totally lytic while prostatic metastases vary with lytic and sclerotic areas. The cellular infiltrates of leukemia tend to give the appearance of lagging destruction.

When a bone has an accessory bone next to it separated by a growth line, the combined mass of the two is greater than you would expect the bony structure to occupy normally (B).

A   B

Where a fragment of bone has been fractured away from its parent bone, you would expect the combined mass of the two to be equal to the expected mass of the bone normally.

One would also expect to see the bed from which the fragment had been torn.

An accessory bone is separated from the parent bone by a radiolucent line.

It is helpful in determining whether a fracture exists to note:

Whether the mass of the parent bone and the bone fragment is greater or equal to the area normally occupied by the undivided bone	46
Whether the parent bone and the bone fragment have a mass less than the area normally occupied by the undivided bone	60

27

YOUR ANSWER: Avascular segments of bone may arise in various ways. The entrance of new blood vessels into the avascular segment is visible roentgenographically as areas of lesser density.

You are correct. The areas of lesser density occur about the newly vascular areas as old bone is resorbed.

There is another important distinction that can be made roentgenographically as an aid in diagnosis. This is the distinction between ossification and calcification.

Ossification has bone structure, and individual bone stria can be seen. Calcification is homogenous and structureless. When examined pathologically it is also amorphous.

Amorphous calcification occurs as a deposit in degenerative areas in bursae, tendons, and in metabolic disease. Ossification may occur as a repair process or as a reaction to tumor or infection.

If an adventitious area of calcific density has definite structure visible in the roentgenogram, it could be termed:

Ossification   55
Calcification   37

28

YOUR ANSWER: Total destruction of the bone area occupied is characteristic of metastases from lung and thyroid carcinoma.

You are correct. Lung and thyroid carcinoma metastases, when present in bone, totally destroy all bone visible in the roentgenogram within the area occupied by the tumor. Little reaction is excited in the host bone and, consequently, bony reaction about the tumor is not prominent.

Metastases such as those from breast and prostate exhibit lytic areas of increased density as well. Here new bone is laid down around the exciting lesion.

1. A metastases from the thyroid would tend to give a totally lytic area in bone.
2. A leukemic lesion would tend to give lagging destruction.
3. A prostatic metastasis might look both more dense and less dense than the surrounding bone.

In the three statements above:

Numbers 1 and 2 are true; number 3 is   49
    false.

Numbers 1 and 3 are true; number 2 is   15
    false.

Numbers 1, 2, and 3 are true   26

29

YOUR ANSWER: The number of visible vessel lines would be decreased with a swelling.

You are incorrect. Vessel lines are normally not remarkable on the x-ray film. It is true that the swelling in its central portion obscures vessel lines by rendering the whole area of water dense and homogeneous. At the periphery, however, in areas of lesser density, the vessel lines caused by vascular dilation become well marked in the presence of inflammation.

Return to number 56 and try again.

30

YOUR ANSWER: Tumor bone tends to a pattern determined by the stress on the bone.

You are incorrect. Since the bone is destroyed, the normal engineering stresses are no longer present and the pattern of the bone that is formed is grossly irregular.

Return to number 59 and try again.

31

YOUR ANSWER: Avascular segments of bone may arise in various ways. The entrance of new blood vessels into the avascular segment is visible roentgenographically as increasing density of bone about the avascular segment.

You are incorrect. Increasing density of the uninvolved bone may indicate greater use of the extremity, but does not necessarily foretell the entrance of new blood vessels into the avascular segment.

Return to number 47 and try again.

32

YOUR ANSWER: Water density is less dense than fat.

You are incorrect. Fat contains no water and its roentgenographic density is less than water as exemplified by the muscle shadows on the x-ray film.

Return to number 1 and try again.

33

YOUR ANSWER: *B* is less dense than *C*.

You are correct. Subcutaneous tissue is less dense than muscle or water density.

If you contrasted gas or air and fat or subcutaneous tissue, fat or subcutaneous tissue would be most dense. If you contrasted water density and fat density, water density would be most dense. Bone has a very dense cortex, but one would expect the interior contents of the bone to have water density if they could be x-rayed isolated from the cortex.

Bone density is the density of the medullary contents of the bone.	2
Bone density is principally formed by the cortex.	19
The interior contents of the bone would be less dense than fat density.	45

34

YOUR ANSWER: A tumor tracks irregularly along the easiest anatomic route.

You are incorrect. An infection tracts irregularly but a tumor grows concentrically. An infection is associated with a poorly defined deep soft tissue swelling, a tumor with a mass with clean-cut edges.

Return to number 61 and try again.

35

YOUR ANSWER: Osteomyelitis can be distinguished from destruction of bone due to malignancy by the area of bone involved.

You are incorrect. It is true that blood-borne osteomyelitis is typically a metaphyseal disease. However a malignant tumor could be a metaphyseal lesion as well.

Return to number 12 and try again.

36

YOUR ANSWER: A tumor expands in concentric fashion into a rounded mass.

You are correct. A tumor will grow in all directions until it meets an anatomic obstacle. This gives rise to a rounded mass with clean cut edges.

A bone tumor with well defined mass producing tumor bone.

A bone tumor producing tumor bone is an osteogenic sarcoma. This tumor destroys bone in the area it occupies. Some malignant bone lesions, particularly those arising from cells in the medullary canal, tend to infiltrate through and around bone trabeculae displacing normal marrow elements. This gives rise to a type of destruction designated as "lagging" destruction. It is found in lesions such as Ewing's tumor.

A tumor that is designated an osteogenic sarcoma:

Infiltrates through the bone marrow giving rise to lagging destruction	62
Always arises from marrow elements	10
Always produces tumor bone	53

37

YOUR ANSWER: An adventitious area of calcific density having definite structure visible in the roentgenogram is termed calcification.

You are incorrect. Definite structure is not a characteristic of calcification. Calcification represents a toothpaste-like deposit occurring particularly in tendons and bursae about joints. It does not have bone formation within it. The ability to distinguish it from ossification is a great aid in differential diagnosis by roentgenogram.

Please return to number 27 and try again.

38

YOUR ANSWER: Avascular segments of bone may arise in various ways. The entrance of new blood vessels into the avascular segment is visible roentgenographically as areas of greater density.

You are incorrect. The new blood vessels remove the avascular bone (dense segments still apparent have not yet been invaded). New bone formation will be of normal bone density.

Return to number 47 and try again.

39

YOUR ANSWER: Water density is more dense than bone.

You are incorrect. Bone contains water and, in addition, mineral. It is consequently more dense than water or muscle density on the x-ray film.

Return to number 1 and try again.

40

YOUR ANSWER:

You are incorrect. The rounded compression of both superior and inferior cortices result in a biconcave vertebra. This is due to compressible bone in the presence of fluid incompressible disc material. Such a compression is secondary to osteoporosis. A fracture principally affects the superior cortex, producing anterior breaking, and the anterior cortex breaks as well.

Return to number 20 and try again.

41

YOUR ANSWER: A swelling obscures fat lines running through the muscle density area because swellings have fat density.

You are incorrect. Fat density would obviously not obscure an area of fat density.

Return to number 9 and try again.

42

YOUR ANSWER: Tumor bone tends to a pattern which is grossly irregular within the tumor.

You are correct. Tumor bone is within the area occupied by the tumor. Since the bone has been destroyed in this area the normal engineering stresses are no longer present and the pattern is grossly irregular.

X-ray features such as a mass or a swelling, benign or active destruction can now be distinguished. We are aware of the fact that a lesion in bone may not be readily distinguished unless it involves the cortex. A simple cyst involving the metaphysis is shown in the figure for frame 42.

Of diagnostic importance also is the location of the lesion. The metaphysis is the portion of the bone converted from the cartilage of the epiphyseal line until it becomes remodeled into diaphysis. The diaphysis serves a supporting function, lying between the metaphysis at either end. The metaphysis is an area of active blood supply, end-arterial loops and formation of blood elements. As an active metabolic area it is more likely to be the seat of embolic disease such as blood-borne infection. The epiphyseal area caps the metaphysis and supports the articular cartilage. It is less likely to be the seat of embolic disease than the metaphysis because its blood supply is frequently limited by the extension of the joint cavity about it. A giant cell tumor tends to arise in the epiphysis; a simple bone cyst, because it arises in the bone laid down from the epiphyseal line, is in the metaphysis.

The metaphysis is more likely to be the seat of disease than other areas of the bone because:

It is the most active portion of the bone 15
from the standpoint of metabolism

It lies midway between the diaphysis 43
and the epiphysis.

Embolic phenomena lodge in the meta- 4
physis due to the formation of end
arterial loops in this area

43

YOUR ANSWER: The metaphysis is more

likely to be the seat of disease than other areas of the bone because it lies midway between the diaphysis and the epiphysis.

You are incorrect. The mere fact of location is not important. Each of these areas of the bone has its own specific function, and, of all the area, the metaphysis is the most active and has a peculiar endarterial loop formation which is typical of it.

Return to number 42 and try again.

44

YOUR ANSWER: Total destruction of the bone area occupied is characteristic of metastases from prostatic carcinoma.

You are incorrect. Prostatic carcinoma may have both lytic and sclerotic areas of bone involvement as the host tissues are excited to varying degrees of reactive bone formation.

Return to number 53 and try again.

45

YOUR ANSWER: The interior contents of the bone would be less dense than fat density.

Your are incorrect. The isolated medullary contents of the bone would have water density of greater density than fat alone.

Return to number 33 and try again.

46

YOUR ANSWER: It is helpful in determining whether a fracture exists to note whether the mass of the parent bone and bone fragment is greater or equal to the area normally occupied by the individual bone.

You are correct. If the combined mass is greater than the expected size of an individual bone, this tends to indicate that this is an accessory bone and the line is a growth line.

In the figure (A) represents a growth line and (B) a fracture line.

A fracture line has sharp angles, irregular edges, and uneven width.

A growth line separating an accessory bone from its parent has even width throughout. Its edges are rounded.

With trauma to the area, soft tissue swelling could be present in either event.

The diagnosis would be fracture line if:

Soft tissue swelling were present   16

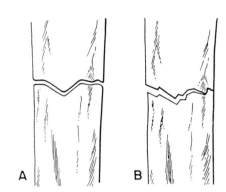

A   B

The radiolucent line was of even width   58
   throughout with rounded edges

The radiolucent line was of uneven   18
   width with sharp angles and irregular
   edges

47

YOUR ANSWER: In order to recognize the avascular state of a segment of bone by roentgenogram a contrasting change in density is necessary in the bone about it.

You are correct. The avascular segment is no longer in contact with the metabolic equilibrium of the body; consequently, it remains at its original density. This will only be apparent if the bone about it loses density. Note the density of the femoral epiphysis on the reader's *right* compared to the femoral neck in the figure.

Areas of lesser density appearing in the previously dense avascular femoral epiphysis.

Bone that exhibits greater than normal density may arise typically at the femoral epiphysis which has a perilous blood supply. As bone is revascularized, areas of lesser density appear due to the invasion of new blood vessels. The extension of infection in bone may isolate segments of its from its blood supply. These fragments are called sequestra. Trauma may divide the blood supply in bones such as the carpal scaphoid. If new blood vessels then invade the avascular bone one would expect it to become less dense.

Avascular segments of bone may arise in various ways. The entrance of new blood vessels into the avascular segment is visible roentgenographically as:

Areas of greater density	38
Increasing density of bone about the avascular segment	38
Areas of lesser density	27

48

YOUR ANSWER: A bone cyst could be smaller than evident on the x-ray film.

You are incorrect. This could not be true since the area seen is the area where the cortex has actually been made thin by the pathologic lesion. Consequently at least the area seen to be involved on the x-ray film must be involved.

Return to number 19 and try again.

49

YOUR ANSWER: Numbers 1 and 2 are true; number 3 is false.

You are incorrect. Metastases from the thyroid tend to be totally lytic, and leukemia tends to infiltrate rather than grow across an area, giving rise to lagging destruction. However, prostatic metastases do tend to be both lytic and sclerotic.

Return to number 28 and try again.

50

YOUR ANSWER: A tumor cannot be differentiated from an infection.

You are incorrect. Both the irregular tracking nature of the bone destruction by an infection and the poorly defined inflammatory swelling in the deep tissues which accompany it distinguish infection from tumor.

Return to number 61 and try again.

51

YOUR ANSWER: A swelling obscures fat lines running through the muscle density area because swellings have air density.

You are incorrect. Air, being less dense than fat, would not obscure it.

Return to number 9 and try again.

52

YOUR ANSWER: An osteomyelitis first is evident on the x-ray film as an area of superficial swelling centered about the metaphysis.

You are incorrect. Superficial soft-tissue swelling is associated with cellulitis. An osteomyelitis involving the bone involves the deep soft tissue of muscle density. It is centered at the metaphysis.

Return to number 4 and try again.

53

YOUR ANSWER: A tumor that is designated an osteogenic sarcoma always produces tumor bone.

You are correct. Tumor bone is bone actually produced by the tumor cells. It is not bone produced by the host tending to wall off the tumor such as the periosteal cuff at either side. Tumor bone is irregular and lacks alignment along stress patterns.

By contrast with lesions which exhibit lagging destruction, in which the advancing destructive edge is poorly visualized, some types of bone metastases totally destroy the bone within the area they occupy. Tumor bone is not formed. Metastases from the lung, thyroid, and kidney have this characteristic, for example. Would you expect leukemia to have this total type of destruction or an infiltrative (lagging) type of destruction?

Other metastases exhibit not only active destruction but tend to excite the host tissues to lay down bone in reaction to it, thereby tending to wall it off.

Total destruction of the bone area occupied is characteristic of:

Metastases from breast carcinoma	11
Metastases from prostatic carcinoma	44
Metastases from lung and thyroid car- cincoma	28

54

YOUR ANSWER: A fracture line is most likely associated with superficial soft-tissue swelling.

You are incorrect. The fracture occurs beneath the deep soft tissues and swelling would appear there first. The superficial tissues may be injured and subsequently swell due to the same trauma.

Return to number 18 and try again.

55

YOUR ANSWER: An adventitious area of calcific density having definite structure visible in the roentgenogram is termed ossification.

The presence of definite bone stria in this area of calcific density is a guideline to ossification. Your ability to distinguish structure as compared to amorphorus calcific density is a useful tool in differential diagnosis of bone and joint disease by roentgenogram.

56

YOUR ANSWER: A swelling would be likely to be associated with an infection.

You are correct. A swelling is caused by inflammatory edema rather than growth. Consequently its edges fade gradually into the other soft tissue densities. The inflammation involves all tissues in the area, which is reflected by their conversion to water density. The *arrow* in the figure for frame 56 indicates a deep soft tissue swelling about the metaphysis consistent with early osteomyelitis.

Because a lesion in bone is frequently hidden until it involves the cortex, it may involve a considerable portion of the bone in which it is not seen. A bone is like a metal pipe: unless the wall of the tube is thinned the x-ray film will not record what is inside. Consequently the soft-tissue shadows may be a very important guide to a lesion in the skeleton.

A swelling, because it is associated with inflammation, often creates a reaction in tissue about it. The vessel lines running through the

fat show a greater contrast with the subcutaneous tissue than is normal.

The number of visible vessel lines would be expected to be:

Increased	12
Decreased	29

57

YOUR ANSWER: In order to recognize the avascular state of a segment of bone by roentgenogram the original density of the bone segment must change.

You are incorrect. The original density of the bone segment cannot change since it is avascular. Contrast is created only by changing the density of the bone still alive.

Please return to number 22 and try again.

58

YOUR ANSWER: The diagnosis would be fracture line if the radiolucent line was of even width throughout with rounded edges.

You are incorrect. These features distinguish a growth line. A fracture line has sharp angles, irregular edges, and uneven width.

Return to number 46 and try again.

59

YOUR ANSWER: Osteomyelitis can be distinguished from destruction of bone due to malignancy by the decision as to whether a mass or a swelling accompanies the destruction.

You are correct. Active destruction is present in both conditions. A swelling with poorly defined edges is typical of the inflammation about an infection. A mass with globular shape and clearly defined edges is typical of a tumor.

Active destruction of bone is distinguished by a fine, spiculated irregular edge. Destruction associated with a benign lesion has a relatively smooth edge. There often tends to be some condensation of bone density about it.

Active destruction is associated with malignant tumor or infection.

An osteogenic sarcoma would have a junction with bone about it which is a fine spiculated irregular edge. An osteogenic sarcoma is also distinguished by the fact that it produces tumor bone. Tumor bone consists of gross bone stria which are laid down in an irregular pattern and do not conform to the stress patterns usually visible in the arrangement of bone trabeculae.

Tumor bone tends to a pattern:

Which is around rather than in the tumor — 7

Which is grossly irregular within the tumor — 42

Determined by the stress on the bone — 30

60

YOUR ANSWER: It is helpful in determining whether a fracture exists to note whether the parent bone and the bone fragment have a mass less than the area normally occupied by the undivided bone.

You are incorrect. In determining whether this is a fracture fragment or an accessory bone the only important consideration relates to the fact that an accessory bone, if combined with the parent bone, would be greater than normal size.

Return to number 26 and try again.

61

YOUR ANSWER: An osteomyelitis first is evident on the x-ray film as an area of deep soft-tissue swelling centered about the metaphysis.

You are correct. The metaphysis is the area of localization for blood-borne bacteria. It is not necessary to wait for the development of bone destruction to make the diagnosis of osteomyelitis. This change occurs so late that considerable damage may already have been done.

Osteomyelitis is associated with active destruction and a deep soft-tissue swelling. It also behaves in a characteristic manner in bone as compared with tumor. An infection tends to track irregularly as if it had pseudopods reaching out to find the easiest way out of the bone. A tumor, on the other hand, tends to expand concentrically until it reaches an anatomic obstacle. It then tends to a globular form. A tumor also tends to be associated with a soft tissue mass rather than a swelling.

A tumor:

Expands in concentric fashion into a rounded mass — 36

Tracks irregularly along the easiest anatomic route — 34

Cannot be differentiated from an infection by roentgenogram — 50

62

YOUR ANSWER: A tumor that is designated an osteogenic sarcoma infiltrates through the bone marrow giving rise to lagging destruction.

You are incorrect. Lagging destruction is typical of tumors such as Ewing's sarcoma. Tumors that destroy in this manner, infiltrating through the bone, tend to arise from marrow cells.

Return to number 36 and try again.

63

YOUR ANSWER: A fracture line is most likely associated with no soft-tissue swelling.

You are incorrect. The nature of the pathology of a fracture with developing hematoma makes this statement impossible.

Return to number 18 and try again.

CHAPTER 2

The Foot

FLAT FEET IN CHILDHOOD

Perhaps the most common orthopaedic problem confronting the physician caring for the growing child is flat feet. The symptoms that may be associated with weak feet are often not recognized. The child who appears lazy, dislikes long walks, and comes indoors while the rest of his age group is still out playing may be suffering from foot strain. The toeing-in or "pigeon-toeing" in a child's gait is frequently due to weak feet. When actual pain is complained of, it frequently is located not in the foot but in the calf. This leg discomfort has two characteristics: it is intermittent; it tends to occur at the end of the day.

On first standing, the infant's feet are almost invariably pronated, spread apart in a wide-based stance for balance as he grips his support. Standing barefoot in this position stretches out the ligaments of the medial side of the foot. Gradually he brings his feet closer together, and they supinate. The infantile fat is redistributed as the child's activity increases. As a preventive measure, the child should be in firm shoes with a heel as soon as he gains upright posture. The child whose foot is not responding to increased activity is ordinarily not recognized until the age of 2 or later

Why does an early walking child wear high shoes? There is really one reason—in order to keep them on. The infant's heel is rounded and not developed posteriorly. High shoes are not worn to support the ankle which is a tight mortise. The stiff counter of the heel holds the os calcis upright and thereby aligns the subtalar joint where inversion and eversion take place. It follows that the time when oxfords can be worn is shown by the ability of the child to keep these low shoes on without walking out of them. This can be determined by trial and error at the shoe store.

Clinical Picture

The child is brought to medical attention because the parents have noted the flat or pronated feet, or because the child toes in (i.e., walks pigeon-toed), or because he limps or complains of foot or leg pain.

A history of intermittent limp with an essentially negative physical examination except for pronated feet suggests foot strain. Calf pain, when due to muscle fatigue from supporting an inadequate foot, tends to be located in the region of the posterior tibial muscle. Foot pain due to ligamentous strain is located by the patient along the medial arch.

Physical Examination

The examiner seeks to find, not a flat foot, but a foot functioning in a position that throws strain on its ligaments and muscles and does not use its bony support. The degree of arch medially and longitudinally is noted in recumbency. Most feet are well arched in this position, but some feet are architecturally flat on non-weight bearing. The tightness of the heel cord is noted by dorsiflexing the foot in inversion while the knee is straight. A foot normally should be able to dorsiflex at least $10°$ above the right ankle when examined in this way.

A tendency to hyperextended knees, elbows, and thumbs gives a clue to the ligamentous laxity of the child. The ability of the foot to roll from full eversion to full inversion should be noted. The inability to invert the foot may be due to peroneal spasm, which can be confirmed by palpating the peroneal muscles as the inversion is attempted. In spasm, these muscles stand out as taut structures limiting inversion. An examination of the complete child, with special attention to all joints, is carried out in every case of suspected foot strain.

When the child is standing, the position of the os calcis in relation to the weight-bearing line out from the tibia, is the degree of pronation of the foot. It is best noted from the posterior view with the foot at eye level. As the os calcis everts beneath the astragalus, the medial side of the foot comes into prominence.

Fig. 2.1. Pronated feet with prominence of the calcaneonavicular area medially and a valgus position of the os calcis in the posterior view.

Fig. 2.2. The foot everted (*left*) dorsiflexes further than the foot inverted (*right*).

Pressure on the medial side of the foot reveals whether or not the os calcis can still be tilted into an upright position. The contrast between the weight-bearing and the non-weight-bearing position is important from the standpoint of strain.

The alignment of the leg affects the foot. Tibia vara with a medial facing of the ankle mortise means that the foot must pronate in order to bring its weight-bearing surface onto the ground. Internal torsion of the tibia may be confused with the tibia vara deformity or may be part of it. Internal torsion is noted by placing the knee facing directly to the examiner and dorsiflexing the foot in line with the ankle joint. It should be in the same plane as the knee. Deviation of the ankle joint medially in relation to the plane of the knee joint may be due to internal torsion. A facing outward or laterally of the coronal plane of the ankle joint in relation to the knee is external torsion.

Internal torsion accentuates a "bowlegged" appearance, but gives rise to "in-toeing," which gives a somewhat stronger weight-bearing position than that produced by external torsion. Here the foot turns outward, carrying it away from direct transmission of body weight, to a position that tends to accentuate pronation.

Valgus at the knee frequently develops in children with pronated feet. This is particularly true in youngsters with chubby thighs, whose legs are widely separated on weight bearing.

Fig. 2.3. The foot with ligamentous laxity is normally constituted without weight bearing (*A* and *B*). With weight bearing, the foot pronates and the os calcis goes into a valgus position (*C* and *D*).

Valgus may be a product of the same relaxed ligamentous structure that allows the foot to pronate.

Gait

One of the most important features of childhood foot strain is the gait. "In-toeing" or walking "pigeon-toed" is frequently a protective gait to guard against foot strain. There may, of course, be mechanical factors in the leg such that no other form of gait is possible, but on the basis of frequency, protection is a much more likely cause. Nor is every child who toes outward without difficulty. Such a gait tends to develop a pronated foot in a growing child.

Treatment

The placing of wedges on the lateral side of the shoe to make an in-toeing child toe outward is contraindicated. This practice pronates the foot still further, increases the strain, and often results in increased in-toeing for compensation.

The treatment of weak mechanical feet consists of providing adequate support to hold the foot in a strong position. Growth taking place while the foot is held in this position should result in relative tightening of the ligaments and prevention of bony deformity. It is not possible to make the worst pair of feet into the strongest, but is should be possible to change the foot mechanics sufficiently so that they do not constitute a point of great weakness as the individual attempts to walk and stand in life. The failure of inadequate treat-

Fig. 2.4. In the tibia vara there is a medial facing of the distal tibial surface at the ankle joint, resulting in the necessity for the foot to pronate to bear weight on its medial side.

ment should not result in wholesale condemnation of the method.

A medial arch pad or support helps to prevent rotation of the foot within the shoe. This increases the effectiveness of a medial heel wedge, which is designed to tilt the hindfoot into inversion. The usual well tolerated medial heel wedge height is 1/8 inch. If the hindfoot is controlled, the forefoot will follow. Medial arch supports that are carried too far forward result in difficulty in fitting the foot over them into the shoe.

The subastragalar area is the point at which

support is needed most. The usual height for a medial arch support in childhood is 3/8 inch. A medial prolongation of the heel may be used in addition to the wedge. This so-called "Thomas" heel is a part of shoes that are sold as "orthopaedic shoes."

Straight-last shoes (Plumb-line) disguise in-toeing by the child and are used when the forefoot tends to turn medialward or to adduct in relation to the hindfoot.

Exercises for the feet of an inverting or

A   B

Fig. 2.5. The weight-bearing line is brought medial-ward by valgus at the knee, as in (A). External torsion of the tibia rotates the foot outward and away from the weight-bearing line (B).

supinating type have been of little help in the author's treatment of flat or pronated feet in childhood. Adults derive much more benefit from them.

There is one exception to this: the case of a tight heel cord. Since the foot can dorsiflex further in inversion, the youngster is forced into a weak mechanical position in order to get his heel on the ground in the presence of tight heel cords. No progress in the direction of improvement of the feet can be expected while the heel cord remains tight. The mother can stretch this tendon when the child is small by inverting and dorsiflexing the foot while the knee is extended. When the child is older, he or she can be taught heel cord stretching exercises as illustrated in Figure 2.17. Such exercises need not be done to the point of boredom, but should be regularly and thoroughly done at least once each day. It usually takes 3-4 months to notice improvement.

Correction of a foot and gait problem does not take place instantaneously when corrective measures are applied, but only with further development and growth of the foot.

Stiff plates of steel or plastic tend to make the foot rigid and to wed the child permanently to their use. Flexible supports appear prefer-able. Pasted-in longitudinal arch supports such as are commonly seen commercially as a general rule are inadequate, since a fully adequate support necessarily gives the child some slight difficulty in getting his foot into the shoe.

This probelm is avoided by not building the

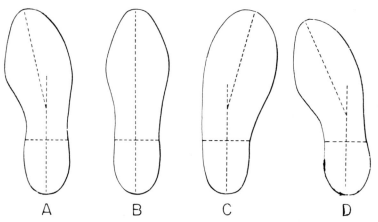

A   B   C   D

Fig. 2.6. Varying types of shoe lasts controlling relation of hindfoot to forefoot: (A) regular, (B) straight, (C) forefoot abduction, (D) forefoot adduction.

A   B   C   D

Fig. 2.7. The effect of various measures on the position of the os calcis is shown. In (*B*), a normal heel alone improves the position, but this effect is increased further by a medial wedge combined with a longitudinal arch pad. A medial wedge alone is not sufficient to keep the heel from the valgus (*C*), but when it is combined with a pad, the full effect of both is felt (*D*).

Fig. 2.8. The effect of a heel alone on foot position. Valgus of the os calcis is largely corrected.

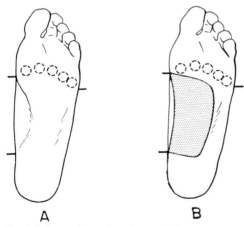

A   B

Fig. 2.9. In tracing a foot for medial arch support, the area just proximal to the first and fifth metatarsal head is marked, as well as the posterior termination of the medial arch. Keeping the anterior end of the pad behind these prominences is important for comfort

pad too far forward. Its most important function in the simple pronated foot of childhood is to control the hindfoot; the forefoot must necessarily fall in line. A longitudinal arch pad ends behind the first metatarsal head and extends posteriorward to the end of the arch and inward (lateralward) from there to tilt the os calcis into an upright position by its support.

PERSISTENT IN-TOEING GAIT

When a child presents with the chief complaint of in-toeing gait over the age of 4, the physician must consider persistent anteversion

and for fitting the pad into the shoe. The pad is brought well toward the middle of the foot posteriorly to support the subastragalar area.

Fig. 2.10. Leather arch supports with felt insert. The extra felt is inserted when the first becomes compressed.

A   B

Fig. 2.11. Location of inner heel wedge to aid in inverting the os calcis.

Fig. 2.12 (*left*). The sitting posture that allows persistent anteversion and subsequent in-toeing gait in the older child. A youngster with this sitting posture characteristically has relaxed ligaments allowing this posture in comfort—of this persists as a habitual posture.

Fig. 2.13 (*right*). On standing the child who has been subject to the sitting posture (Fig. 2.12) stands with external torsion of the tibia, a secondary effect of the posture. In order to bring the foot forward in line with a forward progression, the knee must turn in.

of the femur. This occurs because of a characteristic sitting posture into which the child sinks to play on the floor or look at a center of attention such as the television screen.

The children that get into this habitual sitting posture are those with generally relaxed ligaments. This can be demonstrated by hyperextension of the fingers, thumb, elbows, and knees.

Clinical Picture

The in-toeing gait is symmetrical and involves the entire limb. The knee turns in as well as the foot. The limb itself is well lined up without excessive internal tibial torsion; in fact, there may be considerable external tibial torsion. The ankle and the knee occupy the same rotational plane.

The condition is apparent when the physician places the child in the characteristic posture. The hips readily rotate 90° or more, the knees are then readily flexed so that the heels come under the buttocks. The child sits comfortably in this position.

Roentgen Appearance

The femurs reveal anteversion of over 70°. The femoral head has normal height in relation to the trochanter. In the anteroposterior view the femoral neck angle appears increased. A second view in full internal rotation at the hips confirms the fact that the femoral neck angle is normal in the range of 135°.

Treatment

Although it is true that a correctly performed osteotomy de-rotating the femur would establish a normal relationship, this is generally not indicated by the relatively minor nature of the child's complaint. If the child is to overcome the skeletal alignment through growth it is obvious that the force causing persistent anteversion must be eliminated.

The child must not be allowed to sit with the hips rotated internally 90°.

From a practical point of view the only way to accomplish that is forbid the child from either sitting on the floor or in large furniture. A small child's chair must be presented which makes it impossible to tuck the heels under the buttock. This becomes the child's television viewing chair and play chair. It takes 5 years of growth to achieve correction.

DISABLING FLAT FEET

There are children with severe disability from the utter collapse of the foot as a means of entering into life. This is true despite well founded attempts at support. For the most part, these children fall into the group with excessive ligamentous laxity. Dorsiflexion of the foot comes 45° above neutral. The child's inactivity discourages the parents and affects the child's personality and development.

Rarely in the age group below 10 the symptoms and the effect on the child's activity are such as to justify soft-tissue correction of the deformity. Conservative treatment here has not been successful in changing the course of the child's activity.

Kidner Operation

In such instances, we have employed the Kidner procedure. The Kidner operation excises the accessory navicular or medial tuberosity of the navicular and transposes the posterior tibial tendon into a groove on the inferior surface of this bone. It is primarily for children below the age of 10 with symptomatic feet. In this operation a curvilinear incision over the medial aspect of the foot and outlining the navicular area is made. As the flap is retracted with a silk stitch, the insertion of the posterior tibial tendon is seen. This is carefully outlined in order to save a flap of soft tissue both inferiorly and superiorly over the navicular. The inferior flap is dissected underneath the navicular, and the undersurface of the navicular is exposed. A groove of varying depth will be found here. The tendon of the posterior tibial muscle is now skived from its navicular attachment, care being taken to keep it intact and continuous and its distal portion radiating under the cuneiform. It is then brought under the navicular to act as a slinglike support of it. A stay suture may be needed to ensure that the tendon is held in place. The previously devised flaps are now sewn over the exposed surface of the navicular. This is a relatively simple procedure with an evident purpose—to reconstitute the medial arch.

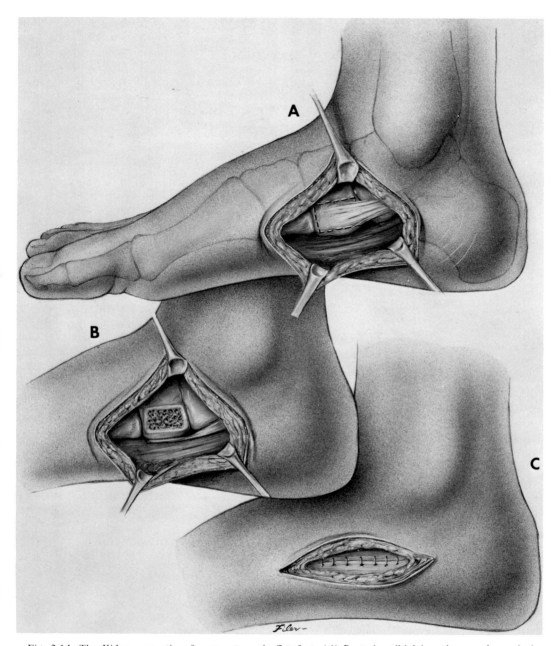

Fig. 2.14. The Kidner operation for symptomatic flat feet. (*A*) Posterior tibial insertion on the navicular tuberosity is visualized. The area to be removed with a thin shell of bone is outlined by the *dotted line*. (*B*) The bare surface of the navicular is visualized above the inferior surface of the navicular where a subcortical flap has been raised. The posterior tibial insertion is placed beneath this flap. (*C*) The soft tissues are repaired holding the posterior tibial insertion in place. A cast is then applied.

Fig. 2.15. Roentgenogram of disabling flat feet. Condition is shown in Figure 2.16 after treatment.

Hypermobile Flat Foot with Short Tendo Achillis

Harris and Beath[1] have reemphasized a type of flat foot that is frequently associated with disability. The disability is often not apparent until the "teen" age is reached. It was noted in Canadian soldiers once in every 145 men examined. This foot has excessive ligamentous laxity and a short tendo Achillis, which are recognizable on physical examination. The foot on non-weight bearing appears to have a good longitudinal arch both medially and laterally. On standing the foot pronates severely.

This foot combines two elements likely to cause disability: (1) function in a position for which the foot was not designed; (2) a mechanical abnormality, which is not necessarily a primary cause, that forces use in this poistion. Harris believed, however, that the primary cause was a structural abnormality: the head of the talus is displaced downward and inward in relation to the os calcis.

Since the severity of this condition varies greatly, treatment varies from mere support and exercises to operation. Stretching of the tendo Achillis is important, and in the "teen" age group a metal type support, perhaps including a lateral flange as in the Whitman plate, may be used. It is hard to get the foot well supported here, and a plaster mold is usually made with the foot in a corrected position as a guide to the making of the support.

Hoke Operation

The Hoke operation for a flexible pes planus involves lengthening the tendo Achillis as the first step. The naviculocuneiform joint is then exposed. The articular cartilage is removed from the articular surface of both navicular and cuneiforms both first and second.

The foot and the distal end of the first metatarsal is then forced into equinus. In this

Fig. 2.16. The foot as in Figure 2.15 treated with subastragalar bone block. The os calcis has been brought under the astragalus, evident in both anteroposterior and lateral views.

Fig. 2.17. In heel cord stretching in the older child, the heel of the posterior limb is kept on the ground. The elbows are flexed, and the child leans toward the wall.

position a rectangular block is removed from both the navicular and cuneiform. A nice piece of carpentry is then involved since an accurately sized bone is needed. This is taken from the tibial cortex and fitted as a inlay graft across the joint and into the rectangle formed in both the navicular and cuneiform. The cast to immobilize the patient postoperatively starts as a plaster slipper holding the foot in equinus and the heel in varus. The foot is then brought up to neutral and a long leg cast incorporates the slipper.

The cast is held for 6 weeks followed by crutch walking for 3-4 months with a medial support shoe and longitudinal arch pad and partial weight bearing. When the fusion appears fully formed and swelling of the operative site gone the crutches are discarded, but the shoes are used for the next several years.

CONGENITAL VERTICAL TALUS

A very disabling and surprisingly common type of foot has been described as due to a congenital vertical talus. This foot is best

Fig. 2.18. In the Hoke operation, a bone graft, in the form of a rectangle taken from the tibial cortex, is placed into a cancellous bone slot made to involve navicular and cuneiform bone. The medial arch is reconstituted before the cuts are made.

thought of as a dislocation of the foot away from its normal relationship with the astragalus. Its treatment consists of the reduction of the dislocation so that the navicular rests in normal relationship to the talus and the holding of the reduction until sufficient adaptive changes have taken place to retain the foot in position and to permit normal function.

Fig. 2.19. Congenital vertical talus. A lateral roentgenogram reveals the forefoot dislocated superiorly in relation to the plantar flexed talus.

Fig. 2.20. A 9-year follow-up of patient seen in Figure 2.19 reveals that the navicular had not been retained in an anatomical relationship to the talar head and the consequent deformity of the tarsal bone is obvious.

Clinical Picture

At birth, children who have a congenital vertical talus are hidden among infants with calcaneal valgus feet. There is one important differentiating feature. The foot with congenital vertical talus cannot be reduced into normal relationship with the astragalus.

The head of the talus produces a marked prominence on the medial side of the foot. The remainder of the foot is drawn lateralward in relation to this prominence. The forefoot is dorsiflexed in relation to the hindfoot. The os calcis is not in normal relation to the talus and does not have the same degree of equinus. However, it is not dorsiflexed to equal the

Fig. 2.21. The hypermobile flat foot with short Achilles tendon results in severe pronation.

Fig. 2.22. Lateral roentgenogram of the weight-bearing foot, showing the plantar-flexed talus, depressed navicular, loss of the medial and lateral arches of the foot, and subluxation of the talar head over the anterior portion of the os calcis. Note, however, that the navicular is still in normal relation to the astragalar head, in contradistinction to congenital talus when this joint is dislocated.

Fig. 2.23. (*A*) Anterior view of foot with superior dislocation of the forefoot carried into supination in a child with congenital vertical talus. (*B*) Lateral view of foot, making the dislocation superiorly more evident with resultant loss of the lateral arch of the foot. (*C*) Medial view of foot with prominence in the center of the medial arch produced by the head of the astragalus.

forefoot position, and this feature becomes more prominent as the infant grows older. It results in an evident "rocker bottom" foot with a prominence beneath the calcaneal cuboid joint caused by the reversal of the lateral arch of the foot.

When the infant starts to walk, the gait is not normal, for the dislocation taking place in the foot deprives the child of a normal take-off.

In our experience, the astragalus is movable through an adequate range of motion in the ankle mortise. This is borne out when treatment is successful.

Treatment

After roentgen examination, the reduction is first attempted by successive plaster casts. The dorsal soft tissues are extremely tight. The forefoot, to be brought into normal alignment with the astragalus, must be brought down into equinus. The navicular must be brought over the astragalus head and placed squarely into anatomic relationship with it. In the author's experience, this has been difficult to do. Should the reontgenogram reveal successful reduction, the position is held with appropriate changes of cast (much as a dislocated hip is held) for several months until sufficient adaptive changes and growth have taken place so that reduction is not lost when the cast is removed. To assure permanent reduction, a Denis-Browne bar may be used to hold the foot inverted in the shoe for several months thereafter.

Fig. 2.24. The difficulty in weight bearing with congenital vertical talus uncorrected is painfully apparent in this older child. Such feet are extremely disabling.

Fig. 2.25. The vertical talus deformity uncorrected in the older child. The navicular and the entire forefoot are dislocated in relation to the hindfoot. The os calcis, the talus, and the cuboid form a triumvirate creating a weight-bearing prominence which is extremely difficult to walk upon.

Operative treatment has often been necessary when conservative treatment has failed.

Operative Treatment

Excision of the navicular has been found to be a very helpful step in securing reduction of the dislocated talar head. It is evident that the soft tissues dorsally and medially are contracted relative to the bony length of the medial side of the foot. Either the soft tissues must be extensively lengthened or the bony length of the medial side of the foot shortened. This may be accomplished by a single incision on the medial side of the foot excising the navicular and reducing the talocuneiform joint, but an additional lateral incision is often helpful to lever the talar head up into position and place the os calcis beneath it.

A lateral incision is made over the anterior portion of the sinus tarsi and brought up on the dorsum sufficiently to expose the head of the talus. The incision is carried directly down through the sinus tarsi to the inferior surface of the astragalar neck.

A joker can then be inserted under the astragalar neck to prevent the astragalus from sinking into further equinus as the rest of the foot is reduced in relation to it.

Over the past 10 years we have used this operation to reduce the head of the talus into normal relationship with the forefoot. It is frequently impossible to accomplish the reduction of the foot without extensive dissection and soft-tissue lengthening of the tendons on the dorsum of the foot otherwise.

A simpler alternative is to excise the navicular through the addition of a small medial incision. The cuneiform can then be brought into relationship with the talar head reconstituting the medial arch and slightly adducting the forefoot. The relationship between these two bones is then secured by a Kirschner wire entering the foot over the first metatarsal, passing through the cuneiform and into the talus. The talar head is held up out of equinus by a blunt dissector from the lateral incision while this is done; levering up in this way brings the os calcis under the talus. A cast is then applied and both cast and wire left in place for 6 weeks.

The wire is then removed and a bivalved cast used to maintain position.

Active exercises into inversion are used twice daily for 2 months and medial support shoes and partial weight bearing with crutches then used, progressing gradually to full activity.

When weight bearing is finally started, a single lateral upright brace with a medial T-strap may be necessary. Later the foot is supported by a medial arch pad for several years. A great deal of work is necessary to correct this foot, but the disability associated with the uncorrected foot justifies great efforts to prevent it.

The talus and the cuneiform adapt with secondary growth into a well formed joint and a normal appearing foot. It is often not realized

A

Fig. 2.26. (*A*) Diagrammatic conception of navicular excision allowing replacement of the talus into a normal relationship with forefoot and abutting on the cuneiform. (*B* and *C*) An 8-year follow-up of a child's foot in which the navicular was excised in infancy to allow the reduction of the forefoot in relation to the hindfoot. The subsequent molding of the tarsal bones is evident with maintenance of the medial arch of the foot (lateral (*B*) and anteroposterior (*C*) views).

that the navicular is missing in later roentgenograms.

PERONEAL SPASTIC FLAT FOOT

Peroneal spastic flat foot is recognized clinically by the patient's inability to invert the foot. On attempted inversion the peroneal muscles are noted to stand out as taut structures. Lapidus[6] notes that rarely the extensor digitorum may join the peroneal in holding the foot in pronation.

There are a number of possible causes for this condition. In children inflammatory lesions, such as those caused by tuberculosis, may be present in the mid- or subtarsal area. Subtalar arthritis of a rheumatoid type may be present, and lesions such as osteoid osteoma have been found. Occasionally the condition

Figs. 2.26*B* and *C*

may be secondary to trauma. It is important to rule out bony anomalies such as calcaneonavicular coalition, which may give rise to midtarsal strain and form the most common etiologic group.

The foot may be rigidly fixed even if there is a contracture of the peroneals. When there is a congenital fusion of the tarsal bones, motion into inversion is obviously impossible, regardless of the guarding action of the peroneals.

Fig. 2.27. The calcaneal-talar bar is easy to miss by roentgenogram. In (A) the abduction of the forefoot due to peroneal spasm is evident. In (B) no definite bar is shown connecting os calcis and the navicular (oblique view). In (C) the union of the medial side of the subtalar joint is shown with the talus and os calcis joined (45° posteroanterior view of the os calcis).

Harris and Beath[5] found the most significant and frequent anomaly to be a talocalcaneal bridge, rather than a calcaneonavicular bar, and are responsible for its clear recognition. Such a bridge is apparently a variation similar to that which produces the os sustentaculum and may actually represent fusion of this accessory bone at either end. A similar bone, calcaneus secondarius, is the basis of the calcaneonavicular bar.

The bridge may be bony or fibrous. The limitation of subtalar joint motion causes a characteristic talonavicular infringement. This gives rise to a characteristic dorsal slipping of the talus. A 45° posteroanterior view of the os calcis is necessary to demonstrate the subtalar joint and its pathology.

Treatment

Peroneal spastic flat feet must be thoroughly investigated as to etiology. The condition usually persists until the underlying cause is cured. Correction sometimes requires a triple arthrodesis. Rest in bivalved casts with daily exercise (non-weight bearing) is part of the treatment of arthritic conditions. This is followed by support of the foot in normal weight-bearing position. Dickson, Dively, and Whitman recommend manipulation under anesthesia and immobilization in plaster followed by physiotherapy.

The underlying etiologic factor usually must be cured to prevent a recurrence of the protective muscle spasm. Local excision of accessory bones and bars in the cartilage state has been attempted in children with some success.

METATARSUS ATAVICUS

In the metatarsus atavicus anomaly described by Morton, the first metatarsal is excessively short. Its length is usually less than that of the second and third. This defect results in a tendency to pronate the foot in order to put the head of the first metatarsal into a weight-bearing position. Feet pronated for this reason should be supported by a prolongation of a longitudinal arch pad beneath the first metatarsal to procure weight bearing.

METATARSUS PRIMUS VARUS

Metatarsus primus varus is seen at birth. The first metatarsal is adducted medialward so that a well defined defect exists between the first and second metatarsal heads.

This results in abnormal weight bearing on the second metatarsal, and the use of footwear carries the first toe into a hallux valgus position. The hallux valgus deformity is the most striking physical aspect.

Treatment

The essential point to note on physical examination is the presence or absence of a defect between the first and second metatarsal heads. This area is filled with soft tissue. In the true deviation of the first metatarsal alone, such a defect is present. When it is not present, the other metatarsals are deviated as well. We have become more and more aware of the necessity of correcting a true deviation of the first metatarsal alone. The base of the transverse arch has been lost on one side; and abnormali-

Fig. 2.27*B*

Fig. 2.27C

ties of the second toe, in the form of hyperextension of the proximal phalanx and flexion of the interphalangeal joint causing a callus to form beneath the second metatarsal head, will soon appear.

Correction of this deformity can only be achieved surgically. Varying the last of the shoe does not result in any permanent improvement.

If the defect is truly corrected a hallux valgus deformity will no longer exist and the space between the first and second metatarsal heads will be obliterated.

Experience in the correction of this deformity has resulted in settling on an osteotomy at approximately the midpoint of the first metatarsal. A wedge of bone based laterally is removed. The base of the wedge faces toward the second metatarsal and should be sufficient to fully correct the deformity when the wedge is closed. It is now necessary to hold this correction—some form of internal fixation is mandatory as the deformity otherwise will readily recur in the cast. We have placed drill holes through the cortex on either side of the operative defect and held the closure by wire sutures. Transferring the adductor tendon in addition greatly increases the surgery in this relatively small area and has not been found necessary if the osteotomy is done far enough distally on the metatarsal.

The correction obtained can be seen in Figure 2.30. The obliteration of the space between the first and second metatarsal heads and the realignment of the great toe secondary to this correction is evident. A short leg cast is necessary for 6 weeks.

Fig. 2.28. (A) In this oblique roentgenogram of the foot, the calcaneonavicular bar is clearly shown. A union such as this may be fibrous, cartilaginous, or osseous. In the young child, resection frequently yields normal foot function, but, in the older child, a triple arthrodeses is necessary to cure the condition. (B) At operation the bar is visualized adjacent to the retractor. The peroneal tendons are retracted by tape, and the skin inferiorly by a rake. (C) The resected portion laid on a diagram of its location.

PAINFUL HEELS IN CHILDREN

Pain located at the superior angle of the os calcis is a common childhood complaint in the 6-12-year-old age group. The causes of such complaints are varied.

There is also a common occurrence in the teen-age group wherein a painful callus and underlying bursa arise. In slang terms this condition has been designated "pump bumps" and is very common when the wearing of a loafer style shoe dependent on a tight heel fit is in vogue.

An excessive prominence of the posterior superior angle of the os calcis predisposes to the development of this bursa which can become very painful. The tight upper ridge of the heel counter sliding back and forth over this prominence is the cause. To remove it either the bony prominence must be removed surgically or the design of the heel counter changed. Obviously the latter alternative is preferable.

The stiff support of the heel counter may be removed or careful attention paid to procuring a shoe with a heel counter of sufficient height that its superior reinforced edge is above the bone prominence.

Occasionally the symptom complex may lead to operation. When this is done the posterior angle is removed without destroying the attachment of the tendo Achillis.

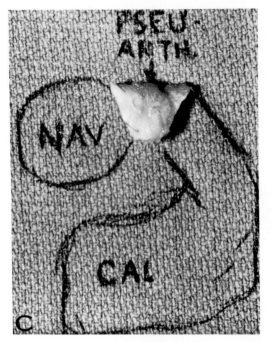

Fig. 2.28C

In the 6-12-year-old age group this postero-superior prominence can often be implicated. The style range that this age group will accept in a shoe is not so narrow, however, and shoes less likely to bring about pressure can be obtained. The stiff heel counter can again be removed.

Tendinitis of the Achilles tendon is revealed by sensitivity or occasionally by swelling or crepitus noted over the tendon on palpation. The roentgenogram reveals thickening of the Achilles tendon shadow. Complete rest, which is readily achieved by immobilizing the heel in a plaster cast, may be indicated until symptoms disappear. Elevation of the heel and Hydrocortone injections may relieve mild cases.

Bursitis of the Achilles bursa (beneath the Achilles tendon) rarely occurs. Such a lesion may form part of the calcaneal apophysitis syndrome, which has been thought in the past to be a process of osteochondritis similar to that of Köhler's disease, Freiberg's disease, and Legg-Perthes disease. Such a diagnosis was based on the density of the apophysis. A review of the development of the os calcis from infancy reveals, however, that the calcaneal apophysis normally passes through an extremely dense stage which is alleviated after union with the parent bone. No unusual fragmentation has been noted.

Roentgenograms have revealed changes in those cases which clinically appeared to have calcaneal apophysitis with tenderness and thick-

Fig. 2.29. A metatarsus primus varus. The medial deviation of the first metatarsal is seen with the great toe lying in a valgus position.

Fig. 2.30. (A) Preoperative roentgenogram showing the deviation medially of the first metatarsal and secondary hallus valgus, with the space between the first and second metatarsal head. (B) Postoperative connection of the first metatarsal by osteotomy. The great toe no longer is in a deformed position as the first metatarsal has been aligned with it. A wire suture holds the osteotomy closed.

Fig. 2.31. The normal development of the os calcis includes a dense stage of the apophysis; (left) 4½ years, (center) 5 years, (right) 8 years.

Fig. 2.32. Diagram emphasising the angle made by the junction of the Achilles tendon and the os calcis. This angle is obscured by inflammatory swelling at the heel. Angle *AOC* is formed by the junction of the Achilles tendon and the superior surface of the os calcis.

ening at the junction of the Achilles tendon with the bone. These changes have consisted of thickening of the soft-tissue shadow in this area and in the angle formed by the juncture of the tendon and the os calcis. Rarely there is ossification of the apophysis at some distance from the parent center.

Both these changes and the syndrome itself have been quite rare in our experience.

Treatment

Elevation of the heel and softening of the heel counter and changing its height have all helped to alleviate symptoms. Rest in a plaster

Fig. 2.33. Congenital duplication of the apophysis of the os calcis. As a result of the excessive superior prominence a bursa formed over it and secondary ossification developed within it. Clinically this resulted in a marked form of the syndrome known as "pump bumps."

cast, Hydrocortone injection, and heel cord stretching may be of some value in resistant cases.

METATARSUS VARUS

In pediatric orthopaedic practice, two variations of the common deformity, metatarsus varus (also termed "metatarsus adductus") are seen. Attention was called to this condition by Kite[5a] and it is known by some as a "third of a clubfoot." This colloquialism emphasizes that the deformity is in one plane only: the forefoot occupies an adducted position in relation to the hindfoot. There appears to be no sex-related variation. The condition may be unilateral or bilateral, and there is often a tendency to turn the unaffected foot out.

Clinical Picture

The deformity is present at birth. An important clinical distinction between the two variations of it should be made. Sometimes the forefoot can readily be pulled into a normal

Fig. 2.34. Inflammatory swelling about the heel in osteomyelitis of the os calcis. This marked inflammation obscures angle *AOC* as shown in Figure 2.32.

Fig. 2.35. Aseptic inflammatory swelling at the junction of Achilles tendon and os calcis.

Fig. 2.36. The patient's right forefoot deviates medially, forming a metatarsus varus. The left foot is carried medialward by internal torsion of the tibia while the knee points forward.

alignment with the hindfoot by passive motion. In a few such instances, the everting muscles of the baby's foot can be stimulated to active contraction, and the foot is thus partially corrected. The baby's foot tends to follow, rather than to pull away from, the stimulating finger that strokes it. The second and less common variety cannot be passively corrected and constitutes a true deformity. It is important to make this distinction as a basis for treatment.

There is usually an accompanying internal torsion of the tibia that accentuates the "turned-in" appearance of the foot. The patients often make their first appearance for treatment at the age of 2 or 3 months. At that time the foot has become troublesome because

Fig. 2.37. Forefoot varus with the heel in neutral position in metatarsus varus. This can be demonstrated as positional by applying passive correction and achieving a normal relation between forefoot and hindfoot.

it has failed to improve, owing either to the patient's sleeping on his abdomen with his feet turned in (in the case of a mobile foot) or to the foot's being of a fixed variety.

Treatment

Mobile Foot

Since it is not desirable to change the baby's sleeping habits, the simplest method of getting the foot in good position during sleep is to use reversed shoes on a Denis-Browne bar. The shoes are placed on the bar in about 45° of external rotation. While the baby is awake, reversed shoes or forefoot abduction shoes without the bar are used to avoid a tendency to develop genu valgus.

In addition, at each diaper change the mother holds the hindfoot and carries the forefoot into abduction with the other hand. She thus lines the foot up in normal position and stretches the structures of the medial side of the foot. The usual time needed to procure correction is 4-6 months. When walking starts, straight-last shoes are used as there is a tendency to recurrence.

Fixed Foot

Here the metatarsus varus must be stretched sufficiently to convert the foot to a mobile

Fig. 2.38. A bar holding the feet forward tends to correct internal torsion of the tibia and holds a corrected metatarsus varus in straight alignment.

foot. This is best accomplished by corrective plaster casts that bring the foot into full overcorrection. Either wedging casts or complete plaster changes may be used. Once the foot is mobile, the Denis-Browne bar with reversed shoes is used, again for a period of months or until the patient is walking. Shoes with a last that carries the forefoot into abduction are then used.

There is a marked tendency to recur, which can be noted particularly when the child is standing and indicates the necessity for prolonged follow-up.

COMBINATION OF POSITIONAL METATARSUS VARUS OF ONE FOOT AND CALCANEAL VALGUS OF THE OTHER

This is a frequently seen positional deformity in infants. The child appears to be deviating to one side; some refer to this abnormality as skiing to one side.

The positional element of the metatarsus varus deformity can be recognized by the fact that the forefoot can readily be pushed into proper alignment with the hindfoot. The opposite foot at birth was pushed up against the tibia; it can readily be brought into proper alignment, but resumes a calcaneous position on release of pressure.

The infant usually perpetuates the deformity by sleeping on his stomach with the feet in this position.

Treatment consists of the use of a Denis-Browne bar attached to shoes to control the deformity. The shoe for the metatarsus varus is sold as a so-called "prewalker"; that is, the toe of the shoe is open. The last is built with forefoot abduction to carry the forefoot into a corrective position. It is turned outward 45° on the bar.

The calcaneous foot is treated with a prewalker type shoe with a regular last, or with a straight last if a regular one cannot be obtained. This shoe is turned inward 45°. The total effect of this apparatus is to hold the feet in positions that deviate in directions opposite to the deviations seen in the examination. This apparatus is usually worn for 4 months during all sleeping hours, night and day. In waking hours, the bar only is removed. The shoes remain on except during the hour of the bath, which is at 10 or 11 a.m. in most families.

After 4 months, the shoes alone are worn during sleeping hours, usually until age 1½.

OVERLAPPING FIFTH TOES

The fifth toe, when structurally overlapped, is held in place by a tight skin fold and a shortened tendon. This deformity is frequently familial. The condition is often bilateral, and accompanying radial angulation of the distal phalanx of the fifth fingers is not uncommon.

In mild degrees of the condition, the toe may be strapped in place with adhesive for many months with the possibility of some success. When the fifth toe is well up over the fourth, however, conservative methods will not correct the deformity. Surgical correction is indicated because the condition has a tendency to cause a soft corn to develop between the fourth and fifth toes and a callus overlying the dorsum of the fifth. Correction includes a Z-plasty in the line of the short skin segment, lengthening of the extensor tendons, and a capsulotomy of the metatarsophalangeal joint. At the conclusion of surgery, the toe should lie naturally in normal position without having to be splinted.

CONGENITAL CLUBFOOT

Congenital clubfoot is one of the oldest known and treated deformities of mankind. Since the days of Hippocrates, various methods of manipulation, strapping, and binding have been used in its correction. The condition occurs once in every 1,000 births and is approximately twice as common in males as in females. The characteristic deformity has three elements: forefoot adduction, inversion, and equinus of the foot. Such a foot has been termed talipes equinovarus. Although some reports have indicated an equal distribution between unilateral and bilateral types, most authorities say that the unilateral type is slightly more common.

Etiology

Duraswaimi produced this deformity in chick embryos after treating the developing embryo by insulin injections into its milieu in the egg. Despite this and other work indicating that perhaps lowered oxygen tension at a critical stage of limb bud development plays a part in

Fig. 2.39. Fifth toes overlapping bilaterally—a fixed congenital deformity. Pulling the toe laterally retreats the contracture of the skin on the dorsum of the foot.

the etiology of clubfoot, the cause of the deformity in humans is not established. Stewart notes a familial and racial predilection in his study of Hawaiian Island inhabitants. Bechtol and Mossman, in dissecting two fetal specimens, found evidence favoring abnormality of muscle growth resulting in failure of the muscles to keep pace with skeletal development. The relative shortening of the muscle fibers was thought to be due to degeneration. Flinchum, in studying a 6½-month, premature infant, found the peroneal muscles on the involved side to be about one-half the size of those on the normal side. This suggested an imbalance between medial and lateral musculature. Stewart, in his dissections of clubfeet, found abnormal insertions of the anterior tibial tendon apparently playing a part in producing adduction and supination of the forefoot. Other authors have emphasized abnormalities of the ligaments (Brockman[2]) and of nerves (Moore), and the older German authors discussed bony anomaly. Perhaps all of this points to the clubfoot as being a faulty and incomplete development involving all structures that control the position of the foot.

It is evident that at least some clubfeet have an intrinsic deformity of the astragalus. This has been shown in postmortem dissection by Sherman, among others. The body of the astragalus is in its normal position in the ankle mortise. From this point the head and neck of the astragalus are deviated medialward. Cartilage covers the head of the astragalus, but when the forefoot is brought into a corrected position

Fig. 2.40. Plantar view of equinovarus deformity revealing forefoot adduction, hindfoot inversion, and equinus.

the navicular is actually further lateral than this cartilage-covered area. This bony deformity helps to account for the peculiar flat-topped outline of the astragalus in a lateral x-ray of the foot, since most of the astragalus is oblique rather than lateral to the x-ray when the film is taken. The external torsion of the lower limb that accompanies clubfoot still further accentuates this position by holding the body of the astragalus in the opposite direction to the deformed position of the head and neck.

Clinical Picture

The orthopaedist hopes to see a patient with a foot in an equinovarus position immediately after birth. The immediate problem is to differentiate the positional foot from the fixed

Fig. 2.41 (*left*). The calcaneus valgus foot with excessive dorsiflexion.
Fig. 2.42 (*right*). Positional metatarsus varus correctable by passive manipulation.

Fig. 2.43. Denis-Browne bar of which there are many types. This one corrects rotation of the leg without foot deformity.

"clubfoot." The clubfoot cannot be passively corrected. Stimulation of the peroneal muscles by stroking the lateral side of the foot reveals a deficiency in their action and an inability to evert the foot. Should the foot be mobile, the expectation is that it can be readily and easily corrected. True clubfoot deformities are fixed. The foot has fixed forefoot adduction, fixed inversion particularly noted in the hindfoot, and equinus of the hindfoot carrying the forefoot with it.

The calf size should be noted. Smallness of the calf may be noted at birth before treatment is begun. It tends particularly to be associated with the more rigid types of clubfoot, such as those seen in arthrogryposis.

The degree of internal or external torsion of the tibia should be noted. Surprisingly, perhaps, when the relation of the medial to the lateral malleolus is accurately determined, it is found that they lie in the position of external torsion in relation to the knee. The medial deviation of the foot apparently is accounted for by the forefoot adduction.

If one is able to appreciate that external torsion is the normal position of the tibia in clubfoot then the truly corrected position will carry the forefoot into further forefoot abduction than initially conceived.

The hips must be carefully checked for associated dysplasia or frank dislocation, which is often seen in arthrogryposis. The opposite foot may be the site of less severe deformity, such as metatarsus varus.

Treatment

Forcible methods of manipulation have been found in the past to be associated with the development of rigid, insufficiently corrected feet. Such manipulation was particularly done by means of the Thomas wrench—a tool found in the hospital instrument cupboard, but now seldom used. Kite[5b] has been responsible for an emphasis on gentle correction and an insistence on fully correcting one portion of the deformity before continuing treatment to other portions. If fundamental principles are followed, most clubfeet can be corrected into pliable, fully useful feet. Ten percent or less prove very resistant and sometimes require other means.

Plaster casts in various forms, constructed either in sections or as a complete unit, are used by some orthopaedists. Others prefer Denis-Browne splints. Whatever method is used, the results should be carefully assessed, both clinically and by roentgenogram, to ensure that full correction of all elements is obtained.

In Kite's method, a plaster slipper is made for the correction of forefoot adduction. Inversion is corrected by everting the slipper. Finally, after the first two elements have been corrected, the foot is brought out of equinus. Such plasters are carefully applied without padding the foot to the point of obscuring landmarks and the true position of the foot.

Wedgings can be used, but greater efficiency is obtained by complete changes of cast at weekly intervals. Some surgeons apply a cast as a unit to foot and calf. The cast is then lengthened to a full leg cast that holds the knee approximately in right-angle flexion. To control the heel so that it will not slip up, the cast is molded in well just above the prominence of the os calcis, and a full leg cast is used.

As Kite has emphasized, holding the foot too long in a valgus position before dorsiflexion is attempted creates a flat foot. Pressure is not exerted on the forefoot to bring the foot into dorsiflexion. This too frequently results in a "rocker bottom" foot in which the forefoot has been advanced into dorsiflexion ahead of the

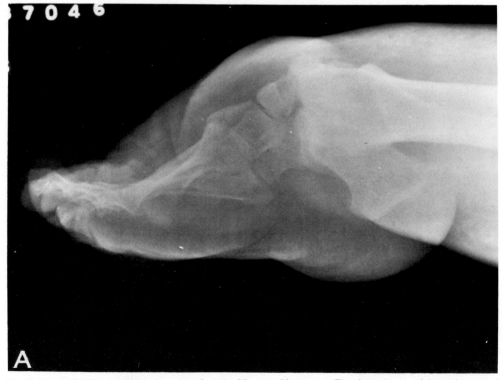

Fig. 2.44 (*A-C*). Untreated equinovarus foot in 30-year-old woman. Fixed equinus and inversion are shown with secondary holding of the bone shapes. The persistent external torsion of the fibula and tibial relationships is clearly evident in the anteroposterior view of the ankle.

Fig. 2.44 (B-C)

Fig. 2.45. Clubfeet, posterior view.

Fig. 2.46. Roentgenogram of uncorrected equinovarus feet with forefoot adduction and fixed equinus.

Fig. 2.47. Multiple congenital anomalies with abdominal wall hernia, absence of cord below the 12th dorsal vertebra, and equinovarus deformities. Paralytic feet such as these are exceedingly difficult to correct. Once corrected, bracing is necessary to hold the correction as the child grows.

Fig. 2.48. Correcting forefoot adduction by wedging cast.

equinus deformity of the hindfoot. Both these conditions are very difficult to correct.

The area beneath the calcaneocuboid joint is

Fig. 2.49. Wedging cast that holds the foot in dorsiflexion is done with axis of wedge at the ankle joint. Placing it still more distally would result in dorsiflexion of the forefoot alone.

well molded, but not overly so, so that the cuboid is displaced medially.

The usual time for correction started at birth is 6-8 weeks. The foot is held in a corrected position to ensure its continuance for a period of weeks. The foot brought merely to neutral will revert to its former position. The corrected foot must have motions corresponding to those of the "normal" foot. The correction should be checked by x-ray. Both os calcis and astragalus should be out of equinus and into 15° of dorsiflexion. The long axis of the astragalus should run down the long axis of the first metatarsal. The supination of both hindfoot and forefoot should be fully corrected so that the shadows of the astragalus and os calcis do not overlie each other: the os calcis should have been brought out laterally from beneath the astragalus. A lateral of the foot should be a lateral of both hindfoot and forefoot.

Stretching into dorsiflexion is done when the navicular has been brought back into normal alignment with the astragalus. The foot in valgus can be readily dorsiflexed, but after this position is secured, the foot must be returned more closely to "neutral." This locks the os calcis beneath the astragalus so that the tendo Achillis is more thoroughly stretched and a plantar-flexed talus is avoided.

Denis-Browne Splints

This method of correction, particularly of forefoot adduction and inversion, is not as efficient as casts in the correction of equinus. Bell and Grice[1a] have described the method of strapping the foot to the splint in detail. Minute attention to method is necessary to avoid loosening of the foot from the plate and skin decubitii. Tincture of benzoin is applied to the foot.

The forefoot is first held to the plate by a circular strap. Bringing the plate to the foot is more effective than trying to hold the foot in a corrected position while applying adhesive.

Two straps then crisscross over the dorsum and attach to the rear flange of the plate to keep the foot from slipping forward, the dorsum being protected by a felt pad. One of these straps comes up under the cuboid area of the foot. The foot is held firmly against the plate as adhesive running down the back of the calf is split just above the heel, carried forward, and attached to the plate. Further straps are added to hold the hindfoot to the lateral flange. There should be no play between plate and foot when the application is finished, and the color of the toes should be normal.

The other foot is also strapped. When the plate is attached to a connecting bar in varying degrees of external rotation, the forefoot adduction and the inversion are corrected. In later stages the cross bar can be bent in a V to achieve still further correction.

The feet are suspended by a cord to the bar so that the baby can kick freely and procure dynamic correction. When the process is correctly done, a very pliable, well corrected foot can be obtained.

Resistant Clubfeet—Surgical Treatment

With the small percentage of feet which are very resistant to correction during the first 6 months of life, great care must be taken to eliminate dorsiflexion of the forefoot ahead of the hindfoot. No operative treatment is entertained until the foot has been thoroughly attacked with corrective plaster casts by an experienced orthopaedist.

The two elements which may prove particularly difficult are inversion and equinus of the os calcis. Release of the medial ligamentous structures, capsulotomy of the ankle joint, and heel cord lengthening or transfer of the medial portion of the Achilles tendon to the lateral side of the os calcis are the usual procedures.

Anatomy of Clubfoot

Turco[11] describes the talocalcaneonavicular joint well as a ball and socket joint separate from the posterior subtalar joint. The socket is formed by the navicular anteriorly, dorsomedially by the talonavicular joint capsule, deltoid ligament, and posterior tibial tendon. The lateral support is the bifucated (Y) ligament and inferiorly the head of the talus is supported by the middle and anterior subtalar articular surfaces of the calcaneus and spring ligament.

The cup formed by these structures moves around the ball (head of the talus) and expands and contracts through the fibroelastic ligaments. The clubfoot has been described as a subluxation of the talocalcaneonavicular joint.

When the talus is in equinus and fixed there, the posterior tuberosity of the os calcis is displaced laterally and superiorly in relation to it. The structures now fixing the position are the posterior talocalcaneal capsule heel cord and the calcaneofibular ligament. Anteriorly the deltoid and spring ligaments, the posterior tibial tendon, and the subtalar interosseous ligament resist correction.

In resistant clubfeet the stressed dorsiflexed lateral x-ray reveals a failure of the calcaneus to dorsiflex. If full dorsiflexion of the os calcis can be achieved at operation and held for at least 4 months, Turco has noted an absence of recurrent deformity.

Medial Release

In the medial release procedure described by Turco, sharp dissection is used through a long medial incision beginning at the base of the first metatarsal and running posteriorly to the tendo Achillis.

The posterior tibial tendon is identified and both its sheath and that of the flexor digitorum longus tendon is divided around and above the medial malleolus. The neurovascular bundle is immobilized and retracted gently. When retracted the flexor hallucus longus tendon is freed from its sheath.

The master knot of Henry is a fibrocartilaginous structure attached to the undersurface of the navicular and enveloping the flexor digitorum longus and flexor hallucus longus ten-

Fig. 2.50. Comparison of the normal foot with treated clubfoot of the same patient (girl, age 5). (A) Lateral normal foot. (B) The external torsion normally present in clubfoot deformity is accentuated by the obliquity of the hindfoot to the x-ray. This also results in a flat topped appearance of the astragalus. The os calcis is in calcaneus, the forefoot in relative equinus, the navicular deformed. The x-ray is a true lateral of the forefoot. This is maximum dorsiflexion for this foot. (C) The normal foot is supple when plantar flexed and motion takes place equally in the forefoot and ankle joint. (D) The old equinovarus foot has limited eccentric motion at the ankle joint as the astragalus hinges out of it in plantar flexion. The forefoot achieves most of the plantar flexion.

Fig. 2.50 (C)

Fig. 2.50 (D)

A

Fig. 2.51. The medial and posterior release of tight ligamentous structures should not be postponed when the foot is evidently resistant to cast treatment. If this is done, immobilization atrophy becomes excessive, the cartilage of the small bones of the foot is deformed, and motion of the joint becomes limited. (These drawings have had a liberal inspiration from both Turco and Bost in their articles on medial release, but have been modified according to our concepts as well.) (*A*) The incision extends posteriorly beyond the peroneal tendons and forward sufficiently to visualize the naviculocuneiform joint. (*B*) The neurovascular bundle can be isolated and drawn to either side to avoid damage to it during the course of the procedure. (*C*) The posterior tibial tendon and the flexor digitorum longus are identified and the sheath of both divided posteriorly around the medial malleolus. The "master knot of Henry" is a fibrocartilaginous structure attached to the undersurface of the navicular and enclosing the flexor hallucis longus and flexor digitorum longus as they cross over one another. This structure is excised. (*D*) The Achilles tendon is lengthened by a Z-plasty. The neurovascular bundle and flexor hallucis longus are retracted anteriorly to bring the posterior ankle and subtalar joint into view. (*E*) Once visualized the capsulotomy of the talotibial and subtalar joint is performed. The calcaneofibular ligament can be divided deep in the wound as well as the talofibular ligament. (*F*) The posterior tibial tendon is cut just above the medial malleolus and allowed to retract. (*G*) The ligaments medially are then divided including those shown plus the spring ligament and the attachment of the posterior tibial tendon inferior to the navicular after it is no longer needed to pull the point toward the surgeon. When the heel is everted, the deltoid ligament can be cut to completely release the os calcis anteriorly and posteriorly. (*H*) When the heel deformity is completely corrected, the navicular is then correctly reduced onto the head of the talus and held with a Kirschner wire. This can project through the cast and be removed 3 weeks postoperatively.

Fig. 2.51 (B)

Fig. 2.51 (C)

D

Fig. 2.51 (D)

E

Fig. 2.51 (E)

Fig. 2.51 (F)

Fig. 2.51 (G)

H

Fig. 2.51 (H)

dons as they cross over one another. This structure is excised.

Once these structures have been mobilized, a posterior, medial, and subtalar release is made.

The tendo Achillis is lengthened by a Z-plasty, detaching the medial half from the os calcis.

Anterior retraction of the neurovascular bundle and flexor hallucus longus tendon brings the posterior aspect of the ankle into view. A posterior capsulotomy of the ankle joint is then done. The posterior capsule of the posterior component of the subtalar joint is divided along with the calcaneofibular ligament. This is seen deep in the wound and is important to reach. Retracting the neurovascular bundle posteriorly the posterior insertion of the deltoid ligaments of the calcaneus is dividing.

Medially the posterior tibial tendon is cut just above the medial malleolus and allowed to retract. The distal portion pulls out the talonavicular joint. The deltoid ligament on navicular and talonavicular capsule is then incised. The posterior tibial tendon attachments to the sustentaculum tali and spring ligament are cut and the spring ligament detached from the sustentaculum tali.

When the foot is then everted the subtalar joint is exposed, permitting release of the superficial layer of the deltoid ligament. The deep portion inserting into the body of the talus is preserved.

Further subtalar release involves the talocalcaneal interosseous ligament and the bifurcated (Y) ligament extending from the calcaneus to the lateral border of the navicular and medial border of the cuboid.

The navicular is then correctly reduced on to the head of the talus. The os calcis must have been released both anteriorly and posteriorly to completely correct the heel deformity.

A Kirschner wire inserted on the dorsum of the foot transfixes the talonavicular joint once it is correctly reduced—avoiding overcorrection. The foot is dorsiflexed to a right angle and the tendo Achillis is approximated with sutures. The Kirschner wire is left in 6 weeks.

Turco recommends cast changes at 3 and 6 weeks, and after 4 months of immobilization a Denis-Browne bar with everted feet for sleeping for 1 year.

A wire through the superior posterior portion of the calcaneus may be used to control the position of the calcaneus as the plaster is applied; it is incorporated in the plaster. The wire is removed at 3 weeks, the plaster at 6.

Follow-Up Therapy

Feet that are fully corrected can be held in bivalved casts or forefoot abduction shoes attached to a Denis-Browne bar. The mother performs eversion and dorsiflexion exercises at each diaper change. She should be carefully instructed not to dorsiflex the forefoot, but to let it be carried by the dorsiflexion of the hindfoot. The forefoot is stretched into abduction daily, however.

The patient is seen regularly by the orthopaedist during the first 2 or 3 years. If the foot begins to lose mobility, it is promptly placed in long-leg plaster casts and wedged out into full correction. Short-leg casts cannot fully control the forefoot adduction or the equinus.

Anterior Tibial Transplant

Recurrence of deformity in apparently well corrected feet may be due to peroneal weakness or imbalance between the anterior and posterior tibia and the peroneals.

As emphasized by Garceau and Manning,[3] if supination occurs on active dorsiflexion, an anterior tibial transplant may be necessary to prevent recurrence of the deformity. The usual age period when the need for transplantation becomes apparent is 4-6 years. The foot should be corrected by wedging casts prior to transplantation.

The anterior tibial tendon, when transplanted to the lateral side of the foot (base of the fifth metatarsal), has been found to be a weak dorsiflexor and to function poorly. The usual procedure is to transplant the tendon to the base of the second metatarsal. This position preserves the action of the anterior tibial as a dorsiflexor while weakening it as a supinator.

The anterior tibial tendon is detached from its insertion and drawn up through a second incision into the calf. It is then rerouted into the common extensor sheath and brought out on the dorsum of the forefoot. Here it is attached to the base of the second metatarsal through a drill hole or trap door.

Posterior Tibial Transplant

Owing to results with the anterior tibial transplant which did not completely satisfy our service, we have turned to the posterior tibial transplant, which has given improved performance as to both correction and function.

In many resistant clubfeet, the posterior tibial tendon appears taut and, when released, allows correction which had not been possible previously. While operating through the medial incision, the surgeon can also perform a capsulotomy at the navicular talar joint and release the medial structures that hold the hindfoot in inversion. A second incision is made on the medial aspect of the calf running proximal from just above the medial malleolus. The posterior tibial tendon can be found just beneath the great toe flexor. The neurovascular bundle is carefully avoided. A linear incision into the interosseous membrane is made from a point at which tibia and fibula come so close together than anything further in that direction is impractical proximally for about 2 inches. The tendon is then passed through this opening into the anterior compartment and distal to an incision made over the base of the second metatarsal. The tendon is not long, but usually just reaches the metatarsal if it has been thoroughly mobilized before detachment. Occasionally it is necessary to attach it proximally to this position. The tendon, once attached at its resting length, holds the foot in good position. A long-leg cast is applied for 6 weeks.

Rocker Bottom Foot

Rocker bottom foot is a product of treatment. The foot has, for practical purposes, been overstretched in the midtarsal region. This results in a prominent cuboid area which becomes the point of weight bearing with resultant callus and disability. There are at least four ways this foot can be produced: (1) pushing the forefoot up out of equinus before the hindfoot equinus is corrected; (2) slipping of the foot up into the cast so that the forefoot must be pushed up; (3) walking on a foot with uncorrected equinus; (4) dorsiflexing the forefoot in exercises.

This tendency in the foot is very difficult to correct, and the foot must be held for a considerable period. The forefoot is pushed back down into equinus until it is lined up with the hindfoot in the cast. The foot is then brought up as a unit until it is corrected.

When the foot cannot be corrected because of persistent equinus of the hindfoot, a heel cord lengthening and ankle capsulotomy posteriorly may be necessary. It is usual also to insert a wire into the posteriosuperior angle of the os calcis to control its position. The wire is incorporated in the cast.

At 6 weeks the cast is removed, but still further holding in plaster may be necessary for perhaps 2 or 3 months, with cast changes at approximately 3-week intervals.

Recurring Clubfeet Below Age of Eight

Wedging casts are resorted to in this period to restore full correction. These feet presumably once were fully correctable and readily tend to wedge out. The forefoot adduction is wedged across the midtarsal area. Equinus is corrected by wedges at the level of the ankle joint and not below it.

Uncorrected Clubfeet After Age of Eight

It is apparent that by the age of 8 considerable bony deformity has taken place in the feet. A triple arthrodesis of the midtarsal and subtalar joints can create a satisfactory foot for useful function without disability. The Hoke arthrodesis with replacement of the astragalar head is also useful. Corrective wedges are removed so that the foot lies in good position without forceful effort. Such an operation is ordinarily not done before the age of 12. It should be remembered that the tibia is

Fig. 2.52. Recurring clubfoot with dorsiflexion in inversion. This foot has unbalanced muscle power controlling it and recurrence can be expected with growth. Either brace control or operative restoration of muscle balance is necessary.

Fig. 2.53. Uncorrected clubfoot walking with hindfoot in inversion.

Fig. 2.54. "Rocker bottom" foot with reversal of the lateral arch and cuboid prominence.

Fig. 2.55. Uncorrected equinus with break at midfoot and relative dorsiflexion of the forefoot in "rocker bottom" foot.

Fig. 2.56. Aseptic necrosis of the body of the astragalus resulting from resection of the anterior portion for equinovarus foot deformity. An osteotomy of the astragalus corrects the deformity but cannot be done without the risk of necrosis.

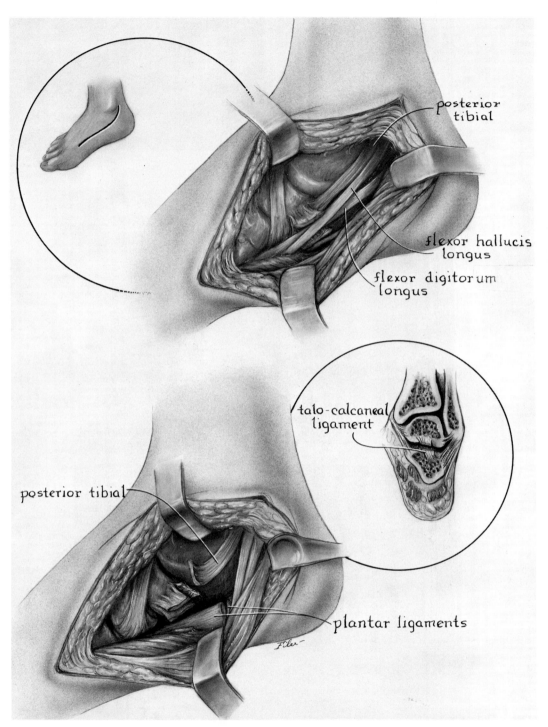

Fig. 2.57. The medial release of Bost, Larsen, and Schottstadt follows the lines of the old Ober ligamentous procedure and is the basis of the still more complete procedure as described by Turco.

externally rotated and the foot should be lined up with it.

Talectomy

As Menelaus[7,8] has suggested, talectomy overcomes some of the inadequacies of soft-tissue release in severe fixed deformity. The situation of inadequate medial soft tissues including skin to allow adequate correction occurs principally in association with arthrogryposis or spina bifida syndrome. Talectomy creates relatively lax soft tissues to allow adequate correction of both equinus and varus deformities. It is an operation that ordinarily is not necessary for congenital talipes equinovarus.

Whitman[12] used the operation for a variety of paralytic deformities, reporting on it first in 1901.

Menelaus used as his indications for talectomy (1) badly deformed equinovarus feet, (2) very rigid feet, and (3) multiple disabilities making prolonged standing unlikely. The usual age at operation is 3 years and is limited to the age group of 1-5 years.

The operation is done through a curved lateral incision. The ankle subtalar and midtarsal joints are opened and the ligaments

Fig. 2.58. Diagrammatic representation of the talectomy with positioning of the os calcis in the ankle mortise.

divided. The talus is grasped with a towel clip and rotated as the soft tissue is stripped from it. The heel cord may be lengthened. The lateral malleolus may abut against the lateral surface of the os calcis—if necessary the tip of the lateral malleolus may be removed. The os calcis is thrust posteriorly in the ankle mortisse to maintain the heel contour.

The low lateral malleolus may project sufficiently to warrant trimming thus avoiding pressure in the shoe. Following operation a plaster cast is applied for 6 weeks—ankle in neutral, heel corrected into valgus.

CALCANEOVALGUS FEET

The calcaneovalgus foot can be recognized at birth from its characteristic dorsiflexed and everted position.

The foot is very hypermobile, except when it is moved into equinus, when it may be noted that the anterior tibial tendon becomes tight. If the foot is fully mobile in all directions and actively corrects, it tends to resume normal alignment in about 2 months.

Some of these feet, when checked by tight dorsal structures, may be stretched out by corrective casts. The use of a Denis-Browne splint with the cross bar inverted to keep the feet in the proper position has been suggested by Thomson.[10] Such treatment over a period of time sufficient to eliminate the excessive dorsiflexion and eversion is of value.

The sleeping position tends to maintain the overstretched ligaments of feet such as these. When weight bearing begins, the foot sags into

Fig. 2.59. Calcaneovalgus foot with excessive dorsiflexion and tight anterior tibial tendon.

severe pronation. A patient who has had feet such as these at birth should be supported by stiff-soled shoes with ½-inch inner heel and sole wedges.

CAVUS FEET

The characteristics of cavus feet—high arched feet with equinus of the forefoot, cock-up toes, and a calcaneous position of the hindfoot—are readily recognized clinically. This foot without a very severe deformity can produce severe disability. It is very rarely seen below the age of 3.

Etiology

Such a foot brings to mind a triad of neurologic diagnoses as possible underlying causes. The first is an anomaly of the lumbosacral spine that may be accompanied by adhesions interfering with foot function. The resultant muscular imbalance is thought to result in the cavus foot. A previous attack of poliomyelitis may result in muscular imbalance. Weakness of dorsiflexors with the posterior tibial still present may result in this situation. Degenerative neurologic conditions such as Friedreich's ataxia may underlie this foot deformity. It is important to recognize that chronic neurologic disturbance may exist and to take appropriate steps to diagnose it.

Clinical Picture

These youngsters are usually recognized in the 7-14-year age group. The changes in the foot by this time are well established. The usual complaint is deformity, which is noted by the parents. Symptoms in this age group are rare. Calluses beneath the metatarsal head or over the proximal interphalangeal joint may be the presenting complaint.

Suspicion of the foot deformity is aroused by equinus of the forefoot in non-weight bearing. Confirming factors are hyperextension deformity of the metatarsophalangeal joints and flexion deformity of the interphalangeal joints, which results in clawtoes. These toes are subluxated dorsalward on the metatarsal heads. The os calcis is not in equinus but in a calcaneous or dorsiflexed position; it thus gives

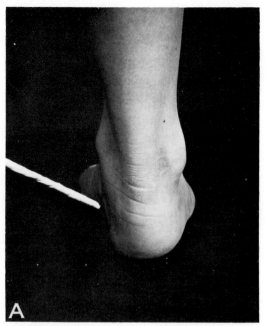

Fig. 2.60. Demonstration of the hindfoot-forefoot relationships in cavus feet. (*A*) The hind foot is in varus and related to the ankle which is in external rotation. The forefoot is abducted. (*B*) When the forefoot is held up the cavus deformity is partially masked. (*C*) Covering the hindfoot makes the equinus deformity of the forefoot apparent as a direct continuation of the tibia. (*D*) Covering the forefoot with a black sheet makes the relative lack of equinus of the hindfoot apparent – actually the os calcis is in calcaneus.

Fig. 2.60 (B)

Fig. 2.60 (C)

Fig. 2.60 (D)

rise to the high arch. Passive elevation of the forefoot in this age group results in straightening of the toes.

Depending on the duration and severity of the deformity, there may be thinning and atrophy of the fat pads over the metatarsal heads so that they may readily be palpated. Calluses may form over these bony processes. The plantar fascia may be palpated as a tight

contracted band on attempted correction of the forefoot and may limit full correction.

Treatment

Conservative treatment consists of passive stretching of the plantar fascia by dorsiflexion of the forefoot and flattening of the medial arch. The toes are brought down from their

Fig. 2.61. Cavus feet (note equinus of forefoot in relation to hindfoot).

The operation that attacks the heart of the deformity is a transplantation of the long extensor tendons to the metatarsal necks. The short extensor tendons are detached at their insertion into the proximal phalanx and sewn

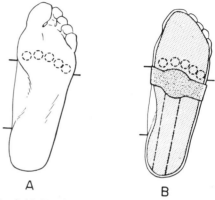

Fig. 2.62. Tracing of pad with Jones bar to elevate forefoot. The transverse bar is felt covered with leather. The *dotted lines* indicate the position of a corset stay to impart stiffness to the pad.

Fig. 2.63. Effect of moving long extensor of toes back to metatarsal neck to correct equinus of forefoot and allowing toes to drop down to correct dorsiflexion of the proximal phalanx.

subluxated position on the dorsum of the metatarsal heads, and the interphalangeal flexion deformity is passively stretched.

A Jones bar pad is either worn as an inner sole, where it is most efficient, or built into the sole of the shoe. This pad to be corrective must be placed so that its elevation is directly behind the metatarsal heads. In the still pliable foot, this elevation restores the toes to their rightful position. The shoe aids in holding them down.

Operation is considered in the presence of progressive deformity as a conservative regime and must be performed before the fat pads beneath the metatarsal heads have atrophied.

into the stumps of the insertions of the long extensors. If necessary, a capsulotomy of the metatarsophalangeal joints is done on the dorsum. An accessory bit of surgery that is sometimes necessary is a division of the plantar fascia. This is done just forward of the origin of the fascia from the os calcis.

The most medial incision is used for the great toe. Two tendons are approached through each of the other two incisions. The result of too few incisions is unnecessary retraction at the expense of the vitality of the skin edges.

A triple arthrodesis is sometimes used for correction of the deformity. While this proce-

Fig. 2.64. Detail of insertion of the long extensor tendon into the metatarsal neck, with insertion of the short extensor tendon into the stump of longus.

dure corrects in part, it does so at only one of the many series of joints involved, and it fails to attack the area causing disability—i.e., the metatarsal necks and toes. Some correction in this area is achieved by shortening the bones relative to the soft tissues by means of a triple arthrodesis. This procedure is sometimes used in the older age groups, but it has not proved as satisfactory as tendon transplant. After tendon transplant, the foot is kept in a short-leg plaster cast for 6 weeks.

KÖHLER'S DISEASE

Köhler's disease is a condition causing pain and swelling in the foot. The roentgenogram reveals abnormal density of the navicular bone. Involved in this way, the navicular can be compressed if it is not protected. Unfortunately this condition, which is quite rare, is often confused with the normal fragmentary ossification of the navicular, which is not associated with symptoms.

Normal ossification of the navicular from multiple centers occurs in the 3-6-year-old age group. Cases showing increased density of the navicular consistent with Köhler's disease usually occur past this stage in the 6-10-year age group.

Etiology

This condition is usually thought of as secondary to circulatory interference. The reason for this change is not clear. It is related presumably to other lesions such as Kienböck's disease, the Legg-Perthes syndrome, and Frieberg's disease of the second metatarsal head.

Clinical Picture

The patient complains of foot pain that tends to be continuous rather than intermittent, as in the case of foot strain. There is tenderness over the area occupied by the navicular bone. Thickening and even frank swelling may be noted in this area. When the condition is active, limping and a tendency to walk on the lateral side of the foot are noted.

Roentgen Findings

The disease can be accurately diagnosed by roentgenogram. Confusion with normal ossification of the navicular can be avoided once it is realized that the navicular normally arises from at least three separate centers of ossification in the 3-6-year age group. These centers coalesce rapidly to form one center. When one overlies another, an appearance of increased density is sometimes given. In Köhler's disease the navicular or a portion of it exhibits increased density and then fragments. The radiolucent areas finally heal in to form normal-appearing bone. While it is going through the dense stage, the navicular may become narrowed and compressed if the patient has been weight bearing.

Treatment

The patient is taken off weight bearing. A protective plaster cast and crutches are used, usually for several months. Before weight bearing protected with crutches is begun, the areas of density should be repaired and the

Fig. 2.65. Diagram to illustrate a simple method of determining wedge resections in triple arthrodeses to correct the deformity. The *long dotted lines* illustrate the axis of forefoot and hindfoot as in (*A*). All cuts in the forefoot side are made at right angles to the forefoot axis. All cuts on the hindfoot side are made at right angles to the hindfoot axis. All cuts should come out at the apex of the triangle at the junction of cartilage of the joint surface and of bone. In this way, no more bone will be removed than is absolutely necessary, and a normal looking foot will be maintained. In (*C*), the talar cut is made in relation to the axis line of the tibia. The os calcis cut, based posteriorly, will follow the line of the subastragalar joint but will still bear the axis of the os calcis in mind. Triple arthrodeses ordinarily require 8 weeks in a long-leg plaster cast followed by several weeks in a short-leg walking cast before fixation is terminated. Crutches are usually required for at least 4 weeks thereafter

Fig. 2.66. Roentgenogram of compressed and dense navicular in Köhler's disease with associated soft-tissue swelling.

soft-tissue thickening relieved. Full weight bearing is gradually achieved as the lesion heals.

FREIBERG'S DISEASE

Although patients with pain beneath the second metatarsal head and with roentgenographic evidence of deformity of the head of the second metatarsal are often first seen as adults, the onset of this disease is in adolescence. The disease appears to be an aseptic necrosis of the epiphyseal area of the second metatarsal occurring about the time of epiphyseal line closure. There is often a history of chronic trauma caused by such activities as ballet dancing. The disorder is much more common in female patients.

Clinical Picture

There is a complaint of pain with use in the region of the second metatarsal head. Swelling about the area is appreciated by palpation and is often visible. Tenderness may be acute.

Roentgen Picture

The epiphyseal area is originally dense; then rarefied areas appear at the base of the metatarsal head, and irregular replacement follows so that the density is eventually completely removed. If, during this period, the area is unprotected, the joint surface becomes flattened. This deformity is a permanent, residual one.

Fig. 2.67. Anteroposterior view of the foot in a 12-year-old girl. Flattening of the surface of the second metatarsal head (*arrow*) has already taken place. There is increased density distally and a line of rarefaction proximal to it as vascular penetration takes place.

Treatment

When seen at the onset of the disease, the youngster is immobilized in a walking plaster cast molded to bring the pressure of weight bearing behind the metatarsal heads. After the swelling has subsided, a carefully molded foot plate is worn so that the metatarsal head does not take weight directly. The elevation of the plate in the midmetatarsal area must be sufficient to accomplish this and can be checked by lateral roentgenogram of the foot in the shoe. A Jones metatarsal bar in the sole of the shoe may be an additional safeguard. Once deformity has occurred, the metatarsal head cannot be reconstituted. Persistent pain may lead to resection of the proximal portion of the proximal phalanx in order to procure a new joint.

References

1a. Bell, J. F., and Grice, D. S.: Treatment of congenital talipes equinovarus by modified Denis-Browne splint, *J. Bone Joint Surg., 26:* 799, 1944.

1. Bost, F. C., Schottstaedt, E. R., and Larsen, L. J.: Plantar dissection, an operation to release the soft tissues in recurrent and recalcitrant talipes equino-varus, *J. Bone Joint Surg., 42A:* 151, 1960.

2. Brockman, E. P.: Modern methods of treatment of clubfoot, *Br. Med. J., 2:* 572, 1937.

3. Garceau, G. J., and Manning, K. R.: Transplantation of the anterior tibial tendon in the treatment of recurrent congenital clubfoot, *J. Bone Joint Surg., 29:* 1044, 1947.

4. Harris, R. I., and Beath, T.: Hypermobile flat foot with short tendo Achillis, *J. Bone Joint Surg., 30A:* 116, 1948.

5. Harris, R. I., and Beath, T.: Etiology of peroneal spastic flat foot, *J. Bone Joint Surg., 30B:* 624, 1948.

5a. Kite, J. H.: Congenital metatarsus varus, *J. Bone Joint Surg., 49A:* 388, 1967.

5b. Kite, J. H.: Congenital talipes equinovarus, *J. Bone Joint Surg., 39A:* 282, 1957.

6. Lapidus, O.: Spastic flat foot, *J. Bone Joint Surg., 28:* 126, 1946.

7. Menelaus, M. B.: *The Orthopaedic Management of Spina Bifida Cystica,* Edinburgh: E. & S. Livingstone, 1971.

8. Menelaus, M. B.: Talectomy for equinovarus deformity in arthrogryposis and spina bifida, *J. Bone Joint Surg., 53B:* 468, 1971.

9. Osmond-Clarke, H.: Congenital vertical talus, *J. Bone Joint Surg., 38B:* 334, 1956.

10. Thomason, J.: Treatment of congenital flat foot, *J. Bone Joint Surg., 28:* 787, 1946.

11. Turco, V. J.: Surgical correction of resistant clubfoot, *J. Bone Joint Surg., 53A:* 477, 1971.

12. Whitman, R.: The operative treatment of paralytic talipes of the calcaneus type, *Trans. Am. Orthop. Assoc., 14:* 178, 1901.

CHAPTER 3

The Knee

It is well to mention at the outset that knee pain in children may not be a symptom of pathology centered at the knee. Hip joint pathology frequently gives rise to knee pain. Foot strain may sometimes appear to give rise to knee symptoms.

Lesions of the knee in children include entities such as osteochondritis dissecans, discoid meniscus, and Osgood-Schlatter disease. Popliteal cysts or Baker's cysts cause swelling posteriorly at the knee. Monarticular arthritis, a rheumatoid-like lesion, occurs most commonly at the knee. Foreign bodies sometimes give rise to a chronic swelling at the knee. Septic arthritis and tuberculous synovitis are not uncommon.

POSITIONAL DEFORMITIES

Apparent Bowlegs

The infant with an almost constant flexion of the hips and knees can give an appearance of bowleggedness to the family. The internal tibial torsion that accompanies this flexion accentuates the appearance because it turns the soft tissues lateralward and the foot inward. If the examiner hides the foot with one hand and pulls the soft tissues of the calf medialward and then fully extends the knee, it can be appreciated that the knee actually gives a position of valgus to the tibia. The tibia is straight, and it is safe to tell the family that, by the age of 3 years, the youngster will actually be somewhat knock-kneed.

It must also be noted that when the infant first stands, the hips are in external rotation while the foot is straight or turned in, and the apparent bowleggedness is thus further accentuated. Because of the wide-based stance of infancy, the viewer situated in front of the child actually sees the medial aspect of the flexed leg. Telling the family this in advance helps to allay their fears.

Aside from prescribing corrective shoes, the physician should refrain from treating the infant. He should persuade everyone concerned to wait for growth to occur. One often suspects that the hardest principle to observe in raising children is that of allowing them to grow out of difficult stages, whether the difficulty is physical or psychologic.

The internal tibial torsion results in a varus facing of the ankle joint. Secondarily, the child must pronate when he attempts to stand. During this period, shoes with Thomas heels and 1/8-inch inner heel wedges to carry the foot in line with the ankle joint are important. They prevent overstretching of the ligament of the medial side of the foot.

Uterine-Packing syndrome

The name that is given this bowing deformity of the lower extremities implies that the etiology is known. It has been thought that this particular deformity was the result of intra-uterine crowding because of its spontaneous tendency to correct and a lack of associated anomalies.

Clinical Findings

It is important to distinguish just what deformity is included in this syndrome. Clinically, a varus bow of the distal tibia and fibula is evident. The lower leg is not the only site of involvement, however, for the thigh may exhibit an isolated bow. The lower leg and thigh deformities do not ordinarily occur together.

Roentgen Appearance

The important diagnostic feature is readily evident on the roentgen film of the lower extremities. Both tibia and fibula are bowed symmetrically at the same level. There is no associated abnormality of the bone such as increased density or widening of the cortex to obscure the medullary canal. Such narrowing of the medullary cavity as may occur is only that brought on by the physical deformation. The curve of the bow is rounded, not angular.

Treatment

The most important aspect of treatment is accurate recognition of the condition. Once the physician is certain of the diagnosis it is fundamental to understand that active use of the limb will correct the deformity. Casts or braces are not indicated. If the limb is left free, and the infant allowed full activity, the deformity will correct itself over the first year of growth.

Developmental Genu Valgum

Valgus at the knee is a natural and normal phase of development. Although often present at birth, it is masked by internal torsion of the tibia and flexion at the knee and hips in the first 2 years of life. When internal torsion of the tibia is combined with a wide and externally rotated stance of the lower extremities, the child may appear to have bowlegs. After walking starts, by holding the legs straight and rotating the knee so that it faces forward, one can appreciate the true genu valgum.

Developmental valgus at the knee is most marked in the age group of 2-5 years. It has a

Fig. 3.1. The difference in position of the tibia relative to the femur is apparent when standing in children with positional tibia vara. (*A*) Recumbent film shows accentuated medial cortex on tibia. Epiphyseal growth centers are normal. (*B*) On weight bearing, the knee joint opens up laterally due to the tilt of the tibia medialward. The foot pronates secondarily.

Fig. 3.1B

natural tendency to improve, except in children who are the victims of underlying growth disturbances. Some valgus remains into adult life owing to the medial deviation of the femur from its lateral position at the side of the pelvis.

Valgus at the knee of this type is recognized by its symmetry. It rarely exceeds 20° at each knee. Its presence in children 2-5 years old is to be expected.

An x-ray of the knee helps to separate from the group with symmetric valgus those rare individuals who have an underlying disease affecting growth, such as rickets. Asymmetric or unilateral valgus demands a thorough search for the underlying cause.

Treatment

Pronated feet often accompany the genu valgum. Medial arch pads combined with 1/8-inch inner heel wedges are indicated in an attempt to keep the heel inverted and to prevent the development of further valgus. These simple measures often seem but a small obstacle to put in the path of the obvious stress of weight bearing. It is perhaps fortunate that

Fig. 3.2. Stance with tibia vara–external rotation at the hips, internal tibial torsion with medial inclination of the ankle joint, and secondary pronation of the feet to bring the foot flat on the floor and straight ahead.

Fig. 3.3. Intrauterine packing syndrome. There is no abnormality at either metaphysis of the tibia and the bowing is gradually straightening out with growth and full activity.

improvement is in most cases naturally indicated. Osteotomy for the correction of symmetric developmental valgus has not been indicated in our experience. Braces with built-in correction that bends the knee over a medial pad seem to us nothing but a means of crowding an emotional disability on top of a normal difficulty of growth.

OSTEOCHONDRITIS DISSECANS

Osteochondritis dissecans is known in adults but, in the presence of intermittent disability at the knee, it must be considered in children. It is most common in males, at least one-third of the cases are bilateral, and it has a tendency to be symmetric. The lateral aspect of the medial femoral condyle is the most common site, although rarely it can occur in the lateral condyle and in the patella. Osteochondritis dissecans occurs at the ankle, hip, and elbow, but is so frequent at the knee that it is rarely thought of prior to roentgenogram at other joints. It has not been reported below the age of 4 and may be confused with irregular ossification of the condyle in young children.

Pathology

From the pathologic point of view, the lesion appears to be an aseptic necrosis of the subchondral bone for a variable, but usually quite shallow, depth. The cartilage is not primarily involved, but becomes so when its underlying support is weakened. It is possible on viewing the lesion to find that the articular cartilage is intact and yet that typical roentgenographic changes are present. The cartilage overlying the lesion secondarily develops fibrillation and cleaves from the cartilage areas which are well supported by normal subchondral bone. The fragment which separates includes subchondral bone and cartilage.

Etiology

It is assumed that the lesion develops because of localized interference with the blood supply

Fig. 3.4. The effect of weight bearing at the knee is a child with ligamentous laxity: (*A*) weightbearing, (*B*) recumbent.

to the area. The lesion has been likened to that which would occur if a small area of a hollow sphere were indented and then allowed to spring back into place. If the lesion is allowed to heal on a conservative regime, it does so by creeping substitution. The etiology is not clear, but trauma appears to be the initiating factor.

Clinical Picture

Most characteristic perhaps is the intermittency of the symptoms. Recurrent pain at the knee is the presenting complaint, and there is a further history of clicking, giving way, and intermittent swelling at the knee. If a fragment has become detached, previous mild symptoms may be unnoticed in the acute and sudden onset of pain and swelling at the knee.

Depending on the duration of symptoms, a variable degree of atrophy of the thigh may occur. Such atrophy reflects the disability that the patient has undergone. Fluid may be noted in the knee, but diagnostically most pertinent is localized tenderness on the lateral aspect of the medial condyle. The intermittent symptoms may be the only reason for clinical attention, for there may be no signs of apparent disability.

Roentgen Findings

There is involvement of the subchondral bone. A radiolucent line separates a small dense

Fig. 3.5. (*Left*) Developmental genu valgum with fairly severe deformity. The child stands with pronated feet as well. Surgery is not indicated at this age, but the feet should be supported with medial arch pads and medial heel wedges in the shoes. (*Right*) Lateral view of a child with developmental genu valgum. The hyperextended knees are seen. The general posture is typical of a child with excessive ligamentous laxity.

fragment of this bone from the parent area. A minimal amount of reactive bone may be found about the lesion. The lesion may not be clearly visualized in the usual anteroposterior view of the knee. A so-called "tunnel" view—taken posteroanteriorly—with the knee flexed approximately 30° is helpful in throwing the area most commonly involved into relief. When the patella is involved, a tangential view of it may be helpful. Irregular ossification of the medial condyle is a normal finding in the 2-6-year-old age group.

Treatment

Green and Banks[1] have called attention to the fact that the lesion may be treated conservatively with a non-weight-bearing regime with good results. Such treatment, which uses a non-weight-bearing splint or brace, involves a healing period of approximately 4-6 months and perhaps longer. The opportunity it offers of achieving an intact articular surface makes this conservative regime the treatment of choice, as compared to surgical excision, which of necessity leaves a cartilage defect. For patients under 10, in whom detachment is unlikely, this is the treatment of choice.

Operative treatment has been frequently advocated and is followed by good results. It has the advantage of requiring a shorter period of convalescence—usually about 6 weeks. If the fragment of subchondral bone and cartilage has become detached, its removal is indicated. If it is still partially attached, the lesion, when visualized, can be readily eased from the surrounding bone. A cleavage plane of fibrous tissue exists between the fragment and the parent bone.

When the cartilage is completely intact, the area of subchondral weakness can be recognized by palpation and by a slight grayish discoloration. The lesion is cored out so that it has smooth edges and so that no unattached cartilage or bone remains. Drilling the base of the lesion may result in unwelcome exuberant

Fig. 3.6. Diagram of characteristic site of osteochondritis dissecans slightly toward the lateral aspect of the medial femoral condyle.

Fig. 3.7. A large osteochondritic fragment involving the lateral surface of the medial condyle. Fragments of this magnitude are seen in the older age group, in this case at 16 years.

repair; it is not recommended.

Actual detachment of a separate fragment is so rare below age 10 that operative therapy is ordinarily done in the teen-age group.

Reference

1. Green, W. T., and Banks, H.: Osteochondritis dissecans in children, *J. Bone Joint Surg., 35A:* 26, 1953.

DISCOID MENISCUS

Congenital "discoid" meniscus is a lesion of the cartilaginous meniscus of the knee occurring primarily in the lateral meniscus.

Normal Development

It has been stated that the meniscus originally consists of a complete disc. Kaplan[1] disputes this as a result of his fetal dissections, stating that the meniscus assumes its adult form immediately on differentiation of the structure. The intermediate zone between the femur and tibia that appears early in embryologic develop-

ment is called the intermediate disc. The disc does not break up into two separate discs, according to Kaplan, but directly into two semilunar menisci. The theory that the central portion of the originally disc-shaped structure wears away thus becomes untenable. Normally (in man) both the lateral and the medial meniscus are attached to the tibia both anteriorly and posteriorly on the intercondylar ridge.

Etiology

Dissection of animals enabled Kaplan to point out that none of the animals has a discoid meniscus except those in which the lateral meniscus normally is not attached posteriorly to the tibia, but instead continues via the ligament of Wrisberg to attach posteriorly to the lateral face of the medial femoral condyle (meniscofemoral ligament). Knees in animals are adapted to the flexed position, whereas, in man, knees are used primarily in extension. The lateral meniscus in anthropoids is almost completely circular, but never discoid.

Fig. 3.8. Air injection of knee reveals a defect in the medial femoral condyle with a fragment loose in the center of the joint.

In man, lack of attachment of the lateral meniscus to the tibia is an anomaly that leaves the ligament of Wrisberg the sole posterior attachment. In extension, this short ligament fails to allow the meniscus to glide forward. As extension takes place, the lateral meniscus is pulled into the intercondylar area. Persistent action of this type wears a groove in the center of the cartilage as the meniscus is drawn into the joint. Secondary thickening of the meniscus due to hyperplasia and the formation of fibrocartilage results in a deeper than normal cartilaginous meniscus with a ridge on either side of the groove. The original depth of the meniscus is not greater than normal, but development and use of the knee secondarily results in increased apparent depth.

Clinical Picture

Classically, as emphasized in the literature, the primary complaint is a "snapping knee." In the early years of childhood such complaints are vague indeed, and the diagnosis is usually not made until the eighth or ninth year. By this time the displacement of the cartilage that occurs as the knee is extended results in a very

Fig. 3.9. Photomicrograph of a fragment from the case shown in Figure 3.8 shows dead bone and articular cartilage.

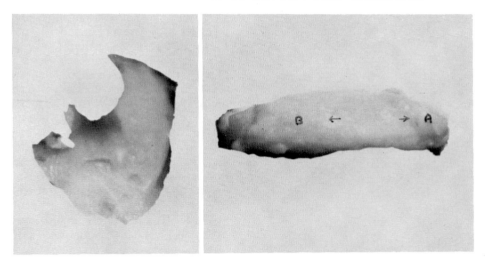

Fig. 3.10 (*Left*). Discoid lateral meniscus with ridge due to fibrocartilaginous hypertrophy beginning at the periphery.

Fig. 3.11 (*Right*). Lateral view with free edge of the meniscus toward the reader. A ridge forming both anteriorly (*A*) and posteriorly (*B*) can be discerned.

audible "clunk" in the knee, and an anterior prominence can be felt when the "clunk" is heard. The motion of the cartilage can be palpated anteriorly at the joint line. Older children may complain of a "giving way" of the knee. Rarely there may be episodes of swelling at the knee, and fluid may be palpable on examination. The author has never seen this lesion in the medial meniscus. It is a rare condition usually found only once a year in a large children's orthopaedic service. As time goes on the symptoms are sufficiently severe to curtail the youngster's activities.

Treatment

Excision of the disc is justified on the basis of the abnormal mechanics it introduces at the knee. The recovery period following such an excision is greatly shortened if the youngster has been taught quadriceps-setting exercises prior to surgery. It is difficult to teach these exercises immediately after the operation when the child has a painful knee.

Kaplan,[1] in his excellent article, points out that an abnormal meniscus of the lateral joint compartment in children, compared to the same lesion in adults, is difficult to excise. He recommends making two incisions: a posterior one to divide the meniscofemoral ligament of

Wrisberg, and an anterolateral one. The posterior incision needs to be really posterior if it is going to be done at all. Coming down on the lateral head of the gastrocnemius, the operator, standing posterior to the biceps tendon, retracts it. The joint is entered, and the posterior attachment via the meniscofemoral ligament is divided. To compromise by remaining lateral and anterior to the biceps tendon results in poor visualization of the ligament. The anterolateral excision is simple and usual. An attempt to remove the meniscus by means of an anterior approach alone is unsuccessful because the usual more proximal posterior attachment is not present and because the posterior meniscofemoral attachment cannot be visualized when the anterior incision alone is made.

Crutch-walking is begun when the foot can be lifted from the bed while the knee is extended. Full activity is allowed in the presence of full motion and a strong quadriceps, and in the absence of swelling at the knee. The approximate period of convalescence for a child is six weeks.

References

1. Kaplan, E. B.: Discoid lateral meniscus of the knee joint; nature, mechanism and operative treatment, *J. Bone Joint Surg., 39A:* 77, 1957.
2. Smillie, I. S.: The congenital discoid meniscus, *J. Bone Joint Surg., 30B:* 671, 1948.

OSGOOD-SCHLATTER DISEASE

Osgood-Schlatter disease, a disease of adolescence, causes pain anteriorly at the knee. Osgood first called attention to the enlargement of the tibial apophysis in 1903. The entity is best understood when thought of as a tendinosis, rather than as an apophysitis, however. Hughes notes that the common feature by roentgenogram is calcification within, or enlargement of the ligamentum patellae. The disease is self-limited and runs a 2-3-year course. The age of incidence is from 10 to 16 years. It is slightly more common in males, and unilateral cases occur twice as often as bilateral ones.

Etiology

A history of an extremely rapid growth spurt in the year preceding the onset of symptoms is to be expected. One suspects that the increased soft-tissue tension produced by very rapid growth causes abnormal stress at the apophysis of the tibia. Such stress is directly transmitted by the ligamentum patellae. There is a resultant swelling of the tendon at its insertion and, secondarily, an irregular ossification. Changes very similar to those caused by Osgood-Schlatter disease can be produced in the rat by shortening the patellar tendon. The disease in man ceases with fusion of the apophysis to the parent bone, if it is still active when this fusion occurs. Growth plays an important part in the etiology by producing abnormal stress at the tibial apophysis. It is possible that trauma to the tibial tubercle may also produce such stress.

Clinical Picture

The history reveals that the discomfort is experienced with activity and decreases with rest. Sports which involve much running and jumping are particularly likely to produce exacerbations of the disease. A rapid growth spurt is common in the year preceding onset. Discomfort and swelling are located anteriorly in the region of the tibial apophysis. There is no swelling that involves the joint itself. Thickening and enlargement of the tibial tubercle are characteristic.

Careful palpation reveals tenderness at the point of insertion of the tendon into the bone,

Fig. 3.12. Swelling in the area in which the patellar tendon inserts into the tibial tubercle in a case of Osgood-Schlatter disease.

but not over the apophysis itself. Extreme flexion is painful. Atrophy of the quadriceps is not remarkable unless the symptoms have been severe.

Roentgenogram

The apophysis ordinarily appears at the age of 11 and fuses with the parent epiphysis at 15, in males. It is most hazardous to base the diagnosis on irregular ossification of the apophysis because this kind of irregularity may be part of normal development. The one constant finding is swelling of the tendon shadow where the tendon inserts into the bone. The swelling frequently obliterates the angle formed by the tendon and the bone. In some cases adventitious ossification may proceed into the tendon itself.

Treatment

The discrepancy in functional length between soft tissue and bone may take 2-3 years

Fig. 3.13. Swelling at the patellar tendon insertion and fragmentation of the tibial apophysis, as seen by roentgenogram. The soft tissue reaction seen here is characteristic of Osgood-Schlatter disease.

to adjust. If the abnormal stress on soft tissues disappears, the symptoms may cease even before fusion of the apophysis with the parent bone takes place. When the symptoms are severe, rest is enforced by strapping the knee with adhesive. If necessary, a walking plaster cast in the form of a cylinder may be applied.

Voluntary limitation of activities may often be obtained in this age group, particularly when the relationship between activity and symptoms is pointed out to the patient and his parents. The patient may remain ambulatory, but he should abstain from sports, running, and long walks. The relationship between activity and symptoms is a very direct one and is readily appreciated by the patient once it is pointed out. Limitation of activity is usually necessary

for a period of only approximately 6 months. Once the functional length of the soft tissues has caught up with that of the bone, the patient can enter into full activity with impunity. Hydrocortone injected into the swollen area may give symptomatic relief in cases of acute inflammation.

Thickening and enlargement of the apophysis persist even after the disease heals and symptoms subside. The enlargement itself may be a source of discomfort in kneeling which persists after the disease is no longer active.

POPLITEAL CYSTS

Popliteal cysts have also been named "Baker's cysts." Baker[1] in 1877 described cases

Fig. 3.15. Popliteal cyst, posterior view.

Fig. 3.14. Diagram of the area of swelling in Osgood-Schlatter disease. The swelling of the distal portion of the patellar tendon appears to precede the bony changes.

of swelling in the popliteal space and thought that perhaps they were herniations of the knee joint space, which had been chronically distended by fluid. Faucher, in 1856, had described 11 dissected specimens under the impression that they represented distension of bursae located in the region of the medial head of the gastrocnemiosemimembranosus bursa, which had become filled with fluid as a result of chronic irritation.

These cysts are not uncommon in children, for about one-third of the cases occur in the 1-15-year age group. They are most common in males (by a ratio of 2:1) and are ordinarily unilateral. The etiology of these cysts in adults may be quite different from that in children. Most children have a history of no previous effusion or symptoms at the knee when the cyst is discovered.

Clinical Picture

The complaint, in children, is the swelling itself. There are no symptoms of the knee joint dysfunction. In the adult, these cysts are often associated with osteoarthritis. The symptoms referable to the knees are usually based on the arthritis, and these symptoms are due to the arthritis itself.

Because it is very difficult to palpate the popliteal area, the physician may often be misled into believing that a cyst exists. In general, when one does exist, there is no doubt. The swelling tends to lie distal to the knee crease and on the medial side of the posterior aspect of the knee.

Roentgenogram

The x-ray picture should be of help in confirming the clinical impression. A smoothly outlined swelling of fluid density is present in the popliteal space and can be noted particularly in contrast with the picture of the other

Fig. 3.16. Diagram of popliteal cyst location—medial posterior aspect of knee, inferior to knee crease.

knee. The fact that the cysts are rarely bilateral is of great help.

Treatment

Excision is recommended in the usual case. Wilson et al.[2] dissected the gastrocnemiosemimembranosus bursa in 1938 and pointed out the anatomic relationship of this bursa to the popliteal cyst. Invariably there is an intimate attachment of the bursa to the tendinous portion of the medial head of the gastrocnemius and semimembranosus muscles, requiring a partial resection of these structures in order to maintain the cyst wall. The cysts often communicate with the knee joint capsule through an opening on the proximal portion of the medial condyle beneath the medial head of the gastrocnemius. Wilson states that this connection was found in 15 of 21 operated cysts and in 17 of 30 anatomic specimens of the bursa.

Examination of the cyst walls after removal reveals fibrous thickening, areas of retained hemosiderin, and areas of metaplasia into cartilaginous and osteoid elements.

References

1. Baker, W. M.: On the formation of synovial cysts in the leg in connection with disease of the knee joint, St. Barth. Hosp. Rep., 13: 245, 1877.
2. Wilson, P. D., Eyre Brook, A. L., and Francis, J. D.: A clinical and anatomical study of the semimembranosus bursa in relation to popliteal cyst, J. Bone Joint Surg., 20: 963, 1938.

MONARTICULAR ARTHRITIS

Monarticular arthritis consists of chronic synovial thickening. The joint fluid findings are similar to those in rheumatoid arthritis, but are limited to one joint. The anomaly may occur at other areas, such as the ankle, hip, and elbow, but is so characteristic at the knee that it is fully described in this chapter. The age group affected is not well defined, but most cases occur between 5 and 10 years of age. The disease is slightly more common in females.

Etiology

The etiology is very closely related to that of rheumatoid arthritis—so closely that some cases under observation are noted to develop other involvement. Imperceptibly, thickening and fluid develop at other joints and obtain the more typical rheumatoid distribution. Aspiration of fluid from the joint reveals cellular chemical changes similar to those found in rheumatoid arthritis. Nonetheless, this entity is very frequently limited to one joint and remains so. Amelioration of symptoms is possible with intelligent care.

Clinical Picture

The child presents chronic swelling of the knee often of several weeks' or months' duration. Pain is not a prominent feature, but a limp is usually noted by the parents. The knee reveals synovial thickening, and fluid in the suprapatellar pouch produces a ballottable patella and a fluid wave in examination. There is increased heat and moderate tenderness of the anatomic area occupied by the joint. The knee lacks 10-20° of full extension. Full flexion is also limited. There is palpable and measurable atrophy of the quadriceps.

Fig. 3.17. Popliteal cyst, lateral view.

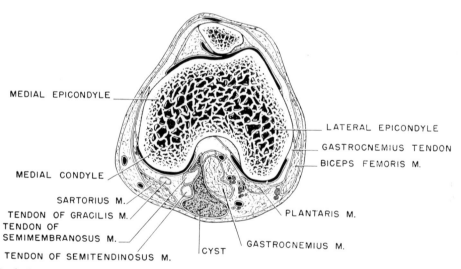

MEDIAL EPICONDYLE

LATERAL EPICONDYLE
GASTROCNEMIUS TENDON
BICEPS FEMORIS M.

MEDIAL CONDYLE

SARTORIUS M.
TENDON OF GRACILIS M.
TENDON OF
SEMIMEMBRANOSUS M.
PLANTARIS M.

TENDON OF SEMITENDINOSUS M.
CYST
GASTROCNEMIUS M.

Fig. 3.18. Diagram showing location of popliteal cyst in anatomic site of semimembranosus bursa. (*Redrawn from* P. D. Wilson, A. L. Eyre-Brook, and J. D. Francis: Clinical anatomical study of semimembranosus bursa in relation to popliteal cyst, *Journal of Bone & Joint Surgery, 20:* 963, 1938.)

Laboratory Findings

Laboratory work reveals an increased sedimentation rate and occasionally a mild leukocytosis. Aspiration of the joint may reveal a considerable elevation of polymorphonuclear cells, and the total cell count may reach 3,000-4,000 cells per cubic millimeter. The joint sugar may be depressed in relation to the blood sugar taken at the same time—that is, by more than 20 mg/100 ml. A positive tuberculin test (in the absence of a clear-cut clinical differentiation from tuberculosis) may necessitate biopsy of the joint to establish the diagnosis.

Fig. 3.19. Lateral and anterior view of knee in monarticular arthritis. There is thickening of the capsular shadows about the joint and posterior subluxation of the tibia.

Treatment

The child often walks with a knee flexion contracture. This position of strain in weight bearing does not help a low grade condition of this type to clear. Traction is often advisable to secure full extension. Bivalved plaster casts may be used with non-weight-bearing exercises to secure the same result.

Rest is still the therapy of choice for monarticular arthritis, although Hydrocortone injected into the joint may be of some help. Absolute rest from weight bearing is achieved by means of a bivalved cast or a removable splint holding the knee just off full extension.

It is important that the parents understand the chronicity of the lesion. The child is usually

Fig. 3.20. Knee flexion contracture in ambulant child.

Fig. 3.21. Swelling of the suprapatellar area due to synovial thickening and fluid.

at rest for 4 months and gradually resumes weight bearing (with crutches) in the following 2 months. Signs of recurrence of fluid are regularly sought, and the sedimentation rate is checked.

The joint, handled tenderly and slowly, responds first by losing its fluid and thereafter by a gain in the range of motion, loss of heat, and subsidence of most of the synovial thickening. Some slight thickening may remain. Rest during the early months includes complete bed rest, and a home teacher should be arranged for if the patient is of school age.

A careful and gradual resumption of activity of the joint is usually rewarded by complete cure, except in those cases which pass gradually over into rheumatoid arthritis.

FOREIGN BODY KNEE

A picture very similar to that of monarticular arthritis is sometimes seen in a patient with a history of marked trauma in the months immediately preceding consultation. The trauma is such that pieces of glass, wood, cinders, or clothing might have been driven into the knee.

The patient has a unilateral chronic, swollen knee. X-ray may reveal small bits of foreign body, but often does not. The joint fluid often contains an unusual amount of fibrin clot.

Incision into the joint reveals a large fibrin clot filling the suprapatellar pouch. This knee

may require synovectomy of the accessible portions of the joint to effect a cure. The synovectomy must be followed by traction and physiotherapy, including range-of-motion exercises and active exercises of the quadriceps

Fig. 3.22. Air arthrogram of knee with pieces of glass present laterally and in the femoral notch.

musculature, to effect a good result. Synovectomy should not be undertaken until it has been demonstrated that removal of the fibrin clot and accessible foreign material will not effect a cure.

SEPTIC ARTHRITIS OF KNEE

Septic arthritis is not as common in the knee as in the hip because the metaphyseal area of the knee is not enclosed within the joint.

Etiology

When acute, it is most often blood-borne—a complication of a severe childhood septicemia. In patients below the age of 1, the most likely etiologic agent is the streptococcus; the older age group is more often involved with the staphylococcus. Direct involvement of the knee by foreign bodies following puncture wounds gives rise to a low grade type of septic arthritis that is frequently a puzzling diagnostic problem.

Clinical Picture

The acute septic knee gives rise to apprehension, pain at the knee, and elevated temperature and increased pulse, the signs of sepsis. The swollen joint is extremely tender to palpation. The knee is held in a flexed position, and there is marked hamstring spasm. Swelling is most apparent in the region of the suprapatellar pouch.

Joint Fluid Findings

Aspiration reveals a white, cloudy to thick, purulent fluid. Cells usually number more than 4,000 per mm^3, and almost all of them are polymorphonuclear. Smear with a Gram stain frequently reveals the organism.

The fluid clots on standing; it contains increased protein and frequently clumps of fibrin. The joint sugar is depressed more than 20 mg/100 ml below the blood sugar taken at the same time.

Aspiration is performed from the lateral side into the suprapatellar pouch just proximal to the upper pole of the patella. A needle (at least 19 gauge and preferably 18 gauge) such as that used for spinal puncture is most valuable. The aspiration is likely to be more successful if pressure is exerted on the joint and the fluid is milked out rather than withdrawn by suction. Chemotherapeutic agents in appropriate concentration may be inserted into the joint following aspiration. Both anaerobic and aerobic cultures should be made of joint fluid. In a small percentage of joints, the suprapatellar bursa does not communicate with the joint space, and aspiration must be done into the joint space on either side of the patella at its lower pole.

Treatment

The patient is made comfortable by traction in line with the flexion deformity of the knee. Such traction is most simply accomplished by means of both a sling under the knee and a foot strap; this method is called split Russell traction.

Following aspiration, chemotherapy of the sort indicated for the suspected organism is instituted. As a rule the symptoms tend to subside rapidly. Intra-articular insertion of the chemotherapeutic agent may be continued. In some cases the suprapatellar pouch and joint remain thick and boggy. The temperature continues to hover at a slight elevation, and the sedimentation rate remains elevated. It may be

Fig. 3.23. Aspiration of knee from suprapatellar pouch. In a small percentage of cases, the pouch does not communicate with the knee joint itself.

necessary to drain the joint if symptoms do not rapidly subside. Incision into the joint reveals it to be filled with fibrin clot. Once the joint is emptied, the synovia is repaired with plain catgut. A catheter for the instillation of appropriate chemotherapy may be left in place, but the remainder of the wound is repaired per primam. The expected course is subsidence of symptoms.

TUBERCULOSIS OF KNEE

Tuberculosis at the knee in childhood occurs in a typical form which must be differentiated from other causes of chronic joint effusion.

Etiology

The disease is metastatic to the knee following primary involvement of the lung and is due to the tubercle bacillus originally described by Koch in 1882.

Pathology

It is most common for the synovia to be involved initially. Rarely the epiphysis of either the femur or tibia is first involved, and the synovia is involved secondarily. In the typical early case the synovia, which is markedly

redundant, tends to fill the joint space. There is an increased amount of joint fluid. The synovia tends to have a grayish discoloration, but when

Fig. 3.25. Thickened capsular shadows and filling of suprapatellar pouch area with shadows of soft-tissue density in synovial tuberculosis of the knee.

Fig. 3.24. Synovial tuberculosis of the knee. The normal anatomic outlines proximal to the patella have deen obliterated by swelling of the suprapatellar pouch on the right.

viewed at operation under tourniquet, it appears plum-colored. Tubercle formation is usually not visible in the gross, but is seen microscopically. The articular cartilage appears uninvolved, although this appearance may be deceptive. The portions that are involved are usually covered with adherent synovial membrane.

It should be remembered that tuberculosis has a tendency to extend subchondrally, leaving the cartilage relatively uninvolved but separated from the subchondral bone by underlying granulation tissue. Rheumatoid arthritis, on the other hand, extends suprachondrally, covering the cartilage with pannus.

In late cases there is extensive involvement of the ligamentous structures. The result is great disorganization of the joint. Such progression of the disease leaves little hope for

preservation of the joint as a functioning structure. There is ordinarily a history of exposure to an individual suffering from tuberculosis or a record of previous involvement, which may include tuberculous glands or meningitis, as well as disease of the lungs.

Clinical Picture

It is usual to see the patient after swelling of the knee has been noted for several months. Pain is not a prominent feature in the synovial tuberculosis seen at the knee.

Palpation reveals a plastic type of protuberance in the suprapatellar region. Areas in which the synovia can be palpated are thickened and tender. A fluid wave can often be demonstrated. There is usually a flexion contracture of the joint.

Fig. 3.26. Synovial tuberculosis of the knee. The joint surface is at the top; tubercle formation, mononuclear phagocytes, lymphocytes, and giant cells are seen below.

The tuberculin test is positive. Where the disease is suspected, it is best to begin testing with a dilution of 1:100,000. The sedimentation rate is elevated, and the white blood cell count, though not markedly elevated, frequently reveals a lymphocytes-to-monocytes ratio of well over 5 or 6 to 1.

Aspiration of the joint reveals white cells ranging from about 1,000 to 2,000 per mm^3 and preponderantly polymorphonuclear. The fluid is slightly cloudy to turbid and may contain flecks of fibrin. The joint sugar is usually more than 20 mg/100 ml lower than a blood sugar count taken at the same time.

Roentgenogram

There is a shadow of water density filling in the suprapatellar pouch area and rounding out the normal anatomic shadows of the joint. Signs of chronicity are apparent in the demineralized bone. In cases of fairly long duration, the joint space is narrow. Rarely an area of bone destruction may be seen in the epiphysis. However, areas of bone destruction may usually be seen in the subchondral region running linearly.

Treatment

The absolute rest of joints that has been enforced on tuberculous patients since the disease was first recognized remains a dominant treatment to the present day. Joint fusion was developed to aid in obtaining complete rest and healing of the disease. Such fusions save the epiphyseal discs, but in children they sometimes cause progressive deformity at the knee. The soft bone in this area allows considerable flexion to develop.

A unilateral hip spica is necessary to secure rest for the knee and should be applied after biopsy is performed. Biopsy is usually necessary to confirm the diagnosis. The current tendency is to try to preserve knee motion under the cover of the chemotherapy of tuberculosis. There is no reason to abandon rest as a principle, however, and to do so leads to recurrences of the disease.

The spica is bivalved and affixed with canvas straps; the leg is removed from it twice daily for exercise. The usual duration of treatment with chemotherapy and spica is 7 months for synovial disease of the knee. Synovectomy of the knee results in considerable impairment of motion and, in view of the excellent possibility of healing tuberculosis of the knee in childhood, is not thought necessary.

Para-Aminosalicylic Acid

This drug is inadequate when used alone because the organism ordinarily develops a resistance to it after 6 months. Its greatest value is in preventing the emergence of strains resistant to streptomycin when it is used in conjunction with that drug.

Streptomycin may affect the eighth nerve in such a way as to leave permanent deafness and troublesome vertigo.

Isonicotinic Acid Hydrazide

The use of this drug with streptomycin delays the development of resistance, which occurs with greater rapidity when either is used alone. Isonicotinic acid hydrazide, when used alone, causes resistant strains to develop in the second 3 months of treatment. This drug apparently has the ability to penetrate cells and to affect the tubercle bacillus. It is very definitely synergistic with streptomycin, for the bactericidal property of both is enhanced when they are used together.

Para-aminosalicylic acid, isonicotinic acid hydrazide, and streptomycin are apparently most effective when they are used together, since a drug is usually used for a period longer than 3 months. Persistent strains tend to die out when streptomycin is discontinued, and second courses may be given with effect.

Chemotherapy allows a period of conservative therapy to be shortened and results in greater likelihood of obtaining a cure and a functioning joint. Traction can be used as an adjunct to rest in a bivalved spica to obtain motion at the knee once the disease is controlled. There should be a normal sedimentation rate and restoration of a normal lymphocyte-monocyte ratio. The resumption of weight bearing should be gradual; it should be delayed for a 6-month period after chemotherapy and the cessation of signs of activity of the disease. During these 6 months, the patient may walk in a non-weight-bearing splint. Afterwards, progress may be made in the absence of signs of recurrence to partial, and finally full, weight bearing. The patient should have 90° of flexion and full extension of the knee and a good quadriceps before weight bearing is resumed.

References

1. Bosworth, D. M., Della Pietra, A., and Farell, R. F.: Streptomycin in tuberculosis bone and joint lesions with mixed infection and sinuses, *J. Bone Joint Surg., 32A:* 103, 1950.
2. Hughes, F. S., Mardis, R. E., Dye, W. E., and Tempel, C. W.: Combined intermittent regimens in the treatment of non-miliary pulmonary tuberculosis, Transactions of the Tenth Conference on Chemotherapy of Tuberculosis, Washington Veteran's Administration—Army-Navy, p. 67, 1954.

CONGENITAL DISLOCATION OF THE KNEE

This is an apparent congenital deformity consisting of a subluxation of the tibia anteriorly on the femur and a hyperextension of the knee.

There is some confusion as to whether this is an intrauterine positional deformity or a true congenital deformity. In some cases, usually unilateral ones, anterior subluxation is not marked and correction is readily and permanently obtained. More commonly, however, the deformity occurs in both knees. The incidence of breech presentation in cases of congenital dislocation of the knee is well above the expected 4% of the population. Associated dislocation of the hip has occurred in 50% of some series. An occasional patient has multiple deformities involving the upper as well as the lower extremities.

Deformities of the condyles of the femur and tibia appear to be secondary changes seen in older infants, but not evident, at least by roentgenogram, in the newborn.

In a 25-year period Curtis and Fisher[1] reported 16 patients with resistant congenital hyperextension of the knee who were admitted to Newington Children's Hospital. In the same period there were 650 cases of congenital dislocation of the hip.

In resistant cases the principal obstacle to reduction is a tight anterior capsule and contracted quadriceps mechanism.

Fig. 3.27. The hyperextended position of both knees is evident in this infant. Genu recurvation may actually include dislocation of the tibia in relation to the femur and secondary changes in the soft tissues. This infant has evident hand and foot deformities as well.

Clinical Picture

The positional type does not reveal any fibrotic feel in the quadriceps area. The quadriceps readily responds to gentle stretching and active exercise. Progressive flexion casts may be necessary to regain flexion. Even though it does regain flexion, it is necessary to hold the knee in 90° of flexion for a 6-week period in early infancy in order to prevent a recurrence of the hyperextended position. Once stabilized, there is no tendency toward recurrence of the hyperextended position, since the quadriceps is not involved in a fibrotic process.

Those with fibrosis of the quadriceps, loss of suprapatella pouch space, and more severely lateral dislocation of the patella represent a more difficult treatment story.

Other musculoskeletal deformities are common—of 11 patients reported by Curtis and Fisher, 7 were felt to have arthrogryposis multiplex congenita, 10 had congenital dislocation of the hip, and 7 had congenital foot

Recurvatum   Sublaxation   Dislocation

Fig. 3.28. Congenital hyperextension of the knee runs the gamut from a positional deformity to actual dislocation and a fibrous remnant of the quadriceps tightly binding down the deformity.

Fig. 3.29. Lengthening of the quadriceps to allow reduction of the tibia on the femur and knee flexion by achieving increased length.

deformities. Other organ systems were not involved.

A tight extensor mechanism with fibrous replacement of the quadriceps is a virtually constant finding in the operative cases. This occurs predominantly in the lateral portion of the muscle. Displacement of the entire quadriceps mechanism and patella occurred to the lateral side in over one-half of the cases operated by Curtis and Fisher.

Treatment

Repeated use of flexion casts that bring the knee joint into corrective flexion at each application is usually a successful method of reduction.

If the more resistant cases after at least $90°$ of flexion are obtained it is important to hold the knee in a flexed position over a 3-month period. The cast may be bivalved for active exercise of the quadriceps and hamstrings, but never allowing hyperextension.

Kirschner wire traction may be necessary in some cases to achieve a conservative reduction. Should the more conservative methods fail, an open reduction that frees the anterior capsule, replaces the quadriceps mechanism over the anterior aspect of the knee, and where necessary lengthens the quadriceps is a desirable procedure. It is desirable before secondary deformities of the proximal tibial and distal femoral epiphysis occur.

Even after open reduction, however, a holding period of many months is important in order to avoid ligamentous instability—not only in the plane of flexion, but also laterally and medially.

Niebauer and King[3] have described lengthening of the patella ligament and quadriceps and advancement of the insertion of the anterior cruciate ligament in the tibial plateau.

References

1. Curtis, B. H., and Fisher, R. L.: Congenital hyperextension with anterior subluxation of the knee, *J. Bone Joint Surg. 51A:* 255, 1969.
2. Leveuf, J., and Pais, C.: Les dislocations congenitles du genou, *Rev. Orthop., 32:* 313, 1946.
3. Niebauer, J. J., and King, D. E.: Congenital dislocation of the knee, *J. Bone Joint Surg., 42A:* 207, 1960.

GENU VALGUM

It is important to know that children pass through a stage of fairly marked genu valgum in the process of growth and development. This natural "deformity" is most noticeable about age 2; it becomes less noticeable with increased height by the age of 6. Because of the natural tendency toward improvement, surgical correction is not indicated in this age period.

The lateral condyle of the femur normally bears the most weight in the human. Valgus is a normal position for the knee and is built into the normal femur. The distance between the femurs at the hips is greater than the distance between the knees. Intrinsic valgus corrects for this discrepancy and results in apparently straight limbs.

In the younger age groups, pronation of the feet is frequently present as well. In some, pronation reflects a loose ligamentous structure which can be demonstrated at wrist and elbow by hyperextension. Roentgenogram examination may reveal that the valgus is greater in weight bearing than in recumbency in these children.

Treatment

In the 2-6 year age group, treatment consists of increasing medial arch support in order to invert the heel, separate the knees, and shift pressure from the lateral to the medial femoral condyle.

Where the valgus is marked, use of a longitudinal arch support and a 1/8 inch inner heel wedge with a prolongation of the medial heel (Thomas heel) seems a puny effort in relation to the deformity. High shoes will increase the efficiency of this apparatus somewhat, and rarely a long-leg brace with a medial pad at the femoral condyles and a built-in overcorrection to the knee may be indicated. We are concerned here not with a pathologic growth disturbance but only with a normal stage of development, and bracing is usually too limiting to the child for the slightness of the condition.

Surgical Correction

Surgical correction of a genu valgum may be indicated, for example, in cases of unilateral

Fig. 3.30. Diagrams to illustrating the fact that valgus may arise above (A) or below (B) the knee joint. The location of the anomaly determines the area selected for surgical correction, since it is desirable to have both the plane of the knee and that of the ankle at right angles to the straightened weight-bearing line.

genu valgum secondary to trauma or to a growth abnormality such as may occur in achondroplasia or Ollier's disease. Poliomyelitis may be implicated by the development of contracture laterally at the knee.

Trauma includes scarring laterally at the knee when the soft tissues have been lost owing either to traumatic avulsion or to burns. The scar may have a stapling effect that hinders the rate of growth laterally at the epiphyseal line compared to that of the medial aspect.

There are some clinical considerations in determining whether the correction should take place above or below the knee.

The desirable end result is an anatomic alignment of the plane of the ankle and that of the knee joint. Both planes should then be at right angles to the weight-bearing line. When the deformity has taken place principally in the distal femur, in which case the plane of the knee joint is oblique, correction should take place in the distal femur. When the deviation takes place in the proximal tibia, the plane of the knee joint is unaffected, but the plane of the ankle joint is oblique on weight bearing. Here correction must be done in the proximal tibia to ensure the desired result.

Roentgenograms of both knee joint and ankle joint are important in evaluating the individual case.

Since the abnormality seldom occurs in only one place and often includes a rotary deformity as well, wedge resections are seldom used. A transverse cut of the bone results in an unstable situation that is difficult to place accurately in plaster. Incidentally, a single hip spica, not merely a long-leg cast, is necessary to be certain of maintaining position.

A dome-shaped or telescoping V osteotomy gives more stability and increases the bone surface available for healing. It also allows correction in more than one plane. When the osteotomy is done in the tibia, the fibula must always be divided to allow accurate correction.

RECURRENT DISLOCATION OF PATELLA

A good illustration of the effect of body mechanics and growth on the production of disease is afforded by the entity known as recurrent dislocation of the patella. The patella may be dislocated at birth and may remain dislocated unless it is surgically corrected. Simple dislocation may follow trauma. Recurrent dislocation is a result of an abnormal direction of pull of the quadriceps muscle and may or may not be accompanied by other structural abnormalities which render dislocation easy of accomplishment. It is twice as common in females and tends to be familial.

Etiology

In order to produce a recurrent dislocation, the quadriceps musculature—which contains the patella in the manner of a sesamoid bone— must, when contracted, tend to pull the patella laterally. The factors that bring about a lateral force rather than a force running straight through the condyles of the femur include structural abnormalities which carry the patella tendon insertion in a lateral direction. This is

Fig. 3.31 (*Top*). As this 10-year-old extends the knee, the knee to the reader's left exhibits lateral displacement of the patella—an abnormal mechanism giving rise to damage of the opposing cartilaginous surfaces.
Fig. 3.32 (*Bottom*). With flexion, the patella is drawn back into the intercondylar notch.

true in genu valgus and in external rotation of the tibia. Both of these structural deviations may result from abnormal growth secondary to unequal muscle pull, as in poliomyelitis, or from congenital anomalies of the lower legs.

Absence of the vastus medial is from whatever cause, underdevelopment of the lateral condyle of the tibia, failure of the intercondylar groove to form—these all aid in the production of dislocation. An unusually long patellar tendon allowing the patella to lie above the intercondylar groove also promotes lateral displacement.

Mechanism

For functional purposes the quadriceps musculature may be visualized as contracting in a straight line between the origin of the rectus femoris or the anterior inferior spine of the ilium and the insertion of the quadriceps via the patellar tendon into the tibial tubercle or apophysis. This line should run directly between the condyles of the femurs in the intercondylar groove. Either valgus or external rotation of the tibia in relation to the knee may carry the tibial tubercle lateralward. When the patient is unusually long limbed, even a small lateral displacement may produce lateral motion of the patella.

The lateral condyle of the femur ordinarily provides a bony hindrance to lateral movement of the patella. The vastus medialis and the medial capsule provide a ligamentous hindrance. Underdevelopment of the lateral condyle, paralysis or absence of the vastus medialis,

Fig. 3.33. The line of quadriceps pull. (*A*) Normal, (*B*) valgus at the knee (*C*) external rotation of the tibia. Lateral displacement of the patella tendon insertion tends to carry the patella laterally on contraction of the quadriceps.

Fig. 3.34. Dislocated patella in six-year-old girl. The *apparent* patella prominence is due to a fat pad. The *actual* prominence can be seen above and lateral to it.

and laxity of the medial capsule eliminate these check reins. Any, all, or none of these features may be present.

A patella tendon that allows the patella to ride above the intercondylar notch eliminates the lateral condyle as a buttress in preventing lateral dislocation and may be a contributing mechanism.

Fig. 3.35. Roentgenogram of bilateral dislocated patellae. Anteroposterior view (*top*) and view with ray directed tangential to the patellae as the knee is flexed (*bottom*).

Clinical Picture

The child is usually more than 6 years old and tends to be in the early adolescent group. A period of rapid growth of the extremities often precedes the development of the condition. The rather tall, long-legged, early adolescent girl with genu valgum of moderate severity is the typical subject.

The dislocation is usually not seen. The child is brought to the physician because of recurrent pain or swelling at the knee. The actual dislocation which occurs when the knee is flexed ordinarily reduces itself when the knee is extended. The history usually contains several episodes of difficulty. These are most likely to occur after periods of prolonged sitting, for example, when the child has been entertained. On arising, inability to straighten the knee is noted, and the displacement of the patella may actually be appreciated, although often it is not.

When the patient is seen within 48 hrs of the dislocation, the knee usually contains fluid. The medial capusle of the knee in the parapatellar area is tender. Atrophy of the thigh is variable and dependent on the degree of previous disability.

A helpful sign for diagnosis, whether the child is seen immediately after the dislocation or many months later, is acute apprehension on an attempted lateral displacement of the patella. When the knee is extended and the quadriceps relaxed, passively pushing the patella over the lateral condyle of the femur gives rise to acute apprehension as the patient feels the patella about to slip out of control.

Structural abnormalities are noted. A mild valgus position of the tibia results in considerable lateral displacement of the tibial tubercle in a tall, long-limbed child. There may be external rotation of the tibia, again with lateral displacement of the tibial tubercle.

When the patient is seen at a time well removed from the acute episode, examination of the knee while the patient is sitting and the knee is flexed 90° is frequently very revealing. As the knee is extended, the patella may be seen to sublux laterally. Now, when the knee is flexed, the patella first has to track over into the intercondylar groove. This movement is accompanied by a palpable, and often audible, clicking, from which damage to the opposing cartilaginous surfaces may be inferred. Pressing the patella so as to rub it against the femur frequently reveals crepitus secondary to the cartilage changes.

Destruction of the patella and the condylar surface has been seen to be secondary to recurrent dislocation of the patella so often that surgical correction of the mechanism is urged as a preventive measure against further trauma.

Roentgen Findings

The anteroposterior view of the knee may reveal dislocation of the patella, if it is present. A tendency of the reduced patella to ride more lateralward than usual and valgus at the knee may be noted. A lateral film may reveal the patella to be proximal to, or at the superior edge of, the femoral condyles. A view taken tangential to the condyles to show the intercondylar notch and the relation of the patella to it may reveal dislocation or underdevelopment of the lateral condyles.

Treatment

The fundamental aim in treatment is to correct the line of pull of the quadriceps so that it runs through the intercondylar area. Since a lateral force produces the dislocation, it follows that correction of this force will result in a cure of the condition.

The reasons for attempting cure are alleviation of episodes of discomfort, production of normal function, and protection of the undersurface of the patella from further injury. Chondromalacia of the patella seen in later life often gives a history of recurrent or chronic dislocation of the patella in childhood.

The treatment may be complicated by the patient's age. Before the age of 14 in girls and 16 in boys, interference with the growing apophysis forming the tibial tubercle may give rise to growth deformity. After this age, the mechanical line of pull of the quadriceps can readily be corrected by transference medialward of the patellar tendon insertion. The age of election for surgery for any individual patient varies.

In the young age group, when the recurrent dislocations are frequent and productive of fluid in the knee, temporizing measures may have to be undertaken. However, to prevent the development of chondromalacia of the patella in the "teen" age period, an attempt at surgical correction may be made in young patients, even though the results are not as satisfactory as those of moving a bone and the attached tendon in the later age group.

In the child with the epiphyseal line still open, the incision is made laterally above the patella and is brought medialward below the patella to cross the tibial tubercle and to extend far enough to allow for easy reimplantation. The tight lateral capsule, as well as the fascia, is divided over the distal vastus lateralis. The infrapatellar fat pad is exposed, and the patellar tendon is delineated. The tendon is skinned from the tibial tubercle area in such a way as to leave some of its fibers still covering the tubercle. Great care must be taken to avoid scarring or damaging the cartilage of the tubercle, which is continuous with the epiphyseal line. The distal end of the patellar tendon is sewn subperiosteally just distal to the epiphyseal line. The fact that there is some slack in the patellar tendon when it is in full extension allows this. It is not wise to try to advance the tendon further than just beyond the line, however, as to do so would secondarily put considerable pressure on the cartilage surfaces related to the patella. A cylinder cast that holds the knee extended is worn for six weeks.

A

Fig. 3.36 (A). Changing the line of the quadriceps pull and the patellar tendon alignment requires some careful attention to significant details in order to be successful. When done for dislocating patella the bone block should never be advanced. The bed into which the patella tendon and its attached bone block from its point of insertion is put in immediately adjacent to the site of the original insertion. The new bed is angled slightly to avoid torque in the tendon. Lateral bands are divided as high as need be to allow the patella tendon to pull in a direct line with the quadriceps. The proximal cortex of the new bed is undercut with a curette to allow a projection superiorly of the bone block attached to the patella tendon to go beneath it. When the fascia and tendinous insertion of the pes anserinus is then sewn back over the block and patella tendon are firmly held without the need of screw fixation. (B) Anteroposterior and (C) lateral view of the proximal tibia with bone block fashioned for a patellar tendon transplant visible. Note that patella is not advanced, block is sunk beneath cortical level and angled in line with the patella tendon pull.

Fig. 3.36B

Fig. 3.36C

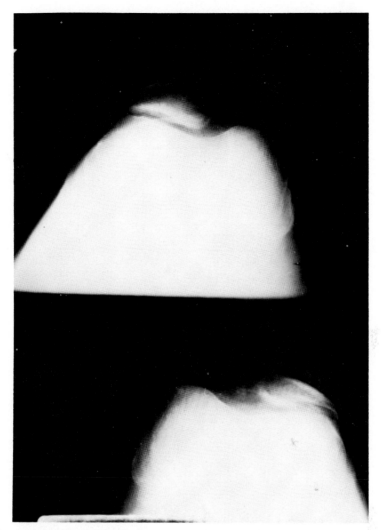

Fig. 3.37. The lateral riding patella leads to patello-femoral arthritis. The narrowing of the joint space, sclerotic and irregular subchondral bone are evident in this skyline roentgenogram of the patellofemoral joint (45 year old male).

Green[1] has advocated extensive reconstruction of the quadriceps mechanism in relation to its pull on the patella. This includes division of the lateral insertion and advancement of the insertion and advancement of the insertion medially of the vastus medialis.

If is, of course, preferable to wait for closure of the epiphyseal line at the proximal tibia to perform the operation. In such a case, the incision is again lateral and curves medialward over the tibial tubercle. The patellar tendon is separated from the infrapatellar fat pad. The area of the patellar tendon insertion is outlined by drill holes, and a bone block having a superior edge approximately 1/8 inch above the beginning of the insertion is removed. Drill holes now outline the bed into which this bone block is to be placed. This bed is tilted so that its long axis lies in line with the expected pull of the patellar tendon. This position brings the superior lateral corner of the bed close to the area from which the first bone block was removed. No attempt is made to advance the patellar tendon unless it is excessively relaxed.

Fig. 3.38 (A). Swelling of the proximal end of the patella tendon as it arises from the patella in Larson-Johannson's disease. There is some irregular ossification extending out into the center of the tendon shadow from the accessory center at the lower pole of the patella. (B) Normal irregular ossification of the projecting anterior surface of the patella as ossification becomes complete and the accessory center forms at the lower pole of the patella.

Fig. 3.38B

The superior lip of the new bed is cleared infracortically by a curette so that the bone block can be hooked under it. A single screw is inserted through the center of the bone block, and the block is now securely held. A cylinder cast supported by straps running over the contralateral shoulder is worn for 6 weeks. Quadriceps-setting exercises are used while the patient is in the cast. Active motion and quadriceps exercises are begun as soon as the cast is removed.

Reference

1. Green, W. T.: Recurrent dislocation of the patella; its surgical correction in the growing child, *J. Bone Joint Surg.*, 47A: 1670, 1965.

LARSON-JOHANSSON DISEASE
(OSTEOCHONDRITIS OF PATELLA)

The lower pole of the patella normally has an accessory ossification center. There is however a syndrome of pain, swelling of the site of origin of the patella tendon from the patella, and local tenderness at this site. It occurs principally in boys running through the age groups of 7-14 years. It is most often bilateral, but can occur unilaterally or be considerably more symptomatic on one side. Larson and Johansson separately described this disease in 1921.

Activity increases symptoms and rest relieves them. Although painful on occasion there is no implication of destruction of the infrapaellar surface as a result of continued activity. It acts in a manner similar to Osgood-Schlatter's disease but at the proximal rather than the distal end of the patella.

As the accessory center fuses with the parent bone, the symptoms subside.

Roentgen Features

The normal infrapatella ossification center is linear, regular, and separated from the patella by a thin, dark line. When the area is the seat of Larson-Johansson disease, the proximal pole of the patella tendon exhibits swelling of the soft-tissue shadow outlining it. There may be irregular ossification extending out into the center of the tendon area.

Treatment

Explanation to the parent and child is an imporant form of therapy. The symptoms are ordinarily not severe enough to justify cast immobilization. Although the symptoms will subside with immobilization they can be expected to recur with activity until approximately age 15 or when fusion of the accessory patella center is complete.

CHAPTER 4

THE HIP

CONGENITAL HIP DISEASE

Primary congenital dislocation of the hip without any associated nerve or muscle lesion is one of the most common congenital malformations. It can be found in the newborn child if looked for specifically within the first few days of life. The instance has been variously reported as from 1 to 15 per 1,000 live births. This instance would be consistent with that found in Europe and in the United States. It is more common among the Navajo indians in North America, and it may be simplistic to say that this is because they swaddle their young. It is relatively rare among Negroes and Chinese. It cannot be clearly related that carrying the infant on the hip with legs spread is the feature that reduces the incidence.

Abduction splints are not found among these races. It may be that the abduction is accomplished more slowly and gracefully. There is no question that there is an increased instance of breeched presentations among those children having congenital dislocation of the hip (17-20%) as compared to the normal instance of 2-4%.

Two surveys have investigated the relationship of social class to congenital dislocation of the hip. No effect of the social environment was noted in either investigation in terms of uncovering late diagnosis of the disease as resulting in an increased instance. Upper social class patients have an increased instance of neonatal congenital dislocation of the hip, and there is an increased proportion of siblings in these families compared with lower income groups. A significantly greater number of children with this deformity are born during the winter months than during the summer. There has been no real explanation for this, but it has been pointed out by Wynne-Davies.

We have been able to divide children with dislocation of the hip in its various forms exclusive of those with neurologic disease into three types:

1. *Neonatal type.* Dislocation is found with the femoral head separated from its seat in the acetabulum by a tight iliopsoas and capsular constricture. This is by far the most common. It is important to realize that this type has all the elements that it should have for a normally constituted joint with a fully formed acetabulum, a normal capsule, a normal ligament, and a normal femoral head. Secondary changes in these structures result from the position in which the femoral head is maintained relative to the acetabulum.

2. *Dislocation associated with lax ligaments.* In this type the hip slides in and out of the acetabulum due to excessive distensibility of the capsule; and if the life style of the infant is such as to promote dislocation, the incidence of this type can go up. It is relatively rare compared to the first type and occurred once in 45 incidences of congenital dislocation of the hip in our series. It should be emphasized again that all the elements that the hip joint should have are present in this type, including acetabulum, labrum, femoral head, and ligamentum teres capsule.

3. *Teratologic dislocation.* The important distinction here is that there has been a definite intrauterine disturbance at the time of formation of the hip joint and some portion of the hip joint is actually missing at birth. This may include any of the elements of the proximal third of the femur and may include various portions of the acetabulum including complete failure of the acetabulum to form. This type is exceedingly rare and is often associated with other extremity anomalies.

The very noticeable limp due to weakness of the hip abductors when the hip is unstable has been with mankind since the first civilizations. Hippocrates (460-370 B. C.) wrote:

There are persons who, from birth or from disease, have dislocations outward of both thighs; in them, then, the bones are affected in a like manner, but the fleshy parts in their case lose their strength less; the legs, too, are plump and fleshy, except that there is some little deficiency at the inside, and they are plump because they have the equal use of both legs,

Fig. 4.1. The normal hip is well formed at birth. The acetabulum is not shallow at birth but a deep, rounded cartilaginous cup. The femoral head is a section of a perfect sphere and fits congruously within the acetabulum.

for in walking, they totter equally to this side and that.

An enlightened medical community has succeeded in recent years in recognizing states which predispose to dislocation and, thereby, has grealty reduced its incidence. Hart[20,21] has emphasized the preventive nature of treatment undertaken within the first year of life to form an adequate hip joint in an individual who might otherwise develop dislocation of a previously dysplastic hip joint. Hart has also shown that the end result of an uncorrected subluxated hip may be degenerative arthritis in adult life.

Dislocation may be present at birth, but it also may occur in the first years of development. Dysplasia or presubluxation may be the first indication of abnormal mechanical forces which may eventually result in dislocation. The work of Hart, of Hass, and of the Italian orthopaedic surgeons such as Putti,[30] Scaglietti, and Poli[28] has been responsible for the recognition of anomalies of the hip other than frank dislocation.

Gill[18,19] and Crego and Schwartzmann[11] and others have noted that the age at which treatment is begun may be correlated with the excellence of the end results in terms of percentages. The percentage of failures rises with the age of the patients at initial treatment.

The sex incidence of congenital dislocation in various reported series has varied from 81 to 87% females. Hass states that female infants are affected 6 times as frequently as male. Unilateral dislocations are twice as common as bilateral ones, when frank dislocation is spoken of. When various forms of hip dysplasia are included, however, the incidence of bilateral involvement, particularly in the age group

Fig. 4.2. Dislocation of the hip present at birth can be easily missed on roentgen examination. An increased slant to the acetabulum when present as the only sign means little. The femoral head rides in the lateral one-third of the acetabulum without riding upward and signs of this location should be looked for. An attempted abduction x-ray is helpful.

Dysplasia

Subluxation

Dislocation

Dislocation plus
weight bearing

Fig. 4.3. Diagram of the features of dysplasia, subluxation, dislocation, and dislocation plus ambulation. In dysplasia the hip is actually centered in the acetabulum but forces are at work preventing the development of the hip from equaling the other side. The most common situation is a positional trunk contracture at birth elevating the pelvis on one side and adducting the hip. In subluxation the hip is not truly centered in the acetabulum but lies in the lateral third and is beginning to make a plastic impression on both the cartilage of the acetabulum and of the hip. In dislocation, the hip is not centered—a line running centrally up the femoral neck will not bisect the triradiate cartilage. The lateral one-third of the acetabulum is permanently deformed either by pressing the limbus up along the ilium or, if the leg has been maintained abducted, it could press the limbus inward. The cartilage of the femoral head is fibrillated and deformed. Ambulation causes the femoral head to progress superiorly, causing the formation of a groove in the lateral cartilage of the acetabulum.

under 1 year, is more nearly equal to that of unilateral difficulty.

Congenital dislocation of the hip becomes extraordinarily frequent in some areas. Localities have been reported in France, Holland, and Italy—the northern provinces of Italy, for example—in which the incidence of the disease appears to be greatly increased. It seems, however, that the disease is exceptionally rare among Negroes. In Asiatic countries, where the mother characteristically carries her child balanced on her hip with its legs in abduction, the incidence of poor hip development is much reduced.

Congenital dislocation of the hip is a poor term for a lesion that often begins with the hip fully formed, but with the femoral head laterally displaced, and further pathology developing as a result of this position.

Etiology

A review of the many scholarly attempts to determine the etiology of congenital dislocation of the hip leads to the conclusion that there is not just one but many causes of this condition.

The possibility that primary acetabular dysplasia is the cause has been supported by many. It has been thought that the posterior superior, buttress-like acetabular roof may

Fig. 4.4. A femoral head located in the lateral third of the acetabulum leads to early osteoarthritis and will not get better with use but instead will regress. (*A*) Seven-year-old girl with previously treated congenital dislocation of the hip. The lateral position of the femoral head and secondary acetabular cysts are seen. (*B*) Despite attempts at repair of the acetabulum, the femoral head has progressed still further.

Fig. 4.5. Old uncorrected subluxation of the hip with degenerative changes.

Fig. 4.6. Unilateral dislocation of the hip. Note increased acetabular slant, diminished size of the epiphyseal growth center, lateral and superior position of the femur, and anteversion as shown by the externally rotated position of the proximal femur in relation to the anteroposterior view of the distal femur.

Fig. 4.7. Development of the normal hip joint, viewed from the rear and as if the femur were flexed 90°. Note the progressive deepening of the acetabulum as the limb bud changes from a lateral to a parallel position. There is progressive development of anteversion from 0° at 3 months to 35° at birth. (Redrawn from C. E. Badgley: Etiology of congenital dislocation of hip, *Journal of Bone & Joint Surgery, 31A:* 352, 1949.)

genetically be prevented from forming. This does not fit the pathology that we have observed.

The femoral head originally must have been in relationship to the acetabulum since the joint develops as a cleft in the primordial cell block. Embryologic studies by Strayer reveal that this cleft does not become complete until the embryo reaches the 35-mm stage. Joint clefts have formed, however, even in the absence of the distal bone. It is obvious that, although the cleft may develop as the result of primary differentiating factors, the later development of the joint becomes more and more subject to other factors.

Badgley,[2] beginning with the 8-mm embryo, reviewed the embryologic development of the hip joint. The following comments are drawn from his article. Only nerves and vessels are added from the trunk to the original limb bud in its development. At the stage of 14.8 mm, the predestined site of the hip joint can be seen as a dense accumulation of mesenchymal cells. These undifferentiated mesenchymal cells are still present at the 25-mm stage between the femoral head and acetabulum. The capsular structures and glenoidal labrum have begun to form.

At the 33-mm stage, the ligamentum teres has appeared, and the joint space is completely differentiated. The glenoid labrum is prolonged over the head of the femur. The limb bud has developed during this period in marked abduction, which is decreased considerably by the time the 58-mm embryo is reached. During this developmental period, the limb bud is also undergoing rotation.

It seems reasonable to assume that, up to the point of innervation of the musculature of the limb, development of the joint is predestined. As Badgley points out, delay in rotation of the limb bud or in innervation of the muscles at a period of rapid embryologic growth may produce alterations in the development of the acetabulum or in the head and neck of the femur. Adaptive changes to malposition can occur in intrauterine as well as in postnatal life. Breech births have been noted frequently to be the subjects of adduction contractures at the hip joint.

Underdevelopment of the limbus may encourage dislocation of the hip. The cartilaginous acetabulum and limbus cover the femoral head at birth. Elongation of the capsule, allowing subluxation and dislocation, has been mentioned as a contributing factor by Howorth.

Anteversion, which may be the result of inward rotation of the limb bud as an angle of 90° is traversed to bring the patella forward, is a factor in poor presentation of the femoral head to the acetabulum. It may be one of the adaptive changes responsible, at least in part, for dislocation. The hip, developing in the flexed position and extending after birth, is aided in its tendency toward dislocation by the anteversion. Anteversion is more evident after conventional treatment than at birth.

Dislocation of the hip sometimes occurs in association with other anomalies, such as clubfeet, clubhands, metatarsus varus, and arthrogryposis. That dislocation may not be present at birth and yet develop, presumably through the stages of dysplasia to subluxation to actual dislocation, has been noted by many. Such hips may, however, already have joint development changes which allow dislocation such as displacement laterally into the outer third of the acetabulum.

The development of dislocation after birth is similarly due to many factors. The classic direction of dislocation is said to be posterior, although McCarroll[24] states that primary anterior dislocation of the hip occurs in approximately one-fifth of the cases. The presence of an adducted position of the femur relative to the pelvis, with a myostatic contracture of the adductors maintaining this position, stands out from a clinical point of view. Enlargement of the ligamentum teres and of the Haversian pad of fat lying in the acetabulum depths has been implicated but appears secondary to the lateral position.

The acetabulum appears to have the ability to respond to correct seating of the femoral head within it and is slow to develop when these forces are not transmitted to it. Anteversion, as well as adduction, of the femur is important in this regard.

Weight bearing is regarded by some as a factor influencing a hip that is subluxated toward dislocation.

The forces of heredity may be instrumental in delaying rotation of the limb or its innervation and, as such, may accomplish the sequence of events outlined by Badgley. How-

Fig. 4.8. Development of congenital dislocation of the hip and acetabular dysplasia. (*A*) The 35-mm fetus without anteversion of the femur. (*B* and *C*) Development of normal and then excessive anteversion. (*D* and *E*) Progressive dislocation with increasing anteversion and lack of normal pressure resulting in acetabular dysplasia. (*F* and *G*) Development of anterior dislocation. There is delay in proper timing of the rotation of the head into the acetabulum with both anterior and posterior dislocation, as illustrated in the series from *D* to *G*, so that at no time does it actually point into the acetabulum. Depending on the degree of the developmental error, either dysplasia or dislocation may be the result. (Redrawn from C. E. Badgley: Etiology of congenital dislocation of hip, *Journal of Bone & Joint Surgery, 31A:* 353, 1949.)

Fig. 4.9. View of the acetabulum from child with dislocated hip on the *left* and, for contrast, the normal side on the *right*. On the *left* the limbus or cartilaginous rim has been pressed toward the acetabulum. This is the result of forcibly abducting the hip without connecting the tight iliopsoas contracture. As a result, the limbus, by being pushed in, appears enlarged (*A*) and partially obscures the acetabulum. The femur must be pulled down by traction in line with the trunk before being abducted in order to avoid the production of this pathology. Forcible abduction without correction of the iliopsoas leads not only to deformity of the acetabular rim, but also to degeneration of the cartilage of the femoral head which is the seat of this localized pressure.

ever, this is difficult to prove. Many factors appear to play a part in producing congenital dislocation of the hip.

Mechanics of Iliopsoas

This discussion of etiology has included all types of dislocated hips from so-called dysplasia to the teratologic dislocation, excluding neurologic dislocation. It should be emphasized, however, that despite the fact that the acetabular index may appear slanted excessively by x-ray the reader should bear in mind that he is looking only at the ossification center. In the normal hip at birth the cartilage components of the acetabulum form a deep cup just as in the adult, and it may be very misleading to assume nonexistence of these components from viewing the ossification center alone. Position obviously plays an important role in etiology—witness the increased incidence in breech births, in higher social class environments, and in winter months. These factors may lend some credence to the fact that the heavily swaddled child has no opportunity to spontaneously correct the dislocation that is present at birth.

The author's own feeling heavily implicates a positional contracture of the iliopsoas and occasionally the hypertrophy of this muscle as a cause of congenital dislocation of the hip. The

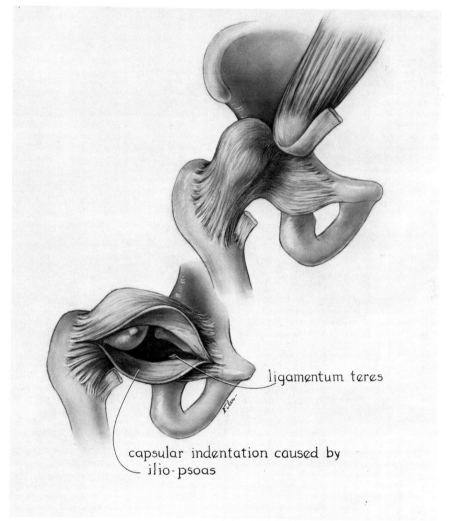

ligamentum teres

capsular indentation caused by ilio-psoas

Fig. 4.10. Drawing of the capsular defect caused by the iliopsoas. As the capsule is drawn up the opening for reduction of the femoral head is reduced.

Fig. 4.11. Forcible abduction on the acetabular rim can result in an apparent two-headed femur. In (A) the femoral neck is short, the head height diminished. In (B) the deep cleft between the two segments of the head is clearly evident.

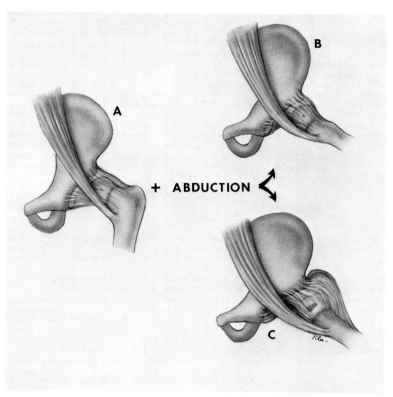

Fig. 4.12. Abduction of an improperly seated femoral head yields either acetabulum deformity (*A*) or femoral head deformity (*B*).

hip forms fully in all its components in this disease. The flexed intrauterine position may allow the femoral head to wander into the lateral third of the acetabulum. The iliopsoas is not stretched with growth and tends to lie medial to the femoral head. The infant is born with the hip flexion contracture. As the youngster extends the hip in the first 6 weeks of life, if the femoral head is lying deep in the acetabulum rather than in the outer third, the iliopsoas will stretch, and the youngster will have a normal hip. If it happens to be slightly laterally displaced, further progression of the pathology of congenital dislocation of the hip may be expected to take place with medial migration of the iliopsoas tendon. If not diagnosed in the neonate it may go on to the frank dislocation with which we are familiar. McKibbin[24a] has shown that with a contracted iliopsoas the hip cannot be seated in extension.

The importance of the iliopsoas contracture as an etiologic factor in congenital dislocation of the hip helps to explain the influence of life style in terms of swaddling the baby since that increases the incidence of congenital dislocation of the hip.

Of all the factors that have been reviewed here the iliopsoas appears to us to be by far the most prominent in effecting what is otherwise a normal hip. The other factor which may be of importance is the excessive laxity of the ligaments allowing the femoral head to easily lie in the lateral third of the acetabulum. We have seen no evidence for enlargement of the ligamentum teres, the filling of the acetabulum with soft tissue of various types, or failure of the limbus to develop (except in teratologic dislocation). Bear in mind in considering etiology that all elements of the hip are fully formed at birth in this disease.

Acetabular Index

If one uses the acetabular index as the sole feature of determining that a hip is dysplastic, one will be markedly misled. This has been

Fig. 4.13. The iliopsoas in hip dislocation pulls the inferior capsule across the acetabulum effectively blocking the placement of the femoral head with the joint. The capsule can be easily mistaken for fibrous tissue in the depths of the acetabulum.

emphasized by Caffey, and it is perfectly possible for a normal youngster with normal hips to have an acetabular index as recorded by our usual measurements of over 40° and to develop the hips normally. When this occurs, it is usually bilateral. It is more important to appreciate the development of the outer third of the acetabulum than it is to appreciate the slanting edge to the ossification center of the ilium that is forming the acetabulum. When one measures this ossification one has not measured the actual formation of the acetabulum which is cartilaginous in infancy and cannot be seen. The outer third of the acetabulum can be contrasted with the inner third and, when the outer third slants in relation to the inner third, this is significant.

Severin[32],[33] has reported a means of measuring the acetabular angle that was originally devised by Hilgenreiner. This generally accepted and simple method serves to emphasize the importance of the acetabular obliquity in congenital dislocation of the hip. Kleinberg and Lieberman report the angle to be 27.5° at birth and 20° between ages 1 and 2. The normal acetabular angle is considered to be 23-25°, and any greater measurement is taken as indicating abnormality, particularly in the patient more than 6 months of age. A line is drawn between the tips of the ilia at the triradiate cartilage in the depth of the acetabulum. A second line drawn from the tip of the ilium to the outer edge of the acetabulum creates the angle known as the acetabular index. The significance of an acetabular index that is apparently higher than normal is easily misinterpreted.

Remember that it is the outer third of the acetabulum that is significant in congenital dislocation of the hip. Caffey's study of children constituting a well child population helps to bring this out. A higher than normal index occurred with infants who were shown as they developed in later life to have had normal hips. It is true that children with dislocation in the older age group will have deficiency of ossification of the lateral third. This is secondary to the cartilage deformity that develops in this disease, but one cannot use the high acetabular index as the sole feature on which a diagnosis of dislocation of the hip is based. The diagnosis must also rest on other features of acetabular development, such as irregular ossification in the outer third, alteration of the head of the femur to the acetabulum, the delayed development of the capital femoral epiphysis, and then finally of course on physical examination as well. In this regard we have found it most helpful to have an anteroposterior roentgenogram made with the hips in neutral, and another one with the hips abducted, which helps to bring out the malalignment of the femur in relation to the acetabulum. This will not occur in the presence of high acetabular indexes if the hips are normally located.

C-E Angle

Wiberg has established an objective method of evaluating the position of the femoral head in relation to the acetabular roof. The measurement is called the C-E angle (center of the capital femoral epiphysis to the lateral edge of the acetabulum).

A line is drawn from the center of the head of the femur to the lateral edge of the acetabulum. This line forms an angle with a vertical line running through the center of the head. A transparent circular protractor placed on the x-ray film so that its central point is at the center of a circle enclosing the head of the femur readily enables this angle to be read.

The angle is less than normal when either the acetabular roof is underdeveloped or the femoral head is laterally displaced. It is helpful in determining both acetabular dysplasia and subluxation of the femoral head.

Severin[32,33] gives figures for this angle based on a study of 136 children between 6 and 13 years. He believes that a C-E angle of less than 15° is definitely pathologic, of 15-19° is equivocal, and of more than 20° is consistent with normal development.

Anteversion

Anteversion may be defined as the relation of the long axis of the femoral neck to a line

Fig. 4.14. A curved clamp has been inserted beneath the iliopsoas and its tendon as it runs over the medial capsule of the hip joint on its way to the lesser trochanter. The capsule enclosing the femoral head lies to the right of the muscle. The tendon is often severely shortened in dislocation of the hip.

Fig. 4.15. Ludloff's article in the 1912 edition of the *American Journal of Orthopedic Surgery* contained this illustration comparing the normal and the dislocated hip. On the dislocated side the iliopsoas muscle and tendon have been drawn in. Many of the features of the pathology of dislocated hip have been drawn in—the capsule drawn up by the iliopsoas, the acetabulum bent up in its outer one-third, etc.

drawn through the femoral condyles in the coronal plane.

Anteversion at birth is approximately 25°, but it has a tendency to decrease with growth to 5-15°. The anteversion normally present is approximately 15°, and it is associated with about 45° of internal rotation in flexion at the hip joint. When anteversion is increased, internal rotation is correspondingly increased. Thus excessive anteversion may permit internal rotation as great as 90°.

Anteversion of the femur is recognized by the fact that a roentgenogram of the hip taken with the knees straight ahead reveals the hip to be in external rotation. It is differentiated from valgus of the femoral neck by the fact that the height of the femoral head is not increased over the trochanter. A roentgenogram taken with the femur in internal rotation is also helpful in differentiating anteversion from valgus.

Anteversion of the femur may play a part in poor development of the acetabulum after the femoral head has been placed in the acetabulum. In internal rotation the femoral head is placed well beneath the overhanging roof of the acetabulum. With the limb in the neutral position and the knee pointing forward, ante-

version of the femur tends to bring the femoral head to the anterior lip of the acetabulum and to cause the femur to subluxate outward.

Relation of Hip to Spine

Routine spinal x-rays of patients suspected of congenital dislocation of the hip are illuminating. Two types of spine curvature are often revealed.

1. *Curvature of the spine secondary to adduction contracture of the hip.* The patient, when aligned in the anatomic position for the roentgenograms, develops a pelvic tilt as the result of the adduction contracture. The pelvis is "high" on the adducted side, and there is a secondary curve in the low lumbar area to compensate for this tilt and to align the occiput with the pelvis.

2. *Primary curvature of the spine.* This curve is a total curve involving the entire spine in a single long curve. It results in a tilted pelvis and an adducted position of the hip. Clinically, affected babies will have a limitation of lateral bend in the direction correcting the curve. There may or may not be an accompanying adduction contracture of the hip. Primary spinal curve is presumably the result of position in utero.

When there is no adduction contracture, the hip may be quite well developed by x-ray, which accounts for the baby who is thought to have a congenital hip problem; and yet little is revealed by roentgenogram. The thigh folds are often asymmetric in such a child.

When there is an adduction contracture, the hip is usually underdeveloped; i.e., there is an increased slant to the acetabulum and a delay in mineralization of the growth center of the proximal femoral epiphysis. Improvement of such a hip is markedly aided by trunk-stretching exercises at the hip. Failure to correct the trunk curve delays return of the hip to a normal appearance by x-ray.

There are various forms of underdevelopment of the hip. In the first year of life the hip may not develop into the stable, functioning joint that it should be. This may be owing to actual congenital deformity or to neurologic conditions, but much more commonly it is owing to a persistent adduction and anteversion of the hip. The earlier such abnormal stresses are recognized, the easier it is to correct the hip and to promote its further growth.

Fig. 4.16. (*Left*). Dislocated hip in newborn infant; capsule opened from the anterior and superior aspects. The cartilage of the acetabulum, instead of shelving over the femoral head, is opposed to an enlarged ligamentum teres which intervenes between the cartilage and the femoral head. Here the femur has been displaced from the acetabulum.

Fig. 4.17. (*Right*). The normally developed hip–contralateral side of same patient. The head has been detached from the joint. The cartilage of the acetabulum runs horizontally and shelves out over the femoral head.

Fig. 4.18. (*Left*). The dislocated hip. The enlarged ligamentum teres has been partially torn from its insertion. The acetabulum runs vertically rather than horizontally. An enlarged limbus was not seen. The inability to seat the femoral head without division of the inferior capsule is quite evident.

Fig. 4.19. (*Right*). The lower clamp is attached to the ligamentum teres, which has been pulled inferiorly. The joint space for acceptance of the head is minimal, the acetabulum is vertical, and the capsule tents across the joint just inferior to either end of the acetabular cartilage.

Fig. 4.20. (*Top*). View of superior aspect of femoral head, neck, and greater trochanter showing deformity of head on left and increased anteversion.

Fig. 4.21. (*Bottom*). Comparison of normal hip, on left, and dislocated hip, on right, with enlarged ligamentum teres on the right hip pulled laterally.

The various stages of failure of the hip joint to develop may be designated as: (1) the dysplastic hip, (2) the subluxated hip, and (3) the dislocated hip. The relationship between the underdeveloped hip joint and malum coxae senilis in later life has been pointed out by

Hart.[21] The severe disability that degenerative arthritis of the hip may impose on the adult makes the goal of normal hip development in the child a very worthwhile one to pursue.

DYSPLASTIC HIP

The mother frequently brings the child with dysplastic hip for inspection because she has noted difficulties with one of the legs while placing diapers on the child. The dysplastic hip is recognized clinically by asymmetry of the thigh folds, an adduction contracture of the hip, and an apparent shortening of the leg. The infant is examined for an adduction contracture in recumbency. In this position, the thighs are flexed 90° and then abducted. A limitation of full abduction is very evident by this examination.

A persistent adducted position of the femur relative to the pelvis may be due to a contracture of the adductor muscle group. The adducted position may, however, be secondary to an elevation of one side of the pelvis and a curvature of the spine.

The adducted position results in apparent shortening of the extremity. The hip appears more prominent laterally on the involved side. The knee and popliteal creases are at different levels. The inguinal fold is deepened on the

Fig. 4.22. Measurement of the acetabular angle by the method of Hilgenreiner. The *Y line* connects the triradiate cartilages. *Line h* indicates the tendency of the diaphysis to ride superiorly as compared with the normal position on the other side. *Line d* indicates the lateral displacement from the acetabular floor. (Redrawn from V. L. Hart: *Congenital Dyplasia of the Hip Joint and Sequelae in the Newborn and Early Postnatal Life*, p. 39, Springfield, Ill.: Charles C Thomas, 1952.)

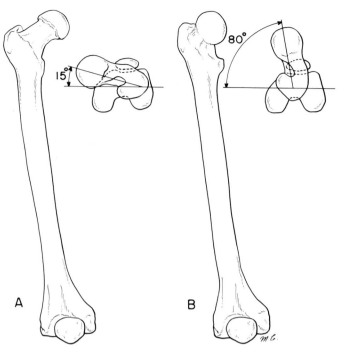

Fig. 4.23. Anteversion of the femur illustrated diagrammatically as the relation between the axis of the neck and the axis of the femoral condyles. In the anteroposterior view, the anteverted femoral neck appears shortened and straightened in relation to the shaft.

involved side so that the labia are partially hidden by it.

Roentgen Signs

The acetabular roof has an angle greater than 25°. The hip is not markedly displaced either laterally or superiorly. There is usually recognizable anteversion of the femur. A delay in development of the hip joint is evident. The ossification center for the femoral head is late in appearance. Ossification of the acetabular roof and closure of the ischiopubic juncture are delayed.

Treatment

The treatment attempts primarily to eliminate the adducted position of the femur relative to the pelvis. The inability of the trunk to bend equally to both sides, if present, must be corrected by stretching exercises.

We no longer use abduction splints either of plastic or of soft felt. Even in the normal hip there is a significant incidence of avascular necrosis (3-6%) and pressure effect on the epiphyseal line such that it starts off as a minimal disability and becomes a severe one through treatment. Abduction exercises done by the mother do not hold the hip in the abducted position and are used instead. The bulk of the ordinary diaper is sufficient abduction with which to treat this condition. The child's own activity will tend to stretch this final contracture. If all of these persist the child has been underdiagnosed, and there actually is a dislocation of the hip with the hip lying in the lateral third of the acetabulum. For this condition a more radical treatment approach is indicated.

SUBLUXATED HIP

Subluxation of the hip, both as a stage in the development of dislocation and as an individual entity, has been studied by Hart,[20,21] who notes that the subluxated state, if not treated, may not progress to dislocation but that it remains, along with an underdeveloped, slanting acetabular roof and a tendency of the femoral head to progress still further laterally and superiorly in the joint.

In this condition the acetabular roof again has a marked slant that is greater than the usually acceptable angle of 25°. The appearance of the epiphyseal growth center is delayed. This hip is distinguished from the dysplastic hip,

however, in that it rides laterally in the joint to the point of actual dislocation. These criteria form a triad enunciated by Putti[30] that enables determination of the so-called "preluxation" state.

From the pathologic point of view, the head of the femur may have pressed the cartilaginous rim or limbus of the acetabulum upward and toward the ilium. As brought out by Leveuf,[22] the limbus may remain attached in this position and be a serious detriment to the formation of the acetabular roof.

The subluxated hip, so-called, is but one stage of the disease of congenital dislocation of the hip. The hip is lying in the lateral third of the acetabulum and abduction x-rays bring out the malalignment of the femur in relation to the triradiate cartilage centrally in the acetabu-

Fig. 4.24. Anteversion (*A*), valgus (*B*), and varus (*C*) of the femoral neck can be differentiated in the anteroposterior view by the relative height of the femoral head above the greater trochanter.

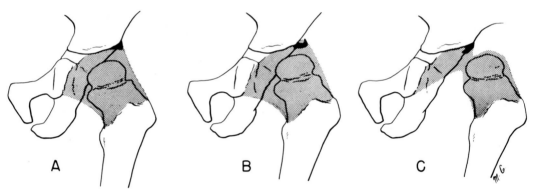

Fig. 4.25. Dysplasia (*A*), subluxation (*B*), and dislocation (*C*) of the hip. The limbus in subluxation is pushed superiorly against the ilium; in dislocation the femoral head may press the limbs inferiorly into the acetabulum.

Fig. 4.26. On attempted abduction in flexion, an adduction contracture is demonstrated, particularly on the right.

lum. These children are those who have not walked, but because of the lateral position of the femoral head are developing increasing changes consistent with dislocation as a result of this position. These changes include pressing the cartilaginous rim or flattening of the femoral head opposite this area. The outer third of the acetabulum is often underdeveloped so far as the ossification center is concerned in the ilium. As compared to so-called dysplasia it is quite evident that the hip rides laterally in the lateral third of the acetabulum, and the abduction x-ray will bring this out. The ossification center of the femoral head is delayed in its appearance and development. Since subluxation is actually the first stage of dislocation, if untreated the development of the joint can be expected to be abnormal and become more evident with later roentgenograms as the skeleton matures.

We believe it is very important to treat this condition fully and radically. By x-ray there is lateral displacement of the femoral shaft in relation to the ilium. A line drawn through the center and neck no longer points toward the center of the triradiate cartilage and the depth of the acetabulum. Clinically there is often asymmetrical thigh and buttock folds. Prominence of the trochanter on the involved side and the adduction contracture can be demonstrated. Palpation of the femoral head beneath the femoral artery and just below the inguinal ligament may still give some feeling of fullness due to the fact that lateral dislocation is not marked at this stage.

Fig. 4.27. Inguinal fold obscuring labia on the involved side. Note the asymmetric folds.

Fig. 4.28. Dysplasia of hip with underdevelopment of acetabulum.

Treatment

If the abduction film on a child of this type fails to reveal that the femur sits normally in relation to the acetabulum, a line drawn through the femoral neck should transect the triradiate cartilage. If it does not do so when the hip is abducted, those measures must be undertaken to accomplish correction of these findings by x-ray. We no longer use simple abduction as a means of accomplishing this because of the high morbidity accompanying the use of fixed abduction devices. Traction in line with the trunk may pull the iliopsoas sufficiently to allow it to stretch and not form a limitation when the hips are abducted. This is primarily true in the youngster with relaxed ligaments, and in these individuals the correction of the abduction x-ray is so quick and easy that it is no problem. For the rest, however, division of the iliopsoas tendon and underlying capsule which will be discussed under the treatment of dislocation of the hip is recommended. It is recommended because the pathology is actually that of a dislocated hip without the development of marked cartilage deformity, and the factor preventing normal seating of the femoral head must be quickly corrected.

PATHOLOGY AND RECOGNITION OF CONGENITAL DISLOCATION OF HIP

The clinical recognition of congenital dislocation of the hip is confused by the fact that an adduction contracture and asymmetrical thigh folds can exist in infants with normal hips. It is further confused by fascial snaps, clicks, or jerks in the region of the hip. These may occur as a result of tight tendons snapping over bony prominences; medially, the likely culprit is the iliopsoas; laterally, the tensor fascia lata.

The frank jolt of a truly dislocated hip during abduction in flexion (described by Ortolani) does not occur in all dislocated hips and when it does occur the entire examination is usually classic and the dislocation frank.

There are two parts to the pathology of congenital dislocation of the hip. One is the fact that it exists at birth. The second are the deformities that develop with growth as a result of the dislocated position of the femur relative to the acetabulum.

The pathology of dislocation of the hip at birth reveals the importance of the iliopsoas muscle in providing a fundamental contracture that causes the femoral head to ride with pressure on the lateral third of the acetabulum. The femoral head has not risen cephalad, but only laterally. The cause of this lateral position is the block to full medial seating of the femoral head found by tight hypertrophied iliopsoas and secondarily the capsular contracture.

The inferior capsule is pulled up by the iliopsoas tendon to cover between 40 and 50% of the acetabulum. There is no way in which the dislocated hip examined on the autopsy table could be seated without pressure on this deformed capsule.

At birth the femoral head is deformed to accommodate to the pressure coming from a medial direction. The cartilage of the femoral head does not reveal any fibrillation at first but if the hip has undergone treatment—particularly casted in abduction—this evidence of pathology may exist.

The capsule is not abnormally thickened, but the capsular deformity is permanent in nature.

In a study of 240 hips of 120 stillborn infants and dead newborn infants, Stanisavjevic and Mitchell found two dislocated hips and three subluxated. In 9 of their normal hips a click or Ortolani's sign was noted as the thighs were abducted. This was found to be produced by the interposition of an unusually large ligamentum capitis femoris in 4 and by sliding of the iliopsoas tendon over an enlarged iliopectineal bursa in 5. In the abnormal hips, hypertrophy of the iliopsoas tendon was found in every instance.

The hip, when dislocated, lies superior to the acetabulum and separates the gluteus medius and minimus from the ilium. The cartilaginous limbus forming the rim of the acetabulum lies inferior to the femoral head. The limbus is often indented by pressure from the head. It is normally largest posteriorly and superiorly. The capsule is stretched so that it continues to enclose the head in its position distant from the acetabulum. There tends to be a constriction of the capsule between the head and the acetabulum. This constriction is the result of pressure from the iliopsoas tendon. The capsule is often adherent, at least in part, to the ilium, where it is held against the bone by the pressure of the

Fig. 4.29. (*A*) Apparent dislocation of the hip accompanied by soft-tissue swelling. (*B*) The arthrogram outlines the callus surrounding a birth fracture with displacement of the femoral shaft, but a located femoral head.

head. It may also be adherent inferiorly where it tents across the acetabulum.

Anteversion of the femur of some degree is a virtually constant accompaniment. Normal anteversion at birth is about 25°, it decreases with growth to about 15°. The acetabulum may be filled by an enlarged Haversian fat pad. The ligamentum teres, which is greatly elongated in actual dislocation, may appear hypertrophied.

In late dislocations the head may lose its round full shape, become flattened in the area pressed against the ilium, and assume a more conelike appearance. The cartilage of the head may become pitted and fibrillated.

Clinical Picture

The patient is usually a female with inability to abduct the hip. This is often noted by the mother when she puts on the diaper. Some asymmetry of the thigh and buttock folds may also be noted. Apparent shortening of the leg on the affected side is a frequent complaint.

The adductors are apparently short in rela-

Fig. 4.30. In the arthrogram of the laterally placed femoral head, the groove in the capsule formed by the iliopsoas tendon is seen. (*A*) Anteroposterior, (*B*) lateral.

Fig. 4.31. Child, age 2, with bilateral dislocation of the hips, wide perineum, and prominent trochanters.

tion to the other musculature about the hip when the hip is dislocated. This is best demonstrated with the leg in 90° of flexion at the hip when abduction is attempted. Whereas infants with normal hips can usually achieve 45° or more of abduction, those with subluxed or dislocated hips are limited to 20° or less. However, the real obstacle to reduction is the iliopsoas.

The buttock fold tends to be higher on the side of the adducted hip than on the unaffected side, and the thigh folds beneath it are frequently asymmetric. There is some apparent shortening of the side involved, and a high pelvis can be demonstrated on that side by palpating the anterior superior spines of the ilium. The inguinal fold runs into the labia so that it appears smaller on the involved side.

With actual dislocation, the femoral head is absent from its normal position beneath the femoral artery just distal to the inguinal ligament. The trochanter is unduly prominent and lies above Nélaton's line, which connects the anterosuperior spine and the tuberosity of the ischium. In unilateral dislocation, Galeazzi's sign is positive; when the femurs are flexed to 90,° one knee, owing to the shortening of the thigh with dislocation, lies below the level of the other. Internal rotation is usually increased to 70° or more owing to anteversion of the hip. The "sign of the jerk" is the click that is felt when the thigh is abducted in flexion and the femoral head slides over the acetabular rim. The adductors must be relaxed to elicit this click, which may be felt on both exit and entry in the dysplastic acetabulum.

When the dislocation is bilateral, the perineum is widened. It may be possible to detect telescoping of the hip by applying traction with one hand while the other grasps the pelvis and, with a finger, palpates the trochanter.

X-rays reveal the hip to have slipped superiorly in relation to the acetabulum and Shenton's line, therefore, to be discontinuous. Shenton's line is formed by the inferior border of the neck and the superior border of the obturator foramen. Discontinuity of it, when it is the only finding, is not a reliable sign of hip difficulty, but as an adjunct finding, it aids in the interpretation of the x-rays. The dislocation may have begun either anteriorly or posteriorly.

Fig. 4.32. In unilateral dislocation, flexion of the thighs to a right angle may reveal shortening on sighting along top of knees (Galeazzi's sign).

Fig. 4.33. Diagram of Nélaton's line, which runs from the anterior superior spine of the ilium to the tuberosity of the ischium. In dislocation, the greater trochanter is palpated above this line.

Acetabular views of the hip reveal the anterior or posterior relation to the acetabulum. The signs of underdevelopment of the joint and proximal femur previously discussed are also present.

In so-called unilateral dislocation, the contralateral hip is worthy of study. A roentgenographic study by DiPrampero[14] has brought some interesting facts to light in this regard. Of 200 patients with unilateral dislocation, subluxation or dysplasia of the hip on the contralateral side was found in 108 cases.

Signs Due to Weakness of Hip Abductors

The displacement upward of the femur and the lack of a stable joint result in weakness of the hip abductors; of these the principal one is the gluteus medius. Shortening of the func-tional length of the muscle results in weakness.

When the patient stands on one leg, inability of the abductors to elevate the pelvis on the opposite side results in a positive Trendelenburg's sign. The pelvis on the opposite side drops. This can be made quite apparent by marking the posterior superior spines of the ilium before the test is performed.

This inability to elevate the pelvis results secondarily in inability to clear the opposite leg on walking. In order to clear the leg when walking, the patient compensates for the abductor weakness by bringing the body weight over and beyond the femoral head. This allows the lateral trunk musculature to aid in elevating the pelvis.

Such a gait, which transfers the trunk over the involved hip with each step, results in a medius limp. If both hips are involved, the trunk is transferred first over one hip and then over the other. The symmetry of such a gait makes it less noticeable than the gait in cases of unilateral involvement and accounts for the fact that, among children who are not found to have hip dislocation until they are walking, unilateral is discovered earlier than bilateral involvement.

Differential Diagnosis

Since the adducted position of the femur relative to the pelvis is responsible for most of the clinical signs that make us suspect dysplasia, subluxation, or dislocation of the hip, it is helpful to review other conditions, of which there are a surprisingly large number, that might cause the same adduction. All of these conditions, of course, have other characteristics that allow differentiation. They are listed here in an order that suggests their relative incidence.

The attempt to adduct the hip on either flexion or extension may reveal a limitation in this plane. Such a limitation could be due to:

1. Voluntary resistance, which can be overcome by thoroughness and persistence in examination.

2. Spina bifida, with weak hip abductors and adduction contracture, which develops with persistent maintenance of the adducted position.

3. Hip joint infection—pyogenic, tuberculous, luetic, etc.—which also limits motion in other places.

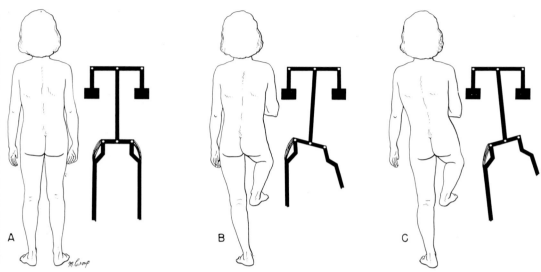

Fig. 4.34. Signs of weakness of the gluteus medius such as may be associated with congenital dislocation of the hip. (*A*) Normal standing, (*B*) dropping of pelvis of contralateral side when standing on affected leg, (*C*) compensation for weakness when walking by shifting center of gravity of trunk in order to elevate pelvis on opposite side.

Fig. 4.35. Possible obstacles to reduction include: (*A* and *B*) adherent capsule, (*C* and *D*) capsule lining the joint with hourglass constriction. This hourglass constriction follows from pressure of the over-riding iliopsoas tendon. (Redrawn from V. L. Hart: *Congenital Dysplasia of the Hip Joint and Sequelae in the Newborn and Early Postnatal Life*, p. 48, Springfield, Ill., Charles C Thomas, 1952.)

4. Obstetrical trauma—contusion, fractures of the epiphyseal area, or dislocation—which may result in resistance to abduction while the hip is tender.

5. Chondrodystrophy—Morquio's disease or Hurler's syndrome—which may limit abduction but also cause other obvious stigmata.

6. Scurvy or rickets, which may result in painful limbs and limited motion (scurvy occasionally is associated with the reverse of this—a flaccid pseudoparalysis).

7. Developmental coxa vara with deformity of the femoral neck, which apes congenital dislocation well on examination, but is unusual before the age of 4 (in this condition, the femoral head is still in the acetabulum and there is no telescoping).

8. In newborns, the limitation of full extension at the hip and knee that is present at birth and with which limitation of abduction is associated (the examiner should be able to abduct each hip 20°, however).

9. Cerebral palsy with spastic paralysis, which characteristically causes a stretch reflex in the adductors that limits abduction.

10. Still's disease (rheumatoid arthritis involving the hips in children), which limits motion in other places as well as abduction.

11. Poliomyelitis, from which an adduction contracture may develop, although an abduction contracture is more usual.

12. Congenital scoliosis, which may result in an elevation of the pelvis on one side and an adducted position of the hip, but which is ordinarily not associated with an actual limitation of motion of the joint.

The age of the patient when he is presented for treatment largely determines both the severity of the treatment and the prognosis of its effects. An awareness of the condition on the part of the medical community results in early presentation of the patient for treatment and is preventive medicine in the highest sense of the word. Throughout treatment tightness of the iliopsoas muscle must be overcome. It is more important than adductor tightness.

Fig. 4.36. Dislocated hip on the left with high buttock fold, asymmetric thigh folds, prominent trochanter, and positive Trendelenburg. The opposite side of the pelvis drops when the patient stands on the affected leg.

TREATMENT OF CONGENITAL DISLOCATION OF HIP UNDER AGE TWO

Rationale: Both closed and open reductions of the dislocated hip in infancy have well recognized complications in the form of avascular necrosis of the ossification center of the femoral head, necrosis of the epiphyseal plate, and stiffness of the hip.

Avascular necrosis and cessation of growth of the proximal femoral epiphysis are two of the major complications of conservative treatment. Massie (1951) reported abnormal epiphyseal changes in 75% of 62 dislocated hips after closed reduction. Of these abnormalities 72% were found to be troublesome. Bost[4] and associates found that 52% of 112 hips were involved. Ponseti[29a] (1966) found changes in 46.2% of 173 hips treated by closed reduction. Massie and Howorth[23a] (1951) and Judet (1958) reported a higher incidence of these changes after closed as compared to open reduction. The lower incidence of epiphyseal changes after open reduction can be explained by the release of soft tissues necessitated in the surgical exposure and the consequent elimination of constricting pressure.

Nicholson and associates in 1954 demonstrated by angiography performed in children

Fig. 4.37. Further development of congenital hip disease with riding upward of the femur.

Fig. 4.38. Some of the causes of poor seating of the femoral head in the acetabulum. (A) Adduction, (B) anteversion, (C) improper alignment.

postmortem that the frog leg position interfered with arterial filling of the medial and lateral circumflex and the profunda femoris arteries. Ogden (1973) demonstrated in anatomic specimens that the limbus as a projecting edge entered the angle at the base of the neck between it and the trochanteric epiphysis. This shut down the lateral epiphyseal vessels in the abducted position.

At the American Academy of Orthopaedic Surgeons meeting in 1972, Gage and Winter reported 6 cases of avascular necrosis of the normal hip in 154 patients treated for congeni-

tal dislocation. Hoyt reported the lowered incidence of avascular necrosis following preliminary traction. Less extreme positions are helpful in reducing the incidence of complications. Wilkinson and Carter found that the femoral head appeared to be fragmented and deformed in 24 of 108 patients after using neutral rotation in a plaster cast or a Denis-Browne harness.

The use of abduction splints causes sufficient difficulty if the hip is kept abducted to negate their use. There is considerable variation in the definition of a dislocated hip amongst various authors. Von Rosen[35] used the Ortolani click as a diagnostic test and reported that all of 31 hips became stable in an abduction-lateral rotation splint and only 3 failed to have a normal appearance at follow-up. If the dislocation is defined as those in whom the femoral head has moved to the lateral third of the acetabulum, the abduction must confront soft tissue obstacles interfering with vascularity in the abducted position even when the femur is flexed rather than fully extended.

Since the iliofemoral approach can be expected to leave some residual stiffness of the hip, a surgical approach must be used which relieves the soft-tissue obstruction without leaving a residual limitation of motion. After the iliofemoral approach Scaglietti and Calandriello found normal motion in only 50 of 171 hips followed for 6 months to 10 years.

The importance of the tight iliopsoas and the

Fig. 4.39. Undercorrected subluxation tends to progress, not to regress.

capsule as the seat of soft tissue obstruction to seating of the femoral head is stressed. Since this can be relieved simply through a medial adductor approach, we have used this surgical relief as the first stage of treatment for infants below age 2. Over age 2, further development of the pathology with growth and or unsuccessful treatment necessitate further measures and a different approach.

Median Adductor Approach

A medial incision in line with the posterior margin of the adductor longus is used. The patient is supine with the hip flexed 90° and abducted, a position that brings out the abduction contracture of the unreduced hip.

A straight incision is made along the course of the adductor longus distally from the iliac crease. After division of the deep fascia the approach goes posterior to the adductor longus, separating it from the adductor magnus and gracilis by blunt dissection. The adductor magnus with the obturator nerve lying on it is then exposed. The dissection thereafter proceeds posterior to the adductor brevis where the lesser trochanter is readily palpated. Any precapsular fat can now be pushed medially so that the iliopsoas tendon is readily visualized. A curved hemostat is inserted beneath the tendon, which when divided transversely retracts superi-

Fig. 4.40. Avascular necrosis and growth arrest of the capital femoral epiphysis secondary to treatment—overgrowth of the trochanteric epiphysis occurs secondarily.

Fig. 4.41. Series of roentgenograms in an infant girl from age 1 month to age 3 years, 9 months. (*A*) At 1 month of age, a line drawn along the femoral shaft deviates from the triradiate cartilage. (*B*) This is still more marked at age 3 months. (*C*) The patient was treated with preliminary traction and abduction cast and readily located. (*D*) At age 9 months the ossification center appears delayed. (*E*) At age 3 years, 9 months, bone is ossifying irregularly and with diminished height—secondary to an interruption of the blood supply to the capital femoral epiphysis.

Fig. 41.1 (*C* and *D*)

Fig. 41.1 (*E*)

orly. Fat can then be pushed superiorly off the anterior capsule so that the hourglass constriction along the former course of the tendon is seen. A retractor can now be passed along the anterior surface of the capsule and superior to the femoral head. The capsule can then be incised along the axis of the femoral neck, the incision proceeding medially and anteriorly far enough to allow the femoral head to be brought into the empty acetabulum, where it is in view. When the head is located the capsular incision is spread and cannot be closed. The adductors, however, fall back together and the skin edges are readily approximated. After reduction, both hips are held in 10-20° of internal rotation, 30° of abduction, and 10° of flexion.

When the spica cast is applied it must be molded on the dislocated side to maintain medially directed pressure over the trochanter to keep the head in the acetabulum. The dislocated position creates a pocket into which the femur will fall by gravity unless this is done. The adduction contracture present when the hip was dislocated vanishes with reduction. It is not necessary to divide the adductors, nor is it necessary to remove soft tissue from the acetabulum. The extent of the deformity of the acetabulum can readily be evaluated by palpation during the operation.

It is evident that this procedure removes the obstacle to reduction without pressure but does nothing to alter the deformed cartilage acetabulum except to relieve the pressure of the femoral head on it. The door to the acetabulum is opened but the roof must still form. Recovery of the cartilage is possible once the mechanical forces acting on it are changed. If the pressure is not relieved in children over 2 months of age, this deformity becomes progressively more serious with advancing age so that, in children more than 2 years old, secondary changes have occurred with capsular adherence to the ilium above the acetabulum as well as to the inferior half of the acetabulum. The operation is used in children in the newborn period and up to 2 years of age with success, provided the hip is immobilized in the functional position of 30° of abduction, 10-20° of internal rotation, and little or no flexion for at least 4 months after the operation.

Evaluation of Reduction

Roentgenograms of the hip should include anteroposterior and acetabular views, and review of them should be exceptionally discerning. Failure to find a perfect reduction in both views should result in open reduction, but this is seldom necessary in the infantile group.

Some infantile hips readily reduce when the patient is under anesthesia, but forceful maneuvers should never be used to achieve this result.

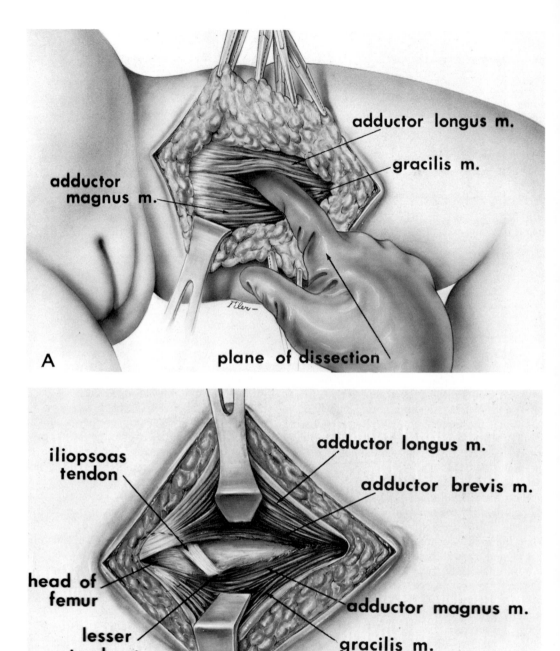

A

adductor longus m.

gracilis m.

adductor magnus m.

plane of dissection

B

iliopsoas tendon

adductor longus m.

adductor brevis m.

head of femur

lesser trochanter

adductor magnus m.

gracilis m.

Fig. 4.42. (*A*) Diagram of the medial adductor approach to the hip. This differs from the Ludloff approach in that the adductor longus and brevis are carried superiorly. (*B*) Finger dissection readily palpates the lesser trochanter—the gracilis and adductor magnus are inferior. There will frequently be some fat lobules about the capsule which must be pushed aside to visualize it and the iliopsoas tendon. (*C*) The iliopsoas tendon and the inferior capsule are divided. The iliopsoas will ascend superiorly—the capsule once opened cannot be brought together with the hip in its located position. (*D*) Photograph of the anatomy of the median adductor approach by John Ogden. (*AL*, adductor longus; *IP*, iliopsoas tendon, *AB*, adductor brevis; *AM*, adductor magnus; *G*, gracilis.) The superior forceps are on either side of the iliopsoas muscle as it descends to the lesser trochanter.

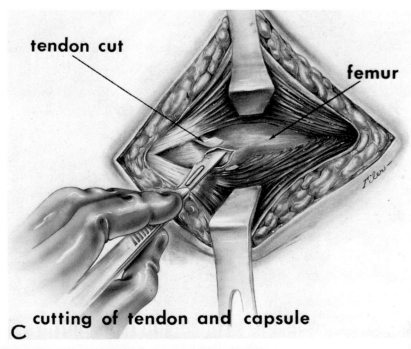

cutting of tendon and capsule

Fig. 4.42 (*C* and *D*)

Fig. 4.43. Girl, age 6 months, with dislocation of the hip treated by median adductor approach. (*A*) Anteroposterior view shows lateral riding of femoral shaft on left. (*B*) Abduction anteroposterior view emphasizes the lateral riding femoral shaft. No ossification center is visible on the left for the capital femoral epiphysis. (*C*) At a period of 4 months postoperative, the ossification center for the epiphysis of the femoral head is ossifying well. (*D*) At 2 years postoperative, the hip is developing well with minor irregularities in ossification of the acetabulum secondary to the old dislocation and deformation of the acetabular cartilage. (anteroposterior view). (*E*) Abduction (anteroposterior view) revealing alignment of femoral shaft to the triradiate cartilage.

Fig. 4.43 (*C* and *D*)

Most patients with dislocated hips have excessive anteversion, which prevents normal seating of the femoral head when the knee is foreward and the limb in line with the trunk. With infants less than 6 months old, there is no need to rush into an anteversion osteotomy since there is great opportunity for corrective growth in the period of rapid growing that they are in. Once the infant is past this early period, the need for osteotomy may be demonstrated by a comparison of roentgenograms of the hip taken anteroposteriorly while the hip is abducted and neutrally rotated with films taken in internal rotation and abduction. Such a comparison may reveal the femoral head to point out of the joint in neutral rotation and to

Fig. 4.43 (*E*)

be in perfect alignment in internal rotation. When osteotomy is necessary, it should not be delayed.

Despite the apparent ease of treating hips in early infancy, difficult cases are found and careful roentgenographic examination must be made in order to procure a well developed joint with the femoral head in normal position.

In evaluating end results it is frequently not appreciated that the femoral head is damaged in varying degrees when the child first presents for treatment. The head may be flattened from pressure against either the acetabular rim or the ilium. The cartilage of the femoral head may also be fibrillated. The shape of the femoral head may not be fully appreciated for several years when the ossification center finally begins to form. It frequently begins ossification eccentrically and may form from a number of separate centers. This irregular ossification has been interpreted as aseptic necrosis although there is no pathologic proof that this is true. The same can be said for delayed ossification of the femoral head. This may not actually be aseptic necrosis but rather a reflection of the abnormal physical forces which have been placed on the femoral head in the past.

An additional aid in determining the adequacy of reduction when it is questionable consists of contrast injection. Approximately 3 ml of an appropriate contrast medium to which the patient is not sensitive and which does not irritate the joint can be inserted into the joint cavity. The approach can be lateral to the femoral artery and anterior, or beneath the femoral artery through the hip adductors.

The dye gives most information if it is inserted just prior to reduction and films are taken. After the hip has been reduced, the position of the limbus can be determined as well as the presence of soft tissue in the joint.

Closed Reduction

If traction and closed reduction is the surgeon's choice then traction should be continued sufficiently long to allow an easily closed reduction. The percentage of hips considered for open reduction can be expected to rise if the use of force is limited and criteria for reduction are exact.

After closed reduction, the hip is placed in a plaster hip spica that holds the involved side to the foot and the uninvolved side to the knee. At the end of 6 weeks, the long side of the cast is shortened to the knee so that rotation of the hip is possible. Such spicas usually last 2-3 months before the child outgrows them. When to discontinue the spicas is a matter of judgement based on a study of x-rays showing the progress of the hip. The acetabular roof should develop into the normal range, and the epiphyseal growth center should appear. The ability of the acetabular roof to respond to the

Fig. 4.44. Subluxation of hip; note malalignment on abduction.

femoral head placed in normal position within it usually continues, at least in part, to age 4.

While in the cast the patient is kept on a Bradford frame, which eases the care of the child and keeps the cast clean. The frame has an opening beneath the genitalia and is kept at a slight downward slant so that urine will not run into the cast but into the bedpan beneath the frame.

Closed reduction, when it is done, should only be done gently. Bost et al.[21] gives the incidence of aseptic necrosis of the femoral head following closed reduction as 12% of reductions done in the first year of life, 59% in the second year, and 62% in the third year. Aseptic necrosis following hip reduction does not always run the protracted course sometimes associated with Legg-Perthes disease.

TREATMENT OF DISLOCATED HIP AT AGE TWO TO FOUR

In this group skeletal traction and open reduction of the hip becomes the treatment for the majority, rather than the minority, of patients. These youngsters are often affected bilaterally, for a unilateral dislocation presents more obvious physical signs in the gait and is therefore recognized earlier. Because these children have been walking for some time, a considerable upward displacement of the hip is likely. Telescoping of the hip as a physical sign is more easily elicited in this group than in any other.

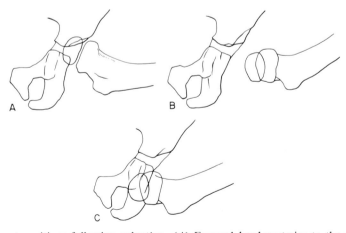

Fig. 4.45. Incorrect positions following reduction. (*A*) Femoral head posterior to the acetabulum, (*B*) too great lateral displacement remaining, (*C*) femoral head inferior to the acetabulum in the region of the obturator foramen. (Redrawn from J. Hass: *Congenital Dislocation of the Hip*, p. 167. Charles C Thomas, Springfield, Ill., 1951.)

Fig. 4.46. Congenital coxa vara in this child mimics most of the physical signs of congenital dislocation of the hip: increased lumbar lordosis, trochanters above Nélaton's line, and gluteus medius weakness. The femoral head, however, is palpated in normal position.

It becomes more important than ever to pull the femoral head into a position opposite the acetabulum. From this position, regardless of the mode of therapy, it can be placed in the acetabulum with relative ease if there is no obstruction. The efficiency of the traction becomes very important. A well leg spica to hold the child in place is necessary, with skeletal traction on the femur.

In this age group, some hips can be replaced by closed reduction so that there is perfect alignment—the centers of the head and neck point directly toward the triradiate cartilage—and no persistent widening of the joint.

The majority of youngsters over 2 have developed changes in the capsule in the the shape of the head and in adherence of the capsule to the acetabulum, so that a perfect reduction is not obtainable. Probably the most important barrier to a reduction is the iliopsoas

tendon. Open reduction is necessary to correct these difficulties. The surgeon should be aware that he will have to carry his dissection to the medial side of the ilipsoas or he will not adequately visualize the acetabulum.

Iliofemoral Incision

An anterior iliofemoral or Smith-Peterson incision is often used. The cartilaginous apophysis of the ilium is carefully spared as the gluteus group is removed from the ilium by subperiosteal dissection. The femoral head, on opening of the capsule, is found to have varying degrees of fibrillation of the cartilage and flattening of the surface opposed to the ilium. The capsule is adherent to the side of the ilium and needs dissection to be brought down to the level of the actual acetabular rim. The psoas muscle may run across the joint in a manner preventing reduction and may need lengthening

Fig. 4.47. Constriction of the hip joint capsule by the tendon of the iliopsoas in dislocated hip riding superiorly. This is a major obstacle to reduction, and traction in line with the trunk is necessary to overcome it—not in abduction. (Redrawn from J. Hass: *Congenital Dislocation of the Hip*, p. 70. Charles C Thomas, Springfield, Ill., 1951.)

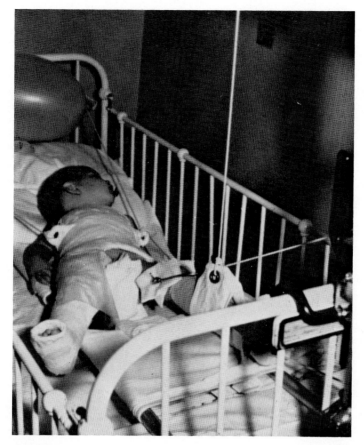

Fig. 4.48. Traction preliminary to reduction of a dislocated hip. A well leg spica is used with eyelets so that the cast can be tied to the Bradford frame. A pin is placed through the femur and traction is axial in line with the trunk, not in abduction, which forces the femoral head against the ilium. The lower leg is supported by a sling underneath the proximal tibia and adhesive traction to the calf.

or transplantation to be removed as an obstacle. The hourglass constriction of the capsule will be formed just beneath it. The femoral nerve will be found just medial and superior to the iliopsoas. The hip usually appears most stable in internal rotation.

The femoral head, when placed in the acetabulum, is held in the position which is most stable. The capsule is repaired in this position.

A spica is applied and bivalved postoperatively at 3 weeks, and gentle, active, guided exercises to obtain further internal rotation and abduction are begun. If the hip is placed in a position of extreme internal rotation, the capsule tends to be wound about the neck, constricting the circulation to the femoral head. Such a position may be responsible for aseptic necrosis of the femoral head following open reduction.

Anteversion Osteotomy

Osteotomies to correct anteversion are only done in the presence of excessive internal rotation at the hip. When done in the subtrochanteric region, a Steinmann pin is first placed in the femoral neck to hold the hip in internal rotation. The distal fragment is then rotated until the knee joint is in line with the anatomic position of the body. When the patient stands with the knee joint pointing straight ahead, the hip is in internal rotation by comparison with its previous position. Excessive internal rotation is no longer possible. The use of osteotomy to correct anteversion is a matter of judgment in

Fig. 4.49. Dislocated hip at age 6 months treated by abduction–cast method. (*A*) Dislocation on right with lateral displacement of the shaft and smaller ossification center. (*B*) Abducted in cast in located position. (*C*) Anteroposterior view 10 years later with diminished head height slanting acetabulum. (*D*) Lateral view with diminished height of capital femoral epiphysis and delay in ossification anteriorly.

Fig. 4.49 (*C* and *D*)

Fig. 4.50. (*A*) The iliopsoas muscle and tendon have been released and retracted superiorly. Branches of the femoral nerve can be seen coursing just above the femoral head. The anterorsuperior iliac spine projects to the reader's left and the limb extends to the reader's right. The capsule is seen on the femoral head as it nestles in the false acetabulum. (*B*) A close-up of the femoral head reveals the damaged cartilaginous surface. (*C*) The femoral head has been retracted slightly from the false acetabulum revealing the acorn shape of the head, the result of persistent pressure in an abnormal position. The false acetabulum frequently leads the operator astray at this point. The elongated ligamentum teres can be seen disappearing into the depths of the wound. The capsule has been striated after having been divided superiorly. It is pulled to the reader's right. (*D*) Persistence in obtaining good exposure reveals the true acetabulum as a dark shadow just to the right of the false acetabulum. The ligamentum teres disappears into it. The apparent acetabular rim to the left is related to the false acetabulum only and not the actual acetabulum, the lines of which can be seen coursing over it underneath the femoral nerve branches.

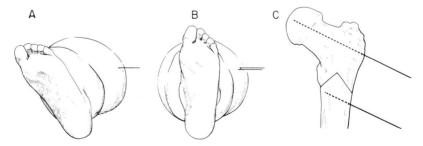

Fig. 4.51. Anteversion osteotomy. (*A*) The leg is internally rotated for the desired degree of correction, and a Steinmann pin is placed in the proximal fragment. (*B*) The bone is divided, and the distal fragment is rotated until the knee is upright; a second pin is inserted in the distal fragment parallel to the first. (*C*) Anterior view of the final situation with parallel pins in place and incorporated in plaster.

each individual case since the degree of anteversion varies in each. Osteotomy can also be performed in the supracondylar region.

Hips that tend to redislocate after open reduction need correction of the factor allowing the redislocation. An acetabular shelf or buttress may have to be built and anteversion, if a factor, corrected at a later date.

Treatment of Primary Anterior Congenital Dislocation

McCarroll[24] has emphasized primary anterior dislocation of the hip as constituting 22.5% of a series of congenital dislocations of the hip. Such dislocations may be the result of rudimentary development of the anterior portion of the acetabulum or of a tendency of the acetabulum to face forward and thereby to diminish the anterior buttress in relation to the head. Dega, in a review of 100 fetal specimens, noted that the angle of foreward inclination of the acetabulum was 29.5°.

McCarroll advocates for this condition preliminary skeletal traction followed by attempted closed reduction. Should the closed reduction be unsuccessful, open reduction is in order. While an effort has been made to form either a shelf or buttress at the anterior margin, the results have not been entirely satisfactory. The innominate osteotomy developed by Salter appears to be an excellent answer for this condition.

Salter's Osteotomy

Robert Salter[31] in 1962 described a method of overcoming frank dislocation or subluxation of the femoral head in children over 18 months. This method used an osteotomy of the innominate bone extending into the sciatic notch. The fragment was then rotated, with the pubic joint used as a hinge, to redirect the angle of the acetabulum without changing its shape. Pemberton in 1958 had reported an osteotomy of the ilium which was hinged on the triradiate cartilage. Salter's method has considerable appeal because it changes, not the shape of the joint, but its location in relation to the femoral head.

The hip is exposed through a Smith-Petersen anterior iliofemoral approach. The ilium is exposed both medially and laterally, and the osteotomy is carried out in a straight line from the anterior inferior iliac spine to the sciatic notch. A Gigli's saw is first passed through the sciatic notch, and the bone is cut toward the operator. A full-thickness graft is removed from the anterior part of the ilium and trimmed in the shape of a wedge, the base of which is equal to the distance between the anterior superior and the anterior inferior spines. If open reduction of the frankly dislocated hip is necessary, it is carried out as a first step of the procedure, and obstructing bands of adipose tissue are removed. The abnormal facing of the acetabulum can usually be appreciated at this time.

The principle of this procedure is to ensure that a reduced subluxation or dislocation previously stable only in abduction and flexion is made stable in the position of function. This stabilization allows early weight bearing once the osteotomy has healed.

The patient is immobilized in a unilateral hip spica that holds the hip in slight abduction, flexion, and internal rotation for 6 weeks.

TREATMENT OF DISLOCATED HIP AFTER AGE FOUR

Dislocated hips in this age group have a poor prognosis, so far as development of the hip is concerned, after a mere replacement in the acetabulum, even when the replacement is done openly. The joint must be maintained in abduction for many months, and frequently there is little or no improvement in the acetabulum itself.

Here again Salter's osteotomy offers great promise, but other procedures which may be used are described here. They have the disadvantage of changing the shape of the acetabulum rather than its relationship to the femoral head.

An acetabular osteotomy has been helpful in cases in which the femoral head is centered laterally in a shallow and slanting acetabulum. Anteversion of a fairly marked degree is usually still present in such cases.

Osteotomy of Acetabulum

It is most important in this procedure, as in the Colonna[7,8] operation or acetabular shelf

Fig. 4.52. The iliofemoral approach exposing both the anterior ilium and the hip joint. It must be carried medially enough to visualize the femoral nerve by retracting or dividing the iliopsoas muscle and tendon.

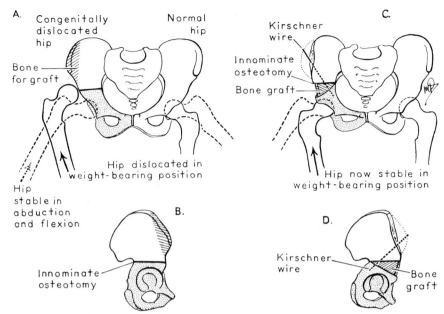

Fig. 4.53. The principle of the innominate osteotomy. A Gigli's saw is inserted in the sciatic notch and drawn forward to the anteroinferior spine. The distal fragment hinged at the symphysis pubis can now be tilted by opening the osteotomy anteriorly and laterally. This carries the acetabulum over the femoral head so that a stable hip is achieved once the osteotomy is healed. It is not necessary to wait for acetabular development to allow the patient to begin weight bearing. If the hip is frankly dislocated, an open reduction is carried out at the same operation, prior to the osteotomy. (Reproduced from R. B. Slater: Innominate osteotomy in the treatment of congenital dislocation of the hip, *Journal of Bone & Joint Surgery, 43B:* 524, 1961.)

procedure, that the femur be pulled down by skeletal traction so that it is well centered in the area normally occupied by the acetabulum. This means a displacement of several centimeters distally from the previous position of the femoral head. Success in all these procedures is possible only if the pressure of the femoral head against the reconstructed area is relieved. In order to achieve the required displacement, excellent mechanical efficiency of the traction is necessary. A well leg, single spica is applied to secure good countertraction. A wire or pin is passed through the distal femur, and traction is applied through this pin by means of a horseshoe clamp holding the pin. The traction is directly in line with the trunk so that it pulls against the iliopsoas, which must be lengthened if the head is to be seated in its normal position.

Traction usually requires between 3 and 4 weeks. When operation is performed, a traction table is used and traction is applied. The proximal two-thirds of a Smith-Peterson incision is used without stripping the ilium medi-

ally. The cartilage apophysis covering the iliac crest is also left intact. After the glutei are stripped from the ilium subperiosteally, the capsule is visualized. It is attached well above the actual acetabular rim and is stripped down by sharp dissection. A small linear incision is made into the joint to make certain of the location of the acetabular rim and the femoral head. The previous location of the head, now uncovered by its downward excursion, is adequately visualized. A curved osteotomy line is begun around the acetabular rim deep within the joint, but exterior to it and within the bone. This entire area is now pried down so that it covers the femoral head, which is held in internal rotation and abduction. A triangular space is now opened up by the descent of the articular flap. A suitable graft is taken above and posterior to the ilium, which may be very thin in areas so that care must be taken to avoid complete penetration. The bone is packed into the defect, which is held open by a periosteal elevator. Once completed, the new acetabular rim should be very close to the femoral head,

Fig. 4.54. Technique of innominate osteotomy. (From R. B. Salter: Innominate osteotomy in the treatment of congenital dislocation of the hip, *Journal of Bone & Joint Surgery, 43B:* 524, 1961.)

and the femoral head should no longer be visible. After wound closure a spica is applied to hold the leg in abduction and internal rotation. An osteotomy of the distal femur is often necessary 1-2 weeks later to bring the knee out of anteversion and into a neutral position. After a total of 8 weeks, the spica is removed for active exercise at both hip and knee. A period of recumbency is now necessary for a further 8 weeks, following which motion is well developed and partial weight bearing with crutches is begun. It is usually possible to discard the crutches 6 months after the operation itself. Pemberton has described a very complete osteotomy of the ilium just above the acetabulum in order to develop an adequate mold for the femoral head.

Acetabuloplasty

Where the fundamental feature of the pathology of the dislocation that remains is a misshapen acetabulum, a direct surgical approach on this feature is possible. Redirecting the acetabulum by iliac osteotomy by the method of Salter, Pemberton or Chiari does not fully answer this problem since the acetabulum remains enlarged and flattened in its lateral third. In a sense this is the residual of the so-called subluxation which in reality is an intra-acetabular dislocation with the lateral third hollowed out and pressed back by the femoral head.

As a clinical problem the hip often appears only minimally displaced. However a gluteus medius lurch and positive Trendelenberg test is a common accompaniment. Internal rotation is often increased by residual anteversion of the femur.

Operation

There are two stages necessary to secure a successful result for this procedure.

First Stage. Skeletal traction is used with a Steinmann pin placed through the distal femoral metaphysis. A well leg spica incorporates the other lower extremity and trunk.

Traction is continued until there is a definable space between acetabulum and femoral head. The femoral head should be drawn down sufficiently to bring the femur into a normal relationship with the original medial third of the acetabulum. There is now sufficient space to pry down the outer one-half of the acetabulum and have it stay down without pressure from the femoral head.

Second Stage. The cast is removed, the pin may remain in place covered with sterile drapes to provide a convenient means of putting traction on the leg during the operation.

The patient is positioned three-fourths of the way up on the opposite side since it is necessary to see the posterior as well as the anterior portion of the acetabulum.

An anterior iliofemoral approach is used going well posteriorly. The capsule is divided from the lateral edge of the acetabulum after running an anterior incision in the capsule in line with the femoral neck.

The portion of acetabular cartilage bent

Fig. 4.55. Acetabuloplasty prying down the lateral one-half of the acetabular rim in order to reshape the acetabulum.

Fig. 4.56. Coming to the hip from the lateral approach, the juncture of the capsule and acetabular rim can readily be visualized. (*A*) The lateral one-third to one-half of the acetabulum is turned down liberally and as far anterior and posterior as possible (*B*). Bone chips are used (*C*) to hold the reshaped portion of the acetabulum in its new position.

superiorly is clearly seen once traction is applied to the femur. This acetabular cartilage must be brought down in symmetrical fashion around the relocated femoral head.

In order to accomplish this an incision into the ilium is begun just superior to the acetabular cartilage and carried anteriorly and posteriorly in rounded symmetric fashion staying outside the acetabular cartilage, but carrying the osteotomy deep enough to carry the deformed portion of the head. A periosteal elevator keeps it pried down as the subchondral bone is backed by graft from the ilium. This maintains the lateral one-half of the acetabulum in its new position. Traction is maintained on the femur as the child has a long leg spica applied. The unoperated thigh is encased to the knee. The cast remains on for 6 weeks.

After x-rays to verify graft incorporation the child is started on range of motion exercises. Although crutches are used for ambulation no weight bearing is permitted for a minimum of 3

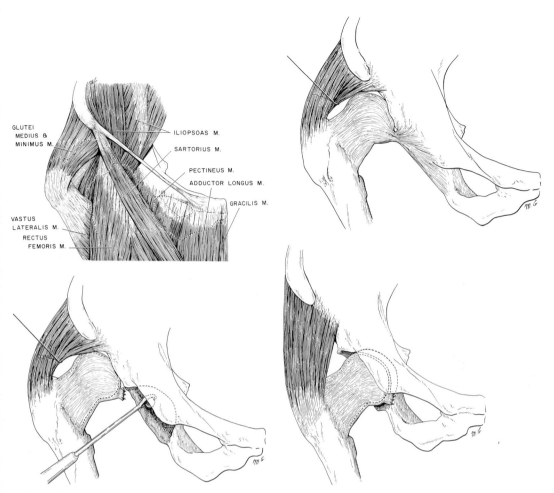

GLUTEI
MEDIUS &
MINIMUS M.

ILIOPSOAS M.

SARTORIUS M.

PECTINEUS M.
ADDUCTOR LONGUS M.

GRACILIS M.

VASTUS
LATERALIS M.
RECTUS
FEMORIS M.

Fig. 4.57. (*Top, left*) In a capsular arthroplasty developed by Colonna, the intact capsule is exposed by a Smith-Peterson incision. (*Top, right,* and *bottom, left*) The acetabulum is refashioned by curetting, and the femoral head enclosed in the capsule is placed within the new joint. By preliminary traction, the femoral head was brought down opposite the acetabulum so that it could readily be reduced. (*Bottom, right*) The femoral head enclosed in the capsular sac is in place in the newly fashioned acetabulum (Redrawn from P. C. Colonna: Congenital dislocation of the hip, *Instructional Course Lectures: American Academy of Orthopaedic Surgeons,* 8: 175, 1951.)

Fig. 4.57.1. Traction applied to the hip to bring it down to a point opposite the acetabulum. Efficient countertraction is necessary to achieve results. Skeletal traction on the femur may be used.

months. A three point type of gait with crutches is used to encourage use of the hip joint in the gait.

Other Procedures

There are several other procedures for developing the joint to the point at which the hip is maintained in position. Colonna has developed an operation for the dislocated hip in the age group of 4-8 years. After preliminary traction has placed the hip opposite the acetabulum, an open reduction is performed. In this procedure, the joint capsule is carefully dissected free of the ilium and surrounding structures. The acetabulum is curetted so that a deep and adequate cavity is produced. In this process, the acetabular cartilage is removed, and the cartilage line at the junction of pubis, ischium, and ilium is visualized.

The capsule, which was left attached at the base of the neck, is sewn at its open end so as to enclose the femoral head. The head and enclosing capsule are then replaced in the joint.

The patient is kept in a cast for 4 weeks thereafter. Following this period, motion is begun at the hip in flexion, abduction, and internal rotation with traction. There follows a very gradual and carefully guarded return to full weight bearing.

If traction preliminary to operation has brought the head opposite the acetabulum so that it is not forced into the newly made joint, the procedure usually produces a good result.

A third procedure to create an adequate joint consists of building an acetabular shelf. This procedure is of value also in treatment of the subluxated hip which is progressing to further subluxation. The insertion of a shelf may be enough to produce stability and prevent progression. Again, to ensure a good result, the hip must be pulled down by traction.

At operation the femoral head should lie opposite the acetabulum. In Ghormley's[17] procedure the anterior iliac crest and acetabular margins are exposed by a lateral hip incision. The capsule is kept intact and bone chips are turned down over the head from the ilium, leaving a bony notch. The anterior superior spine and anterior portion of the ilium are freed subperiosteally. This section of the ilium is then osteotomized on a level. The leveled edge of this bone graft is then placed into the supra-acetabular groove. Traction is maintained for 8 weeks with the patient in a spica to the ankle. Crutch-walking is then permitted. When the procedure is being done for a hip drawn down opposite the actabulum, failure to recognize the true acetabular rim at operation may be a pitfall. Not infrequently the capsule is turned up on the ilium and adherent to it. The capsule frequently has to be dissected from the ilium until the true rim is reached. Occasionally, as suggested by Anderson and Bickel, the capsule may be opened and the acetabular margin visualized.

Variations of the method of building an acetabular shelf have been described by Alber, Gill,[18,19] Phemister, and Lowman. Both tibial grafts and sections of the ilium may be used as grafts after the superior, posterior, or anterior portions of the acetabulum are pried down over the femoral head by osteotomy.

There remains a small group of patients, who are becoming quite rare in recent times, in the older age group with a severely dislocated hip that is well removed from the original acetabulum. These hips cannot be pulled down by traction to a point opposite the acetabulum. Here the general aim is to secure greater stability for the hip and thus to aid elimination of the medius limp.

Exercises to develop greater strength in the gluteus medius are used. When the dislocation is bilateral, these patients are perhaps best left alone. When it is unilateral, some stabilizing procedure is often used. Such a procedure is the building of a shelf with the hip brought to a position just above the acetabulum, after the suggestion of Dickson.[13] Osteotomies have been devised by Lorenz and Schanz which procure increased bony support by displacement of the proximal portion of the distal fragment medially. In the case of the Lorenz osteotomy, there is an actual placing of the shaft in the acetabulum.

Criteria of Reduction

Clinical criteria of reduction are:

1. The prominence of the trochanter is diminished.

2. The femoral head is palpated beneath the femoral artery one finger's breadth below the inguinal ligament.

3. The previously extending knee no longer

Fig. 4.58. There are many methods of performing a shelf procedure to stabilize the femoral head in the true acetabulum. The operation basically pries down ilium and outer portion of the acetabulum and maintains the shelf in position by a bone graft, which may be taken from the ilium. (Redrawn from J. Hass: *Congenital Dislocation of the Hip*, p. 288. Springfield, Ill.: Charles C Thomas, 1951.)

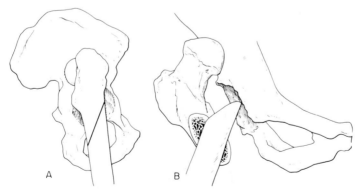

Fig. 4.59. Osteotomy may be used to increase stability in a dislocated hip of long standing. In the Lorenz osteotomy, the shaft of the femur is displaced into the acetabulum. (Redrawn from J. Hass: *Congenital Dislocation of the Hip*, p. 295. Springfield, Ill.: Charles C Thomas, 1951.)

extends.

X-ray criteria include:

1. There is no widening of the joint space.

2. The line through the center of the femoral neck and head runs through the center of the triradiate cartilage in all views.

NEUROGENIC DISLOCATION OF HIP

Such hip dislocations occur following both spastic and flail paralysis of the lower extremities. The underlying etiologic factor is often a combination of events associated with each form of difficulty.

A principal factor in association with spastic paralysis is the persistent adducted position. Shortening of the adductors with use, and reinforcement of the adducted position with growth, may cause the limbus gradually to bend superiorly and the femoral head to ride out. Such a dislocation is aided by valgus of the femoral neck and uncorrected anteversion.

In flail paralysis, valgus of the femoral neck with non-weight bearing is a very common finding. Uncorrected anteversion of the femur may accompany it. One is hard put to weigh properly the relative importance of valgus and anteversion in any one case. In poliomyelitis, where the muscles may not be completely flail and contractures may arise, these may also play a part. The tightness of the fascia lata with contracture in abduction is important because it results in a flexed position with the hip in neutral. Extension then tends to drive the hip posteriorward and over the acetabular rim. Poor seating of the femoral head due to valgus or anteversion aids the progress of the hip laterally. Again, however, the condition must usually be accompanied by factors such as anteversion or valgus to result in actual dislocation. The tightness of the iliopsoas when a flexion contracture is present is a major factor in neurogenic dislocation.

Neurogenic dislocations are seen particularly in connection with myelomeningocele, cerebral palsy, or poliomyelitis.

Fig. 4.61. Anteversion osteotomy on right to aid in keeping femoral head in normal relation to acetabulum.

Fig. 4.60. Neurogenic dislocation on right with excessive anteversion and valgus in both hips.

Treatment

Maintenance of an abducted position helps to counteract the progression of the femoral head toward dislocation. It also aids in reinforcing reduction, once this has been achieved. The forces which originally drove the femur into a dislocated position must be corrected, however, to guard against recurrence. Keeping the patient in plaster spicas over the years may be too costly from the point of view of mental and physical health, and other means must be sought.

In the presence of a well developed acetabulum, correction of anteversion and valgus by femoral osteotomy may be all that is necessary. In cases in which the acetabulum is deficient, shelf procedures to create a stable abutment may be indicated. Levering down the acetabular rim and blocking it in position will be successful only if the hip has been pulled down by traction so that it is not exerting a strong pressure on the reconstructed area.

This procedure has been described in the preceding section. The innominate osteotomy also described in the preceding section may well answer the requirements here better than any other procedure when an acetabulum that covers the femoral head is desired. It has the advantages of maintaining congruity of acetabulum in relation to the femoral head, of requiring a relatively short convalescence, and of bringing about an immediate change in the stability of the hip.

The preliminary of achieving reduction is essential. The hip can be tested for stability at the time of open reduction through a Smith-Peterson approach. The line of the osteotomy runs from the sciatic notch to the anterior inferior spine and is done with a Gigli's saw. A graft is removed from the anterior portion of the iliac crest. It is trimmed to the shape of a wedge the base of which is equal to the distance between the anterosuperior and anteroinferior spines.

The distal segment is shifted forward, downward, and outward so that the osteotomy site opens up anterolaterally. The wedge-shaped graft is fitted into this opening. A Kirschner wire is inserted across the osteotomy site and through the graft; it is buried in the subcutaneous fat as the skin is closed. Salter found displacement of the distal fragment (which is

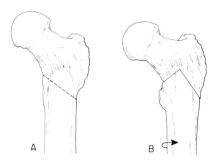

Fig. 4.62. A type of osteotomy for anteversion which also corrects valgus and is of special help in neurogenic dislocation.

hinged on the symphysis pubica) easier when the femoral head was dislocated at the time. He recommends retaining the limbus by wide exposure and reduction of the femoral head deep to it, and he warns against backward or inward displacement of the distal segment. The patient is placed in a hip spica in a position of slight flexion, slight abduction, and slight medial rotation. The spica remains in place for 6 weeks, after which the patient actively exercises to regain muscle function. When this goal is achieved, partial weight bearing is allowed for several weeks, and full weight bearing follows.

Other methods of treating neurogenic dislocations, including Mustard's iliopsoas transplant, are discussed under "Spina Bifida Syndrome."

References

1. Adams, F.: *The Genuine Works of Hippocrates,* London, 1849.
2. Badgley, C. E.: Correlation of clinical and anatomical parts leading to a conception of the etiology of congenital hip dislocation, *J. Bone Joint Surg., 31A:* 341, 1949.
3. Barlow, T. G.: Early diagnosis and treatment of congenital dislocation of the hip, *J. Bone Joint Surg., 44B:* 292, 1962.
4. Bost, F. C., Hagey, H., Schottstaedt, E. R., and Larsen, L. J.: The results of treatment of congenital dislocation of the hip in infancy, *J. Bone Joint Surg., 30A:* 454, 1948.
5. Bradford, E. H.: Treatment of congenital dislocation of the hip, *Boston Med. Surg. J., 108:* 73, 1883.
6. Bradford, E. H.: Congenital dislocation of the hip—results of treatment at the Boston Children's Hospital, *Am. J. Orthop. Surg.,* 7: 57, 1909.
7. Colonna, P. C.: An arthroplastic operation for congenital dislocation of the hip—a two stage procedure. *Surg. Cynec Obstet., 63:* 777, 1936.

8. Colonna, P. C.: Arthroplasty of the hip for congenital dislocation in children, *J. Bone Joint Surg., 29:* 711, 1947.

9. Compere, E. L.: The shelf operation for congenital dislocation of the hip, *Am. J. Surg., 43:* 404, 1939.

10. Crego, C. H., Jr.: Preliminary skeletal traction in the treatment of congenital dislocation of the hip, *South. Med. J., 26:* 845, 1933.

11. Crego, C. H., Jr., and Schwartzmann, J. R.: Follow-up study of the early treatment of congenital dislocation of the hip, *J. Bone Joint Surg., 30A:* 128, 1948.

12. DeNuce, M.: Luxation congenitale de la hanche; operation de Hoffa, *Rev. Orthop., 1s.4:* 108, 1893.

13. Dickson, F. D.: The shelf operation in the treatment of congenital dislocation of the hip, *J. Bone Joint Surg., 17:* 43, 1935.

14. DiPrampero, A.: Morfolojia radioghica dell'ance cosi detta sana nella lussazione congenita laterale, *Chir. Orgi. Mov., 25:* 1, 1939.

15. Frejka, B.: Prävention der angeborenen Juftörrenburg durch das Abduktionspolster, *Wien. Klin. Wochenschr., 91:* 523, 1941.

16. Galeazzi, R.: Esiti lontani della crura incrimenta della lussazione congenita dell'anca, *Arch. Ortop., 32:* 191, 1915.

17. Ghormley, R. K.: Use of the anterior superior spine and crest of the ilium in surgery of the hip joint, *J. Bone Joint Surg., 13:* 784, 1931.

18. Gill, A. B.: Plastic construction of an acetabulum in congenital dislocation of the hip, *J. Bone Joint Surg., 17:* 48, 1935.

19. Gill, A. B.: The end results of early treatment of congenital dislocation of the hip, *J. Bone Joint Surg., 30A:* 442, 1948.

20. Hart, V. L.: Primary genetic dysplasia of the hip with or without classical dislocation, *J. Bone Joint Surg., 24:* 753, 1942.

21. Hart, V. L.: *Congenital Dysplasia of the Hip Joint and Sequelae,* Springfield, Ill: Charles C Thomas, 1952.

22. Leveuf, J.: Primary congenital subluxation of the hip, *J. Bone Joint Surg., 30A:* 875, 1948.

23. Lorenz, A.: La riduzione della lussazione congenita dell'anca, *Arch. Ortop., 14:* 1, 1897.

23a. Massie, W. K., and Howorth, W. B.: Congenital dislocation of the hip. *J. Bone Joint Surg., 33A:* 171, 1951.

24. McCarroll, H. R., and Crego, C. H., Jr.: Primary anterior congenital dislocation of the hip, *J. Bone Joint Surg. 21:* 648, 1939.

24a. McKibbin, B.: Action of the iliopsoas muscle in the newborn. *J. Bone Joint Surg., 50B:* 161, 1968.

25. Mitchell, G. P.: Problems in the early diagnosis and management of congenital dislocation of the hip, *J. Bone Joint Surg., 54B: 1972.*

26. Muller, G. M., and Seddorn, H. J.: Late results of treatment of congenital subluxation of the hip, *J. Bone Joint Surg., 35B:* 342, 1953.

27. Nélaton, E.: *Elements de pathologie chirurgicale edit, Vol. 3,* p. 328, Paris: Pean, 1874.

28. Poli, A.: Contributo alla cura precoce della lussazione congenita dell'anca, *Arch. Ortop., 52:* 749, 1936.

29. Ponseti, I.: Causes of failure in the treatment of congenital dislocation of the hip, *J. Bone Joint Surg., 26:* 775, 1944.

29a. Ponseti, I. V.: Nonsurgical treatment of congenital dislocation of the hip. *J. Bone Joint Surg.. 48A:* 1392, 1966.

30. Putti, V.: Early treatment of congenital dislocation of the hip, *J. Bone Joint Surg., 11:* 798, 1929.

31. Salter, R. B.: Innominate osteotomy in the treatment of congenital dislocation and subluxation of the hip, *J. Bone Joint Surg., 43B:* 518, 1961.

32. Severin, E.: Arthrography in congenital dislocation of the hip, *J. Bone Joint Surg., 21:* 304, 1939.

33. Severin, E.: Contribution to knowledge of congenital dislocation of the hip joint; late results of closed reduction, *Acta Chir. Scand., 84:* Suppl. 63, 1941.

34. Somerville, E. W.: The direct approach to congenital dislocation of the hip, *J. Bone Joint Surg., 39B:* 632, 1957.

35. Rosen, S.: Diagnosis and treatment of congenital dislocation of the hip joint in the newborn, *J. Bone Joint Surg., 44B:* 284, 1962.

36. Wilkinson, J. A.: A post-natal survey for congenital dislocation of the hip, *J. Bone Joint Surg., 54B:* 40, 1972.

DEVELOPMENTAL COXA VARA

Developmental coxa vara has been related to the congenital short femur by Golding.[3] It is not unusual to find the two coexisting. Congenital coxa vara results from anomalous ossification of the proximal femur. The deformity thus produced gives rise to a medius type limp and to marked limitation of abduction, which, when bilateral, is especially disabling.

The lesion results in progressive deformity. Abnormality of the gait does not ordinarily become noticeable before the age of 3 or 4. Thereafter, the gait difficulty caused by the mechanical abnormality of the proximal femur is increasingly noticeable.

There is a gradually decreasing amount of anteversion of the femur as the coxa vara increases. When the varus is well established, retroversion is the rule.

There is no hereditary or familial incidence.

The deformity is more commonly unilateral (3:1) but, when bilateral, tends to be symmetrical. The condition affects both sexes equally. Other anomalies are not ordinarily present

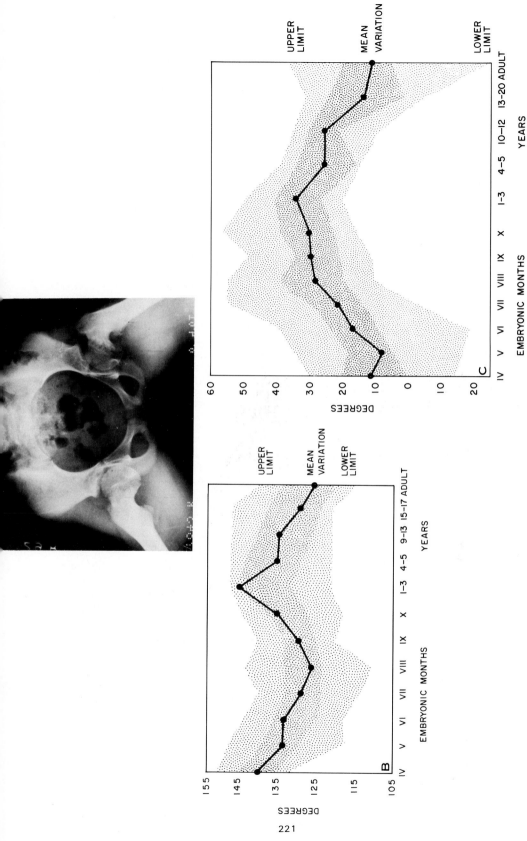

Fig. 4.63. (A) Retroversion is a prominent feature of coxa vara. (B) Variation of the neck-shaft angle with age. (C) Variation of femoral torsion angle with age. (B and C are redrawn from T. von Lanz and A. Mayet: Die Gelenkkor per des Menschlichen Huft gelenkes in der Progredienten Phase Ihrer Unwegiglen Ausforming, Zeitschrift für Anatomie und Entwicklungsgeschichte, 117: 317, 1953.)

helping to differentiate the condition from congenital short and bowed femora which frequently are associated with other anomalies.

Roentgen Findings

The usual angle formed by the femoral neck with the shaft of the femur is 135°. Some change in the direction of increasing varus is always present, and if the patient is first seen between the ages of 4 and 7, the neck of the femur usually forms a right angle with the shaft. The area occupied by the epiphyseal line is usually wide in the young age group. This increased area of radiolucency apparently results from the epiphyseal line plus a gap just distal to it, which occasionally branches away from it as it nears the base of the neck. A triangular segment of bone is thus isolated, as emphasized by Le Mesurier.[4]

In later cases the area occupied by the epiphyseal line becomes quite thin, irregular, and fragmented. The neck appears shorter than it is normally expected to be. The line tends to close prematurely. It becomes evident that there is a decreased rate of growth at this line.

The trochanteric epiphyseal line appears to be normal.

Clinical Picture

The child is brought to medical attention because of a waddling gait due to the medius limp. The limp is progressively more noticeable as the age of the child advances. Pain is not a symptom.

The limitation of abduction is most strikingly effective on the hip motion itself, since the other planes of motion are usually less affected, except in cases of severe deformity. There is a positive Trendelenburg when the patient stands on the involved side. With weight bearing, the trunk shifts over the involved hip in order to clear the opposite leg and to elevate the pelvis, and this movement gives rise to the gait associated with weakness of the gluteus medius. The trochanter is above Nélaton's line. The condition may be confused with dislocation of the hip on physical examination, for actual dislocation is a much more common lesion. The femoral head is palpated in normal position. Telescoping, however, cannot be elicited in coxa vara. Shortening to measurement would depend on the degree of coxa vara present.

Course

If the case is untreated, progressive deformity of the femoral neck-to-shaft relationship to at least a right angle can be expected, and more often there is an even more severe change in the direction of varus.

Since premature closure of the epiphyseal line is the rule, it is unusual to see progression after the age of 12. Once the line is closed, the neck is composed of bone of apparently normal tissue.

Pathology

There has not been a good opportunity to study the actual pathology involving the femoral neck. Study of the x-ray picture yields the principal information about the disease. It is presumed to be a form of anomalous ossification of the proximal third of the femur.

Treatment

Traction has not been shown to affect the deformity. The treatment chosen depends on the degree of deformity at the time the patient is first seen, the amount of growth left, and the gap present in the femoral neck.

Early Cases

Where the deformity present is compatible with good function of the hip and further progression can be expected, attention may be directed to attempting to gain rigid fusion of the epiphyseal line. Le Mesurier[4] has advocated both nailing with a Smith-Peterson nail inserted across the gap and actual bone grafting. Bone grafts may be inserted from the lateral cortex and passed up the femoral neck. Patients treated in this manner should be followed through the growth period thereafter, since continued growth of the trochanteric epiphysis may still result in sufficient varus deformity to need osteotomy.

Late Cases

An abduction osteotomy which obtains adequate correction does not give an ab-

Fig. 4.64. Bilateral developmental coxa vara. Note widened epiphyseal line and filling in of inferior neck angle with triangular area of ossification.

Fig. 4.65. Child with bilateral developmental coxa vara and clinical signs of widened perineum and prominent trochanters.

solutely perfect hip so far as motion is concerned, but results in improvement in gait and abduction at the hip. Where the condition is bilateral, such improvement may be essential. The osteotomy is done just below the level of the lesser trochanter through a lateral incision.

Haas (1933) and White (1946) and most recently Macewen[5] have used an oblique trochanteric osteotomy to correct this condition. The oblique osteotomy is performed in a coronal plane. If the osteotomy runs obliquely from the anterior surface of the femur distally and posteriorly and the distal fragment abducted it will correct coxa vara and retroversion. Since retroversion is the most common accompaniment of the condition this is the cut most often used. A screw is placed across the osteotomy line to stabilize the fragments. A Steinmann pin progressing through the femoral neck stabilizes the proximal fragment and protrudes through the skin to be incorporated in the plaster. The pin should be introduced to the femoral neck through the skin, not through the wound.

Borden et al.[2] reported on a technique of subtrochanteric osteotomy end to side which was fixed with an infant-size blade plate. The plate is present at an angle of 140°. The lateral cortex of the proximal fragment is placed in apposition to the end of the distal fragment.

Fig. 4.66. Progression in developmental coxa vara. There is an 8-year interval between the roentgenogram on the left and that of the same hip on the right with marked increase in deformity.

Fig. 4.67. Congenital short femur and developmental coxa vara in combination.

Fig. 4.68. An oblique intertrochanteric osteotomy of the proximal femur can accomplish various combinations of changes in neck-shaft angle and anterversion or retroversion rotational correction. The degree of obliquity determines the amount of correction of rotation that can be obtained in relation to angulation. Since in most cases the change in angulation desired is greater than that needed for rotation, a cut approaching the axis of the femoral shaft is used as in the drawing at 30°. Above, the abduction of the distal fragment produces internal rotation of the fragment and an increase in the neck shaft angle. To the right, above, adduction of the distal fragment produces external rotation of the distal fragment and a decrease in the neck shaft angle. (Redrawn from G. D. MacEwen and A. R. Shands, Jr.: Oblique trochanteric osteotomy, *Journal of Bone & Joint Surgery, 49A:* 345, 1967.)

Fig. 4.69. Correction of coxa vara in children is difficult to achieve and to hold. One alternative proposed by Borden used a small blade plate and an end-to-side position when the proximal fragment was tilted up.

The plate is inserted parallel to the neck prior to accomplishing the osteotomy. It is preceded by a guide wire fixing the capital femoral epiphysis.

The osteotomy position to bring plate to the lateral cortex of the distal femur is accomplished by traction. It has not been necessary to do an adductor myotomy. There is need for a second procedure to remove the plate and screws. Length is increased by this procedure, the blade is carefully inserted below, the trochanteric epiphysis to avoid injuring this growth structure.

Fig. 4.70. Amstutz devised a type of osteotomy to correct coxa vara using intrinsic carpentry to hold the position. The lateral cortex is extended into the trochanteric area as a spike to hold the valgus position when it is inserted into the medullary cavity of the femoral neck.

Fig. 4.71. The telescoping V osteotomy offers another means of achieving intrinsic stability.

Good healing is obtained before the cast is removed, and the hip is then mobilized with the aid of traction and exercises.

References

1. Barr, J. S.: Congenital coxa vara, *Arch. Surg., 18:* 1909, 1929.
2. Borden, J., Spencer, G. E. and Herndon, C. H.: Treatment of coxa vara in children by means of a modified osteotomy, *J. Bone Joint Surg., 48A:* 1103, 1966.
3. Golding, F. E.: Congenital coxa vara, *J. Bone Joint Surg., 30B:* 161, 1948.
4. Le Mesurier, A. B.: Developmental coxa vara, *J. Bone Joint Surg., 30B:* 595, 1948.
5. Macewen, G. D., and Shands, A. R.: Oblique trochanteric osteotomy, *J. Bone Joint Surg., 49A:* 345, 1967.

SLIPPED CAPITAL FEMORAL EPIPHYSIS

The essence of slipped capital femoral epiphysis is a mechanical change from normal of the relationship of the femoral neck to the capital femoral epiphysis. The anomaly occurs primarily in adolescents.

The results of treatment in cases in which a minimal change has taken place are better than those in cases of marked change in the relationship. An early diagnosis is thus of great value.

The usual age range is 10-17 years; females, by virtue of their approximately 2-year advancement in skeletal maturation, are seen in the early years of this range. Rarely cases are seen in even younger children. The disorder is much more common in males (5:1), and bilateral cases occur in approximately 20% of those affected. Klein et al.[4] state that x-ray signs of bilateral involvement exist in 40% even though clinical symptoms may be confined to one side only.

Etiology

Two general body types are frequently involved by this disease. One is the so-called Fröhlich type, in which there is female fat distribution and underdevelopment of the genitalia; the other is the type of the thin individual whose extremities are long and whose adolescent growth has been very rapid. Approximately one-half of the patients with this disease fall into one or the other group.

The epiphyseal line in the femoral neck is perhaps more subject to a shearing type of stress than any other. Although it is perhaps possible to visualize the onset and progress of the disease on the basis of shearing stress on this line alone, it is as yet unproved that this is sufficient evidence.

An endocrine basis for this disease is suggested by the growth abnormalities. Both growth hormone and sex hormone affect the rate of proliferation of cartilage cells at the epiphyseal plates, which, in turn, may exert a profound effect on the rate of skeletal growth.

Harris tested the shearing force necessary to detach the proximal tibial epiphysis from the shaft in rats. In growth hormone-treated rats with epiphyseal plates thickened principally in the layers of proliferating and maturing cartilage cells, a lesser than normal average force was required. In estrogen-treated rats with thinner plates at the epiphyseal line, a greater average force was necessary than that required in the normal controls.

Although all epiphyses presumably react to endocrine changes, the placement of the proximal femoral epiphysis, which subjects it to shearing stress, may cause this area to become involved to the exclusion of others.

Ghormley[2] emphasized the fact that the epiphyseal plate changes from a horizontal to an oblique position during preadolescent and adolescent periods.

In view of the lack of clear-cut evidence for endocrine factors, some favor the idea that trauma taking place at this point of low resistance to shearing stress is the only etiology.

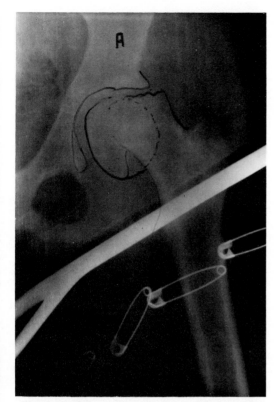

Fig. 4.72. An anterior slip of the capital femoral epiphysis in relation to the femoral shaft is unusual, but possible. When it occurs it is usually acute and traumatic.

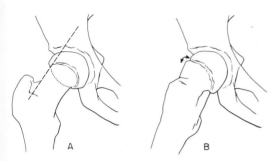

Fig. 4.73. Diagram of the normal relation of the capital femoral epiphysis to the extension of a line drawn along the superior aspect of the neck. (*A*) Anterior view, (*B*) lateral view. (Redrawn from the *American Journal of Roentgenology, Radium Therapy, and Nuclear Medicine, 46:* 386, 1951.)

Pathology

Irritation of the hip joint results in edema and hyperemia in the synovia. In the earliest stage of slipped epiphysis these changes, plus some perivascular lymphocytic infiltrations and villous formation, are all that are noted. In the cases of actual slipping, the epiphysis is not completely detached from the neck but remains attached by periosteum and fibrous tissue. The epiphyseal disc remains attached to the head, the slipping taking place in the more distal layers. The epiphysis is downward and posterior to the neck which slips foward and upward. The angles between neck and epiphysis tend to fill in with callus. The articular cartilage appears normal. The bluish fibrous tissue covering that part of the neck formerly contiguous with the epiphyseal line is smooth and glistening and tends to hide the true location of the epiphyseal line. During a period of several years, the head and neck gradually form a bony union incorporating the epiphyseal line. Late changes in this disease reveal a firm, sclerotic, and

Fig. 4.74. Diagram of slip visible in the anteroposterior view only. No slip is seen in the lateral view. (Redrawn from the *American Journal of Roentgenology, Radium Therapy, and Nuclear Medicine, 46:* 386, 1951.)

Fig. 4.75. Diagram of slip recognizable in the lateral view only. (Redrawn from the *American Journal of Roentgenology, Radium Therapy, and Nuclear Medicine, 46:* 386, 1951.)

thickened capsule and conversion of the callus at the inferior angle of the epiphysis to bone.

Clinical Picture

The typical patient has noted pain in the hip, thigh, or knee, often for several months, and has developed an antalgic limp. Since the hip capsule may not always be markedly irritated, it is not uncommon for the patient to have a history of low grade symptoms of considerable duration.

If the symptoms and the limp are acute, one suspects a slip that has caused the neck and shaft to rotate outward and upward in relation to the head.

On examination the appearance of the patient may be so typical as to allow suspicion of the diagnosis on sight. A large frame, heavy thighs, underdeveloped genitalia, and external rotation of the leg point to the slipped epiphysis. When the thigh is flexed, the leg tends to ride into external rotation and frequently cannot be brought to neutral.

If the hip is irritated, other motion is also limited and a hip flexion contracture is present. If hip irritation is minimal, the patient may actually have increased hyperextension consistent with the degree of slip.

When slipped femoral epiphysis is suspected, the patient should leave the examining room in recumbency, since further slip complicates treatment and jeopardizes the end result.

Roentgen Signs

The earliest manifestation of slipping consists of widening of the epiphyseal line and irregular demineralization of the area immediately adjacent to it. The capsular shadow is rounded and more prominent than normal.

Klein et al.[4] have emphasized the fact that a line drawn along the superior surface of the neck to the outer edge of the acetabulum normally leaves the lateral angle of the head outside it. Medial slipping can be detected in the anteroposterior view of the hip when the head is not transected by this line but lies within it. Posterior slipping, in which the change in relationship is more obvious because the axis of the neck leaves the epiphysis, is detected in the lateral view. A generalized atrophy or demineralization of the head and neck may be apparent.

The epiphysis does not always lie both posterior and medial to the neck. In the anteroposterior view in Klein's cases, a medial slip was apparent in only 68%. In the lateral view of these cases, posterior displacement was evident in 98%. In speaking of the degree or distance of slip, the lateral view is ordinarily used.

Fig. 4.76. A well defined epiphyseal slip with widened epiphyseal line and a build-up of bone beneath the head on the inferior neck on the right are seen.

Treatment

Treatment begins immediately upon suspicion of the diagnosis. The external rotation maneuver performed on the x-ray table to procure the lateral view should be gently and not forcibly done. Once the diagnosis is made, the patient is placed in traction in abduction, and an internal rotation strap is added to his thigh. A considerable improvement in the range of hip motion can often be obtained by traction prior to operation.

Slipped epiphysis of minimal degree may be treated conservatively by a plaster spica and immobilization of the hip until the epiphyseal line is obliterated. The immobilization should be interrupted by periods of traction to maintain good hip motion.

Internal fixation in situ is generally thought to be preferable. There is a generally accepted rule that displacement of the 1 cm or less can be internally fixed in situ. A minimal slip of this type is compatible with good function of the hip if no further slip occurs.

Fixation in situ is done through a lateral proximal femoral incision in a manner similar to that used in treating transcervical fractures of the hip in the adult. A cassette is placed beneath the hip, and a second portable x-ray machine is placed under the contralateral thigh and aimed so as to take a lateral view of the neck with the anterior superior spine of the ilium in the direct line of the rays. The first machine is moved over the hip for the anterior posterior view when necessary. Accurate and firm fixation with the device placed well into the femoral head is necessary.

If a nail of the triflanged Smith-Peterson type is used, it should have an especially sharp point, and the possibility of displacing the head in the process of driving in the nail should be borne in mind. If a screw is used, the head should be fixed by an external wire in the process of insertion so that rotation of the head does not result in further displacement. It is possible that the impaction produced by a screw at the epiphyseal line will result in earlier fusion. In general, the insertion of one or two screws is preferable to the use of a nail or pins.

The use of grafts of the match stick type placed across the epiphyseal line has been advocated by Howorth[3] to hasten closure of the line.

Approximately 1 out of 4 cases of slipped epiphysis seen are afflicted by a severe degree of slipping and by reposition of the epiphysis in relation to the neck. It is necessary to procure a functioning hip which will not degenerate later into the marked limitation brought on by arthritic changes.

A very few patients with severe cases have an acute history. There is no rounding of the corners of the neck or buildup of callus about the slipped epiphysis by x-ray in cases of acute slip. When the slip has been associated with acute trauma, it is sometimes possible to

Fig. 4.77. Acute slip of the femoral epiphysis without ossification at the inferior neck.

Fig. 4.78. (*Top*) Slipped femoral epiphysis treated by screw fixation on the right, and apparently normal hip on left. (*Bottom*) Same patient 4 months later with filling in of the epiphyseal line on the right, but widening and radiolucency of the epiphyseal line developing on the left.

manipulate the hip with internal rotation and abduction of the lower extremity. When gentle manipulation is successful, the hip may be nailed in situ. The remaining cases of acute slip require open arthrotomy for correction of the mechanical derangement and internal fixation.

Southwick Biplane Osteotomy

Southwick[5] has noted that if the capital femoral epiphysis has left its anatomic position by 30° or more in any one plane the function of the hip will be seriously affected. He has devised a method of correction that leads to accurate restoration of the position of the slipped capital femoral epiphysis through an osteotomy at the level of the lesser trochanter.

The physical examination of the patient is used to aid in determining the degree of correction required. If the normal hip flexes to 130° and the affected hip to but 70° with no external rotation, a 60° correction of posterior tilt would be required. A similar estimate of the limitation of abduction is made. These estimates are used in conjunction with the x-ray measurement.

Anteroposterior films are obtained with the hip in neutral positions. A frogleg lateral view is taken with the hip in maximum abductor and external rotation with the knees flexed and the feet facing each other while their lateral surfaces rest on the table. Measurements are made on the films to determine the varus deformity and degree of posterior tilting. A tin template bent at 90° to wrap around the femur and giving both the anterior and lateral osteotomy outline is made. The more bone that is removed the more shortening will occur—it should be as little as possible and with exact accuracy as to the angles.

Fig. 4.81. In this diagram of subluxation existing with slipped epiphysis of the proximal femur, the abutment of the uncovered neck against the acetabular rim is emphasized. Considerable improvement in cases of old healed slips in a malunited position may be gained by surgical excision of the shaded area, as emphasized by Heyman.

Fig. 4.79. Slipped epiphysis, anteroposterior and lateral roentgenograms. Displacement is visible in the lateral view.

Fig. 4.80. The use of the internal rotation strap aids in reducing the external rotation contracture. The adhesive is kept from pulling on the lateral side of the leg by felt placed between it and the skin.

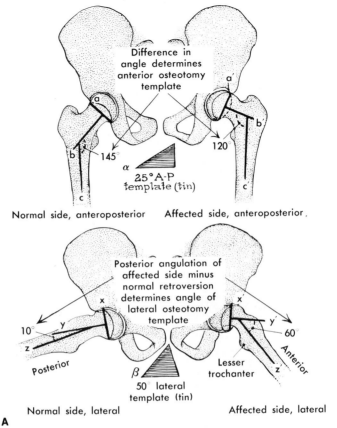

A

Fig. 4.82. Southwick has devised a biplane osteotomy accurately designed to correct the degree of malalignment of the capital femoral epiphysis to the femoral shaft in two planes. (*A*) Diagram of the calculations for the template guiding the osteotomy. (*B*) Operative site. (*C*) Wedge removed at operative site. (*D*) Placement of internal fixation. (Reprinted from W. O. Southwick: Osteotomy through the lesser trochanter for slipped capital femoral epiphysis, *Journal of Bone & Joint Surgery, 49A:* 807, 1967.)

The operation is done through a lateral incision exposing the anterolateral aspect of the femoral shaft at the level of the lesser trochanter. The iliopsoas tendon is released. The anterolateral edge or corner of the femoral shaft is marked with an osteotome. Another orientation mark is made at right angles to the first at the level of the lesser trochanter. This mark is transverse to the femoral shaft. The template is superimposed in relation to these orientation and transverse marks. The appropriate outline is marked with an osteotome. It will lead to a laterally based wedge looking at the anterior surface of the femur and an anteriorly based wedge looking at the lateral aspect.

A Steinmann pin is inserted to control the proximal femur prior to making the biplane osteotomy cuts.

As the wedge of bone is removed, a flat surface will be left on both upper and lower fragment. The osteotomy wedge need not occupy the entire transverse diameter of the bone, the remaining bone can be divided transversely. Sufficient bone should be removed, however, to provide broad bony contact. Tilting of the osteotomy site by more than 60° shortens the femur excessively. The osteotomy is closed bringing the cut bony surface together. Southwick holds his osteotomy in position by multiple pins inserted through a pin-holding device into the proximal and distal fragments. Plates may be used. A plaster spica is also necessary after this preliminary support is applied. The cast ordinarily holds the patient for 8 weeks. The epiphyseal line is normally fused by the time the osteotomy is healed.

Fig. 4.82*B*

Fig. 4.82*C*

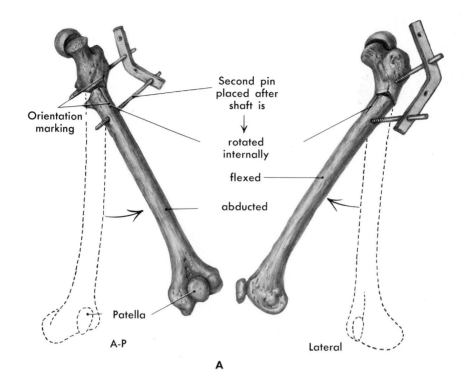

Orientation marking

Second pin placed after shaft is

rotated internally

flexed

abducted

Patella

A-P

Lateral

A

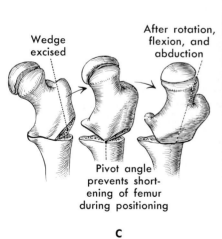

Wedge excised

After rotation, flexion, and abduction

Pivot angle prevents short-ening of femur during positioning

C

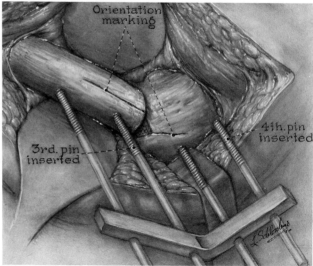

Orientation marking

3rd. pin inserted

4th. pin inserted

D

Fig. 4.82D

Wedge Osteotomy and Klein Procedure

The hip may be approached anteriorly through the Smith-Peterson incision, as advocated by Klein,[4] or posteriorly through a Gibson incision.

The displacement of the epiphysis may be corrected by a wedge osteotomy of the neck. Another method concentrates on the area of the epiphyseal line. This area is divided without removal of a wedge, and the neck is slid back into place beneath the epiphysis.

The first method results in shortening of the neck and thereby relieves stress on the stretched neck vessels. The fact that this method does not interfere with the retinaculum of Weitbrecht and maintains circulation to the femoral epiphysis has been noted by Green. The second method has produced excellent results in the cases treated by Klein et al.[4] When a wedge of bone has been removed prior to replacement of the head, an absolute anatomic reduction cannot be reacquired.

The operation, whether it is performed through an anterior or posterior approach with or without the removal of a wedge, has certain underlying principles.

These include gentle handling of the epiphysis and maintenance of the blood supply to it. Both the internal and external femoral circumflex arteries provide branches running up to the femoral neck. The posterior, superior, and inferior portions of the capsule are particularly important. The capsule should be divided parallel to the lip of the acetabulum and next to it. A further incision should be made only if it is absolutely necessary and should split the capsule in line with the femoral neck so that there is as little interference as possible with the blood supply.

After the head is divided from the neck, the reduction is carried out with the aid of a bone skid and is followed by internal fixation from the lateral cortex of the femur.

Postoperative Treatment

The patient is placed in traction until the postoperative discomfort and muscle spasm have subsided. When the hip can be moved freely, the patient is allowed partial weight-bearing with crutches. Fusion of the epiphysis is noted in 2-8 months after open reduction and in 6 months to 2 years following nailing in situ. Once the epiphsyis has fused, the internal fixation apparatus is removed.

The possibility of involvement of the contralateral side must be constantly kept in mind, and nailing in situ must be performed if the diagnosis is made. Postoperative films should always include both hips. Involvement of the other hip usually takes place within the first year and a half after the initial diagnosis, but may not occur until two or more years later.

The results following nailing in situ for mimimal slips are excellent. The results following open reduction are good if the basic requirements of care are well attended to. These requirements include sparing the vascular supply to the epiphysis during the operation, anatomic repositioning, and early mobilization.

The development of aseptic necrosis of the

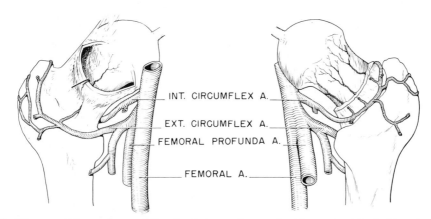

INT. CIRCUMFLEX A.

EXT. CIRCUMFLEX A.

FEMORAL PROFUNDA A.

FEMORAL A.

Fig. 4.83. Diagram of the anatomy of the circulation to the proximal femoral epiphysis. Note that transverse division of the capsule proximally (acetabular side) does not jeopardize the circulation.

Fig. 4.84. Measurement of the amount of slip is made along the arc of slip, as indicated by the *arrows* in the anteroposterior views (*A, B*) and lateral views (*C, D*).

Fig. 4.85. Equipment to procure roentgenograms of the hip is necessary when treating slipped epiphysis operatively. Films must be taken in two planes. The placement of the tube for anteroposterior and lateral views is shown. (Redrawn from A. Klein et al.: *Slipped Capital Femoral Epiphysis,* Springfield, Ill., Charles C Thomas, 1953.)

head threatens a successful result. Such complications are rare, but they occur in all series. Badgley reports three instances in seventy-five hips. The initial displacement may predeter-mine aseptic necrosis regardless of the method used and the care taken in handling the case.

Cartilage Necrosis

Narrowing of the hip joint cartilage space as seen by x-ray is a complication of slipped epiphysis. It occurs in approximately 10% of the cases. It appears to be related to a severe synovitis of the hip accompanying the disease. Clinically it is manifest by markedly limited motion in all planes and by muscle spasm and pain. It can result in a severe hip disability. Not all cases are irreversible, however. Some will recover a considerable portion of the joint space and joint function if followed on a conservative, non-weight-bearing regime with preliminary traction.

For the others the disease represents a severe complication. It can be seen after both minimal and severe slips of the capital femoral epiphysis.

References

1. Ferguson, A. B., and Howorth, M. B.: Slipping of the upper fermoral epiphysis, *J.A.M.A., 97:* 1867, 1931.

2. Ghormley, R. K., and Fairchild, R. D.: Diagnosis and treatment of slipped epiphysis, *J.A.M.A., 114:* 229, 1940.
3. Howorth, M. B.: Slipping of the upper femoral epiphysis, *J. Bone & Joint Surg., 31-A:* 734, 1949.
4. Klein, A., Joplin, R., Reidy, J., and Hanelin, J.: *Slipped Capital Femoral Epiphysis,* Charles C Thomas, Springfield, Ill., 1948.
5. Southwick, W. O.: Osteotomy through the lesser trochanter for slipped capital femoral epiphysis, *J. Bone & Jone Surg., 49A:* 807, 1967.
6. Waldenstrom, H.: On necrosis of the joint cartilage of epiphysiolysis capites femoris, *Acta Chir. Scand., 67:* 936, 1930.
7. Wilson, P. D.: Treatment of slipping of the upper femoral epiphysis with minimal displacement, *J. Bone & Joint Surg., 20:* 379, 1938.

SYNOVITIS OF HIP*

Acute synovitis of the hip is one of the most common orthopaedic conditions seen. It is an infammatory condition of the hip of short duration, relieved by rest. It looms in the forefront of every differential diagnosis of childhood limp. Although this condition is so common, it seldom has been described. It is

* This section, "Synovitis of Hip," is reprinted from A. B. Ferguson, Jr.: Synovitis of the hip and Legg-Perthes disease, *Clinical Orthopaedics, 4:* 180, 1954, by permission of J. B. Lippincott Co.

related to Legg-Perthes disease in that it is potentially preliminary to it.

A review of the cases admitted to the Children's Hospital (Pittsburgh) over the last 4 years reveals that the age distribution is very similar to the 3-10-year-old group found in coxa plana. Occasionally, a case as old as 12 may be seen. Four out of 5 cases are males.

Acute synovitis of the hip is sometimes so mild that its symptoms attract little attention; sometimes it is so severe that it is mistaken for a septic hip joint. Occasionally, cases are recognized by roentgenogram only as synovitis which go on to develop the typical changes of coxa plana.

Etiology

Very frequently, there is a history of respiratory illness from 10 days to 3 weeks prior to the onset of hip symptoms. The relationship of these predominantly strepto-coccal infections to the inflammatory changes of the hip is not clear. When trauma looms large in the history, the presence of free blood in the joint is postulated. Occasionally, this has been confirmed by aspiration. Despite this occasionally clear implication, it is apparent that no single etiologic agent exists; whether or not

Fig. 4.86. Synovitis of the hip. The outline of the capsular shadows is rounded and increased in width on the right; the normal straight outline is seen on the left.

such a joint is an allergic manifestation is uncertain.

Clinical Features

The patient is typically a male about the age of 5. Pain usually begins at the knee in the previous 24 hr. The pain tends to become more localized at the hip as the disease progresses. Frequently, the temperature at the height of the symptoms is as high as 101F, occasionally, 103F. However, the leukocytes ordinarily are not increased. The failure of an increase in the leukocytes aids in differentiating the condition from a septic hip when the temperature is high. The sedimentation rate may be slightly elevated.

Motion of the hip always is limited. There is temporary flexion contracture and limited rotation, particularly internal rotation in flexion, together with limited abduction. Palpation of the hip joint reveals both anterior and posterior tenderness.

Fig. 4.87. Diagrams of the capsular shadows from the accompanying roentgenograms. (*Top*) The hip is that of a patient with symptoms and signs of synovitis with bulging capsular shadow. (*Bottom*) The hip is normal.

Fig. 4.88. Boy, age 3 years, 7 months, with growth arrest of the capital femoral epiphysis on the reader's right (*A*). In (*B*) 8 months later, deminerilization of the epiphysis has occurred. (*C*) Growth restoration is evident 14 months after onset; (*D*) 25 months after onset, the epiphysis is restored.

Roentgenographic Findings

There are two definite x-ray findings. The most obvious of these is swelling of the capsular shadows about the hip. The rounded, increased prominence of the capsular shadows about the hip is seen best superiorly and laterally. Accompanying this is a minimal widening of the hip joint. Although slight and often found only by measurement, still it is commonly seen. Widening of the hip joint space is recognized more easily in the medial inferior portion of the joint. The anteroposterior view of the hip is most instructive. There are no bone changes suggestive of coxa plana.

Fig. 4.88 C and D.

Differential Diagnosis

The hip inflamed because of tuberculous involvement has a chronic history which acute synovitis does not have. Septic involvement of the hip must be differentiated by the more definite signs of sepsis—elevation of the white count and shift to the left. Aspiration may be necessary but in practice rarely turns out to be so. Other possible underlying causes of inflammation of the hip, such as rheumatic fever or rheumatoid arthritis, are evident on general physical examination or future course.

Fig. 4.89. (*A*) Growth arrest and metaphyseal demineralization followed by bone resorption in (*B*).

Treatment

The inflammation about the hip tends readily to subside when weight bearing is eliminated. Traction in line with the flexion contracture is the most certain method of obtaining rapid subsidence of symptoms. While relief from pain is almost immediate, it usually takes from 36 to 72 hr to regain full motion at the hip. Failure to regain full motion at the hip within 4 or 5 days leads to a suspicion that a more serious etiology underlies the condition.

The patient usually is given 1 week of non-weight bearing after full motion has been regained to guard against recurrence. Recurrences lead to a suspicion of coxa plana.

LEGG-PERTHES DISEASE

Although synovitis of the hip may be preliminary to coxa plana, aseptic necrosis of the proximal femoral epiphysis may start without any previous difficulty at the hip. It is known variously as Legg-Perthes disease, osteochondritis deformans coxae juvenilis, or coxa plana. The condition may be defined as a disease of the hip limited by age group and largely by sex; it results in changes in the femoral head apparently secondary to a loss of adequate vascular supply. Its duration is self-limited, but its course may result in irreversible mechanical impairment of the hip. The age group runs predominantly from 3 to 10 years old, with occasionally a case as old as 12. As in synovitis of the hip, the disease occurs predominantly in males (80%). Although Legg-Perthes disease can be bilateral, it is most often unilateral (90%).

Etiology

A good understanding of coxa plana can be achieved if it is considered as a disease of the soft tissues rather than of the bone; then the swelling of soft-tissue shadows about the hip, present on the roentgenogram, is not lost to observation in the presence of rather striking bone changes. Ferguson and Howorth[7] have noted the presence of thickened blood vessel walls and thickened capsule in surgically observed cases. They postulated a relationship between previous simple synovitis of the hip or other causes of inflammation at the hip joint and coxa plana. Many have tried to implicate thyroid deficiency because of the occasional occurrence of a similar x-ray change at the hip in cretins. Conditions resulting in irregular ossification of the femoral head, such as chondrodysplasia, bear a superficial resemblance by roentgenogram but are not associated with capsular swelling about the hip or with clinical symptoms and usually have other stigmata of the underlying condition. It is possible to have an aseptic necrosis of the proximal femoral epiphysis in medical embolic disorders. This includes infections and physiologic variations such as caisson disease.

Aseptic necrosis of the femoral head is seen in patients with congenital dislocation of the

Fig. 4.90. (A) Onset of Legg-Perthes disease, with growth arrest and central involvement. (B) Lateral view reveals fracture of living peripheral (cortical) bone from the present avascular bone as described by Caffey (on left). (C) Later roentgenogram from anteroposterior view, blocking out dead central segment which has collapsed. The living bone laterally is evident and uninvolved.

hip. It has been noted particularly when the hip has been fixed in marked internal rotation.

The importance of abduction as a means of shutting off the vascular supply to the proximal femoral epiphysis has lately been appreciated in studies of the effect of the iliopsoas and capsule in congenital dislocation of the hip (Ferguson) on the limbus superiorly (Ogden).

Pathology

There is a difference between aseptic necrosis of a segment of the femoral head in a child as compared to an adult. Many of the pathologic features are the same including the area of involvement. The differences are occasioned by the epiphyseal line. A lateral fracture at the epiphyseal line can allow displacement of the lateral viable segment. The epiphyseal line itself can be fractured into the metaphysis and of course growth of the epiphysis itself is affected. The epiphyseal line fracture, fibrous metaplasia invading metaphysis and epiphysis, and lateral epiphyseal fracture of a segment of the epiphysis all occur following separation of the avascular central segment.

First Stage

Both Legg-Perthes disease and aseptic necrosis of the femoral head have a similar area of involvement. This area is superior to the fovea and the major portion is anterior. It is the area supplied by a branch of the lateral epiphyseal

Fig. 4.90 C.

Fig. 4.91. The fracture of living cortical bone segment from the avascular central segment. (Courtesy of Robert Clark, M.D.)

Fig. 4.92. The dead segment centrally replaced by fibrous tissue. The periphery is vital and living bone. The cartilage is overgrown.

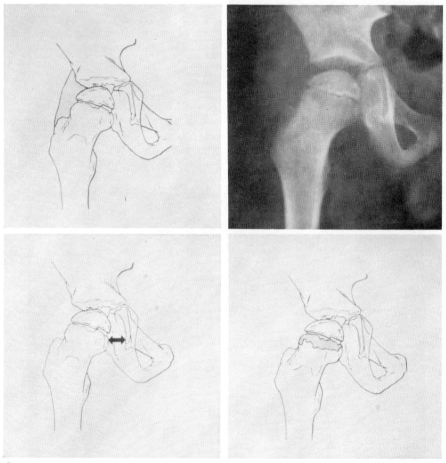

Fig. 4.93. Early signs of Legg-Perthes disease of the hip by roentgenogram. Bulging capsular shadows, increased density of epiphysis, widened joint space, and demineralized metaphysis adjacent to the epiphyseal line are shown.

Fig. 4.94. Prediction of expected result in coxa plana from the roentgenogram when first seen. The predicted flattened outline of the head is diagrammed at *top, right*. (*Bottom*) The follow-up roentgenogram of the same case and accompanying diagram.

artery described by Brodetti.[1a] Brodetti's artery enters the femoral head laterally and slightly posteriorly. The extent of the infarction secondary to its interruption can be variable, but never involves the entire head with one exception. This exception is the younger age group (below 2 years), when the ossification center occupies a small central segment of the cartilaginous head.

The first change in terms of roentgen features is obvious cessation of growth of the ossification center. It is smaller on the involved side. This may be true over 2 years of age as well when the involvement of the artery and the infarction affects growth in height of the ossification center of the femoral head in its central portion.

At this time cartilage proliferation continues unimpeded. Bone growth has stopped. Equatorial growth of the cartilage makes a contribution to widening of the femoral head and neck eventually.

In the younger age group below age 5 years the ossification center is contained within the femoral head sufficiently that the acetabular lip is lateral to it in abduction. Weight-bearing pressure is widespread and not localized. The possibility of infraction and separation of the

Fig. 4.94.1. Dead segment of bone (dark area) in center of femoral head. A lateral viable segment and a medial viable segment are on either side. The superior cortical fracture is composed of cartilage and viable bone and is visualized at the onset of Legg-Perthes disease. The fracture of the dead segment from the living bone on either side represents further progression of the disease. The lateral edge of the acetabulum must be supported by the lateral viable segment or compression will occur.

dead segment from the viable area about it is reduced. This accounts for the improved outlook in terms of clinical involvement in the younger age group.

Second Stage

There is evidence of two processes occurring. One is in growth of new vessels laying down bone on the old trabeculae. At this stage there is no infraction of trabeculae. The new bone that is laid down increases the radiodensity of the segment. Careful visualization of the roentgenogram leads to recognition of a large and wide medial, posterior segment which is not involved, as well as a small lateral segment with a varying progression anteriorly of uninvolved bone.

The importance of this second stage new bone formation was shown by Clark. He tested revascularized femoral heads with a standard trauma. Deformation occurred secondary to the trauma once the head was revascularized.

The second process that is evident at this stage is a fracture of viable subchondral bone and cartilage from the dead segment beneath it. This occurs in the weight-bearing area of the femoral head and extends for a varying distance anteriorly. It is visualized as a thin radiolucent line and may be seen in either the anteroposterior or lateral view (or both) of the femoral head. From this point onward progression of the disease can lead to a lateral epiphyseal fracture and extrusion of the femoral head laterally from the acetabulum. Once the preliminary signs are recognized the lateral extrusion can occur within a 2-month period.

Third Stage

The separation of the avascular segment from the medical and lateral viable areas causes the subchondral bone and cartilage overlying it to float free without support. The area becomes depressed and flattening of the femoral head is evident superiorly. With the lateral epiphyseal

Fig. 4.94.2. Further progression in Legg-Perthes disease occurs with weight bearing. The central necrotic fragment when revascularized is deformed, the epiphyseal line is fibrillated and fractured into the metaphysis and fibrous metaplasia occurs. The lateral viable segment is displaced laterally by a fracture at the epiphyseal line allowing further pressure on the dead segment.

fracture the weight-bearing load abraids the cartilage and the force transmits without distribution to the epiphyseal line. The line fractures into the metaphysis beneath the avascular segment. Fibrous metaplasia occurs streaming in through the breaks in the epiphyseal line to replace the dead bone. The fibrous tissue adds little support to the femoral head and further loss of height occurs. The fibrous metaplasia occurs well into the metaphysis and is visualized radiographically as extrusion radiolucent areas from the epiphyseal line into the metaphysis.

The area of involvement is principally anterior but extends linearly posteriorly about twice the distance of the involvement between the medial and lateral segments.

Fourth Stage

With fibrous metaplasia entering the picture, the femoral head becomes a poor weight-bearing organ. The lateral epiphyseal fracture is accompanied by widening of the bone of the

neck as it grows into the area of chondrogenesis which has extended down the neck. Further flattening of the femoral head occurs as fibrogens of the metaphysis extend into the formerly viable medial and lateral segments. This process occurs due to stress bringing about trabecular fractures in these previously unaffected segments. This occurs principally laterally and the lateral segment may decrease in size as visualized roentgenographically.

The end result of a thin, flat femoral head epiphysis can be prevented if the lateral epiphyseal segment is contained within the acetabulum before it fractures and is extruded and prior to fracture and extrusion of the epiphyseal line into the metaphysis.

Lateral Epiphyseal Fracture

In an older child of 9 years the flattening of the central dead segment is apparent as it fractures and displaces downward from the original joint outline. A lateral viable segment can be seen as well as a medial viable segment can be seen at this juncture with varying degrees of involvement of the radiolucent extension into the metaphysis. At this juncture the end result is still recoverable providing extensive lateral displacement of the lateral viable fracture has not occurred. This epiphyseal line fracture is caused by descent of the dead portion and its lateral extrusion into the ossification center exuding this viable fragment laterally. When this occurs osteotomy may be necessary to get coverage of the proximal femoral epiphysis. X-ray frequently portrays the lateral viable segment being moved laterally by descent of the central dead segment. At times in the lateral view the lateral fragment is not visualized and only appears in this incorrect position when ossification occurs in this area.

Clinical Picture

Legg-Perthes disease covers an age group roughly from 3 to 12 years. Those below the age of 6 at onset may be discovered late in the disease when deformity and synovitis finally occur, or incidentally when x-ray examination is conducted for some other reason.

Characteristically, there is a history of limp and pain at the knee, usually for a period of 3 weeks to 2 months before being seen. The patient is usually a boy and most often 4-6 years old, although he may be anywhere in the 3-12-year-old group. There is a hip flexion contracture readily elicited, and further testing of the motions in flexion develops the limitation of internal rotation and abduction. The hip will come to neutral in rotation. There may be tenderness both anteriorly and posteriorly to external palpation of the hip joint. Measurement of the midthigh often reveals atrophy of ½-1 inch. Even if not measurable, atrophy is regularly recognizable by palpation of the thigh and the gluteal area. The child may be in acute distress. In contrast with this picture, occasionally and rarely there are children who present such mild features that the disease is recognized only by detailed and thorough examination of the motions of the hip. Only by taking the time to make a detailed recording of hip motion, particularly in flexion, will the examiner avoid the embarrassment of having the case diagnosed more successfully elsewhere.

Not all cases of Legg-Perthes disease have symptoms immediately at onset. Some cases first are seen when there is already in existence considerable widening of the neck and the joint space, with no history of previous symptoms; then there are changes which are irreversible. These are not apparent when the femoral head is radiolucent, but study of the roentgenogram will reveal that the shape of the head can be predicted. The stages of coxa plana are discerned best by roentgenogram.

Roentgen Findings

First Stage (Incipient)

There is swelling of the capsular shadows about the hip, widening of the joint space, and demineralization of the femoral metaphysis in the neck immediately adjacent to the epiphyseal line.

Growth stoppage of the proximal femoral epiphysis is an early sign. The bony epiphysis will be smaller on the involved side when this occurs. This may be evident before increased density is evident.

Second Stage (Aseptic Necrosis)

The changes of the first stage are present; in addition, there is definite increase in density of the femoral head in its entirety or in some portion. The area supplied by vascular channels from the ligamentum teres may be spared. Often cases are seen first at this stage. If no widening of the neck has taken place and the head is outlined fully, then no irreversible changes occurred, and treatment has the possibility of restoring a good hip.

A radiolucent line is often seen running from the area of the fovea beneath the subchondral bone. This was described by Caffey[1b] as a fracture line. Experimental pathology studies reveal this as a fracture extending between a dead subchondral segment and the live bone beneath.

Third Stage (Regenerative)

Here, revitalization of the head is taking place, as evidenced by the presence of radiolucent areas. Widening of the femoral neck also may be evident. One can outline, on the basis of the neck width and joint space remaining, the area of the head not visualized. Often to do so is illuminating. It may be evident that considerable mechanical malformation already has taken place. Such malformation still may be compatible with good hip function, but the anatomic outline will not be normal. Still further severity in flattening and widening of the head may be present, so that a poor result is foreordained. However, treatment should not allow any further progression if it is to be of value. In the last portion of this stage, regeneration of the femoral head takes place until the head is filled in completely.

Relation to Coxa Magna

Coxa magna is a frequent end result of coxa plana. Its development can be ascribed to the cartilage overgrowth that apparently takes place under conditions of impaired vascularity at the hip. Widening of the femoral neck becomes evident in the second stage of coxa plana, when conditions of aseptic necrosis are well established. The regenerating head must match this increased width of neck, regardless of whatever other deformity the head may have. The head reformed without deformity other than increased size is consistent with good motion at the hip. However, such increased width results in emergence of the lateral portion of the head from beneath the overhanging acetabular roof. Apparently, coxa magna can occur without the development of aseptic necrosis of the head, that is, as an entity quite separate from coxa plana.

When the coxa magna occurs with incongruity and some lateral flattening of the head and the formation of bone lateral to the acetabulum it leads to limited motion at the hip joint. The lateral bone formation at the epiphysis is a poor prognostic sign. It is often due to lateral extrusion of a viable portion of the epiphyseal ossification center.

Classification According to Area of Involvement

Goff,[11] in a study of 150 children with Legg-Perthes disease, arrived at the following percentages for the various kinds of involvement of the femoral head. His findings have significance in light of the relation of the disease to the area of weight-bearing on the femoral head. This area has been studied by Goff and others in man, the gorilla, and lower forms of animal life.

Thirty-seven percent of the children were found to have total epiphyseal involvement. The epiphyses were involved bilaterally in 13%. Fifty percent, however, had only fractional or partial epiphyseal involvement.

In the cases of partial involvement, the disease practically always involved the anterior two-thirds of the epiphysis. Within 2-6 months there was resorption of this dense bone, indicating a rather rapid return to circulation. In these cases, the weight-bearing zone of the epiphysis was spared.

The clinical problem, then, becomes one of recognizing clearly and definitely just which type of involvement is present. To do so usually requires a 4 months' period of observation during which the hip joint must be protected by a non-weight-bearing splint or by recumbency.

Goff has located the weight-bearing portion of the femoral head in man by stress coat studies. The posterior portion of the head supports the body weight when the body is completely erect. The cortical bone is denser under the articular cartilage in this area. Studies of the blood supply of the proximal femoral epiphysis by Trueta et al. indicate that the posterior portion is more generously supplied than the anterior part. There is considerable variation in vascular patterns with age and genetic factors. Such variations help to explain the rarity of this disease in the Negro. However, in the age group concerned in Legg-Perthes disease and in the Caucasian race, the pattern appears quite constant.

Should the case be an early one, with minimal soft-tissue and bony involvement, it is possible that the time needed to progress to a regenerative stage may be relatively short. These patients regain full motion of the hip quickly and then they may be treated by absolute bed rest with frequent rexaminations to ensure that full motion is being maintained.

In the untreated cases the expected time intervals for each stage are as follows: first (incipient), from 2 to 4 weeks; second (aseptic necrosis), from 1 to 2 years: third (regenerative), from 3 to 4 years.

Coverage of Femoral Head

Emphasis on covering the femoral head with the acetabular outline as visualized on the roentgenogram with hip abducted has been

Fig. 4.95. Development of coxa magna from early coxa plana.

Fig. 4.96. Coxa magna in the adult with degenerative arthritis.

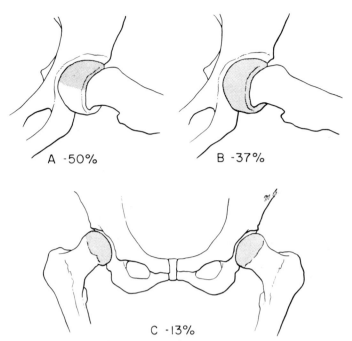

A -50%   B -37%

C -13%

Fig. 4.97. This diagrammatic illustration of the percentages for the various kinds of involvement of the femoral head in Legg-Perthes disease is derived from Goff's figures. *A* shows that 50% of the cases involved the anterior portion only. At least a 6-month follow-up of the patient is necessary to be certain that this is all that will be involved. *B* shows that 37% of the cases involved the entire epiphysis. In *C*, bilateral involvement is shown to be least common, occurring in only 13% of the cases. In this group, the possibility of epiphyseal dysplasia mimicking Legg-Perthes disease must be borne in mind. The differentiation may rest on the failure of the head to go through the various stages of aseptic necrosis.

made in the past decade. Petrie and Cruess brought to clinical attention the maintenance of femoral head outline and joint congruity by the use of a walking hip abduction spica. Despite holding the hip immobilized the anatomical results were good and spoke for the agility of children who mastered walking with crutches in the hip abduction cast.

The fact that the usual patten-bottom splint holding the foot 3 inches off the ground and carrying weight bearing through the ischial tuberosity resulted in an adducted position at the hip joint was also noted.

In order to keep the child in social participation and his hip still abducted, several types of walking hip abduction splints were devised. The simplest had an offset arm on the inside upright of the patten-bottom splint to keep the hip in abduction.

A return to weight bearing is justified when there have been no new dense areas in the femoral head for 2 months and there are no dense areas in the line of the stress trabeculae

of the head. The patient must have full motion at the hip joint. There also must be definite evidence that reconstruction is taking place in the head. It is not necessary to wait for a completely remineralized head, but sufficient bone structure should be present to arouse confidence in the preservation of that structure.

At the Newington home, abduction hip spicas were devised of plastic and bivalved to allow the removal, daily cleanliness, and non-weight-bearing maintenance of motion.

Regardless of the form the device takes, coverage of the femoral head by the acetabulum appears to be an important aid in achieving a good result in patients with this disease. It is particularly important in preventing lateral extension of bone formation of the femoral head.

If it is impossible for the femoral head to get into an abducted position in the acetabulum without pressure on the lateral portion of the acetabulum, a deformity of the acetabulum will occur over the ensuing 4-5 years.

Fig. 4.98. The progression of the maximum weight-bearing surface posteriorward on the femoral head as the monkey progresses into a more erect gait with more extension of the hip is shown. In animals walking with a flexed hip position, weight-bearings is more anteriorward. The areas that soften first as the bone is decalcified admit a marking ink that leaves bare the white area of maximum weight bearing as shown in femurs of the baboon, orangutan, chimpanzee, gorilla, and man. (Courtesy of C. W. Goff.)

Fig. 4.99. Split Russell traction in line with the flexion contracture of the irritated hip.

Fig. 4.100. Legg-Perthes disease in a patient who first presented late in the disease. Time interval: 2 years.

Treatment

The initial discussion of treatment relates to the early stages of the disease.

The primary treatment of Legg-Perthes disease revolves around the principle of containment. By containment is meant achieving location of the acetabular rim outside the femoral head. No matter what ultimate method we are going to choose to maintain this position, we are first going to have to achieve abduction of the hip.

First Goal

A full range of motion of the hip joint must be obtained by alleviating both synovitis and muscle spasm. Do not let a child go with

Fig. 4.101. Legg-Perthes disease in patient who was first seen early in the course of the disease. Time interval: 1 year.

limited hip motion. This leads to local pressure of the lateral third of the acetabulum on the femoral head and collapse and deformity at the junction of the living and dead bone.

In order to achieve a full range of motion, rest is certainly necessary and traction may have to be added. Traction carries with it the connotation of relieving muscle spasm, protecting the hip. This cannot be done by pulling on the hip in extension (as for instance by Buck's extension which is not traction). Traction must be in line with the deformity or contracture. In these cases there is often a flexion contracture of the hip of 45° or more. This requires, at

Fig. 4.102. Effect of osteotomy in Legg-Perthes disease. (*A*) Central collapse with vital peripheral segments; (*B*) 2 months following osteotomy there is a marked rush of vascularity to the area with demineralization of all but the central segment of the head; (*C*) 4 months later revascularization is taking place; (*D*) 13 months later there is reconstitution of the femoral head sufficient for weight bearing.

minimum, a sling beneath the proximal end of the tibia (Russell's traction) often accompanied by a pillow beneath the thigh. The traction must be alive—i.e., watched and changed as the muscle relaxes to gradually bring the hip out of deformity. In Legg-Perthes disease the limited motion may persist beyond the economic feasibility of maintaining the child in the

hospital in traction. Do not be afraid of insisting on bed rest and a home bound instruction (teacher) program for 3 months before embarking on your ultimate therapy of containment.

The full range of motion having been achieved there are a number of therapy choices.

1. *Full activity and full weight bearing.* This

Fig. 4.102 C and D.

is only feasible if the early stage is clearly over and there is minimal involvement of the femoral head so that obviously live bone is available for weight bearing and the head is naturally contained due to failure of the widening of the femoral neck and head to develop. This is most often true in the younger children below age 6. If this program is embarked on its pays to recheck the child at 6-week intervals in the early phase to make certain that synovitis and limited motion does not develop.

2. *Abduction cast* (Petrie and Cruess). The application of an abudction spica followed by containment of the femoral head wholly within the acetabulum gives excellent results in terms of preventing further deformity. It has disadvantages. It is hard to walk with crutches in an abduction spica. That the kids do merely proves how wonderful children are and what good athletes they can become, given a difficult task. The spica obviously limits motion—this is an undesirable feature since local pressure may occur causing fibrillation of cartilage. The

Fig. 4.103. Follow up in Legg-Perthes disease. (*A*) Boy first seen at age 6 with growth arrest and collagen of the central segment of the femoral head. (*B*) Anteroposterior view 15 years later with diminished head height and rounded outline. At this time the boy had become a prominent college basketball player who complained of an aching hip after each game. (*C*) The lateral view is more revealing as to the cause of symptoms with a small anterior projection at the junction of the femoral head and neck.

Fig. 4.103 C.

Fig. 4.104. Irregular ossification of both hips simulating Legg-Perthes disease. No clinical limitation of motion of the hips was apparent.

results as reported speak for themselves, however.

At Newington Children's Hospital, the inevitable immobilization of plaster has been relieved by a bivalved plaster simulation of the abduction spica. This is removable for non-weight-bearing exercise including swimming. This obvious advantage is countered by the fact that it is difficult for this apparatus to stand up to crutch walking—no matter what the fastenings holding the two halves together.

3. *Abduction splint.* There are two types: the ball joint abduction splint used in Toronto by Babechko and the tripod extension of a patten bottom splint (Tachjdian). Of the two, the ball joint abduction splint answers most of the biomechanical analysis eliminating weight-bearing pressure more firmly than the patten bottom splint modification.

How difficult it is for any material, including steel, to stand up to the activities of a child is evidenced by the ball joint abduction splint—it will fail in the face of a boy's activities although it may stand up forever in a Chevrolet cap. There is more freedom, there is hip motion, it is still difficult to get around, but it has some advantages over the spica.

4. *Patten bottom splint.* Holding the foot 3 inches off the ground with a cork elevation of the shoe on the uninvolved side does not prevent adduction of the hip and, therefore, failure of containment. It has the advantage of stretching out tight musculature by making a single lever arm of the leg (no knee hinge), but in the process excessive pressure on the femoral head must occur.

The extension of the patten bottom splint to prevent adduction by holding the splint abducted through a weight-bearing tripod attached on the medial side of the splint answers some of the objections to the splint.

The patten bottom splinting allows the child to enter into the programs of children his own age, an important advantage for his emotional and intellectual growth. Prolonged non-weight-bearing treatment in an institution is mentioned at this point only to be condemned.

Surgical Approach

The advantages of surgery lie in the psychiatry of the child. It gets the child back into the stream of social intercourse and emotional growth—and still preserves the hip joint. There are disadvantages to the approach—the unpleasantness of surgery—compensated for by meeting this brief encounter and finding in oneself the strength to overcome it and win, a confidence-gaining experience that makes the child realize his own strength.

Now the question is, what surgical approach does enough good to justify it and at what stage of the disease is it applicable? Remember enough motion is needed in abduction to get the femoral head fully beneath the acetabulum.

Femoral Osteotomy. It is simpler really to do the femoral rather than the acetabular osteotomy to get coverage of the femoral head. Less surgery is involved. The hip obviously has to be placed in varus so far as the femoral neck angle is concerned. Growth tends to restore the angle. The important consideration once we are past the full motion problem is how are we going to hold it so that the ultimate position accurately reflects our intellectual consideration and x-ray measurements of the problem? An abduction x-ray is necessary before operation to determine (a) that the hip fully enters the acetabulum and (b) the degree of abduction that is desired to hold the hip in and fix it in. The head neck fragment must be fixed before osteotomy. This requires two pins; with one pin, the proximal fragment may flex. (A useful approach in late disease, but not now.)

The osteotomy is done just above the lesser trochanter in order to get a hyperemic flush into the neck and femoral head. Two pins have already fixed the femoral head in the degree of abduction that has been determined necessary. Now the lower extremity is adducted in line with the trunk and weight bearing. How are we going to hold it accurately? A spica incorporating projecting pins is all right if you are confident with it. Otherwise an internal fixation device may be necessary. The usual nail and plate used in the adult may result in epiphyseal line damage. (A small one not holding the epiphyseal line may be practicable occasionally.) A small anterior plate or anterior angled plate (Laing) is probably the easiest answer but will hardly do alone. A hip spica for 6 weeks must be added.

After remvoal of the spica a period of recumbency is necessary to repair hip motion. To keep the child recumbent in prolonged fashion is ridiculous. If this is necessary, you should not have done the operation in the first place. The point of the operation is to get the child out in the world. If this is true, he is ready to go once he has regained hip motion into full activity.

Make sure the lateral aspect of the femoral head is alive, not pushed laterally, before osteotomy. If the head is fully contained, the operation will reward you and the patient.

Acetabular Osteotomy. It occurred to Robert Salter that changing the acetabulum relative to the femoral head and answering the principle of containment was achievable by doing the iliac osteotomy that he devised. It is an important means of containing the femoral head and permitting the child full activity.

The prerequisite is enough abduction to bring the femoral head wholly within the acetabulum. At a youngish age (over 10), there are secondary problems with the anatomical distortion secondary to iliac osteotomy.

There is no point in this osteotomy of the ilium if the acetabular rim cannot fully slide over the femoral head. Make sure this can occur before you start. The techniques of a Salter osteotomy is fully described elsewhere. If you are not a consummate orthopaedic surgeon who can do this osteotomy easily, do not start down this road.

If well done, the results can be excellent. Containment as a principle is observed, motion is quickly regained, and full activity is permitted. Once again, if this is not true, the operation should not have been done in the first place. The wholly contained hip with a good rim of living bone at the edge of the femoral head should sustain itself without the development of further deformity.

Missing will be the hematologic blush secondary to femoral osteotomy; gained is no varus—no limp—no necessity to regain valgus with growth.

Excision of Lateral Aspect of Femoral Head. This is occasionally referred to as bumpectomy—a term that seems too unprofessional for a textbook.

The problem is serious. The hip cannot be abducted and wholly contained within the acetabulum due to projection of a squashed or deformed lateral aspect of the femoral head projecting beyond the acetabulum.

If the motion is otherwise normal including rotation and abduction and the patient is older—over 10—you have a candidate for this procedure whom you can help. If you are going to remove this lateral projection, make sure you are going to do it completely. This requires good exposure, not necessarily iliofemoral. The posterior approach is useful as the lateral aspect of the head is readily visualized and all projections of the femoral head that limit motion can be readily visualizd.

This is rewarding compared to the preoperative state. Do not expect too much out of it—the hip will not regain full motion, but the immediate preoperative limitation will be relieved.

Summary

The lateral and slightly posterior placement of a hip nail can result in localized segmental avascular necrosis. The interruption of the lateral epiphyseal artery gives a picture of involvement which is consistent in both Legg-Perthes disease and in aseptic necrosis in the adult.

Containment becomes a principle in treatment that can be achieved. With evident fracture and hopefully before lateral epiphyseal fracture of the viable segment has occurred, containment must be achieved so healing can occur. If the head and neck begin to widen, osteotomy is indicated. If containment can be done some other way as by bracing—then it may be inicated as well. There is a vascular flush that occurs with osteotomy that may be of some help in addition to the positioning. The rapidity with which serious changes can occur is evident in following serial films. If fracture is present the patient is already at risk to develop lateral extrusion due to epiphyseal fracture: it takes about 2 months for this to occur. Further attempts at abduction in walking in this situation still further laterally extrudes the viable fragment and compresses the dead central fragment.

References

1a. Brodetti, A.: Blood supply of femoral neck and head in relation to the damaging effects of nails and screws. *J. Bone Joint Surg., 42B:* 794, 1960.
1b. Caffey, J.: Early roentgenographic changes in essential coxa plana. *Am. J. Roentgenol. Radium Therap. Nucl. Med., 103:* 620, 1968.
1. Chung, S. M. K., and Moe, J. H.: Legg-Perthes disease: clinical-radiographic correlations, *Clin. Orthop., 41:* 116, 1965.
2. Danforth, M. S.: The treatment of Legg-Calvé-Perthes disease without weight-bearing, *J. Bone Joint Surg., 16:* 516, 1934.
3. Danielsson, L. G., and Heinborg, J.: Late results of Perthes disease, *Acta Orthop. Scand., 36:* 70, 1965.
4. Eaton, G. O.: Long term results of treatment in cosa plana, *J. Bone Joint Surg., 49A:* 1031, 1967.
5. Evans, D. L.: Legg-Calvé-Perthes disease, *J. Bone Joint Surg., 40B:* 168, 1958.
6. Eyre-Brook, A. L.: Osteochondritis deformans coxae juveniles in Perthes disease; results of treatment by traction in recumbency, *Br. J. Surg., 24:* 166, 1966.
7. Ferguson, A. B., and Howorth, M. B.: Coxa plana and related conditions of the hip, *J. Bone Joint Surg., 16:* 789, 1934.
8. Ferguson, A. B., Sr.: Early radiographic changes in Perthes disease, *Clin. Orthop., 1:* 33, 1953.
9. Ferguson, A. B., Jr.: Synovitis of the hip and Legg-Perthes disease, *Clin. Orthop., 4:* 180, 1954.
10. Gill, A. B.: Legg-Perthes disease of the hip; its early roentgenographic manifestations and its cylical course, *J. Bone Joint Surg., 22:* 1013, 1940.
11. Goff, C. W.: Recumbency vs. non-recumbency treatment of Legg-Perthes disease, *Clin. Orthop., 14:* 50, 1959.

12. Haythorn, S. R.: Pathological changes in Legg-Calvé-Perthes disease, *J. Bone Joint Surg., 31A:* 599, 1949.

14. Heyman, C. H., and Herndon, C. H.: Legg-Perthes disease; method for the measurement of the roentgenographic result, *J. Bone Joint Surg., 32A:* 767, 1950.

13. Herndon, C. H., and Heyman, C. H.: Legg-Perthes disease; evaluation of treatment by traction and ischial weight-bearing brace, *J. Bone Joint Surg., 34A:* 25, 1952.

15. Howorth, M. B.: Coxa plana, *J. Bone Joint Surg., 30A:* 601, 1948.

16. Legg, A. T.: The end results of coxa plana, *J. Bone Joint Surg., 31A:* 599, 1949.

17. Levy, L. J., and Girard, P. M.: Legg-Perthes disease; comparative study of the various methods of treatment, *J. Bone Joint Surg., 24:* 66, 1942.

18. Mindell, E. R., and Sherman, M. S.: Late results in Perthes disease, *J. Bone Joint. Surg., 33A:* 1, 1951.

19. O'Garra, J. A.: The radiographic changes in Perthes disease, *J. Bone Joint Surg., 41B:* 465, 1959.

20. Pike, M. M.: Legg-Perthes disease; method of conservative treatment, *J. Bone Joint Surg., 32A:* 663, 1950.

21. Ponsiti, I. V.: Legg-Perthes disease; observations on pathological changes in 2 cases, *J. Bone Joint Surg., 38A:* 739, 1956.

22. Ralston, E. L.: Legg-Calvé-Perthes disease; factors in healing, *J. Bone Joint Surg., 43A:* 249, 1961.

23. Ratcliff, A. H. C.: Perthes' disease, *J. Bone Joint Surg., 49B:* 102, 1967.

24. Waldenstrom, H.: The first stages of coxa plana, *J. Bone Joint Surg., 20:* 559, 1938.

25. Wansbough, M. B., Carrie, A. W., Walker, N. F., and Rukerbauer, M. A.: Coxa plana, its genetic aspects and results of treatment with the long taylor walking caliper, *J. Bone Joint Surg., 41A:* 135, 1959.

26. Zemensky, A. P.: The pathology and pathogenesis of Legg-Calvé-Perthes disease, *Am. J. Surg., 4:* 169, 1928.

EPIPHYSEAL DYSPLASIA

This condition has two elements of importance. First, the epiphysis may be deformed sufficiently that secondary arthritic changes develop, particularly at the hip. Second, the epiphyseal changes may be confused with other anomalies, such as Legg-Perthes disease. Epiphyseal dysplasia may occur as an isolated epiphyseal change or in the form of multiple abnormalities involving particularly the proximal humerus, the distal femur and tibia, and the proximal femoral epiphysis.

It is common for mineralization of the epiphyses to be delayed by arbitary standards, such as those of Todd. Such delay, visualized at the wrist by roentgenogram, often amounts to a 3-4-year deficiency. A familial incidence, visualized by roentgenogram in the parents and siblings, is not uncommon with epiphyseal deformities.

The patients with multiple ossification centers forming their epiphysis vary from those with a normal cartilage anlage for the epiphysis to those in which the anlage is already malformed and as ossification progresses this is evident on roentgen examination and is evident by physical malformation or limited motion.

Another variable are various mesoectodermal disturbances that could be associated in various combinations and possibly so severe as to leave the child with a very limited outlook. It is exceedingly hard to conceive of each of these variations as a clear-cut entity, but to give the reader a concept of the variations involved the classification of Bailey follows:

Multiple Epiphyseal Dysplasia Congenita

Type I.   Normal stature.
Type II. Short stature, saddle nose deformity.
Type III. Short stature, saddle nose, upper limb rhizomelia.
Type IV. Short stature, saddle nose, upper and lower limb inequality in leg lengths, scoliosis, rhizomelia, ectodermal changes, intelligence changes.
Type V.   Same as above plus mental retardation, failure to thrive, and early death.
Type VI. Atypical cases.

The cases are few, but those classified as Type V are the most common and are often reported as Conradi's disease.

Clinical Picture

The youngster is usually short in stature and often among the shortest 10% according to the growth chart. Other outward signs are usually conspicuous by their absence unless gross skeletal deformity at the knee or ankle is evident. In the older age groups, there may be signs of hip disease, such as limited motion in internal rotation, abduction, and flexion and possibly a hip flexion contracture.

Often there are no complaints, the condition being incidentally noted on the roentgenogram after trauma or other disease calls for the examination.

Fig. 4.105. A case of epiphyseal dysplasia showing some of the salient roentgen features. (*A* and *B*) Anteroposterior and lateral views of the hips show irregular ossification of the femoral heads without soft-tissue swelling, bilateral. (*C*) The lower leg shows diminished height medially of the distal tibial epiphysis. (*D*) Delay in mineralization of the lateral proximal humeral epiphysis and of the small bones of the wrists.

Roentgen Findings

The spectrum varies from the mild multiple ossification centers in a normally formed epiphysis to those with deformities of the epiphyseal ends of the bones that gradually become evident with growth. There is often delay in appearance of the ossification centers and restriction of growth in the epiphysis may become clearly evident.

Instability of the atlanto-axial joint may be evident in infancy in the severely affected.

At the wrist, delayed mineralization of the carpal bones is noted. The lateral portion of the proximal humeral epiphysis may be deficient in size by comparison with the medial humeral head. At the hips, the condition appears to be trying to create two femoral heads, and the acetabulum mirrors this contour. Slight degrees of the deformity, causing a central depression in the head, are most common. Relatively minor forms consist of only delayed mineralization of the proximal femoral epiphysis with irregular ossification of the epiphysis. It is this

Fig. 4.105 C.

Fig. 4.105 D.

type that is frequently confused with Legg-Perthes disease. The roentgenogram appearance, however, is not accompanied by signs of limited motion at the hips. The lateral portion of the distal femoral epiphysis is often deficient in height when compared with the medial portion. At the distal tibial epiphysis, a similar type of deformity gives the epiphysis a triangular shape, and the deficiency frequently exists in the lateral portion.

Treatment

For many patients no treatment is indicated or of value. These youngsters have full joint motion and, except for a short stature, are unremarkable. Youngsters are seen who already have limited hip motion and considerable femoral head deformity. The joint space, however, is usually wtill well maintained. Although the need for reconstruction appears inevitable, it is usually not indicated in child-hood. Periods in traction and recumbency to attempt to improve motion at the hips may be indicated. Osteotomy at the knee may be necessary in the presence of gross deformity.

Perhaps most important is the necessity for distinguishing this condition from the conditions loosely termed osteochondritis.

References

1. Bailey, J. A.: Forms of dwarfism recognizable at birth. *Clin. Orthop. 76:* 150, 1971.
2. Christiansen, W. R., Lin, R. K., and Berhaut, J.: Dysplasia epiphysialis multiplex, *Am. J. Roentgenol. 74:* 1059, 1955.
3. Elsbach, L.: Bilateral hereditary microepiphyseal dysplasia of the hips, *J. Bone Joint Surg., 41B:* 514, 1959.
4. Fairbank, H. A. T.: Dysplasia epiphysialis multiplex, *Br. J. Surg., 34:* 225, 1947.
5. Fairbank, T.: *An Atlas of General Affections of the Skeletal System,* Edinburgh: E. S. Livingstone, Ltd., 1951.
6. Freiberger, R. H.: Multiple epiphyseal dysplasia, *Radiology, 70:* 379, 1958.
7. Jackson, W. P. U., Hanelin, J., and Albright, F.: Metaphyseal dysplasia epiphyseal dysplasia, diaphyseal dysplasia, and related conditions. II. Multiple epiphyseal dysplasia, *Arch. Intern. Med., 94:* 886, 1954.
8. Litchman, H., and Chirls, M.: Dysplasia epiphysialis multiplex, *Bull. Hosp. Joint Dis.,* 1957.
9. Silverman, F. N.: A differential diagnosis of adrondroplasie, *Radiol. Clin. North Am., 6:* 223, 1968.

PERSISTENT ADDUCTED FERMURS (POSITIONAL)

A contracture apparently due to intrauterine position causes a number of infants to be seen in the office practice of orthopaedic surgery. These children have many of the physical signs associated with subluxated or dislocated hips. Hip roentgenograms reveal the adducted position of the hip, but there is a normal acetabulum, a normal location of the femoral neck in relation to the triradiate cartilage, and often a normal development of the ossification center of the femoral head (if present). Occasionally this ossification center is smaller than the one on the opposite side.

These infants are normally seen in the first 6 months of life. The birth history is usually normal.

Physical Examination

Asymmetric thigh folds often first call

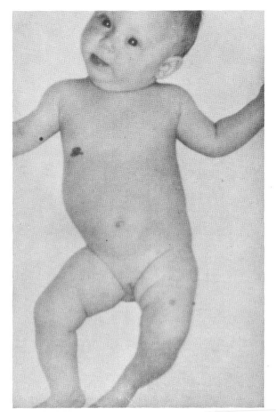

Fig. 4.106. Adduction contracture of the hip. Note the tendency to lie in a total trunk curve as well.

attention to the condition. The infant examined as to total posture is found to lie with the pelvis high on the adducted side and with a total curve of the spine correcting for the adduction. The head and neck tend to assume a posture in line with this spinal curve. When turned on the stomach, the infant maintains this position. It is even possible to be fooled into the recognition of a positive Galeazzi's sign if the position of the pelvis is not carefully compensated for when the thighs are flexed.

Treatment

It is necessary to aid the patient to overcome the adduction contracture despite the fact that much of the normal infant's daily routine stretches these muscles. Adductor stretching with the thighs flexed is taught to the mother. Holding the legs abducted with double diapers for approximately 3 months is all that is ordinarily necessary to overcome this positional disability. Forced abduction should be avoided.

CHAPTER 5

The Spine

POSTURE IN EARLY ADOLESCENT

Posture becomes a common clinical problem with girls between the ages of 10 and 15 years who have no abnormalities. This age group and sex is usually seen purely because of the parents' complaint that "I don't like the way she stands."

It should be recognized that much more than the way the child stands is embodied in the parental concern. The child is beginning to become a young woman of the age of social competition for the female. The mother, impatient that she put her best foot forward, wants the awkwardness of 12 to pass quickly to the poise of 18. The mother is motivated by the desire to obtain the best in life for her child.

The child, on the other hand, is motivated by a desire to cenceal the developing lumps on her chest, which have reached the stage of being embarrassing. Very baggy sweaters and blouses become the rule. In addition, she really does stand poorly. The shoulders slope down and inward, the head protrudes forward, the abdomen is protuberant, and the buttocks are prominent. This posture, in part, is a reflection of an attitude toward life rather than a structural abnormality. The necessity for making oneself as inconspicuous as possible until some measure of understanding or mastery of the adolescent situation is gained is reflected in the stance.

Treatment

It is helpful first to explain to the mother why she is concerned about her daughter in terms of social competition and to assure her that, in any event, the child's stance at 12 will not be her posture at 18, when the motivations become quite different. It is obvious that if she constantly criticizes her daughter's posture, the only result will be the strained mother-daughter relationship that is so common among girls of 13. No amount of nagging correction will make a child stop concealing something she is embarrassed about. Since constant admonition to stand straight accomplishes nothing, it is better omitted.

It is possible to accomplish something with posture in this age group by exercises that tilt the pelvis. Exercises are a definite assigned task, like washing the dishes or doing homework, that it hurts no one's psyche to have and to accomplish regularly. There are two commonly used forms of pelvic tilt exercises. One is the flexed knee sit-up in which the patient lies on the back on a table and flexes the knees on the chest. The head and shoulders are then lifted from the table by the use of the abdominal muscles, and the trunk is held off the table for a moment and slowly dropped back again.

Another form of pelvic tilt exercise consists of flattening the lumbar lordosis against the wall by the use of the abdominal musculature, holding the posture, and then releasing it.

A well tucked-in pelvis is the key to good posture.

BACK PAIN IN CHILDREN— DIFFERENTIAL DIAGNOSIS

The complaint of back pain in a child must always be taken seriously. In our own experience, the underlying cause has always been found to be a serious one, albeit occasionally of psychologic origin. The complaint has sometimes revealed a serious disturbance in the family situation, which, when brought to light early, has offered some hope of solution.

Every orthopaedist should be aware of the fact that leukemia not infrequently presents itself first as back pain. The pain is often fleeting and evanescent in character and gives rise to a generalized complaint referable to the back rather than to one specific area. In difficult diagnostic problems, a sternal puncture and smear should always be included in the work-up.

There are a number of relatively commom possibilities. These include spinal cord tumor (often associated with paralytic bladder and urine retention). Tuberculosis of the spine has

Fig. 5.1. Posture can be affected as illustrated by hip flexion contractures with excessive lumbar lordosis and protuberant abdomen.

well marked soft-tissue abscess shadow in addition would incline the observer toward a diagnosis of tuberculosis. Tuberculosis would, of course, tend to have a more insidious onset and a more prolonged history than osteomyelitis.

Osteomyelitis of the vertebrae occurs as a definite septic process, secondary to generalized sepsis or to the localized introduction of a needle, as in spinal puncture. There is also a type that has no predetermined etiology. The existence of an organism has not been proved in these cases. The disease tends to run a benign course, subsiding after a period of 4-6 months when the patient is immobilized in a cast and put on bed rest. Systemic signs are absent.

Tumor of the spinal cord may be extremely insidious, so much so that considerable time may elapse before sensory symptoms appear. Alertness to this lesion as a possible cause of low back pain when no other cause is evident requires making a lumbar puncture and an examination of spinal fluid, at the very least. It is frequently necessary to make a myelogram in order to rule out definitively the possibility of a spinal cord lesion.

Spondylolisthesis is common enough to receive eminent consideration as a diagnostic possibility. Tight hamstrings that limit straight leg raising are a frequent clinical sign. Localized tenderness at the spine of the fifth lumbar vertebra, or occasionally the fourth, is usually quite marked.

In early childhood, a severe slip of the fifth lumbar or the first sacral is unusual, and many of the so-called classic signs in the examination of the spine are not present.

Back pain due to so-called epiphysitis or Scheuermann's disease arises in the adolescent. Increased dorsal kyphosis is readily evident on physical examination and is confirmed by tenderness in the affected area. Roentgenograms reveal irregularity of the vertebral epiphyseal plates and wedging.

Eosinophilic granuloma may also produce wedging of the vertebra or a wafer-like appearance, as in Calvé's disease. Osteoid osteoma of the posterior element of the vertebra is not infrequently seen in childhood.

Rarely, malignant tumors of the vertebra, such as Ewing's sarcoma, are seen. Postural low back pain is not ordinarily seen in children. Underlying problems of the parent-child rela-

become relatively rare, but it is still seen approximately 3-4 times a year in a children's hospital in a metropolitan area. Perhaps still more common is so-called osteomyelitis of the spine. The affected child presents with localized tenderness at a specific spinal level and a rigid spine due to muscle spasm. Roentgenograms reveal a narrowed interspace between two vertebrae and irregular destruction of the vertebral plate on either side. The presence of a tionship may be suspected when both physical and laboratory examination are negative.

CONGENITAL KYPHOSIS

An important childhood orthopaedic problem is kyphosis of the spine based on either a widespread disturbance of the ossification of the spine or a localized vertebral anomaly.

The patient is seen because of an increased anteroposterior curvature resulting in a rather sharp prominence that usually centers about the 12th dorsal vertebra.

Etiology

There are at least three conditions in which this lesion is frequently seen. Widespread disturbance of the ossification of the spine is often seen in chondrodystrophy. In spines affected by this anomaly, the individual vertebrae frequently have a typical shape caused by lack of ossification of the anterosuperior and inferior angle. Gargoylism and cretinism frequently have associated with them a hypermobility at the 12th dorsal-first lumbar area. The 12th dorsal is often wedge-shaped and irregular.

Individual vertebral anomalies of the type producing kyphosis are most often centered at the junction of the dorsal and lumbar spines. Such anomalies consist of partial absence of the vertebra involved; the posterior portion is present, the anterior absent.

Clinical Picture

Morquio's Disease

Morquio's disease is a syndrome constituting the form of chondrodystrophy in which the changes are most prominent in the spine. It often is not recognized until the child is walking. The trunk is short beyond proportion to the shortening of the extremities. Skull changes are minimal. The kyphosis is diffuse; there is wedging of the vertebrae is addition to localized changes at the 12th dorsal. The extremities reveal widened epiphyses and bizarre bone shapes. Bone that is laid down has normal texture, however. There may be associated deformities, such as knock-knees. There

Fig. 5.2. Lateral roentgenogram of the spine in a cretin, revealing hypermobility between the 12th dorsal and 1st lumbar vertebrae.

is an epiphyseal disturbance of the vertebrae, as well as of the extremities. The epiphyseal line reveals a lack of cartilage column formation and, as a corollary, a lack of a provisional zone of calcification. There is no disturbance of membranous ossification.

The hand in chondrodystrophy is broad, and the fingers are short and have a tendency, when outstretched, to diverge, not at the metacarpophalangeal junction, but at the proximal interphalangeal joints.

Hurler's Syndrome

Hurler's syndrome, also known as gargoylism and dysostosis multiplex, resembles Morquio's disease closely. Many of the features of chondrodystrophy are found in this condition. Hurler's syndrome is associated with mental deficiency and clouding of the cornea. The

Fig. 5.3. The spine in chondrodystrophy with kyphos at the 12th dorsal vertebrae. The anteroposterior diameter of the vertebral body is increased, and ossification is deficient at the anterorsuperior and inferior angles of some vertebrae.

hands sometimes exhibit an inability to extend the distal phalanges, resulting in a clawlike deformity.

The stored substance in gargoylism is not a lipid but a glycoprotein. At least three types of Hurler's syndrome have been delineated, as judged by various types of mucopolysaccharide found in large amounts in the urine and tissues. Greenback and Meyer found that chondroitin sulfate B predominated in 7 of 9 patients. Heparitin sulfate was found in varying lesser percentages. Neither of these compounds has been found in the urine of normal persons although they are normal constituents of connective tissue.

In 2 of these 9 patients heparitin sulfate predominated and in 1 it was the sole constitu-ent. In this patient the intelligence quotient was normal.

A third category of Hurler's syndrome is one in which chondroitin sulfate B is found without heparitin sulfate.

Kyphosis Associated with Single Areas of Bony Anomaly

When kyphosis is associated with single areas of bony anomaly, it is usually sharper and mentality is normal. It results in slight diminu-tion in trunk height. Neurologic involvement has been reported in one-quarter of the published cases, according to Bingold.[1]

The most common site of involvement is the area between the 10th thoracic and the second lumbar vertebrae. The anomalous condition varies from complete absence of the posterior elements or body to a state in which some portion of these elements is present.

Treatment

In many orthopaedic clinics, considerable time and effort have been spent trying to maintain the patient's spine in a corrected position. Plaster shells, turnbuckle anteroposterior wedging jackets, and simple body casts and braces are all used.

In cases in which a considerable change takes place in the kyphos in flexion and extension in the upright posture, holding the spine in a corrected position has some merit. Such a condition frequently exists in various forms of chondrodystrophy. Where there is a single anomaly and the occiput is well centered over the pelvis, the follow-up films indicate that, while the condition enlarges with growth, the angle of the deformity remains the same.

Cosmetic attempts to reduce the deformity by excising the spine are usually misguided. The spines of the involved vertebrae are often rudimentary and have flat laminae enclosing the dural sac.

The consideration of spinal fusion as a means of maintaining the spine in a position of maximal extension through the kyphotic area is a serious one. Growth anteriorly in the presence of fused posterior elements may result in further correction. The posterior elements may be congenitally fused in localized anomalies of the spine. The type of congenital kyphosis most likely to benefit from fusion is that associated with excessive mobility at the area of kyphosis. The outlook in syndromes such as Hurler's, with its associated mental deficiency, must be considered in making a decision for surgery.

References

1. Bingold, A. C.: Congenital kyphosis, *J. Bone Joint Surg.*, 35B: 579, 1953.
2. Lombard, P., and LeGenissel: Kyphosis congenitales, *Rev. Orthop.*, 25: 532, 1938.

VERTEBRAL PLANA (CALVÉ'S DISEASE)

Vertebral plana, characterized by a flattening of the vertebral body which gives a striking x-ray picture, was first reported by Calvé in 1925.[1] It occurs most frequently between the ages of 4 and 10 years, but is occasionally seen in the early "teens." The original etiology postulated by Calvé was aseptic necrosis—a process similar to coxa plana. Compere et al.[2] presented 4 cases which were diagnosed as eosinophilic granuloma. Similar deformities have been noted in patients who have widespread areas of involvement with eosinophilic granuloma.

Clinical Picture

The usual complaint is back pain. There is no radiation ordinarily. The symptoms are of short duration. If progression has taken place, there may be a gibbus, muscle spasm, and limited spine motion.

X-ray Picture

When seen early, the process may be osteolytic and may be gradually producing the thin, collapsed, "wafer-like" body which has been thought characteristic of this disease. The picture is quite different from that of tuberculosis.

Calvé noted that the discs adjacent to the involved vertebrae were intact, that ordinarily only one vertebra was involved, and that the flattened vertebra remained as a dense cortical disc.

Treatment

Rest in recumbency during the acute stage of

Fig. 5.4. Vertebral plana with preservation of the disc spaces, but reduction of the single involved vertebra to waferlike thinness.

symptoms followed by the wearing of a spine brace until the lesion is well healed and recalcified is the usual program. The brace is gradually discarded. The usual course varies between 1 and 3 years. Fripp[3] reported several cases for intervals as long as 22 years. He noted considerable reconstitution of the vertebra. A line of sclerosis was frequently left centrally as a ghost of the old collapse.

References

1. Calvé, J.: A localized affection of the spine suggestive of osteochondritis of the vertebral body with the clinical aspect of Pott's disease, *J. Bone Joint Surg., 7:* 41, 1925.
2. Compere, E. W., Johnson, W. E., and Coventry, M. B.: Vertebral plana (Calvé's disease) due to eosinophilic granuloma, *J. Bone Joint Surg., 36A:* 969, 1954.
3. Fripp, A. J.: Vertebra plana, *J. Bone Joint Surg., 40B:* 378, 1958.

SPONDYLOLISTHESIS

Spondylolisthesis, a low back condition, although most frequently noted as sympto-matic in the age group from 30 to 40 years, is also often seen in childhood.

The essential part of this lesion is a defect in the pars interarticularis of the involved vertebra at the junction of pedicle and lamina (spon-dylolysis). When the condition is bilateral, the body, pedicles, and superior articular processes are separated from the laminae, spine, and inferior articular processes (spondyloschisis). This situation may allow a forward slip of the body (spondylolisthesis).

The most commonly involved vertebra is the fifth lumbar, but rarely the fourth lumbar may be involved.

Etiology

Ossification of the vertebra springs from three centers—one for the body and one for each half of the neural arch. Ossification starts in the pars interarticularis where the vessels originally penetrate the cartilage anlage.

Willis noted the "spondylolisthesis defect" in 6% of dissecting room subjects; 25% of these cases were unilateral. In no reported instance,

Fig. 5.5. Cleared specimen of lumbosacral spine from the newborn. The dark ossification centers of the posterior elements of the lower three lumbar vertebrae are seen coming down to the sacral spine and a portion of each ilium. The isthmus is the point of entrance of the vessels at the junction of pedicle and lamina. There is only one center on each side for the posterior elements, but the isthmus is the thinnest part of it.

not even in the unilateral type, has any evidence of bone repair been found. Hitchcock[5] notes that despite a 5% incidence in the population at large, none has been found in fetal material. He found, in stillborn and infant cadavers, that hyperflexion of the spine fractured the neural arch in the lower lumbar region and tended to support fracture as the basic etiology. The hypothesis that the anomaly is a congenital defect is supported by a high incidence of associated defects, such as spina bifida, in the presence of the lesion. The argument as to whether the defect is a fracture or is of congenital origin in still open.

A third possibility exists, however, in that absorption may exceed accretion at the pars interarticularis. Such a situation would account for the failure of the lesion to be found in newborns, as congenital defects are, and for the lack of bone repair, which occurs in a fracture. It would also account for the high incidence in a group whose occupational habits include prolonged flexion of the spine, but the theory is as yet unproven.

Clinical Picture

The patients presenting in childhood are usually first seen in early adolescence. The male and female population appear to be equally involved. Low back pain with occasional radiation to both thighs posteriorly is the principal complaint. Unilateral leg pain, which is seen in one-third of the cases in adults, is rare in

Fig. 5.6. Spondylolisthesis with defect posterior to pedicle. The fifth lumbar vertebra has slipped forward, and there is cupping of the sacrum around the posteroinferior angle of this vertebra.

children. The low back pain is made worse by activity and is relieved by recumbency.

Hamstring spasm that limits straight leg raising is often present and symmetric. Forward flexion of the spine is limited and painful if the child is having symptoms. Excessive forward flexion has been found by us only in children who are asymptomatic and in whom spondylolisthesis was only an incidental finding. Tenderness over the spine of the involved vertebra is almost invariably present and localized. The trunk, when the patient is examined from the lateral view, appears to be displaced forward in relation to the pelvis.

Roentgen Findings

Forward displacement of the fifth lumbar on the sacrum can be recognized in minimal cases by drawing a line between the inferior angle of the first sacral and the superior angle of the fifth lumbar. A second line is drawn between the superior angle of the first sacral and the inferior angle of the fifth lumbar. These two lines should normally be parallel. Forward slip is indicated by a deviation of these lines.

The defect in the pars interarticularis may be seen in either the lateral or the anteroposterior views of the lumbosacral joint. When it is not visualized, oblique views or a 45° anteroposterior view of the lumbosacral joint will flatten out the lamina so that it may be visualized, if present.

In long-standing spondylolisthesis, the anteroposterior view is often diagnostic, since there tends to be considerable atrophy of the

Fig. 5.7. Marked atrophy of the laminae of the fifth lumbar vertebra in spondylolisthesis. The apparent laminae of the fifth lumbar vertebra are actually of the fourth. The fifth vertebra is represented by the vestiges of posterior elements below it.

laminae involved. A concavity in the inferior surface of the fifth lumbar vertebra, apparently due to excessive lumbosacral motion, may exist. The disc space may be narrowed more than is normal. Spina bifida of the neural arch is frequently seen.

Treatment

Gill[4] has recommended excision of an overgrowth of fibrocartilaginous tissue present beneath the defect and intruding on the fifth lumbar root. He has demonstrated this in his cases, but we have found fusion necessary to relieve both symptoms and root pressure from whatever cause.

In general and depending on the individual patient, the attitude has been taken that the basic cause of the symptoms is lumbosacral instability and motion of the detached fragment directly over the roots.

A lumbosacral joint weak enough to give symptoms in the presence of the healthy musculature of childhood will almost certainly cause adult disability.

Excision of the spine and laminae and fusion of the first sacral to the fifth lumbar vertebrae, as recommended by Barr, have been carried out in our cases. The result has been relief of pain, elimination of hamstring spasm, and good spine motion. The area between the fourth lumbar and first sacral is bridged by a continuous iliac graft on which bone chips are laid so that there is no danger of a reparative reaction involving the roots. Patients so treated are ordinarily kept in a double hip spica for 4 months.

Asymptomatic patients are followed, but not operated on unless they become symptomatic. Strangely enough, mild degrees of slip seem more productive of symptoms than extensive slips involving the total vertebral surface.

References

1. Batts, M.: The etiology of spondylolisthesis, *J. Bone Joint Surg., 21:* 879, 1939.
2. Caldwell, G. A.: Spondylolisthesis, analysis of 59 cases, *Ann. Surg., 119:* 485, 1944.
3. Friberg, S.: Studies on spondylolisthesis, *Acta Chir. Scand. 82:* suppl. 55, 1939.
4. Gill, G. G., Manning, J. S., and White, H. L.: Surgical treatment of spondylolisthesis without spine fusion; excision of the loose lamina with decompression of the nerve roots, *J. Bone Joint Surg., 37A:* 493, 1955.
5. Hitchcock, H. H.: Spondylolisthesis; observations on its development, progression, and genesis, *J. Bone Joint Surg., 22:* 1, 1940.
6. Roche, M. B., and Bryan, E. S.: Spondylolisthesis; additional variations in anomalies in the pars interarticularis, *Arch. Surg., 53:* 675, 1946.
7. Shore, L. R.: Report on a specimen of spondylolisthesis found in the skeleton of a Bantu native of South Africa, with further specimens

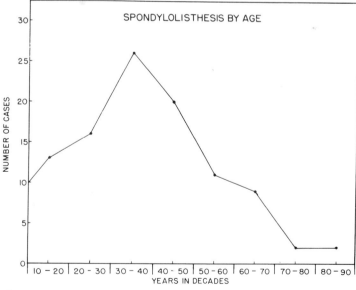

Fig. 5.8. Series of symptomatic spondylolistheses illustrating the age at which symptome bring the patient to medical attention.

Fig. 5.9. Severe spondylolisthesis slipping forward the entire width of the sacrum.

illustrating an anomalous mode of development of the lower lumbar vertebrae, *Br. J. Surg., 16:* 431, 1929.

TUBERCULOSIS OF SPINE

Tuberculosis of the spine, although its incidence has decreased, is still frequently found on orthopaedic children's wards. It continues to account for a formidable percentage of all bone and joint lesions.

In former times, patients ordinarily were not seen until the lesions were well advanced. The fact that they are now seen in earlier stages demands a clinical awareness on the part of the examining physician of the nature of the disease. Tuberculosis does not affect only one localized area, but must be, at least potentially, a generalized infection. Even when the lesions are at first confined to the spine, the involvement there is often multiple. The causal organism, in order to have infected the spine, has been blood-borne at some stage.

Potts first described the disease in 1779. After examining patients with well advanced cases and marked deformity, he noted that, in the histories, symptoms in the spine preceded the development of the deformity.

Etiology

Now that the incidence of bovine tuberculosis has been much reduced, the great majority of tubercular infections of bone appear to be caused by the human form of Koch's bacillus.

Fig. 5.10. Postoperative view of the case seen in Figure 5.9, showing partial reduction of the slip, removal of the posterior element, and fusion posteriorly.

The disease spreads by means of respiratory rather than alimentary infection, and it is most usual to find that the patient has had a close family association with an infectious individual. Although the possibility that infection spreads via the thoracic duct to the dorsal spine has been suggested, a blood-borne infection seems more likely and is supported by the initial localization in the vertebra. A primary lung complex is commonly found on a roentgenogram of the lungs in children.

Pathology

The involvement is most often in the center of the area supplied by the posterior spinal artery. From there the lesion spreads to the disc edge and then to the disc itself. Its progress encompasses the anterior and posterior ligaments but tends to spare the posterior elements, including transverse processes, spines, and facets.

Doub and Badgley note three types of lesions: intervertebral, central, and anterior. The rare anterior localization apparently reaches its destination via branches of the intercostal arteries; it involves a large number of vertebrae, but often causes little deformity.

There may be several or many discrete lesions in the vertebra rather than mere direct extension. The initial lesion, after causing acute inflammation and lymphocytic infiltration, brings about central degeneration, caseation, and calcification. The bone is increasingly destroyed, and there is further debris and caseation and eventually the formation of an abscess. Dorsal abscesses tend to run along the ribs, lumbar abscesses to run down the psoas sheath and to point either posteriorward in the lumbar triangle or anteriorward beneath and

Fig. 5.11. Tuberculosis of the spine at the dorsolumbar junction with destruction in opposing vertebrae, collapse, and deformity, but without marked calcific reaction.

distal to the inguinal ligament. In cervical lesions, the abscess usually gravitates into the mediastinum.

Cave,[2a] reported on a series of 162 cases, noted 7 in the cervical spine and 115 in the dorsal spine. The dorsal spine is by far the commonest site. In this area, the normal dorsal round back accentuates anterior stress and, as contrasted to the cervical and lumbar areas, is more easily deformed.

The majority of initial infections of the spine occur between the ages of 3 and 10, although they also occur in adults.

Clinical Picture

Pain and stiffness in the back are the first symptoms. The parents note wasting, loss of appetite, night cries, withdrawal from activity, and easy fatigue. A low grade temperature elevation frequently accompanies the disease. A chronic, slowly developing course is typical.

The sign which immediately arouses suspicion of a tuberculous infection of the spine is a gibbus. This localized prominence in the back is tender to pressure and may only be minimal to observation. There is accompanying muscle spasm and limitation of motion of the spine in all planes. Patients seen before the development of a gibbus exhibit dislike of jarring activity such as jumping, and some limitation of motion may usually be elicited. Further progression of the disease results in kyphos in the dorsal spine, shortening of trunk height, and descent of the ribs into the pelvis.

Abscesses radiating from the lumbar spine down the course of the iliopsoas may be palpable by abdominal examination posteriorly in the iliolumbar area, anteriorly in the thigh, or anteriorly. Abscesses and infections of the rib may be noted. Abscesses may be accompanied by flexion contracture of the hip.

Laboratory Findings

The sedimentation rate is elevated and becomes of value in following the patient's course rather than in diagnosis. The tuberculin test is positive and should first be used in dilution of 1:100,000. Those at 1:10,000 are virtually always positive. Failure to obtain a positive test in a suspicious case should result in reevaluation of the tuberculin used. The blood count may be unremarkable, but some authors have drawn attention to the lymphocyte-monocyte ratio. A rise in monocytes relative to

Fig. 5.12. Soft-tissue shadow of abscess on left with minimal evidence of vertebral involvement.

lymphocytes above a ratio of 1:3 correlates well with activity of the disease and is one additional guidepost to the appropriate time for surgery, if it is indicated.

Roentgen Findings

In the stage at which the patient is most often seen today, narrowing of the intervertebral disc area is an outstanding sign. Active destruction in the vertebrae, both above and below the narrowed interval between them, may often be found. When these findings are coupled with the visualization of a soft-tissue mass adjacent to the involved area, the diagnosis of tuberculosis becomes most likely. Such a mass should show a gravity effect; that is, it should be largest in its most distal portion and should gradually narrow in a cephalad direction. Obviously granulomatous masses show this effect less than masses composed of encased fluid pus.

In relation to its chronicity, a tubercular lesion, as compared to a pyogenic spondylitis, exhibits very little calcifying reaction. Infections caused by organisms such as brucella may mimic the picture very well, however.

In late stages of the disease, there may be such complete destruction of vertebral bodies that deformity, particularly dorsal kyphos, is marked and a clear recognition of structure in the involved area is unobtainable. Abscess shadows may become especially prominent. In the lumbar area, the iliopsoas shadow may be obliterated by the developing abscess. The entire spine should be x-rayed, as unsuspected silent lesions may be found.

Treatment

One must be quite certain of the diagnosis, and those cases which are thought possibly to

Fig. 5.13. Gibbus in dorsal spine marking the early development of deformity.

Fig. 5.14. Very early tuberculosis of the spine in which thinning of the disc space at the fourth lumbar vertebra is the most striking feature. There is also involvement of the vertebral plates abutting the disc.

have another etiology should be constantly reappraised.

Needle biopsy is not thought to be indicated. Johnson et al.,[6] however, noted that direct surgical biopsy should be done wherever possible as a considerable percentage of cases may be misdiagnosed without it.

The patient is suffering from a systemic as well as a local disease. The ideal treatment includes institutionalization so that bed rest can be enforced and the patient's progress readily reevaluated. Immobilization in hyperextension is not advocated because it unnecessarily prolongs the healing process of a disease which is attempting to heal by bony union. Various types of frames that hold the patient in a more normal position, but one which does not aggravate the deformity, have been used; the simplest type is an anterior and posterior plaster shell, which permits nursing care but aids immobilization. The patient may be turned from front to back in these shells.

A high calorie, high vitamin diet is instituted. Good nursing care is an important adjunct. Sunshine and fresh air, though aids to good health, do not occupy the center of the stage of treatment as they formerly did.

Chemotherapy has now become an important adjunct. The use of streptomycin, p-aminosalicylic acid, and isonicotinic acid hydrazide is discussed in Chapter 3, under "Tuberculosis of Knee." Other antibiotics helpful in tuberculosis are already on the scene. It has not been possible to supplant surgical measures with them, but under their cover the approach has become bolder.

A safe program to pursue includes observation of the child on a regime until definite progress in the direction of healing is obtained. This progress includes elimination of fever, weight gain, declination of the sedimentation rate, and a normal lymphocyte-monocyte ratio.

Fig. 5.15. Spine fusion for tuberculosis of the third and fourth lumbar vertebrae.

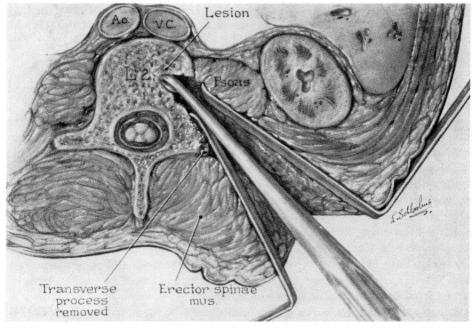

Fig. 5.16. Approach to the lumbar spine. Removal of detritus and sequestra as part of the surgical approach to tuberculosis of the spine is becoming increasingly important. (From W. Southwich and R. Robinson: Surgical approaches to the cervical and lumbar regions, *Journal of Bone & Joint Surgery, 39A:* 631, 1957.

When these signs are manifest, it is thought that the course can be influenced by fusion of the involved vertebra.

Since it has been shown that the disease frequently involves adjacent vertebrae that exhibit no pathology by roentgenogram, a safe rule is to add two vertebrae above and two below the lesion to the fusion. Such a rule can be varied according to anatomic location, deformity, and activity of the disease. Fusion posteriorly is usually followed by fusion anteriorly and eventual cure of the disease. After the fusion the patient must remain on the general measures instituted until the disease is cured. Fusion by itself does not substitute for the general treatment of tuberculosis.

Fusion of the spine as a treatment for tuberculosis was instituted by Hibbs[5] in 1911. By Hibbs' method multiple small chips were raised from the laminae, the articulations were curetted and denuded, and the spinous processes were split and bent over the interspinous area. Albee[1] also reported a spinal fusion operation the same year in which an autogenous cortical tibial graft was inserted between the split spinous processes. Many variations have subsequently been described, but fusion based on Hibbs' original concept has proved most successful.

To a Hibbs' type fusion an osteoperiosteal shaving which is continuous has been added with benefit, particularly when the area of

Fig. 5.17. Soft-tissue abscess causing a paraplegia. Note that the pressure is anterior. (From S. J. Garceau and T. A. Brady: Pott's paraplegia, *Journal of Bone & Joint Surgery. 32A:* 87, 1950.)

attempted fusion involves a deformity with an apex that, to be fused, needs much support.

Sinus formation, particularly when there is a secondary infection in addition to the tuberculosis, has proved responsive to chemotherapy. In general, abscesses are watched conservatively. However, large abscesses pointing so that fluctuation is readily elicited may be drained, and an attempt to collapse the walls by compression may be made. Streptomycin is introduced into the cavity at the time of drainage. Abscesses requiring drainage are usually from lumbar, rather than dorsal, tuberculosis of the spine.

Paraplegia

This distressing complication of tuberculosis of the spine appears to originate in extradural pressure due to abscess formation. Lesions are most likely to be mid-dorsal. Bony deformity, although undoubtedly contributing to the mechanics of the complication, has not been implicated to the degree that granulation tissue, debris, and purulent material have. Purulent material pressing on the cord in the form of a tight abscess sac has resulted in the slow development of paraplegia in 23.9% of cases in a series reported by Bosworth et al.[2] These authors noted that small abscesses tightly bound down by ligaments were of greater danger than large unconfined sacs.

Sustained clonus is a most reliable sign in the presence of a known tuberculous spinal lesion. It may be accompanied by sensory changes, muscular weakness, spasticity, and a positive Babinski sign.

Most authors are agreed that little improvement follows a posterior decompression by laminectomy. Conservative treatment alone results in improvement in many cases. Spine fusion is sometimes helpful. The operative approach of costotransversectomy with drainage of the abscess appears most likely to result in prompt improvement of the paraplegia. The ability of the cord to recover from pressure of this type with dramatic improvement or complete cure is remarkable in recorded cases of paraplegia of more than two years standing.

References

1. Albee, F. H.: Transplantation of a portion of the tibia into the spine for Pott's disease, *J.A.M.A.,* 57: 885, 1911.

2. Bosworth, D. M., Dell Pietra, A., and Rahilly, G.: Paraplegia resulting from tuberculosis of the spine, *J. Bone Joint Surg., 35A:* 735, 1953.

2a. Cave, E. F.: Tuberculosis of the spine in children. *Instruct. Lect. Amer. Acad. Orthop. Surg., 5:* 114, 1948.

3. Garceau, C. J., and Brady, T. A.: Pott's paraplegia, *J. Bone Joint Surg., 32A:* 87, 1950.

4. Girdlestone, S. R.: The operative treatment of Pott's paraplegia, *Br. J. Surg., 19:* 121, 1931.

5. Hibbs, R. A.: An operation for progressive spinal deformities, *N. Y. State J. Med., 93:* 1013, 1911.

6. Johnson, R. W., Hillman, J. W., and Southwick, W. O.: The importance of direct surgical attack upon lesions of the vertebral bodies, particularly in Pott's disease, *J. Bone Joint Surg., 35A:* 17, 1953.

7. Ordell, S., and Blacklund, V.: Diagnosis and exact location of lesions by planigraphy in surgical treatment of tuberculosis, spondylitis under cover of streptomycin, *Acta Chir. Scand., 106:* 61, 1953.

PREADOLESCENT AND ADOLESCENT KYPHOSIS

Preadolescent and adolescent kyphosis leads to the deforming and functional disability due to dorsal wedging round back that arises in the adult. The underlying condition exists in childhood, however. Kyphosis juvenilis, Scheuermann's disease, and vertebral epiphysitis are other names for the condition.

Severe end stages of the condition are recognized in adolescence when wedging of the vertebra, irregular ossification of the vertebral epiphyses, and irregularity of the superior and inferior cortical plates of the vertebra may be striking x-ray features.

Youngsters below the age of 12 who are developing round back deformity should be treated with preventive measures in order to deter further deformity. Persistent anterior vascular grooves, recognizable by roentgenogram, leave the patient susceptible to further wedging.

Etiology

A number of factors have been implicated in the past. These include osteochondritis of the epiphyseal plates with deficient and irregular growth.

Schmorl's nodes have been implicated by some. These nodes appear as cartilage herniations into the vertebra. Associated with deficient growth of the vertebra, they may actually represent a form of chondrodysplasia. In this

Normal Spine Development

In reviewing unselected normal lateral chest films in the age group from 6 to 11 years, certain observations were apparent. There is a normal dorsal kyphos, the curvature of which takes place in the area of the fifth, sixth, and seventh dorsal vertebrae. The time of development of this kyphos varies considerably, some youngsters still having a straight dorsal spine at age 10.

The anterior vascular groove, which is originally present in lumbar as well as dorsal vertebrae, is closed in more than 60% of the children reaching 6 years of age. The wedging that develops in the fifth, sixth, and seventh dorsal vertebrae to form a so-called normal kyphos results in closure of the grooves in the upper dorsal area.

By the time the age of 10 is reached, only 17% have some vestige of a groove remaining. Seventy-one percent have developed a round back in the area of the fifth, sixth, and seventh dorsal vertebrae. The vestigial grooves are below this area in the dorsal spine. The lumbar spine grooves have long since been closed.

The indentation in the anterior border of the vertebra seen by the roentgenogram has been found by dissection to be occupied by a large endothelium-lined vascular lake formed by the confluence of veins at this point. Some cartilage is also present in the younger children. If the soft tissues are removed from the vertebral body, the groove depth varies, depending on the degree of closure.

Fig. 5.18. Developing dorsal wedging round back.

area, bone formation has failed to take place. The edges are vertical and the base flat. Wedging of the vertebra may accompany their presence.

A third implicated factor is the anterior vascular groove. This groove has been observed to close with anterior wedging and appears to be associated with the development of round back in preadolescents.

Whatever the underlying cause, stress appears to bring about the wedging in the defective vertebra. The upright posture forms stress enough. The mechanics that enter into upright posture, such as tight hamstrings, put further stress on the dorsal spine in forward bend (Lambrinudi).

Clinical Picture

The patient is often first seen as a posture problem. There may be a tired, aching sensation in the region of the dorsal spine. The round back due to accentuated dorsal kyphos is noted. There may be tenderness of the spine in this area. Accentuated forward bend may be painful. Tenderness may be localized to the region of the interspinous ligaments. The hamstrings may be tight and may limit straight leg raising.

The use of plaster body jackets and even spinal fusion is necessary in some cases to relieve the symptoms.

Fig. 5.19. Persistent anterior vascular grooves in the dorsal spine.

Roentgen Picture

Before the age of 10 and before the appearance of the epiphyses of the vertebrae, there may be wedging of vertebrae below the fifth, sixth, and seventh dorsal vertebrae. Such wedging added to the wedging above produces the accentuated round back. The anterior vascular grooves may persist or they may have closed, leaving a linear area of increased density in their wake. After the age of 10, the superior and inferior plates of the involved vertebrae may appear irregular. The epiphyseal plates tend to ossify irregularly in the affected area of wedging.

Treatment

The child who appears to be developing an excessive lumbar lordosis and an accentuated dorsal round back posture and who is then found, by lateral film of the dorsal spine, to have wide, open anterior vascular grooves becomes the object of special consideration.

There are preventive measures to relieve dorsal spine stress. Sleeping posture is important; any positions which flex the dorsal spine should be avoided. Sleeping on bed boards and without a pillow helps to maintain a flat surface. Relaxation flat on the back on the floor for 20-min periods relieves dorsal spine stress when the child is tired. Exercises to tilt the pelvis, to obliterate lumbar lordosis, and to stretch tight hamstrings are helpful.

As a constant means of relieving stress in the upright posture, we have used a low back brace which flattens the lumbar spine and thus causes

Fig. 5.20. The central vertebra in this dorsal round back is wedged and has evidence of persistent anterior vascular groove.

a tendency to extend the dorsal spine on looking forward. In the case of the preadolescent, this is used until the anterior vascular grooves are closed. In the adolescent it is used until the epiphyses are joined to the parent vertebra and the symptoms relieved.

"CAST SYNDROME"

In 1950 Doeph used the term "cast syndrome" to describe acute gastric dilatation after application of a body cast. When unrecognized severe hypokalemic alkalosis, hypovolemia and death may result.

Evarts points out that the term is a misnomer since the traction causing the syndrome may be exerted without a cast. The traction exerted by distraction rods, halo-femoral apparatus, correction jackets, and the Milwaukee brace in some patients can result in vascular compression of the duodenum. The horizontal or third portion of the duodenum passes between the aorta and vertebral body posteriorly and the root of the superior mesenteric arterial trunk anteriorly. This anatomic situation gives rise to the possibility of the third portion of the duode-num being caught and partial or complete obstruction thereby resulting. Minimal pressure is needed to flatten the duodenum in this area. Persistent nausea and vomiting is the most common symptoms. Tenderness in the epigastrium occurs early. Severe metabolic alkalosis and dehydration result. Oliguresis, ruptured stomach, and death can ensue.

CONGENITAL SPINAL DEFORMITIES

BY CHARLES S. STONE, M.D.

Malformation of vertebrae originating during the 4th to 6th week of embryonic development can produce malignant progressive deformity leading to paralysis and to death if not properly evaluated and treated. This has been conclusively shown by Winter et al.[37,38] It is, therefore, imperative that congenital spinal anomalies be evaluated properly and not assumed to be benign entities. The fallacies that congenital curves do not progress and that little improvement can result from treatment must be put to rest. Every orthopaedist must be aware of the potential danger in congenital scoliosis and kyphosis.

Fig. 5.21. Dorsal spine flexion on forward bend with tight hamstrings. (Reprinted with permission from *Pediatric Clinics of North America,* W. B. Saunders Co., Philadelphia, 1955.)

Embryology

Failure of segmentation and/or failure of formation of vertebrae results in the abnormalities of congenital absences, congenital scoliosis, congenital kyphosis, and spina bifida syndrome. An understanding of the embryologic development of the spine may give helpful clues to understanding spinal deformities. The development of the neural axis precedes that of the surrounding mesodermal structures but is closely related to that of the bony spine. It is, therefore, not surprising that with congenital spinal deformities there coexists anomalies of the neural elements both grossly and microscopically. These congenital anomalies make the patient's cord more susceptible to either mechanical or vascular injury during natural progression of deformity or during treatment.

There are three stages in vertebral development—membranous, cartilaginous, and osseous. First a neural plate forms from the dorsal ectoderm and a group of endodermal cells form the notochord. The neural plate then invaginates toward the notochord becoming a solid cylinder called the neural tube at 21 days following fertilization. During the later period of invagination, the first pair of primitive somites appear as segmental accumulations of mesenchyme in the mesoderm beside the notochord. A group of cells, sclerotomes, derived from the ventromesial portion of each somite, migrates to each side of the notochord as the primordium of the vertebral body. Each sclerotome pair, aligned beside the notochord, divides into a denser cephalic and a less dense caudal half. The cephalic portion of each sclerotome combines with the caudal portion of its neighbor causing the intersegmental artery

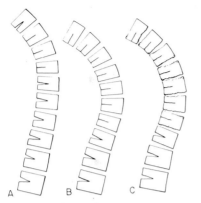

Fig. 5.22. The effect of wedging due to persistent anterior vascular grooves when added to that normally expected in the upper dorsal spine. (A) The normal situation of wedging in the proximal dorsal spine to produce the normal dorsal kyphosis. (B) Persistent vascular grooves allowing wedging in the distal dorsal spine and creating a round back deformity. Such grooves should be closed by the age of seven and certainly by age ten. (C) The effect of wedging and round back deformity is to produce irregularity in the epiphyseal plate ossification consistent with the diagnosis of Scheuermann's disease in the 13- to 16-year olds.

to become situated in the middle of the vertebral body. By the 6th week, the caudal to cephalic combined quarters fuse side to side across the midline, undergo chondrification, and form the vertebral body. The cephalic-caudal cleavage creates the disc space, the center being occupied by the notochord which becomes the nucleus pulposus. Further maturation occurs, ribs grow out from the somites, and by the 12th week ossification centers appear in the ribs and vertebral bodies.

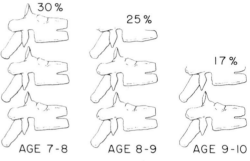

Fig. 5.23. Diagram of decreasing incidence of persistent anterior vascular grooves in the dorsal spine. (From A. B. Ferguson, Jr.: The etiology of preadolescent kyphosis. Dorsal wedging round back in preadolescents, *Journal of Bone & Joint Surgery, 38A:* 149, 1956.)

Transverse Section

Saggital Section

Fig. 5.24. Vertebral embryology. (A) 3 weeks, (B) 4 weeks, (C) 6 weeks, (a) 3 weeks, (b) 5 weeks, (1) notochord, (2) myotome, (3) sclerotome, (4) segmental artery, (5) costal process, (6) disc space, (7) neural tube, (8) posterior elements.

Failure of vertebral formation probably results from lack of original sclerotome migration. Failures of segmentation can be related to lack of cephalic-caudal cleavage. Rib anomalies are closely related to vertebral development and frequently coexist.

After each vertebral centrum takes shape at the 5th week, paired mesenchymal cell concentrations extend dorsally and laterally to form the posterior elements. If normal neural tube formation has not taken place, it will negate dorsal closure of the posterior elements and, thus, create spina bifida syndrome.

All congenital vertebral anomalies probably occur by the 6th week of embryonic life. Experimental deformities of the spine of the congenital type have been produced in chicks by injecting insulin into the yolk sac of the fertile egg. Hypervitaminosis E in pregnant rats and hypoxia or injection of 6-aminonicotinamide to pregnant mice produce scoliosis of the congenital type.

Classification

A classification of congenital spine deformities is given in Table 5.1.

Congenital Scoliosis

Congenital scoliosis is a lateral curvature of the spine due to anomalous vertebral development. Any child with scoliosis requires adequate and complete x-rays to determine the vertebrae involved and to identify vertebral anomalies.

Scoliosis is a physical finding. Establishing the correct diagnosis of this physical abnormality is required of any physician who will undertake its treatment. Treatment in its broadest sense includes as little as giving advice concerning prognosis and need for further follow-up. Correct and accurate diagnosis is particularly necessary in the area of congenital scoliosis. X-ray evaluation of the scoliotic vertebrae is difficult because ossification may not be complete, vertebral rotation may be present, and high quality radiologic technique may not be available. A full history and physical examination must be carried out looking particularly for indications of associated neurologic abnormalities such as small, club, or cavus feet, short extremities, calf

Table 5.1. Classification of Congenital Spine Deformities

I. Congenital Scoliosis
    A. Failure of formation
        1. Wedge vertebrae
        2. Hemivertebrae
    B. Failure of segmentation
        1. Unilateral bar
        2. Bilateral (fusion)
    C. Mixed
II. Congenital Kyphosis
    A. Failure of formation
    B. Failure of segmentation
    C. Mixed
III. Congenital Lordosis
IV. Associated with Neural Tissue Defect
    A. Myelomeningocele
        1. Vertebral body anomalies
        2. Neuropathic type
        3. Kyphosis
        4. Lordosis
    B. Meningocele
    C. Spinal dysraphism
        1. Diastematomyelia
        2. Other

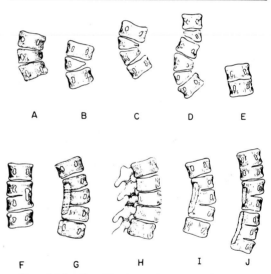

A   B   C   D   E

F   G   H   I   J

Fig. 5.25. Classification of congenital scoliosis: (*A-D*) failure of formation: (*E*) failure of segmentation, bilateral; (*F-J*) failure of segmentation, unilateral. (From R. B. Winter, J. H. Moe, and V. E. Eilers: A study of 234 scoliosis patients treated and untreated, *Journal of Bone & Joint Surgery, 50A:* 3, 1968.)

atrophy, or skin lesions in the dorsal midline of the trunk. X-rays must be of high quality to show bony detail and at a minimum should include anteroposterior and lateral standing and supine views of the entire spine. Spot films and laminagrams may be required to determine the exact anatomy of the scoliotic vertebrae and, thus, a correct diagnostic classification. At the initial visit, bone age should be determined from hand x-rays that are compared with the standard Greulich and Pyle[11] *Atlas.* Other causes of vertebral body abnormalities should be ruled out such as osteochondrodystrophy, postirradiation changes, metabolic diseases, infection, tumor, and trauma. Only by correct diagnosis can the natural history of the patient's curve be known and adequate advice given.

Natural History

Anomalies with a unilateral unsegmented bar between two or more vertebrae are associated with severe progression. This unilateral failure of segmentation may be between the bodies alone, between the posterior elements alone, or between bodies, pedicles, and posterior elements. The next most severe group are those with multiple hemivertebrae one after the other on the same side of the spine. Common sense would lead us to analyze the balance of growth potentials in each anomalous spine. An absolute prediction of progression cannot be made except in the cases of unilateral tethering of bone (unsegmented bar). Thoracic and thoracolumbar curves in general have progressed to the most severe deformities. Any spine with congenital scoliosis can progress anytime during the growth period. Seventy-five percent of congenital curves are progressive. The average progression is 5° a year. Except in those cases with associated neurologic deficit, no progression has been noted after closure of the vertebral ring apophyses.

Treatment Plan

Ideally, any child with spinal deformity will be seen early and a diagnosis made by complete history, physical examination, and radiographic study. Unless the child has a unilateral unsegmented bar and/or neurologic deficit, he should be reexamined and x-rays taken every 6 months.

Initial work-up should include anteroposterior and lateral sitting, standing, and supine x-rays of the entire spine, spot films, and

Fig. 5.26. Unilateral unsegmented bar—a dangerous sign.

laminagrams, if needed. Repeat anteroposterior standing and sitting films should be obtained at 6-month intervals. The limits of each curve should be determined, the curve measured in degrees by the Cobb method, and each measurement recorded on a chronologic chart. This way the degree of original curve can be seen at a glance and compared with all subsequent measurements. The so-called eyeball technique will fail to note the 2-4° progression at each visit. In the 234 cases reported by Winter et al.,[37] failure to appreciate subtle but relentless progression was the most common error. Failure to act on this information was the second most common error. Congenital curves tend to progress and tend to be rigid. The lack of flexibility negating easy correction leads to the recommendation for early fusion. Any patient who is being followed either in a Milwaukee brace or by observation whose curve is nonprogressive must be checked until the vertebral ring apophyses fuse. If progression occurs during growth, arthrodesis is indicated regardless of age.

Classical arguments for not proceeding with early fusion of congenitally deformed spines have been retardation of growth and causation of lordosis. Certainly, in congenital scoliosis the growth potential of the concave side is already diminished or absent. Further growth of the spine will only result in more deformity and not contribute to vertical height. Lordosis has not been shown to increase in those patients who did not have a lordotic component prior to arthrodesis. Early spine fusion with massive bone is the only way to prevent deformity. Once deformity is established, it may be irretrievable. For those patients who have not consulted a physician knowledgable in the field of spinal deformities until their curves are severe, treatment is more involved, more dangerous, and less satisfactory. However, if these patients are abandoned, many will develop cardiopulmonary and neurologic complications leading to death. Operative treatment is the only choice.

When the patient with congenital scoliosis is seen in infancy and a correct diagnosis is made, the following plan is recommended. If the child has an unsegmented bar and the curve is under 35°, a spinal fusion should be performed from at least one segment above to one vertebra below the area of segmentation failure. The child must be kept recumbent in a localizer for 10 months. We now ambulate the patient in a Milwaukee brace and continue biannual follow-up. If the curve increases, the fusion should be reinforced with bone graft and extended to the vertebrae which have been added to the curve pattern.

The patient with the unilateral posterior bar and a curve over 35° should have an osteotomy of the bar, then localizer or traction correction followed by posterior fusion. The unilateral failure of segmentation may involve the vertebral bodies. Anterior osteotomy for correction is considered only with curves over 70° because of the high risk of neurologic complications. Prior to surgical treatment, a myelogram is performed on all patients with congenital scoliosis. If anterior resection is necessary, preoperative selective spinal angiography could be helpful.

The remainder of infants with diagnosed congenital scoliosis are followed biannually with serial x-rays, careful measurements, and good records so that initial and present curve measurements can be noted. It is also important that the same level be measured each time. With any change in levels, the entire series of x-rays should be remeasured. If progression is noted in situ, spinal fusion is performed over the major portion of the curve. The patient is maintained in a Milwaukee brace until after the teen-age growth spurt when fusion may be extended to include a parallel vertebra at the top of the curve to a parallel vertebra at the bottom of the curve.

Frequently, the child with scoliosis is not referred to an interested orthopaedist until the deformity is quite severe. The goal is for all patients with congenital scoliosis to be seen, a diagnosis made, and treatment instituted before even cosmetically unattractive deformities occur. However, enlightened treatment is not yet available to all people, and some children will be seen with rather severe congenital scoliosis. Curves over 70° and decompensated curves in which T1 is no longer over the gluteal crease in the erect position should be corrected. Their treatment may involve osteotomy of unsegmented bars posteriorly or anteriorly, vertebral resection, halo-femoral traction, and spinal arthrodesis.

Milwaukee Brace

The Milwaukee brace has a place in the total treatment plan for congenital scoliosis. Mainly, it is useful following a short fusion in the young child to prevent progression of the curve above and below the fusion area. The brace can also be used for the rare mildly progressive but flexible scoliosis and for more severe flexible curves in children with congenital heart disease of the type rendering operative risk too great. The Milwaukee brace should not be used prior to spine fusion in unilateral unsegmented bars, nonflexible curves, and when the iliac crest skin is anesthetic. Serial x-ray examination and measurement must be carried out when a patient is undergoing nonoperative treatment. Nonoperative treatment should be abandoned in all cases in which satisfactory correction cannot be maintained or progression occurs. At this point spine fusion is indicated at any age.

Surgical Treatment

Posterior in Situ Fusion. Preoperatively, the routine admission work-up should include pulmonary function studies with blood gases. Myelography is done on all patients with congenital scoliosis prior to surgery. The embryologic development of the bony spine and neural elements are so closely related that associated unsuspected intraspinal anomalies such as diastematomyelia, developmental tumors, and tethered cord must be discovered and treated prior to fusion. Intravenous myelography is needed to rule out genitourinary anomalies. Preoperative marker films are obtained by taping a segment of paper clip transversely across the spine at the level of intradermal methylene blue skin markers on appropriate spinous processes. At surgery the skin incision is outlined between the markers using a Steinmann pin as a guide for a straight line incision. Local pressure and self-retaining retractors are used to control hemorrhage during the skin incision and subcutaneous dissection. Subperiosteal stripping of the paraspinal musculature is facilitated by packing gauze sponges along the spinous processes and out onto the laminae with Cobb elevators. Meticulous soft-tissue removal is carried out prior to decortication. The cortex is removed out to the tips of the transverse processes in both the thoracic and lumbar areas. Strip grafts obtained from one iliac crest are placed across the prepared bed. Supplemental homologous bone may be used if the patient's crests do not yield enough volume. In patients below the age of 3, definite provision for bone bank bone must be made. Postoperatively, the patients are kept at complete bed rest for 10 months. The first 6 months are spent in a well fitting localizer cast and the last 4 months in a body cast. If postoperative films at 6 months show evidence of pseudoarthrosis, exploration of the fusion mass is performed, and pseudoarthrosis is repaired with iliac crest bone.

When plaster is removed and the short fusion is solid, it is helpful to fit the patient with a Milwaukee brace in an attempt to prevent the addition of vertebral segments to the curve and to prevent bending of the solid spinal fusion in the plastic bone of a young child. Fusions that were solid at exploration 6 months postoperatively can undergo gradual loss of correction as the patient grows, indicating plasticity in the fusion mass. At the time of corrective osteotomy of the fusion mass, no pseudoarthroses have been identified.

Extension of the fusion may be required after the adolescent growth spurt to maintain a cosmetically and functionally good spine. However, severe rigid deformity will be prevented by the early fusion in all patients with an unsegmented bar and other categories of congenital scoliosis in which progression has been documented.

Fusion in situ is reserved for those patients whose deformity can be accepted and is too rigid for localizer correction. In children, Harrington distraction rods may be used as internal fixation devices, if the instrument size and bone size are compatible. Harrington rods are not to be used for intraoperative correction in these patients because the risk of neurologic damage is great even if a preoperative myelogram is normal.

Cast Correction and Posterior Fusion. Localizer cast correction and fusion with Harrington rods is the mainstay of operative treatment in scoliosis today. If the major curve can be corrected to 30° or less on forced lateral bending films, this method is used. Under adequate sedation a preoperative localizer cast is applied and cut out posteriorly as well as anteriorly for tracheal and abdominal windows.

Spine fusion is carried out over the major curve extending to the neutrally rotated vertebrae above and below the curve. Meticulous fusion technique is used taking care to adequately remove the soft tissue from transverse process to transverse process and decortication over the same area. Harrington rods are inserted in a careful manner. Ten days postoperatively, a new localizer is applied and the patient is ambulated. At 6 months, the localizer is removed and anteroposterior, lateral, and oblique x-rays are obtained of the fusion area. If there are any signs of pseudoarthrosis (loss of correction over 10° or radiolucent defects), the fusion mass is explored and all areas of motion decorticated and packed with iliac crest bone. When no defects are found, a body jacket is worn for an additional 5 months. These patients are then followed clinically and by x-ray until after skeletal maturity.

Selected patients whose curves do not correct to 30° or less on forced bending films are placed in Risser turnbuckle jackets for preoperative correction. Arthrodesis is done in this jacket. Postoperatively, a localizer jacket is applied and the patient is ambulated if Harrington rods have been used.

Halo-Femoral Traction and Posterior Fusion. When forced bending films give poor correction, halo-femoral traction is the method of choice. However, the pelvic-halo distraction method may be substituted. The halo and femoral pins are applied in the operating room under neuroleptic anesthesia. After 24 hr, correction is begun with the patient awake. Four pounds of weight are added initially, 2 lb at the head and 1 lb on each femoral pin. When the patient tolerates this weight, daily additions of 2 lb are made. The added weight should not exceed 50% of body weight. Twice daily neurologic examinations must be carried out. Paralysis of the sixth cranial nerve with loss of lateral rectus muscle function is the most common neurologic complication. This can be quickly reversed by removing the traction weights. Anterior thigh pain is a common prodrome of paraplegia and should alert the physician to decrease the traction force. Inability to void is an early sign of cord dysfunction. In short, any sudden onset of pain, weakness, numbness, or bladder or bowel disturbance is the indication for removing all weights and waiting for complete recovery before again applying traction. Weekly x-rays of the spine are obtained and measured. As long as correction is occurring and twice daily neurologic examination is normal, traction may be continued. Three weeks is the usual time but traction may be continued until maximum correction is achieved. The patient is taken to the operating room in traction. General anesthesia is induced and the patient intubated. One-half to two-thirds of the weights are removed and the patient placed in the prone position. The usual careful posterior fusion is carried out. Harrington rods are used if possible. Never attempt to achieve correction beyond that obtained in traction. Ten days postoperatively, a localizer cast is applied and the patient ambulated. If rods cannot be used the patient is continued in traction until skin healing has taken place and a cast is applied incorporating the halo frame and femoral pins. Bicycle hoop suspension is supplied for large children to facilitate nursing care. At 6 months the fusion is evaluated by x-ray and a body jacket is applied. Ambulation is begun at 10 months.

Spinal Osteotomy. There are some patients in whom halo-femoral or halo-pelvic traction will fail to gain acceptable correction. Many of these patients will have hemivertebrae producing an intolerable pelvic obliquity. The ideal level for hemivertebrae excision is below L3. Technically, vertebral wedge resection or osteotomy can be done at higher levels. Leatherman[21] has reported 24 cases of vertebral resection without serious complications. Most neurologic complications of scoliosis are due to mechanical injury to the spinal cord or interference with its blood supply. At any level, the anterior spinal artery supplies two-thirds of the cross sectional area of the cord. The remainder comes from the bilateral posterolateral arteries. The blood supply to the cervical, upper thoracic, and lumbar cord including the cauda equina is abundant. The so-called watershed area of the midthoracic spine is the most precarious. Adamkiewicz in 1882 described the arteria radiculomedullaris magna. This vessel supplies the midthoracic cord and appears on the left side from T6 to L3 in 66% of cases. It originates from an intercostal or lumbar vessel near the intervertebral foramen and ascends along the anterior surface of the cord as high as the fifth thoracic vertebra where it makes a

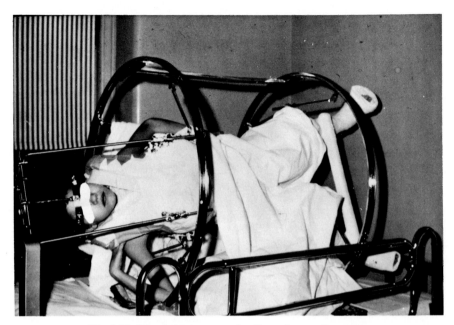

Fig. 5.27. Bicycle hoop suspension for easier nursing care.

hairpin turn and descends as the anterior spinal artery. Doppman et al.[6] have described the technique of selective spinal angiography using a femoral artery catheter passed into the origin of each intercostal and lumbar artery to be visualized. The radiographic technique of subtraction allows the artery of Adamkiewicz to be visualized from its origin.

Paraplegia has been rare in anterior surgery using Dwyer's instrumentation[8] even with the division of 6-10 segmental arteries including the watershed area. Hall[13] has shown arterial bleeding from both ends of the segmental artery if it is divided well away from the intervertebral foramen. This suggests arterial collateral circulation outside the spinal canal.

Selective spinal angiography to determine the location of these arteriae radiculomedullaris magna and strict attention to technique in sparing the arterial supply should reduce neurologic sequelae of vertebral body resection.

Leatherman[21] has described hemivertebrae excision and his technique is applicable to vertebral wedge resection. Following the appropriate transthoracic or retroperitoneal approach, the vertebral body is removed along with the anterior half of the pedicle. Removal of the disc above and below the vertebra to be excised facilitates this resection. For correction

to occur, the body resection must be complete side-to-side. It is safer to resect from the concavity but easier from the convexity of the curve. Care must be taken to follow the neurovascular structures into the intervertebral foramen and protect them during resection. When the anterolateral wound is healed, the posterior spine is exposed through a conventional midline dorsal incision. The posterior part of the hemivertebra and the remaining portion of the pedicle is removed. The wedge may then be closed under direct vision using Harrington compression or distraction rods. Posterior fusion is performed with abundant iliac crest graft.

An alternative method is proceeding with the posterior resection first. Two weeks later the anterior resection is undertaken, the vertebral end plates are removed, and the osteotomy is closed under direct vision by flexing the operating table. The patient is placed in a cast for 3 months, until anterior fusion is solid. Posterior fusion is usually necessary but in the young child the correction can be maintained in a Milwaukee brace proceeding with posterior fusion closer to skeletal maturity.

It is necessary that knowledgable and adequate treatment of congenital scoliosis be carried out. If a unilateral unsegmented bar is present or if the curve shows progression, spinal fusion is indicated regardless of age. The earliest successful fusion has been reported in a child 6 months of age. There should be no hesitation in performing an indicated spinal arthrodesis in the 1-5-year age group.

Congenital Kyphosis

Congenital kyphosis is an abnormal dorsal angulation of the spine due to anomalous vertebral development. Von Rogitansky[34] gave the first description of this condition in 1844. Van Schrick[33] described two groups: Type I—failure of segmentation and Type II—absence of the vertebral body. In 1973 Winter, Moe, and Wang[40] studied 130 patients with congenital kyphosis and described the natural history and treatment of this deformity.

Classification and Natural History

In Type I, failure of formation, nearly all of one or more vertebral bodies fail to form. The posterior elements, spinous processes, and pedicles are present but may be attenuated. Scoliosis frequently coexists in Type I kyphosis because of asymmetric failure of body formation. Type I occurs most frequently and is generally in the upper thoracic area. It is associated with instability during infancy but becomes more rigid and fixed as it progresses past the age of 3. This type has sharp angular deformity, progresses more rapidly than the other two types, and is the only type with associated paraplegia in the Winters, Moe, and Wang series. Progression averages 7° per year.

In Type II, failure of segmentation, the growth plates are absent anteriorly along with

Fig. 5.28. Transverse section of spinal canal and contents with typical segmental artery pattern. Radiculomedullary originates from posterior branch of intercostal artery, supplies small vessel to dorsal root ganglion, and ascends to reach cord above level of entrance. Pattern is similar for posterior radiculomedullary arteries. (*1*) Intercostal artery, (*2*) anterior branch, (*3*) posterior branch, (*4*) muscular branches, (*5*) radiculomedullary artery, (*6*) ganglionic branch, (*7*) anterior radiculomedulary artery, (*8*) posterior radiculomedullary artery, (*9*) anterior spinal artery, (*10*) posterior spinal arteries. (Reprinted by permission from J. L. Doppmen, G. Dichiro, and A. K. Ommaya: *Selective Arteriography of the Spinal Cord*. St. Louis: Warren H. Green, Inc., 1969.)

Fig. 5.29. (A) Diagram of arteria radiculomedullaris magna and anterior spinal artery as opacified by selective intercostal arteriography: (1) catheter; (2) left 12th intercostal artery; (3) arteria radiculomedullaris (B) arteriogram closely corresponding to sketch (A) (Reprinted by permission from J. L. Doppman, G. Dichiro, and A. K. Ommaya: *Selective Arteriography of the Spinal Cord.* St. Louis: Warren H. Green, Inc., 1969.)

Fig. 5.30. Congenital kyphosis—failure of formation type and failure of segmentation. (Reprinted by permission from R. B. Winter, J. H. Moe, and J. F. Wang: Congenital kyphosis, *Journal of Bone & Joint Surgery, 55A:* 255, 1973.)

one or more disc spaces. The kyphosis of this type is symmetrical with the segmentation failure acting as an anterior bar. The curves are more gradual, less severe, and occur within the upper lumbar and thoracolumbar regions. Progression does, however, occur and treatment is necessary.

In a third category, type III—mixed, there is

a combination of Types I and II or the anomalies may be unclassifiable. Mixed kyphosis occurs in the thoracolumbar area, progresses more rapidly, and becomes more severe than occurs in Type II.

All types of congenital kyphosis do progress. Cardiopulmonary, neurologic, and mechanical pain complications occur. Early operative treatment gives the best results. Late operative treatment is better than none at all.

Diagnosis and Preoperative Evaluation

The initial treatment is correct diagnosis. This requires a good history and physical examination with special attention to subtle signs of disturbed neurologic function such as a difference in thigh and calf girth or difference in foot size, early toe clawing and high arch or heel varus, tight hamstrings, and stretch reflexes. A full neurologic examination should be recorded. Radiologic evaluation should include an anteroposterior and lateral standing, sitting, and supine films of the entire spine, spot films from various angles, and laminagrams of the involved area. Lateral x-rays with maximum flexion and extension should be obtained to determine flexibility. If scoliosis accompanies the kyphosis, maximum side bending films are needed. The construction of a perpendicular from the line drawn along the end plate of the maximally tilted vertebra cephalad to the apex of the kyphosis will intersect with a perpendicular line drawn from the end plate of the maximally tilted vertebra caudal to the kyphotic apex. Kyphosis is quantitated by measuring the angle formed by the intersection of these two perpendiculars. All lateral films are measured and compared. Flexibility and/or progression can be determined. Since progression is the rule and bracing of any type is not effective, operative treatment is indicated. Preoperative work-up should include routine preoperative laboratory work, the initial evaluation presented above, pulmonary function studies including blood gases, electrocardiogram, intravenous pyelogram, and complete myelography. A more useful myelogram will be obtained by removing the spinal needle, using a high volume technique, and positioning the patient with the kyphotic and scoliotic deformities in dependent positions. Carelessly done or inadequate myelograms are of no value and cannot be tolerated in patients with this severe deformity.

Early Posterior Fusion

The most successful treatment is posterior spinal fusion in the child under 3 years of age with a kyphosis less than 50°. No rods are used. A postoperative hyperextension type of localizer cast is applied and the patient is kept recumbent for 6 months. Fusion exploration is carried out at 6 months postoperatively and bone graft added even if a pseudoarthrosis is not present. Casting in a horizontal position is continued for an additional 6 months. Clinical and radiographic follow-up are recommended every 3 months, the 2nd year postoperatively, and then biannually unit bone growth proceeds. Type I deformities are unstable in children under 3, and correction may be noted on preoperative bending films. Successful posterior fusion is adequate treatment for most cases of congenital kyphosis regardless of age if bending films measure 50° or less.

In the older child Harrington compression rods may be used. If pseudoarthrosis is present at 6 months, anterior arthrodesis should be done by the technique described in the following sections.

Halo-femoral traction should not be used unless the curve is flexible as demonstrated by hyperextension films. A few patients will require halo-femoral traction and its incorporation into the postoperative cast to hold this correction.

Later Fusion in Moderate Deformity

Posterior fusion alone in the more severe curve is nearly always unsuccessful. This is most likely due to distraction forces on the posterior fusion mass. Any child over 3 years of age and any curve over 50° are best treated by anterior strut grafting arthrodesis followed in 2-3 weeks by posterior fusion. Harrington compression rods are used posteriorly if the patient is large enough. Postoperatively, care and follow-up is the same as described for early posterior fusion in the preceding section. Routine exploration is carried out if the anterior and posterior fusions appear solid on x-rays taken at 6 months. Pseudoarthrosis can occur in spite of both anterior and posterior arthrodesis and should be repaired or the deformity will continue to progress. Postoperatively, Milwaukee bracing has been recommended to prevent loss of correction especially with associated scoliosis.

Severe Kyphotic Deformity without Paraplegia

If hyperextension x-rays show no correction, halo-femoral traction is absolutely contraindicated. Such traction would further stretch the cord over the anterior gibbus leading to cord damage. Anterior spinal decompression and osteotomy with strut graft arthrodesis followed in 2-3 weeks by posterior fusion with Harrington compression rods is the only method to gain correction. The risk of paralysis from anterior resection surgery must be considered. The decision for correction should be based on the experienced surgeon's judgment that in situ anterior and posterior fusion would not prevent the later onset of anterior cord compression and paraplegia.

Paraplegia

Ideally, fusion should be done early in the congenital kyphotic patient to prevent severe deformity and, thus, obviate the cardiopulmonary and neurologic complications. Some patients are not brought for adequate care until spasticity, paresis, or even complete paraplegia have developed. Most have Type I deformity. Posterior decompression by laminectomy alone is useless and contraindicated. Successful decompression requires removal of the anterior gibbus (the posterior portion of the apical vertebral bodies). Lateral rachiotomy and radical posterior decompression with transposition of the cord have been successful. These methods, however, do not effectively treat the entire problem of congenital kyphosis with paraplegia. Recurrence of the neurologic loss can occur. In any salvagable patient with complete or incomplete paraplegia secondary to congenital kyphosis, anterior decompression is indicated coupled with anterior strut grafting to be followed by a second stage posterior fusion with Harrington compression rods. Winter, Moe and Wang[40] report nearly complete recovery in 5 patients undergoing this procedure. Their method is modified from that proposed by Hodgson[16] for treatment of Pott's paraplegia and is applicable to any kyphosis-induced cord compression.

Anterior Decompression and
Strut Graft Arthrodesis

The spine is exposed through a transthoracic or transthoracic-retroperitoneal approach. The rib chosen for removal should be the one above the most cephalad vertebra to be reached. Upon reaching the spine, the segmental vessels will be seen crossing the center of each vertebral body to enter the intervertebral foramina. A number of segmental vessels sufficient to reach all necessary vertebrae should be doubly ligated well away from the foramen and divided between ligatures. An incision is made along the anterior lateral side of each vertebra and disc space. A flap is raised by sharp and blunt dissection to the intervertebral foramen. A second flap is raised anteriorly and around the opposite side. The annulus fibrosus, adherent to each disc space and to the bone, must be raised sharply. The disc material from each space is removed completely back to the posterior longitudinal ligament so that the entire vertebral end plate may be visualized.

The apex of the kyphosis should be removed for decompression and to facilitate a planned corrective osteotomy. Anterior fusion alone does not require decompression. The posterior longitudinal ligament has been identified through the disc space and through the intervertebral foramen. Its absence has been reported in some patients with congenital kyphosis. Begin to hollow out the center of the apical vertebra with a gouge and rongeur. Marked bleeding will occur from the cancellous bone. This is best controlled by bone wax which is preferentially removed prior to strut grafting. Curets and pituirary rongeurs are used to remove the bone posteriorly to the cortex across the entire width of the vertebral body. One or two other bodies are similarly prepared. The spinal canal must be entered either through the disc space most distant from the apex or through a carefully made window in the posterior cortex of a distal vertebra. With removal of the posterior ligament the dura may be seen. At this point, extensive epidural bleeding may occur and it is best controlled by pressure and the use of Gel-foam, topical thrombin, and Surgicil. Once the spinal canal is entered, the dura is identified and a small kerasin rongeur may complete the removal of the posterior aspect of each vertebral body, allowing the cord to move anteriorly into this newly acquired space. With true thoracic kyphoscoliosis, this procedure is most safely done from the concavity of the scoliosis to avoid any stretching of the cord.

After removal of the posterior bodies, a corrective osteotomy may be completed by

Fig. 5.31. Anterior decompression of cord (*a*) Broken lines outline the bone removed for decompression of the spinal cord. *C* is the plane of anterior removal, and *A*, the posterior margin of the bone removed back to the bases of the pedicles. If a scoliosis is present the spine should be approached on the side of the concavity of the scoliosis and the pedicles should be removed (*broken line B*) to allow the spinal cord to move toward the operator forward. After removal of an adequate amount of bone, the cord may not move forward until the posterior longitudinal ligament is excised. The posterior longitudinal ligament, however may not be present in some cases. (*b*) Forward movement of the spinal cord after removal of the posterior longitudinal ligament. The appropriate location for insertion of the strut graft is shown. In this location the graft cannot impinge against the cord even if dislodged. Usually more than one graft is needed. The discs must also be excised and replaced with autogenous bone. (Reprinted by permission from R. B. Winter, J. H. Moe, and J. F. Wang: Congenital kyphosis, *Journal of Bone & Joint Surgery, 55A:* 254, 1973.

Fig. 5.32. Technique of anterior strut grafting. (Reprinted by permission from R. B. Winter, J. H. Moe, and J. F. Wang: Congenital kyphosis, *Journal of Bone & Joint Surgery, 55A:* 252, 1973.)

cutting the remaining anterior vertebral body with an osteotome. In order to obtain correction, the cut must be complete from side to side. Care must be taken to protect the great vessels and segmental vessels entering the intervertebral foramen. Corrective osteotomy is never done without prior anterior decompression.

Anterior strut grafting is always done after osteotomy with decompression as well as after decompression alone. Slots are made in each end vertebra and hollowed out to the vertebral end plate with a curet. A second pair of slots is made in the next adjacent bodies in the kyphotic curve. Autogenous struts are prepared from ribs, fibula, or bicortical iliac crest bone. Each strut is first inserted into superior slots and, with the aid of manual distraction, slipped into the distal slot. The entire exposed cancellous vertebral bone is then cleared of bone wax and packed with autogenous cancellous iliac crest bone. If possible the periosteal flaps and the parietal pleura are closed. Chest tubes are inserted and the chest wound approximated in layers. Postoperatively, the patient is nursed in the horizontal position with frequent turning from side to side. If possible, the complete team of thoracic surgeon, neurosurgeon, orthopaedist, and anesthesiologist should work together in surgery of this magnitude. Blood loss is great. The patient's blood may be recaptured in an auto-transfuser. The blood is heparinized and sent to be washed in a computerized centrifuge. The red cells suspended in saline can be returned to the patient during surgery and in the recovery room.

Several weeks later, a posterior spinal fusion is carried out using Harrington compression rods if possible. A postoperative hyperextension localizer cast is applied. The patient is sent home to bed rest. At 6 months, x-rays are evaluated and, if satisfactory, the patient remains in recumbency with a plaster body jacket for an additional 6 months.

Congenital kyphosis can be successfully managed. Early surgical treatment is best. If the patient's curve is advanced, anterior surgery is necessary. When doing transthoracic and retroperitoneal approaches to the spine, the orthopaedic surgeon must be prepared to treat associated operative and postoperative complications that differ from usual orthopaedic practice.

Myelomeningocele Spinal Deformity

Early in the care of the child with myelomeningocele, attention is directed to control of hydrocephalus, genitourinary infection, and lower extremity deformity. Frequently, the patient has pelvic obliquity associated with hip contracture and dislocation. When the obliquity persists after correction of its infrapelvic cause, attention is directed to the spine. X-rays will show a scoliosis extending into the pelvis causing the fixed pelvic obliquity. Again, a diagnostic classification of the scoliosis must be made. Seventy-five percent of children with myelomeningocele are born with straight spines and their only vertebral anomaly is that of the open posterior elements. At least 50% of these patients will develop a lateral spine curvature, many with associated lordosis. The onset of the curve is usually before the age of 5. The scoliosis is always progressive but at a variable rate. Five percent of children with myelomeningocele are born with scoliosis secondary to associated vertebral anomalies. These lateral curves have a natural history like those with congenital scoliosis alone. Spinal deformities occurring with myelomeningocele are consistently progressive. Early and adequate treatment is necessary to prevent severe deformities from deterring satisfactory levels of achievement. The spinal deformities associated with myelomeningocele are kyphosis, congenital scoliosis, developmental scoliosis, and developmental lordosis. All of these are associated with and contribute to fixed pelvic obliquity which is a dominant factor preventing adequate bracing and adequate sitting.

Pelvic Obliquity

Pelvic obliquity in the coronal plane is present with the transverse plane of the pelvis is not parallel to the floor in the standing position. It may be functional or fixed. Functional pelvic obliquity disappears when the patient is recumbent and may be due to a short extremity or lumbar muscle spasm. Fixed pelvic obliquity persists in all positions. The cause may be infrapelvic due to hip contractures as abduction contractures of the left hip and adduction contractures of the right hip. In order for the patient to stand, a functional type of scoliosis develops to balance the head over

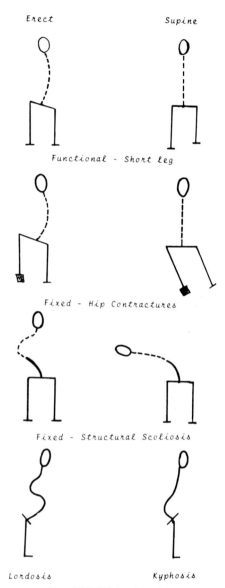

Fig. 5.33. Pelvic obliquity.

the pelvis. This cause may be suprapelvic due to structural scoliosis in which the sacrum is the last vertebra of the structural curve. In order to stand erect, a compensatory scoliosis develops above the major curve. Obliquity of the pelvis is only a physical finding. The cause may be infrapelvic (hips) or suprapelvic (spine). Frequently, the patient with myelomeningocele will have both spine and hip type pelvic obliquity. Fixed pelvic obliquity occurs when the transverse axis of the pelvis is no longer at a right angle to the long axis of the patient and cannot be passively corrected. This describes pelvic obliquity in only the anteroposterior plane.

Saggital plane pelvic obliquity can be fixed or functional. Excessive posterior pelvic tilt is due to fixed lordosis and can produce secondary hamstring tightness and limited hip flexion. Excessive anterior pelvic tilting occurs with fixed lumbar kyphosis.

The third dimension rotation must be considered when the scoliotic curve extends into the pelvis. The pelvis then behaves as a scoliotic vertebra. It may be like a true scoliotic vertebra taking part in the curve and having rotation. It may be like a neutral vertebral body below the curve having obliquity but neutral rotation. This added dimension causes difficulty in getting true anteroposterior x-rays of the hips and lumbar spine, thus confusing the true spatial relationships.

Most patients with myelomeningocele who have motor levels at L3 and above will function best as adults in the sitting position. Their spines must have nearly normal configuration and stability. The pelvis must be level in order to sit with the hands free (independent sitting). In addition the head must be over the pelvis and the shoulders level for good sitting balance. In spite of special fabrication of seats, breakdown of sensory deprived skin will occur when weight distribution is unequal due to pelvic obliquity. The only successful treatment of spinal deformity and pelvic obliquity in the myelomeningocele patient is operative.

Lumbar Kyphosis

Lumbar kyphosis commonly complicates a lumbar myelomeningocele with a motor level of T10 to L3. The posterior prominent spine presents as a subcutaneous mass across two-thirds of the width of the back with a neural plaque stretched over its apex. Lateral x-rays show a kyphotic deformity of the entire lumbar spine with wedged-shaped apical vertebrae. Kyphosis most likely develops from a flexion pull of the paraspinal muscles which lie adjacent to the ventrally everted laminae. The untreated kyphosis is progressive. Kyphectomy is needed to facilitate posterior skin closure, to prevent skin breakdown, and to permit successful bracing. If possible, this procedure should be coupled with myelomeningocele closure during the first day of life.

Kyphectomy

The dura is freed from the skin edges and mobilized anteriorly and laterally in preparation for closure over the neural plaque. The functioning nerve roots are identified and traced to the intervertebral foramina. The lateral tips of the everted posterior elements are identified and the fascial attachments incised. The nerve roots are now identified passing ventrally through the foramina. They can be protected while the posterior elements are removed and blunt dissection is carried to the lateral aspect of the vertebral bodies and a tape passed across the anterior surface of the apical vertebrae. This allows the paraspinous psoas muscles to fall anteriorly and protect the retroperitoneal great vessels and ureters. With careful dissection, successive vertebral bodies can be exposed. Two vertebral bodies are usually removed through the disc spaces. The end plates are then removed from the remaining vertebrae exposing bleeding bone. The pelvis is extended until vertebral apposition is accomplished preferably end to end. A portion of the resected bone is placed at the lateral aspect of the vertebral bodies as bone graft and the remainder is saved in the bone bank. The cord is now relaxed and the dura easily closed. The vertebra can be fixed by passing silk sutures through the vertebral bodies using a heavy cutting needle. Sharrard[28,29] uses cross-

Fig. 5.34. Congenital kyphosis. (*Left*) Normal vertebra with paraspinous muscle posterior; (*right*) kyphotic vertebra with paraspinous muscle anterior. (Reprinted by permission from J. F. Raycroft, and B. H. Curtis: Spinal Curvature in Myelomeningocele: Natural History and Etiology: *Symposium on Myelomeningocele, American Academy of Orthopaedic Surgeons.* St. Louis: C.V. Mosby Co., 1972.)

Fig. 5.35. Kyphectomy.

Fig. 5.36. Preoperative kyphos.

threaded pins. However, the bone is quite soft and metallic fixation devices frequently cut out. The skin can be closed without tension. Care must be taken not to place the pelvis in an excessive lordotic position. Lordotic pelvic obliquity may stop hip flexion short of 90° and, thus, interefere with sitting. The patient is nursed in a plaster shell until the skin is healed and then a double hip spica is applied extending above the nipple line. Plaster immobilization is required for 3-6 months until arthrodesis occurs. Extensive retroperitoneal bleeding accompanies this procedure and leads to fibrosis making later urinary diversion procedures technically more difficult, but not impossible.

If there is no neurologic function in the kyphosis resection area, the dura is oversewn and transected at the upper end of the proposed vertebral resection and removed dis-

tally. The spine may then be dissected free and transected without concern for the neural elements. Operating time is greatly shortened and hemorrhage reduced when dissection and preservation of the nerve roots is not necessary. Posterior interbody bone grafting aids in obtaining solid fusion.

Kyphectomy can be carried out in the older child. Usually there is posterior ulceration over the spine which must first be converted to clean granulation tissue by good nursing care in the hospital. The granulating skin defect is excised when kyphos resection is performed. Skin can be easily closed when the bony ends are approximated. Plaster immobilization must be maintained in the older child for at least 6 months. The cast must extend to the toes to prevent unwanted incidental supracondylar fractures of the femora.

Fig. 5.37. Postoperative kyphectomy.

Congenital Scoliosis

If the patient with myelomeningocele has fixed scoliosis secondary to congenital bony abnormalities, early correction should be attempted with halo-femoral traction followed by spine fusion. A myelogram should be done first to rule out diastematomyelia. Traction is frequently unsuccessful and vertebral resection becomes the method of choice. The pelvic halo has not been found useful in these children because iliac wings are small and flat preventing the seating of iliac transfixion pins. If vertebral resection is carried out above the level of neurologic deficit, the technique described in the section on congenital scoliosis is used. If the major deformity is at the level of the spina bifida and neurologic function is not present, hemivertebra resection or vertebral wedge osteotomy can be carried out from the poster-ior approach in the manner described for kyphectomy. Without the kyphotic deformity, however, greater care must be exercised in protecting the anterior great vessels.

Developmental Lordoscoliosis

These children are born with straight spines. Some have good motor function in the lower extremities. Scoliosis and lordosis begin insidiously around the age of 5 and are relentlessly progressive. Initially, both deformities are supple and correct almost completely with the child supine or suspended. These deformities become clinically important when they interfere with good bracing. Operative treatment is more easily carried out when the deformity is still flexible. The tendency is to delay until after the prepubertal growth spurt. However, we do not hesitate to proceed with correction and fusion at any age if necessary to prevent fixed pelvic obliquity and loss of sitting balance.

At the discovery of scoliosis, anteroposterior and lateral recumbent and erect x-rays of the entire spine including the pelvis are made and measured. Serial examinations are done every 6 months and progression recorded. Correction and fusion are done when the curve is still supple and before the standard myelomeningocele bracing will not accommodate the associated pelvic obliquity.

Treatment

In the child whose scoliosis and lordosis is supple, a posterior approach for spine fusion may be carried out. Special care should be taken to begin the subperiosteal stripping of the paraspinous musculature at the level where normal spinous processes are palpable. Dissection is then carried distally to identify the lateral aspects of the everted posterior elements and stripping is carried out to the posteriolateral vertebral foramen. The open spinal canal is identified and dura protected. Wide decortication is performed and mass bone graft inserted. If no neurologic function is present in the area of wide open spina bifida, the dura may be oversewn, the nonfunctioning neural elements excised, and a posterior interbody decortication carried out. With a flexible spine, preoperative correction is not required. Posterior fusion to the sacrum can be carried out with wide decortication. Graft of iliac crest bone is supplemented with bone bank bone.

A Harrington rod is inserted from the ala of the sacrum to the first neutral thoracic vertebra. The modified deep-seated Moe hook placed on the ala of the sacrum is preferable to a sacral bar because the soft tissue can be more easily closed over the Harrington rod set closer to the vertebra. Postoperative immobilization is maintained in a carefully fitted localizer jacket including the lower extremities for 1 year. The child may stand in the cast to facilitate urinary drainage. On ambulation, the patient is examined and x-rayed every 6 months. Breakage of the Harrington rod indicates pseudoarthrosis and repair must be undertaken. With meticu-

Fig. 5.38. Myelomeningocele with associated congenital scoliosis.

Fig. 5.39. Myelomeningocele developing scoliosis. (*A*) Birth, (*B*) age 5, (*C*) age 10.

lous technique successful posterior fusion can be achieved. Pseudoarthrosis rate as high as 40% is not unusual, but pseudoarthrosis repair is successful.

Anterior Dwyer instrumentation[8] with interbody fusion has been advocated when posterior elements are absent. The technique is especially useful in the child with myelomeningocele, both for correction of supple lordoscoliosis and as a good technique for arthrodesis after preoperative correction. It has been our experience that the paralytic curve in the myelomeningocele must have arthrodesis to the sacrum in order to maintain adequate sitting stability and correction of pelvic obliquity. At the present time, the Dwyer instruments cannot be applied across the L5-S1 joint and the screws

and staples are too large for the younger child. Dwyer instruments can be used over the major portion of the curve if either routine anterior interbody fusion is performed from L5 to the sacrum or complete posterior fusion with Harrington rod fixation is carried out as a second procedure. Combined anterior and posterior arthrodesis will reduce pseudoarthrosis in these neurogenic curves and is frequently indicated with thoracic level paralysis.

If the child's deformity in either or both planes has become rigid and does not significantly correct on forced bending films, operative correction of scoliosis and lordosis is necessary. It is possible to obtain some correction of the rigid scoliosis and good correction

Fig. 5.39B.

of lordosis with one operative procedure using the anterior Dwyer technique. Again, however, the L5-S1 joint cannot be crossed with the Dwyer instrumentation. An alternate method is, therefore, described. Anterior lumbar osteotomy at the apex of the curve is carried out through a midline transperitoneal approach. The abdominal contents are palpated and packed off with the patient in the Trendelenburg position. When lordosis develops, the bifurcation of the aorta and the common iliac veins ascend to lie over the body of L2-L3. The posterior peritoneum is opened and dissection carried down bluntly to the anterior aspect of the body of L4. The great vessels are identified and if necessary mobilized and retracted with tapes for access to the bodies of L4-L5. The osteotomy should be carried out at the apex of the lordosis. Generally, the apex is at the L4-L5 disc space. The disc is excised. The posterior longitudinal ligament is identified and a rongeur is used to resect the posterior lip of the vertebral bodies of L4 and L5. A $35°$ wedge is cut from the body of L5 and the body of L4. The patient is placed in femoral traction with the hips maintained at $90°$ for 2 weeks. When the lordosis is corrected, the patient is maintained in a hip spica with the hips and knees flexed at $90°$ for 3 months until anterior arthrodesis is complete. If the osteotomy does not close, the L4 inferior articular facets and L5 superior articular facets are resected bilaterally via the intervertebral foramina through a posterior laminotomy approach and the patient

Fig. 5.39C.

Fig. 5.40. Anterior lumbar osteotomy.

is returned to traction. When the patient's lordosis is controlled, localizer cast correction and posterior fusion is carried out. Harrington rods are used when possible. Excessive fixed lordosis will not allow the skin to be closed without tension over Harrington rods. Therefore, anterior surgery for fixed lordosis is required prior to rod insertion. If the scoliosis is especially severe, a biplane anterior osteotomy may be done to obtain some degree of concurrent scoliosis correction. When the major fixed deformity is scoliosis, halo-femoral traction is useful for correction prior to fusion.

Developmental lordosis and scoliosis usually coexists in the patient with myelomeningocele, causing fixed pelvic obliquity in both the saggital and coronal planes. Rotational deformity has not been corrected. Successful spinal arthrodesis from the neutral thoracic vertebra above the curve to the sacrum is absolutely essential if these children are to function in society. Enough correction of the deformities must be achieved so that stable unsupported sitting is possible. Any solid fusion that does not fulfill these criteria is a treatment failure and corrective osteotomy may be needed.

References

1. Bailey, H. J., Sister Mary Gabriel, Hodgson, A. R., and Shin, J. S.: Tuberculosis of the spine in children, operative findings and results in 100 conservative patients treated by removal of the lesion and anterior grafting, *J. Bone Joint Surg.,* 54A: 1633, 1972.
2. Blount, W. P.: Congenital scoliosis, transactions, 8th Congress, International Societe de chirurgie orthopedique et traumatolie, New York, pp. 748-762, 1960.
3. Carlioz, H., Dubousset, J., and Guillaumat, M.: Therapeutic Problems of Scoliosis with Pelvic Obliquity. Reunion Commune. "Scoliosis Research Society." Groupe D'etude de la Scoliose. Lyon, France, September, 1973.
4. Compere, E. L.: Excision of hemivertebrae for correction of congenital scoliosis; report of 2 cases, *J. Bone Joint Surg.,* 14: 552, 1932.
5. Dewald, R. L., and Ray, R. D.: Skeletal traction for the treatment of severe scoliosis, *J. Bone Joint Surg.,* 52A: 233, 1970.
6. Doppman, J. L., Di Chiro, G., and Ommaya, A. K.: *Selective Arteriography of the Spinal Cord,* St. Louis: Warren H. Green, Inc., 1969.
7. Duraiswami, P. K.: Experimental causation of congenital skeletal defects and its significance in orthopedic surgery, *J. Bone Joint Surg.,* 34B: 646, 1952.
8. Dwyer, A. F., Newton, N. C., and Sherwood, A. A.: Anterior approach to scoliosis. *Clin. Orthop.,* 62: 192, 1969.
9. Ehrehaft, J. L.: Development of the vertebral column as related to certain congenital and pathological changes, *Surg. Gynecol., Obstet., 76:* 282, 1943.
10. Gold, L. H., Leach, C. G., Kiefer, S. A., Chous, S. N., and Peterson, H. O.: Large volume myelography; an aid in the evaluation of curvature of the spine, *Radiology, 97:* 531, 1970.
11. Greulich, W. W., and Pyle, S. J.: *Radiographic Atlas of Skeletal Development of the Hand and Wrist,* Ed. 2, Stanford, Calif.: Stanford University Press, 1959.
12. Hall, J. E., and King, J. D.: Hyperlordosis following lumbar peritoneal shunts for hydrocephalus, *J. Bone Joint Surg., 53A:* 198, 1971.
13. Hall, J. E.: The anterior approach for spinal deformities, *J. Bone Joint Surg., 54B:* 765, 1972.
14. Hodgson, A. R., and Stock, L.: Anterior spinal fusion, *Br. J. Surg., 44:* 266, 1957.
15. Hodgson, A. R.: Correction of fixed spinal curves, *J. Bone Joint Surg., 47A:* 1221, 1965.
16. Hodgson, A. R., Stock, F. E., Fang, J. S. Y., and Ong, G. B.: Anterior spine fusion; the operative approach and pathological findings in 412 patients with Pott's disease of the spine, *Br. J. Surg., 48:* 172, 1960.
17. Hyndman, O. P: Transplantation of the spinal cord; the problem of kyphoscoliosis with cord. Signs, *Surg. Gynecol. Obstet., 84:* 460, 1947.
18. Ingalls, T. H., and Curley, F. J.: Principles governing the genesis of congenital malformations induced in mice by Hypozia, *N Engl. J. Med., 257:* 1121, 1957.
19. Klebanoff, G.: Early clinical experience with a disposable unit for the intraoperative salvage and reinfusion of blood loss (intraoperative autotransfusion), *Am. J. Surg., 120:* 718, 1970.
20. Kuhn, J. G., and Hormell, R. S.: Management of congenital scoliosis; review of 170 cases, *Arch. Surg., 65:* 250, 1952.
21. Leatherman, K. D.: Resection of vertebral bodies, *J. Bone Joint Surg., 51A:* 206, 1969.
22. Macewen, G. D., Conway, J. J., and Miller, W. T.: Congenital scoliosis with unilateral bar, *Radiology, 90:* 711, 1968.
23. Raycroft, J. F., and Curtis, B. H.: Spinal Curvature in Myelomeningocele Natural History and Etiology. Symposium on Myelomeningocele; American Academy of Orthopaedic Surgeons, pp. 186-201, St. Louis: C. V. Mosby Co., 1970.
24. Riseborough, F. J.: The anterior approach to the spine for the correction of deformities of axial skeleton, *Clin. Orthop., 93:* 207, 1973.
25. Roaf, R.: Wedge resection for scoliosis, *J. Bone Joint Surg., 37B:* 97, 1955.
26. Schneider, R. C.: Transposition of the compressed spinal cord in kyphoscoliotic patients with neurological deficit, with special reference to the vascular supply of the cord, *J. Bone Joint Surg., 42A:* 1027, 1960.
27. Shands, A. R., Jr., and Bundens, W. D.: Congenital deformities of the spine; an analysis of the roentgenograms of 700 children, *Bull. Hosp. Joint Dis., 17:* 110, 1956.
28. Sharrard, W. J. W.: Spinal osteotomy for congenital kyphosis in myelomeningocele, *J. Bone Joint Surg., 50B:* 466, 1968.
29. Sharrard, W. J. W.: Osteotomy excision of the spine for lumbar kyphosis in older children with myelomeningocele, *J. Bone Joint Surg., 54B:* 50, 1972.
30. Simmons, E. H.: Observation on the technique and indication for wedge resection of the spine, *J. Bone Joint Surg., 50A:* 847, 1968.
31. Stiram, K., Bobechko, W. P., and Hall, J. E.: Surgical management of spinal deformities in spina bifida, *J. Bone Joint Surg., 54B:* 666, 1972.
32. Thomas, B. H., and Cheng, D. W.: Congenital abnormalities associated with vitamin E malnutrition, *Proc. Iowa Sci., 59:* 218, 1952.
33. Van Schrick, F. G.: Die angelorene Kyphose, *Z. Orthop., 56:* 259, 1932.
34. Von Rokitansky, K. F.: Hanbuch der pathologiscen. Antomie, Vol. II, Weir Braumuller, 1844.
35. Wiles, P.: Resection of dorsal vertebrae in congenital scoliosis, *J. Bone Joint Surg., 33A:* 151, 1951.
36. Williams, J. M., and Stevens, K.: Recognition of surgically treatable neurologic disorders of childhood, *J. A. M. A., 151:* 455, 1953.
37. Winter, R. B., Moe, J. H., and Eiler, V. E.: Congenital scoliosis; a study of 234 patients treated and untreated. I. Natural history, *J. Bone*

Joint Surg., 50A:, 1, 1968.

38. Winter, R. B., Moe, J. H., and Eiler, V. E.: Congenital scoliosis; a study of 234 patients treated and untreated. II. Treatment, *J. Bone Joint Surg., 50A:* 15, 1968.

39. Winter, R. B., and Moe, J. F.: Anterior fusion of the spine for difficult curvature problems, *J. Bone Joint Surg., 52A:* 833, 1970.

40. Winter, R. B., Moe, J. H., and Wang, J. F.: Congenital kyphosis; its natural history and treatment as observed in a study of 130 patients, *J. Bone Joint Surg., 55A:* 223, 1973.

NONOPERATIVE TREATMENT OF KYPHOSCOLIOSIS

BY WILLIAM T. GREEN, JR., M.D.

Careful clinical and roentgenologic examination of the child permits early recognition of structural scoliosis before severe progressive spinal deformity occurs with growth. Until an effective nonoperative treatment was developed, most children were watched until the deformity became severe enough to warrant major surgery.

In 1958 a spinal distraction brace was introduced by Blount and Schmidt of Milwaukee, Wisconsin. Experience has shown that this Milwaukee brace, complimented by an appropriate exercise program, can halt or even reverse the progression of scoliosis in the growing child when used judiciously.

Milwaukee Brace

In addition to a distractive force, the Milwaukee brace is designed to apply a bending and derotational force for the correction of the scoliotic curve (Fig. 5.41). The distractive force is applied between the pelvic girdle, which rests above the iliac crests, and the occipital rest. The head is held against the occipital rest by a chin piece or more recently by a throat mold. Use of this throat mold has eliminated the bite deformity often complicating use of the chin piece. The bending and derotational force is applied by the use of appropriate pads applied to the convexity of the curves, through the ribs in the thoracic spine or through the transverse processes in the lumbar spine. The brace is constructed in balanced alignment and by the application of these forces gradually brings the wearer into balance also.

The pelvic girdle, fabricated of leather and Monel Metal or thermoplastic, is connected to the neck ring by an anterior upright of aluminum and two posterior uprights of stainless steel. These uprights can be bent or lengthened as correction and growth occur, and they provide attachment for the corrective pads. Hinged laterally at the neck ring and anteriorly at the pelvic girdle, the brace is entered and secured at the back.

Best results are achieved when the Milwaukee brace and the corrective exercise program are supervised by a skilled team of orthotist, physical therapist, and orthopaedist. Under these conditions in children with juvenile or adolescent thoracic kyphosis (Scheuermann's disease), with idiopathic scoliosis measuring less than 40-50° by the Cobb technique, or with congenital scoliosis, brace treatment is often indicated. This is particularly true when the curve is flexible, the child is young, and he is enthusiastic to participate in his own care. Treatment with this brace can be used to supplement surgical fusion. An early short fusion followed by control with a brace is often indicated in progressive congenital scoliosis (Fig. 5.42).

Prescription for a Milwaukee brace should indicate to the orthotist the types of corrective pads desired and their initial placement: shoulder ring or axillary sling for high thoracic and cervicothoracic curves, "L"-shaped thoracic pad for lower thoracic and thoracolumbar curves, and an oval or upright-backed lumbar pad for lumbar curves. Also it is good to note whether there is a pelvic obliquity or other special problems that will be encountered. The selection of the material for fabrication of the pelvic girdle is usually best left to the orthotist, allowing him to work with the material with which he is most comfortable. However, there is a strong preference for thermoplastic in the child who is not toilet-trained.

Prescription to the physical therapist should include general exercises to improve posture; pelvic tilt, spine extension and push-up exercises; also specific exercises to correct spinal deformity: shift of the torso away from the pad controlling the primary curve to restore spinal balance and thoracic flexion into the thoracic pad to derotate the spine and thereby to correct thoracic asymmetry.

Fit is a continuing problem. First the pelvic

A

B

girdle must be fitted correctly. A common problem is failure to tighten the girdle adequately, allowing it to descend and painfully pinch the iliac crests laterally. This can be prevented by having the child grasp the girdle at the sides and hold it up while it is being tightened so it pinches inward above the crests. Once the pelvic girdle is in proper position the height of the occipital rest and throat mold can be adjusted so the former is just below the occiput and the latter is flush against the upper throat (Fig. 5.41B). The trim line of the pelvic girdle should be just above the pubic symphysis anteriorly, the greater trochanter laterally, and the chair surface when seated posteriorly. It should allow enough room for hip flexion so the brace does not ride upward when seated. The anterior upright and the posterior upright on the side contralateral to the thoracic convexity should be adequately away from the thorax so that they make insignificant contact with deep inspiration or with thoracic flexion exercises. In contrast the posterior upright on the side of the thoracic convexity backs the pad against the thoracic prominence. When appropriately placed the wearer ought to be able to shift away from any pad 1/2 inch. A long-cassette standing roentgenogram in the brace is very helpful in adjusting the position of the pads so their force is applied to the convexities of the curves, just inferior to their apices.

Initially it is usual for the child to wear the Milwaukee brace at all times, including sleep, except for twice daily. At these times, a total period less than 1 hr, he can come out of the brace for bathing and skin care with alcohol and powdered talc. The brace is best worn over one layer of underclothing. All activities including non-contact sports are encouraged since, when performed in the brace, corrective forces are applied to the spine with movement.

During the first 3-6 months of brace wear the initial correction is usually achieved. Often it is preferable to apply the primary corrective pad initially alone until spinal balance from C-7 is

Fig. 5.41. (A) Young girl wearing a Milwaukee brace prescribed with a shoulder ring to control an elevated left shoulder and high left thoracic curve, an L-shaped thoracic pad to control a right thoracic curve, and a triangular shaped lumbar pad to control a left lumbar curve. (B) Position of the occipital rest and throat mold.

Fig. 5.42. This boy was born with a severe congenital scoliosis and low thoracic meningocele. The meningocele was closed at 5 days of age. At 7 months he developed a mild asymmetric spasticity in his legs. Spinal roentgenogram demonstrated hemivertebrae at T8 and T9, loss of definition of the pedicles on the concave side of the curve, failure of fusion of the primary ossification centers of the body of T11, fusion of the 10th and 11th rib on the right, and a boney diastema at L1 and L2 (indicated by the *arrow* in *A*). This curve was convex to the left and measured 52° from T7 to L1. The boney diastema was resected and interestingly the spasticity cleared. However, the infant was so badly out of spinal balance to the left that he was unable to sit without support until a localizer cast was applied. At 15 months of age he had a posterior fusion from T7 to L1 utilizing the posterior elements remaining along the convexity of the curve. Five months after the operation he was fitted with a Milwaukee brace which held him in balance (*B*). In a few months he was up walking and playing normally (*C*). This scoliosis will need to be watched carefully, and will probably require further surgery and a Milwaukee brace until spinal growth is complete.

Figs. 5.42*B* and *C*.

corrected or slightly overcorrected, then to add the secondary pads.

The Milwaukee brace, correctly applied in a favorable case, can convert a child who is out of balance with a deforming curve to a child who is in balance with multiple smaller curves, a better physiologic and cosmetic situation (Fig. 5.43). The child's progress can be followed by long-cassette roentgenograms taken standing in the brace at decreasing intervals once correction has been achieved so radiation is minimized. It should be emphasized that if the brace does not adequately correct the scoliosis due to inappropriate selection, brace fabrication or application, then surgical correction should be done promptly. It is wise to advise the child and his parents before use of the Milwaukee brace is agreed upon that surgery may be required if adequate correction is not achieved and maintained.

If satisfactory correction is achieved and maintained by the Milwaukee brace when can it be discontinued? It is generally accepted that most scoliotic curves under 50° do not progress after spinal growth is completed. Risser suggested that the cessation of spinal growth occurs when the iliac apophyses have finished their ossification toward the sacroiliac joints; however, more recently the criterion of the fusion of these apophyses to the ilia or the ring apophyses to the vertebral bodies has been used. Both these events take place at a later age,

Fig. 5.43. This 15-year-old girl was seen with a right thoracolumbar curve from T8 to L3 out of spinal balance to the right. A Milwaukee brace with right L-shaped pad was prescribed (A). One year later standing in her brace, a roentgenogram (C) shows balance has been achieved into multiple small curves and the T8 to L3 thoracolumbar curve corrected from 35° to 12° as compared with her prebraced roentgenogram (B). Importantly, she is an athletic girl who did her exercises enthusiastically and has obtained a good correction despite her relatively advanced bone age as demonstrated by the maturity of her iliac apophyses (B).

Fig. 5.43C.

17 to 20 years. Fortunately in the adequately corrected more mature spine, part-time wear often holds this correction. Standing roentgenograms after the brace has been removed for increasing periods of time will determine whether the correction will be maintained when the brace is worn part-time. Frequently it is possible to gradually discontinue brace wear until it is worn only during sleep until spinal growth has been completed. It is usually necessary to make several pelvic girdles during this period so the fit remains adequate as the child's pelvis changes. Thus the cost with this method of treatment is grossly comparable with surgical methods; however, in the correctly chosen case under favorable conditions the result can be very gratifying.

References

1. Blount, W. P.: Scoliosis and the Milwaukee brace, *Bull. Hosp. Joint Dis., 19:* 152, 1958.
2. Blount, W. P., and Bolinske, J.: Physical therapy in the nonoperative treatment of scoliosis, *Phys. Ther., 47:* 919, 1967.
3. Blount, W. P., and Moe, J. H.: *The Milwaukee Brace,* Baltimore: The Williams & Wilkins Co., 1972.
4. Blount, W. P., Schmidt, A. C., and Bidwell, R. G.: Making the Milwaukee brace, *J. Bone Joint Surg., 40A:* 526, 1958.
5. Blount, W. P., Schmidt, A. C., Keever, E. D., and Leonard, E. T.: The Milwaukee brace in the operative treatment of scoliosis, *J. Bone Joint Surg., 40A:* 511, 1958.
6. Galante, J., Schultz, A., Dewald, R. L., and Ray, R. D.: Forces acting in the Milwaukee brace on patients undergoing treatment for idiopathic scoliosis, *J. Bone Joint Surg., 52A:* 498, 1970.
7. Moe, J. H.: The Milwaukee brace in the treatment of scoliosis, *Clin. Orthop., 77:* 18, 1971.
8. Moe, J. H., and Kettleson, D. N.: Idiopathic scoliosis; analysis of curve patterns and the preliminary results of Milwaukee-brace treatment in 169 patients, *J. Bone Joint Surg., 52A:* 1509, 1970.

SCOLIOSIS

BY WILLIAM F. DONALDSON, JR., M.D.

During the past 15 years, many new workers have made significant contributions to our knowledge concerning the problems of patients with scoliosis. Its many diverse aspects are being given better definition. Certain strides have been made toward understanding the etiology of scoliosis, but there are still many gaps and much work must still be done to solve such questions as: Why does a scoliosis develop? What determines the curve pattern and its progression? Advances in treatment have been more concrete and dramatic. Even so, those involved in the management of these patients realize, all too well, the limitations of treatment currently available. We are still trying to control the effect, not the cause. Although much credit must be given to individual workers for the progress that has been made in recent years, the establishment of the Scoliosis Research Society in 1966 has been of particular importance. This has produced a much needed forum for the presentation and discussion of new and often preliminary ideas. The stimulus from this has resulted in a reevaluation of old ideas, in the development of the new, in cooperative studies, etc. Thus, the care of these patients has become based less on empiric thought[83] and tradition.[90] As a result of the efforts of those involved in the Scoliosis Research Society, there is now a single acceptable method of measuring a curve[38] (Cobb) (Figs. 5.44 and 5.45). There is a standard way of recording rotation and vertebral wedging.[97,135] At one of the most recent meetings, a standard nomenclature was accepted. All of these advances provide a format within which more accurate comparison of patient studies can occur and truly scientific information can be exchanged.

Although numerous methods of conservative therapy have their advocates, the use of the Milwaukee brace has become widespread and is the most widely accepted method of nonoperative treatment for scoliosis. The technique of the construction and use of this brace is described elsewhere in this volume. The necessary accompanying exercise program as described by Blount[8] is an indispensable part of this program. The current modification of the brace, as developed by Schmidt and Blount, are important. Anyone using this method must be conversant with all facets of the treatment program. An appropriate course of nonoperative treatment demands close cooperation between the patient and the patient's family, the orthopaedist, orthotist, and physical therapist.

In the surgical treatment of these patients, we owe a debt to such men as Albee,[2] Hibbs,[56] Cobb,[10-13] Moe,[85-89] and Goldstein[39-41] for their contributions to the development of the surgical technique of spinal fusion for scoliosis. An exciting development has been the introduction and use of a method of posterior spinal instrumentation by Harrington.[49,53-55, 75,121] For many patients this has resulted in a

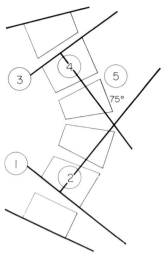

Fig. 5.44. Scoliosis, measurement of a curve (Cobb). *1*, Bottom vertebra: lowest one whose bottom tilts to concavity of curve. *2*, Erect perpendicular from bottom of bottom vertebra. *3*, Top vertebra: highest one whose top tiles to concavity of curve. *4*, Drop perpendicular from top of top vertebra. *5*, Measure intersecting angle. This is the accepted method of measurement of a curve according to the Scoliosis Research Society.

more satisfactory correction of their scoliosis with less morbidity. A more recent innovation, anterior instrumentation as described by Dwyer,[27-29,48,51,116] shows promise but its more exact role in our armamentarium is yet to be determined.

Preoperative surgical correction has undergone many improvements. Although the turnbuckle jacket (Fig. 5.46), as developed and modified by Ferguson,[32-34,117,124,125] Hibbs, Risser,[107-112] and Cobb, still remains one of the most efficient ways of correcting an angular deformity, other methods of preoperative treatment may be used in particular circumstances to improve the results obtained. These include the localizer cast of Risser, halo-femoral traction, halo-pelvic distraction, and Cotrell's cervical-pelvic traction.

We are learning more concerning the natural course of the patient with scoliosis, but most of these advances are concerned with those patients who have a specific etiologic basis for the development of their scoliosis such as congenital scoliosis with an unsegmented bar (Moe and Winter), neurofibromatosis, etc. Cobb's work concerning untreated idiopathic scoliosis[14,98] has not been followed up, and this leaves a

Fig. 5.45. Scoliosis, measurement of a curve (Ferguson). The central points of each end vertebra and of the apical vertebra are marked. The end vertebra are defined as the first nonrotated vertebra identified by the position of the spinous processes. The lines from the central point of the apical vertebra to those of each end vertebra form an angle. The deviation of these lines from 180° is the angle of the curve.

great deficit in our understanding of the natural course of the disease.

Scoliosis has been defined as any lateral curve, tilt, or angular deviation of one or more vertebral segments of the spine from the normal straight position. Scoliosis may be divided into two major and distinct groups: functional and structural scoliosis.

A functional curve is one that the patient can voluntarily correct and that correction can be maintained in the erect position. In this type of scoliosis, there is no intrinsic involvement of the mechanics of the spine. There is no structural abnormality of the bone, nerve, or muscle elements of the spine. Conversely, in structural scoliosis, there is involvement of the intrinsic structure of the spine. This may be bone, neural, muscular, or a combination of any or all of these elements. In a structural scoliosis, complete correction cannot be obtained and maintained by the patient in the erect position.

Functional Scoliosis

Functional scoliosis may be seen in a variety of conditions. It may be due to poor posture alone, or it may represent a compensatory adjustment for an organic angular deformity such as a short leg, a pelvic tilt secondary to either an abduction or an adduction or a flexion contracture of the hip, "sciatic scoliosis", etc. (Fig. 5.47). These functional curves are not precursors of structural curves. Their nature must be understood and their significance appreciated if one is to evaluate appropriately and properly treat the patient with scoliosis.

By x-ray a functional scoliosis has different characteristics from those of a structural scoliosis. For example, in a functional curve, no evidence of wedging or other structural changes in the vertebrae are seen. No treatment is indicated for the functional scoliosis itself. The basic curve pattern, a C-curve, is such that it never crosses the midline in two directions. Therefore, it is a single curve and there are no minor or compensatory curves either above or below it.

Structural Scoliosis

While Cobb's classification (Table 5.2) of structural scoliosis has worked well for us in the past, with the newer knowledge available, it became clear that a more detailed and definitive segregation of patients according to etiology was necessary if we are going to be able to compare like groups of patients. Therefore, the current Scoliosis Research Society classification of patients with scoliosis is preferred (Table 5.3).

The importance of discovering the correct etiologic diagnosis cannot be overemphasized. It must be remembered that scoliosis is only a physical finding and is not, in itself, a diagnosis.

The etiology of the scoliosis has much to do with its characteristics and prognosis. The fact that the largest segment of the group must still be labeled idiopathic[66] does not detract from the value of determining the etiology, but rather emphasizes the importance of recogniz-

Fig. 5.46. (A) Modified Risser turnbuckle jacket with full head piece and thigh extension of the side of the convexity of the major curve. The anterior and posterior hinges and the position of the turnbuckle can be seen. (B) A modified Risser turnbuckle jacket viewed from the side of the convexity of the major curve. Note the eccentric position of the anterior and posterior hinges. These hinges are made of aluminum and are, therefore, relatively radiolucent. (C) An overhead view demonstrating the position of the posterior hinge eccentric to and above the apex of the curve to be corrected. The anterior hinge is directly opposite. (D) M.K. Patient is immobilized in her turnbuckle jacket. The portion over the sacrum is removable so that the posterior window is large enough to permit the taking of bone grafts from the posterior iliac crest.

Fig. 5.46*D*.

Fig. 5.47. (*A*) Functional scoliosis, patient has 2-cm shortening of the left leg resulting in a pelvic tilt and functional scoliosis in the lumbar area. (*B*) With shortening corrected by a wooded block of appropriate height, the patient can maintain a straight spine in the erect position.

Fig. 5.47*B*.

ing the other categories. This classification is based upon the systems and various disease processes that may be involved etiologically in the development of scoliosis.

Idiopathic scoliosis is divided into three separate groups, depending upon the age of onset or recognition.[60] The infantile[35,62,63] age, 3 years and under, while quite uncommon in the United States, composes a significant group of patients in Great Britain. No specific explanation is currently available for the marked statistical difference. There are two subgroups of patients in this category: (1) the resolving type is found in patients who manifest a significant curve (20° or more) that subsequently disappears without specific treatment; and (2) the progressive form is exceedingly

difficult to manage because it has a great propensity for increase in the degrees of angular deformity regardless of the nonoperative treatment program used.

The juvenile patients (Figs. 5.48 and 5.49), ages 4-9, are a relatively small but important segment of patients for whom nonoperative treatment should be considered and enthusiastically pursued. At times it may be necessary, as in the infantile, to perform a limited fusion to aid in halting the progression of the spinal deformity. Secondary surgery may be necessary at a later date depending on the progression of the scoliosis.

The adolescent form is the most common type of scoliosis seen and will be discussed in greater detail (Fig. 5.50).

Table 5.2. Structural Scoliosis (Cobb's Classification)

I. Osteopathic
  A. Congenital
  B. Thoracogenic (postempyema, post-thoraco-plasty)
  C. Postirradiation
  D. Other osteopathic
II. Neuropathic
  A. Congenital
  B. Postpoliomyelitis
  C. Neurofibromatosis, syringomyelia, etc.
III. Myopathic
  A. Congenital
  B. Muscular dystrophy
  C. Other myopathic
IV. Idiopathic

The neuromuscular and myopathic groups of patients deserve special consideration for they emphasize the importance of making the specific diagnosis associated with the clinically noted scoliosis. Appropriate treatment must be rendered for the primary disease and the management of the patient's scoliosis modified.[4]

Many advances have been made in the management of patients with congenital scoliosis, particularly those who have segmental variations and those who have scoliosis associated with a myelomeningocele. These patients are discussed in detail in another section of this text.

The remainder of the classification is directed to patients with specific etiologic classification who have the potential to develop scoliosis as a portion of their disease process.

It is extremely important in the management of the whole patient and, in particular, the existent scoliosis to recognize that these entities coexist. We must always remember that, in treating scoliosis, we are not just dealing with a roentgenograph filled with angular deformities, but rather with a patient who has the physical and roentgenographic findings of a structural scoliosis.

Idiopathic Scoliosis

In the past, a wide variety of etiologies were proposed for idiopathic scoliosis. Old wives' tales, such as carrying a heavy load on one side, the performance of asymmetrical exercise, the adoption of a pattern of a poor sitting or standing position, still persist. To associate these "facts" as cause and effect is to ignore the mechanics of the spine as related to scoliosis. It is mechanically impossible to demonstrate the forces of such suggested etiologies that could possibly produce a structural scoliosis with a three or four curve pattern.

Some have said that idiopathic scoliosis represents the unrecognized effect of anterior poliomyelitis. One can readily demonstrate mathematically that this is not true. Idiopathic scoliosis occurs predominately in female patients, who account for approximately 85% of the cases. Recognizeable postpoliomyelitis scoliosis occurs equally in male and female patients. Idiopathic scoliosis occurs within definite age limits, whereas postpoliomyelitis scoliosis might develop at almost any age. The spine in idiopathic scoliosis is almost always stable (Fig. 5.51). In a large percentage of the postpoliomyelitis scolioses, the spine is unstable. Postpoliomyelitis scoliosis often demonstrates marked telescoping and collapse in the erect position (Fig. 5.52). The characteristic curves of these two forms of scoliosis are different, and the prognosis and behavior of the curve in each instance are different. For example, postpoliomyelitis scoliosis may increase after growth is complete, or it may originate after growth is completed. Further and most significant, since the advent of the poliomyelitis vaccine, there has been no decrease in the incidence of idiopathic scoliosis. Idiopathic scoliosis, on the other hand, usually increases before the completion of growth and only occasionally afterward. Urbaniak and Stelling[122] have shown that some of their patients, followed 2-20 years after iliac crest capping, demonstrated a mild increase in the degree of their curves. Certainly, though, the time for the greatest likelihood of an increase in the degree of angular deformity of a curve in idiopathic scoliosis is prior to skeletal maturity as evidenced by bone age, capping of the iliac apophyses, and, finally, closure of the vertebral ring apophyses. Comparative measurement of idiopathic scoliotic curves in the erect position and recumbent position seldom show a variation of more than 10-15°, whereas postpoliomyelitis scoliotic curves may show considerably more variation than this.

Table 5.3. Classification of Spinal Deformity

I. Idiopathic
  A. Infantile (3 years of age or younger)
    1. Resolving
    2. Progressive
  B. Juvenile (4-9 years of age)
  C. Adolescent (10 years of age or older)
II. Neuromuscular
  A. Neuropathic
    1. Upper motor neuron lesion
      a. Cerebral palsy
      b. Spinocerebellar disease
        (1) Friedrich's
        (2) Charcot-Marie-Tooth
        (3) Roussy-Lévy
      c. Syringomyelia
      d. Spinal cord tumor
      e. Spinal cord trauma
      f. Other
    2. Lower motor neuron lesion
      a. Poliomyelitis
      b. Other viral myelitis
      c. Traumatic
      d. Spinal muscular atrophy
        (1) Werdnig-Hoffmann
        (2) Kugelberg-Welander
      e. Myelomeningocele (paralytic)
    3. Dysautonomia (Riley-Day)
    4. Other
  B. Myopathic
    1. Arthrogryposis
    2. Muscular dystrophy
      a. Duchenne (pseudohypertrophic)
      b. Limb-girdle
      c. Facioscapulohumeral
    3. Fiber type disproportion
    4. Congenital hypotonia
    5. Myotonia dystrophica
    6. Other
III. Congenital
  A. Conigenital scoliosis
    1. Failure of formation
      a. Wedge
      b. Hemivertebra
    2. Failure of segmentation
      a. Unilateral bar
      b. Bilateral ("fusion")
    3. Mixed
  B. Congenital kyphosis
    1. Failure of formation
    2. Failure of segmentation
    3. Mixed
  C. Congenital Lordosis
  D. Associated with neural tissue defect
    1. Myelomeningocele
    2. Meningocele

    3. Spinal dysraphism
      a. Diasetmatomyelia
      b. Other
IV. Neurofibromatosis
V. Mesenchymal
  A. Marfan's disease
  B. Homocystinuria
  C. Ehlers-Danlos disease
VI. Traumatic
  A. Fracture of dislocation (nonparalytic)
  B. Postirradiation
  C. Postlaminectomy
  D. Other
VII. Soft-Tissue Contractures
  A. Burn
  B. Other
VIII. Osteochondrodystrophies
  A. Achondroplasia
  B. Spondyloepiphyseal dysplasia
  C. Diastrophic dwarfism
  D. Mucopolysaccharidosis
IX. Scheuermann's Disease
X. Infection
  A. Tuberculosis
  B. Bacterial
  C. Fungal
  D. Parasitic
  E. Other
XI. Tumor
  A. Benign
  B. Malignant
XII. Rheumatoid Disease
  A. Juvenile rheumatoid
  B. Adult rheumatoid
  C. Marie-Strümpell
XIII. Metabolic
  A. Rickets
  B. Juvenile osteoporosis
  C. Osteogenesis imperfecta
XIV. Related to Lumbosacral Area
  A. Spondylolisthesis
  B. Spondylolysis
  C. Other congenital anomaly
  D. Other
XV. Thoracogenic
  A. Postempyema
  B. Post-thoracoplasty
  C. Post-thoracotomy
  D. Other
XVI. Hysterical
XVII. Functional
  A. Postural
  B. Secondary to short leg
  C. Other

Fig. 5.48. (*Left*) M.W., 8-year-old female with idiopathic scoliosis, 1948. Treatment consisted of the use of exercises and braces. Operative intervention was never suggested. (*Right*) X-ray of same patient taken in 1953; patient now aged 13. Correction and fusion resulted in very definite improvement, but certainly the ideal time for this procedure was missed. Serial x-ray observation at 3-month intervals would have graphically demonstrated the progression of angular deformity and indicated the need for surgical therapy.

The work of Wynne-Davies[123],[133] and that of MacEwen and Cowell[78] have demonstrated that there is more of a genetic factor in many of the families of patients with idiopathic scoliosis. We have all seen patients who have other family members with idiopathic scoliosis. Until these studies, the genetic pattern had not been well established. By examining and x-raying members of patients' families and collecting roentgenograms of persons unavailable for personal examination, MacEwen and Cowell[16,78] were able to construct family trees of their patients and demonstrate the inheritance pattern. Admittedly, many of these angular deformities were small, but their curves did have structural characteristics. The pattern of inheritance they found was sex-linked and dominant, whereas Filho and Thompson[36] concluded that the pattern was multifactorial (polygenetic). As a result, it is now our policy to inform the patients and their families that such potential does exist, that they should make a practice of checking the spines of their children on their birthdays and seek medical

evaluation if there is any evidence of a developing scoliosis. We are equally positive in our recommendation that this factor alone should not influence the decision of the patient concerning future child bearing.

Still others have postulated that a nutritional deficiency is the responsible factor, but this has never been proven even by extensive biochemical studies. It is difficult to prove either a nutritional or endocrine variation. In a study of a large segment of patients with scoliosis at any one time, the vast majority show no increase in their angular deformity while they are under observation. Idiopathic scoliosis tends to increase at irregular and unpredictable intervals; therefore, the variations that might occur would be relatively infrequent and difficult to evaluate and check.

In idiopathic scoliosis, definitive curve patterns[61] can be identified and this is the only category in which such a classification is possible. The most common varieties are the single major or single structural curve with minor or compensatory curves above and

Fig. 5.49. (*A*) A.F. This patient was first seen at age 8 with a typical juvenile idiopathic scoliosis. Treatment was recommended but refused by parents on the advice of the family physician. (*B*) When examined by us in 1966, the 38° curve had increased to 155°. The patient did subsequently undergo surgical treatment, but the end result is certainly far from that desired. She has severe restrictive ventilatory defect and a vital capacity of 33%. Her scoliosis had been allowed to progress to the degree where she is a pulmonary cripple.

below, and the double major or double structural in which there are two structural curves with two minor or compensatory curves, one above and one below. A third pattern is thoracolumbar structural curve, that usually extends from T10 or T11 to L3 or L4 with compensatory curves above and below. This usually has a convexity to the left. The single structural curve usually has its convexity to the right and extends from T5 or T6 to T11, T12, or L1 and the double major structural curve has its convexity to the right from T4 or T5 to T10 or T11 and to the left from T10 or T11 to L3 or L4. There is a fourth pattern of an upper dorsal curve that is the least common. It extends from T1 or T2 to T5 or T6. It is the most difficult of all curve patterns to manage with a nonoperative treatment program.

Much has been written concerning the transformation of a functional scoliosis into a structural one. In spite of all that has been said, no valid proof exists that such a true transition ever occurs. Even the earliest x-rays of true structural scoliosis usually show structural changes.

History

In evaluating the patient with scoliosis, we are interested in having a complete and accurate

Fig. 5.49B.

history, not only of the scoliosis, but also of the general condition of the patient. Care must be taken to try to elicit a history of specific illnesses that have the potential to produce a structural scoliosis. It should be recorded that the family history does or does not reveal that other members of the family (siblings or maternal or paternal ancestors) have a scoliosis. As noted, recent studies in this area suggest that definite genetic patterns do exist.

Physical Findings

Again, the physical examination of the patient must not be limited to the scoliosis, but must be complete and general. If it is superficial or too narrow, the etiologic background of cases of known etiology is missed and, therefore, the proper management of the patient is not determined. We are particularly interested in trying to find evidence of neurologic deficit, muscular weakness, or significant skin lesions.

In a patient with scoliosis, the findings that are directly related to the scoliosis itself are asymmetrical, prominence of the rib cage, an elevated shoulder, a prominent hip and asymmetry of the flank creases (Fig. 5.51). These findings are directly related to the lateral deviation of the spine and its associated rotation. We are also interested in such findings as café au lait spots, subcutaneous or pedunculated neurofibroma, and the various skin lesions associated with congenital malformations of the spine—for example, a hairy patch, a midline hemangioma, a skin dimple, a lipoma, or a myelomeningocele.[17,23]

We have found it useful to grade the degree of rotation, as evidenced by clinical rib promi-

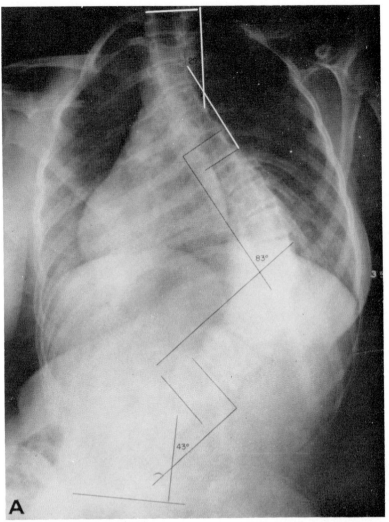

Fig. 5.50. (A) S.T., age 14, with a typical idiopathic scoliosis. Major curve, D6 to L2, 83°. Minor curves, D1 to D6, 29°, and L2 to S1, 43°. (B) Recumbent left bending film. Minor curve, D1 to D6, reduces to 16°; L2 to S1 reduces to 10°. This demonstrates considerable flexibility in the opposite curves and indicates that considerable reduction in the angular deformity of the major curve, D6 to L2, is permissible. (C) Postoperative film. Major curve, D6 to L2, 30°. This degree of correction has been maintained.

nence, depending upon severity. Grade one is the mildest, grade four is the sharp razor back. While this method is empiric and fairly gross, it has been clinically useful. A number of attempts have been made to grade the degree of rib hump and the associated contralateral thoracic valley. The use of a spirit level, (and the recording in centimeters of the difference in height at the apex of the curve) appears to be the most accurate but, in a practical sense, has not resulted in significant follow-up variations of clinical importance. List should be described as that distance to the right or left of the midgluteal crease that a plumbline reaches when dropped from the posterior spine of T1 or in patients with other than idiopathic scoliosis from the occiput down, i.e., list of 1 cm to the right (Fig. 5.53A).

X-ray Findings

The original x-ray studies should include anteroposterior views of the spine (standing, sitting, and recumbent) from the iliac crests up

Figs. 5.50B and C.

Fig. 5.51. (A) M.K. Patient had a right dorsolumbar scoliosis with marked asymmetry of the flank creases and a list to the right of 4 cm. (B) Postoperatively, patient has marked improvement in symmetry, but there is still some asymmetry. In most instances, surgical treatment results in improvement not in elimination of all the physical signs associated with scoliosis. (C) On forward flexion, the right dorsolumbar rib hump is evident preopertively. (D) Postoperatively, it is improved but, of all the clinical stigmata of scoliosis, it is the angulation of the ribs that can be reduced the least. Even in patients in whom it is permissible and obtainable to reduce the angular deformity of the thoracic curve to 0°, there will still be some residual deformity of the rib cage present both anteriorly and posteriorly.

Figs. 5.51*C* and *D*.

to and including the first thoracic vertebra. If there is a cervical component to the scoliosis, the cervical spine must also be included. These studies should be made on large films (preferably 14 X 36 inches but at least 14 X 17 inches) in order that the entire curve pattern, as it exists from the first thoracic vertebra to the sacrum, may be visualized (Charts 5.1-5.3). Segmental films do not permit accurate measurement of the curves. A lateral view of the spine must also be made as part of the original x-ray study. In patients with idiopathic scoliosis, we have been impressed with the higher incidence of spondylolisthesis than that seen in the population at risk. Several studies have documented this. The presence of spondylolisthesis certainly should modify one's approach to the surgical management of such a patient's scoliosis if it should be necessary. Follow-up films need include only anteroposterior standing and sitting x-rays of the spine. They should be made at 3- or 4-month intervals during the period of time when an increase in the angular deformity may be

reasonably expected. The erect films of the standing and sitting positions serve as a mathematical countercheck against each other. By either method of measurement (Figs. 5.44 and 5.45), the variation between these two films usually is not more than 3-5°. This countercheck excludes technician error. However, the variation may be greater if the patient has, for example, atrophy of a buttock and, therefore, a pelvic tilt in the sitting film. If an inequality of leg length is present, it will distort the spine in the standing films. Such deformities must be compensated for when the films are taken, for, depending on their severity, they produce significant changes in the degree of angular deformity and make comparative measurements imprecise.

All the curves must be measured and the measurement should be recorded each time for comparative study in the future. If a change in the degree of a measured curve exceeds 5° in both the sitting and standing films, an increase in the angular deformity can be said to have occurred. Additional views, such as sitting tilt

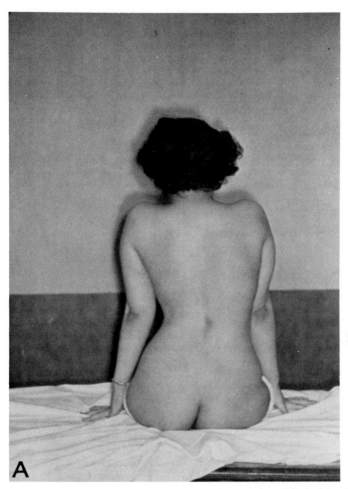

Fig. 5.52. (A) M.W. Patient developed anterior poliomyelitis as an infant. She had involvement of her trunk and lower extremities. Her scoliosis developed within 2 years after onset of her polio. Bracing became increasingly difficult. The patient eventually could sit only with support of her right hand because of the progressive scoliosis and the marked instability of her spine. (B) Patient is able to distract her unstable spine. Correction and fusion resulted in a stable, almost straight spine and the patient became independent of bracing and able to perform most normal activities.

and lateral bending studies, are chiefly of value in the preoperative evaluation of the patient prior to correction and fusion. These studies are of particular value in establishing the flexibility of the major (structural) and minor (compensatory) curves. They are used to determine the amount of correction that is permissible as evidenced by the flexibility of the major curve or curves, thereby indicating how much correction might be obtained (Figs. 5.50 and 5.55). We are using forced bend lateral recumbent films (Fig. 5.56) to give us a better index of the correction that can be expected with the various methods of preoperative correction.

In addition to the degree of angular deformity of the curves, one should also record the amount of rotation and wedging. Both rotation and wedging may be graded from one plus to four plus. Rotation may be determined by the location of the apical posterior spinous process or by the outline of the vertebral pedicles. The former is easier to define, but the necessary landmark is destroyed when a spine fusion has been performed. Therefore, pedicle rotation, as described by Nash and Moe,[97] must be used if we are going to be able to compare preoperative and postoperative rotation as seen in the roentgenograph.

Fig. 5.52B.

Many other things might be measured in the x-rays, but these fundamental findings have proven to be the most significant and valuable aids to an accurate follow up of the patient with scoliosis.

Adolescent Idiopathic Scoliosis

In our large scoliosis service where all degrees of scoliosis are seen and followed, the vast majority of the cases are idiopathic in nature. Idiopathic scoliosis is a self-limited disease characterized by the development of a structural scoliosis for which there is no known etiology. The probable genetic basis for it has already been referred to. Apparently the predisposition is inherited, but its expressivity is delayed. This, however, still does not explain why the scoliotic curve develops. The angular deformity does not progress at a constant rate but, rather, at unpredictable intervals. If an increase occurs, it almost always appears before age 15 in female patients and age 16 in male patients. Progression may or may not occur and, if it does, it may stop spontaneously with or without treatment. Growth is not the only factor associated with an increase in the angular deformity of an idiopathic scoliosis. Many patients show a marked increase in height without any significant change in the degree of angular deformity.

If the curves increase, they most often do so while growth is occurring, but not because of it (Fig. 5.49). These two, then, are concomitant occurrences and not cause and effect. Some patients show an increase in their curves after

Fig. 5.53. (*A*) R.E. This patient demonstrates severe but typical clinical findings of a structural scoliosis. He has a major (structural) right cervical dorsal curve with a higher right shoulder and prominence of the right scapula. His left dorsolumbar curve is a minor (compensatory) curve as is his upper cervical curve. There is marked list to the right (6 cm). This list is a further automatic attempt to balance for the major, structural, curve. (*B*) On forward flexion the marked +4 razor back rib hump is seen on the convex side of the curve. On the left concave side of the thoracic curve, the deep thoracic valley is readily appreciated. The anterior chest mirrors these deformities. As the spine bends laterally, it also rotates bringing the ribs back on the convex side of a curve and forward on the concave side. As a juvenile, this patient had had empyema which was surgically treated. He was not followed for the development of scoliosis and, when recognized, it was ignored.

skeletal maturity and, therefore, these patients must be followed at least to age 21. After skeletal maturity, they may be checked at yearly intervals instead of every 3-4 months.

The observation by Risser[110] that, after the iliac crests are fully capped by their apophyses, idiopathic scoliosis does not usually increase, is of particular value in treating those patients whose spines mature before the age of 15 or 16.

The crest may be considered to be fully capped when the mineralization of the apophysis has progressed from the lateral aspect medially to include the area of the posterosuperior iliac spine.[136] A better index of skeletal maturity is bone age and the maturity of the spine is best determined by the closure of the vertebral ring apophyses.

Approximately 85% of the cases of idio-

Chart 5.1. Scoliosis History

Name	Date	History of Number

Date of Birth	Age	Sex

Complaint: (High shoulder, prominent shoulder blade, high or prominent hip, prominent chest or breast, short leg, curvature, poor posture, awkward walk, pain in back, general fatigue, *etc.*)

Present History: Which deformity noted first
    Age first noted   by whom (patient, parents, doctor, teacher, nurse)
    Age first treated   what treatment (corset, brace, frame exercises, traction)
    Duration of treatment
    Progress of deformity (stationary, increasing, decreasing, rapid, slow)

Family History: Give history of scoliosis or other deformity in each case (other side).
    Maternal grandmother (descent . . . .) Paternal grandmother (descent . . . .)
       "   grandfather (descent . . . .)   "   grandfather (descent . . . .)

			standing height		sitting height	
Father	Age					
Mother	Age		" "		" "	
Brothers	1	Age	" "		" "	
(names)	2	"	" "		" "	
	3	"	" "		" "	
	4	"	" "		" "	
Sisters	1	"	" "		" "	
(names)	2	"	" "		" "	
	3	"	" "		" "	
	4	"	" "		" "	

Past History: Birth difficult or normal. Evidence of trauma?
    General health (robust, weak, normal weight, underweight, overweight, good color, pale, sickly, frequent illness.) Illness—(age and duration) scarlet fever , measles , mumps , chicken pox , whooping cough , polio , rickets , diphtheria , empyema , pneumonia , torticollis , Friedreich's ataxia , chorea , tonsillitis ; menses, age onset , (regular, irregular, scanty, profuse, duration)

Examination   Date
    General posture (good, fair, poor). General development (good, fair, poor). Musculature (good, fair, poor). Nutrition (good, fair, poor). High shoulder (rt., left). Prominent scapula (rt., left). Prominent low ribs (rt., left). Exaggerated flank crease (rt., left). Prominent hip (rt., left). High hip (rt., left). List (rt., left). R.A. L.A. Rotation (no, mild, moderate, severe)
    Standing height   Sitting height   Weight
    Flexibility of spine (flexible, moderately fixed, fixed)
    Curve   (Note muscle imbalance on other side of sheet)
    Curve corrected on forward bending? (No, slight, moderate, complete)
    Curve corrected on suspension? (No, slight, moderate, complete)

Diagnosis—Scoliosis   { A. Functional
(check which)   { B. Structural

I. Osteopathic { 1. Congenital / 2. Thoracogenic / 3. Other osteopathic

II. Neuropathic. { 1. Congenital / 2. Post polio / 3. Other neuropathic

III. Myopathic { 1. Congenital / 2. Muscular dystrophy / 3. Other myopathic

IV. Idiopathic

pathic scoliosis occur in female patients, many of whom have a very early or very late onset of sexual maturity as evidenced by the menarche.[68,103] Many of the male patients who develop idiopathic scoliosis have a fairly feminine type of build, at least during their active growth period.

Chart 5.2. Scoliosis Record

Name ....Doctor ....
Diagnosis ....History No. ....

Date						
Age						
Ht. Standing						
Ht. Sitting						
Weight						
L. A.						
R. A.						
List						
High Shoulder						
Low Hip						
Prominent Hip						
X-ray Date						
Born Age						
( ) Curve { Standing / Sitting / Supine						
Rotation (+, ++, etc.)						
Wedging (+, ++, etc.)						
( ) Curve { Standing / Sitting / Supine						
Rotation (+, ++, etc.)						
Wedging (+, ++, etc.)						
( ) Curve { Standing / Sitting / Supine						
Rotation (+, ++, etc.)						
Wedging (+, ++, etc.)						
( ) Curve { Standing / Sitting / Supine						
Rotation (+, ++, etc.)						
Wedging (+, ++, etc.)						

Nonoperative treatment of these patients is difficult to evaluate because of the lack of predictable progression of the angular deformity. Elsewhere the use of the Milwaukee brace is discussed. Certainly time has shown that exercises alone have no effect on the progression of the degree of the curves. Other forms of bracing have not tolerated the test of time. It is unfortunate that there are so few well documented series of the use of the Milwaukee brace and its associated exercise program.[30,37,91]

Operative treatment of a patient with idiopathic scoliosis must be based upon an accurate knowledge of the mechanics of the spine, both normal and abnormal. Surgical treatment is not indicated in a patient with a mild idiopathic scoliosis whose serial x-rays show that there has been no increase in the angular deformity.[15,47,64] It is indicated in those whose angular deformity, when first seen, is severe enough to warrant correction and in those in whom there has been a rapid and/or a significant increase. The procedure may be relatively contraindicated for patients in whom the amount of correction obtainable is not significant ($20°$ or less) or for those in whom no correction of the major curve is permissible, provided that the scoliosis is not progressive. It may also be contraindicated by the presence of other organic or psychologic conditions that make any surgical procedure unwise.

The ideal time for performing this procedure is between the ages of 12 and 16. However, as we must not fuse unnecessarily in the mild, nonprogressive cases, we must also not allow the young patients to become so progressively deformed that they can no longer be salvaged cosmetically and physiologically.

The preoperative evaluation of the patient must include a complete history, physical, and x-ray studies and certain baseline laboratory studies, not only for initial evaluation but, also, for the postoperative regulation of the patient who may in this period of time develop any disease. We routinely obtain a complete blood count with differential, urinalysis, sedimentation rate, serology for luetic infection, total protein and albumin-globulin (A/G) ratio, electrocardiogram, chest x-ray, and pulmonary function studies.[43,45,67,72,95,106,114,115,126-128] Many of these patients, particularly those with curves of at least $90°$, have significant pulmonary dysfunction. Up to 60°, the pulmonary status is usually satisfactory in patients with stable spines. It is unfortunate but true that significant reduction in the degree of angular deformity by correction and fusion does not result in proportionate gains in pulmonary function. Therefore, patients must not be permitted to develop severe curves. Cor pulmonale secondary to scoliosis has not been seen in patients whose thoracic curve measures 60° or less (Fig. 5.54). In addition, we also require a thorough dental check and, if significant difficulties are found, they are corrected before treatment is begun.

The amount of correction permissible may be determined by the use of standing and recumbent bending films (Fig. 5.55). The amount of correction to be expected is eval-uated by forced lateral bend in recumbency (Fig. 5.56E).

In our hands preoperative correction of the patient with idiopathic scoliosis has undergone significant modification. Essentially, we are using one of three different modalities: (1) Risser localizer cast (Fig. 5.57), (2) turnbuckle jacket (Fig. 5.46),[5,70] (3) halo-femoral traction (Fig. 5.58),[102] halo-pelvic distraction (Fig. 5.59),[19,20,59,99,101,134] or Cotrell traction. The choice of the method depends upon the flexibility of the curve or curves undergoing treatment. For the more flexible curves, the localizer jacket has proven to be most satisfactory. If more correction is permissible than can be obtained by this method, then we resort to the turnbuckle jacket. For the still more rigid curves, we use halo-femoral traction, or at times

Chart 5.3. *Scoliosis File*

Fig. 5.54. P.S. Neuropathic scoliosis with marked progression over a 4-year period. Pulmonary function studies, including blood gases, demonstrated less than 20% of the normal.

halo-pelvic distraction. We have had a very limited experience with the Cotrell method of traction and, therefore, are not in a position to express our own evaluation of its role.

The greater the forces used and the more rigid the curve undergoing correction, the more likely the patient is to develop complications such as pressure sores, neurologic deficit, etc. These patients demand close monitoring while undergoing preoperative correction.

Regardless of the preoperative method of correction used, we try to convert all patients into a localizer type of jacket immediately preoperatively (Fig. 5.57). Great care must be taken in transferring a patient from a turnbuckle jacket or halo-femoral traction so that significant correction is not lost.

The posterior aspect of the localizer cast is cut out exposing the entire length of the spine and both posterior iliac crests (Figs. 5.46D and 5.57).

The spine is marked at two levels, one at either end of the intended fusion area. We have found the methylene blue, metal marker technique, to be most satisfactory (Fig. 5.56F). Correct identification of the fusion levels is imperative (Fig. 5.60).

The selection of a fusion area in an idiopathic scoliosis must be done with extreme care if satisfactory results are to be obtained. Where a complete permissible correction has been obtained, the minimum fusion area in a stable idiopathic scoliosis is the extent of the major (structural) curve or curves. If it has not been possible to obtain the maximum amount of correction permissible, then the inclusion of some compensation by addition to the fusion area of an extra segment from the adjacent

Fig. 5.55. (A) Preoperative film of patient M.K. (See Figs. 51A and B). Major curve, D6 to L1, 89°. Minor, D1 to D6, 53°, and L1 to S1, 36°. (B) Diagram of (A).

opposite curve or curves may be desirable. More recent work has shown in single major curves the extent of the fusion should be increased to include all those vertebrae that are rotated into the curve, that is, from the neutrally rotated vertebrae above (pedicle) to the neutrally rotated segment below the extent of the actual curve (Fig. 5.61). This has obviated apparent loss of correction caused by the angulation of adjacent vertebrae, particularly those inferior to the major curve. They can add to the length of the original curve and increases its angular deformity.

For some years now we have adopted Harrington spinal instrumentation combined with a spine fusion as our standard surgical technique for patients undergoing surgical treatment for idiopathic scoliosis. As a result, we have modified our spine fusion technique and now, in these instances, perform only a complete decortication of the posterior elements. If spinal instrumentation is not feasible, we still perform a modified Hibbs fusion supplemented by autogenous posterior iliac crest bone (Fig. 5.62). In the thoracic area, the fusion bed extends from the tip of one transverse process across to the tip of its counterpart. In the lumbar area, we extend the fusion bed from facet to facet. We have found that, with the use of spinal instrumentation, the

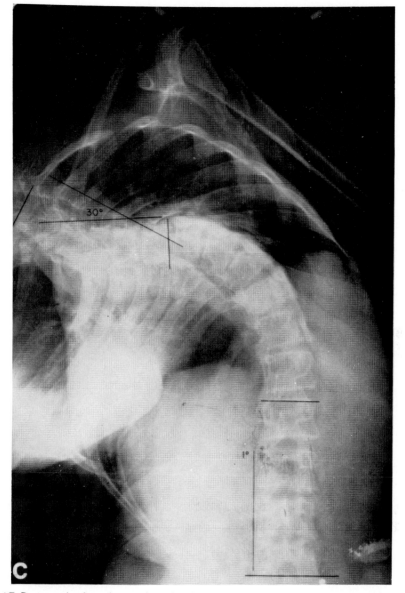

Fig. 5.55. (*C*) Preoperative lateral recumbent bending film. Minor curves, D1 to D6, 30°, and L1 to S1, 1°. (*D*) Diagram of (*C*).

modified Hibbs type of fusion makes it technically more difficult to insert the distraction rod and its hooks. Further, since resorting to simple decortication over this same broad bed, our incidence of successful fusion in the presence of satisfactory instrumentation has not decreased but, rather, improved even though we permitted our patients to become ambulatory earlier.

We have discarded the use of the compression rods (Fig. 5.63) as a part of our standard procedure. In our hands it had not resulted in significantly increased correction or better maintenance of correction. As previously stated, we attempt to gain almost all the permissible correction preoperatively and, therefore, at the operating table we are attempting to gain only another 10-15°. This

D

Fig. 5.55D.

limited goal of additional correction has a most important side benefit in that there is little opportunity for the operator to produce a relatively sudden distraction with the potential for vascular embarrassment of the cord. We limit ourselves to that amount of force which can be applied to the distraction apparatus with one hand (approximately 40 inch-pounds).[93,94] For similar reasons, we do not employ the outrigger to obtain correction.

The distraction hooks are placed into the facetal joint proximally on the concave side and beneath the superior laminal edge of the inferior lumbar vertebrae to be included in the fusion (Fig. 5.64). In a single major curve, the distal hook is placed on the convave side. In a double major curve, it is placed on the opposite side of the thoracic proximal hook, thus causing the rod to cross over to the opposite side.

Autogenous bone graft is obtained from the posterior iliac crest. Most patients have a sufficient volume of bone available from a single posterior crest.[42] Only occasionally is it necessary to supplement the graft volume with bone bank bone. We reserve the opposite crest for use, should a secondary procedure ever become necessary. In a few patients, particularly those with other forms of scoliosis because of the small posterior iliac crest, it may be necessary to rely entirely on bone bank bone. This is strictly second class bone as has been shown in our studies of consecutive patients whose spine fusions were explored routinely 6 months postoperatively (Table 5.4).[21,24,25,82] Since the incidence of pseudoarthrosis was reduced so dramatically by the use of autogenous bone, we feel that routine exploration is not indicated in patients in whom autogenous graft can be used and, particularly, in those in whom spinal instrumentation has been performed. We reserve exploration for those who show a significant amount of loss of correction (10° or more).

With rare exception, all of our patients undergo a one-stage operative procedure. Blood loss is followed by weighing sponges and appropriate replacement is given with either

Fig. 5.55. (*E*) Preoperative x-ray showing reduction in the major curve, D6 to L1, from 89° to 34°. Note the metal markers over the spinous processes of D6 and L1. The film is made through the Risser jacket. The opague discs are the studs in the hinges. The central opaque disc is at the apex of the anterior hinge, the posterior hinge having been removed in excising the window for surgery. It is to be noted that even when the desired correction has been obtained, the apex of the hinges has just reached the concavity of the major curve from its original position eccentric to the convexity and at or about the apex of the major curve. (*F*) Diagram of (*E*).

whole blood or packed cells and plasma. The patient undergoes continuous monitoring with electrocardiogram, central venous pressure, and temperature, and, in the more complicated or prolonged cases, blood gases are determined at intervals.

In spite of the use of spinal instrumentation, it is still the mature fusion that must be counted upon to maintain the corrected position against all the forces that have produced the curve. The necessity for a mature massive fusion is apparent.

Immediately postoperatively the patient is maintained recumbent in the localizer jacket or the turnbuckle jacket, etc., until the sutures are removed on the 10th postoperative day. We routinely have a nasogastric tube in place and it is maintained until bowel sounds are present and the patient is able to tolerate liquids with the tube clamped off. By such a system, we have been able to avoid the "cast syndrome."[31,52,104] The hemoglobin and hematocrit are check the day postoperative and 2-3 days later. Additional blood may be required in

Fig. 5.55F.

the early postoperative period, particularly if the amount of replacement blood and other maintainers of fluid volume has not been adequate. We do not use prophylactic antibiotic coverage in the routine idiopathic scoliosis patient. We emphasize pulmonary toilet and place all our patients on an "intermittent positive pressure breathing" program.

In the immediate postoperative period, it is imperative that the patient be carefully monitored[96] for the presence of or the development of neurologic deficit. We have not resorted to waking the patients during surgery to have them move their feet at the time instrumentation has been completed, as described by Keim, nor do we perform routine preoperative selective angiography.[57] We do closely check the patient in the recovery room for neurologic deficit. The presence of acute anterior thigh pain is a prodromal symptom of impending neurologic deficit. If neurologic deficit is

present or develops, it is an immediate indication for the removal of the rod and one should not try to reinsert it. Time is of the essence if recovery is to be expected. This has become abundantly clear in the reports of the morbidity committee of the Scoliosis Research Society.

Following suture removal and primary wound healing, a new localizer cast is applied and the patient is permitted to become ambulatory. If spinal instrumentation has not been used, the patient is not permitted to get up but, rather, remains recumbent. The vast majority of the patients are suitable for instrumentation and, therefore, are discharged to their homes ambulatory. They may return to school on a limited activity program (no gym, etc.). Six months postoperatively the cast is removed and x-rays are taken to determine the maintenance of correction and the progression of the fusion. The bony mass is best visualized in oblique

Fig. 5.55. (*G*) Composite film showing the eventual angular pattern of the patient on completion of correction and fusion. The top and bottom portions, the minor curves, are taken from Figure 5.55*B*, bending film, Superimposed between these is our preoperative correction film, Figure 5.55*C*. By this means we can determine that our patient is not overcorrected. More correction would have been permissible if it had been obtainable. Serial x-rays taken during correction showed that no further correction was obtainable. (*H*) Diagram of (*G*).

Fig. 5.55. (*I*) Postoperative films demonstrate maintenance of correction obtained. Note the neurologic clips which have been placed on the remaining tips of the spinous processes at the ends of the fusion area, D6 to L1. These readily identify the area fused in the follow-up x-ray studies. (*J*) Diagram of (*I*).

projections of the fusion area. A body cast is then applied for another 4-5 months. If at 11 months follow-up roentgenographs are satisfactory, the patient is permitted to discard the body cast and gradually resume normal activities. We ask our patients not to engage in such sports as tumbling, the use of a trampoline, etc.

It is our experience that, with a solid mature fusion, there is no appreciable loss of correction. Since we have switched to using autogenous rather than homologous bone, the incidence of pseudoarthrosis has markedly

decreased from about 30% to less than 10% in patients with idiopathic scoliosis. With spinal instrumentation this has been further reduced to less than 3% in the patient with idiopathic scoliosis (Fig. 5.65) (Table 5.4).

Postpoliomyelitis Scoliosis

Patients with postpoliomyelitis scoliosis in the past accounted for approximately 10% of

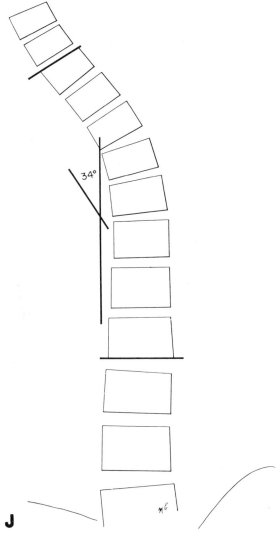

Fig. 5.55J.

the cases of scoliosis seen. However, as we get further and further away from the prevaccine days, their numbers are rapidly diminishing; but there are still some cases being referred for their spinal problems.[9,44,65,76,100] Many of these people have unstable spines and, for them, correction and fusion may be indicated to obtain stability rather than for the amount of correction permissible.

All patients who have had anterior poliomyelitis must be watched for the development of scoliosis. Some of them do not develop a clinically evident scoliosis for as long as 10 years after the onset of the disease. One cannot predict which patients will develop scoliosis by the muscles involved. The muscles attached to the spine are numerous and the possible mathematical combinations in which they may be involved, as well as their effect upon the spine, cannot be comprehended. The use of bracing and casts in the postpoliomyelitis scoliosis may have definite value in providing stability for the trunk, but it must not be felt that they will stop the curve from progressing.

Patients with postpoliomyelitis requiring the use of respirators have been shown to develop

Fig. 5.56. (A) B.E., age 11. Scoliosis first noted 1 year earlier. Received chiropractic treatment. Serial films demonstrated an increase in her major curve of her adolescent idiopathic scoliosis. Her major, structural, curve extends from T4 to T11, 63° standing with minor, compensatory, curves T1 to T4 above, 26°, and below, T11 to sacrum, 32°. She has +4 rotation of the apical vertebrae of the major curve as evidenced by the pedicles. (B) In recumbency, the major curve, T4 to T11, reduces to 54°.

and increase an angular deformity even though their activities are so completely confined and their recumbency so prolonged.

In selecting the area for fusion in these patients, at least the major (structural) curve and a segment or more below it must be included. At times it may be necessary to fuse a more extensive area in order to provide the necessary stability. In some patients it may be desirable to fuse to the sacrum. When the cervical region is severely involved (Fig. 5.68), it may be necessary to include the cervical spine and occiput in the fusion area. In these patients it is usually desirable to use the halo technique. A preliminary tracheostomy may be desirable if

they have severe respiratory involvement. The more severely involved the patients are, the more the spine telescopes and the more the patient needs stability. These patients must be stable sitters. Very early and extensive fusion in some patients has resulted in severe lordosis, but these patients were operated upon before spinal instrumentation was available. As in all cases of scoliosis, each patient must be individually evaluated, and therapy must be adapted to the evaluation.

It may be advisable to use halo-pelvic distraction for correction and immobilization for those patients with marked respiratory embarrassment who would not tolerate a

Fig. 5.56B.

plaster jacket. These patients may be operated upon while in the apparatus by temporarily removing one or two of the uprights during surgery. The avoidance of a prolonged period of immobilization in a plaster jacket may prevent further reduction of their already faulty pulmonary function.

For patients in whom it is necessary to fuse to the sacrum, we have found Harrington's spinal instrumentation in combination with the sacral bar to be of particular value because of the gross instability of their spines.

Congenital Scoliosis

In evaluating a congenital scoliosis, one cannot add up the segmental errors to determine the prognosis. It must be remembered that the x-rays show only the bony variations and not the associated soft-tissue changes. These patients must be closely observed, not only for a change in the scoliosis, but also for the development of neurologic deficits—motor, sensory, or sphincter changes (Fig. 5.67). Any of these suggests the possibility of such lesions as diastematomyelia, extradural lipomas, etc. Patients who have errors in segmentation usually have a trunk that is short in proportion to the extremeties. Most congenital scolioses are stable.[105,118,119] Elsewhere in this text the management of congenital scoliosis is discussed in detail. In general, procedures that shorten the spine and that can be performed in the lumbar area have less chance of producing neurologic embarrassment.[58,73,84,130-132] Other congenital anomalies should be sought for in these patients, i.e., kidney.[80]

Fig. 5.56. (*C*) On lateral bend, recumbent, toward the concavity of the major curve, the minor compensatory curves reduce to 20°, T1 to T4, and 8°, T11 to the sacrum. (*D*) On lateral bend, recumbent, toward the convexity of the major curve, the major structural curve reduces to 40°. This demonstrates very limited flexibility for the age of the patient and the degree of the curve present.

Von Recklinghausen's Neurofibromatosis

The curve pattern in a patient who has a scoliosis associated with a neurofibromatosis is usually characteristic (Fig. 5.68). The curve presents a short, sharp angular pattern by x-ray (Fig. 5.69) and the structural changes are usually greater than those usually associated with the amount of angular deformity present.[113,129] This is particularly evident in the milder curves. Many of these patients show the cutaneous manifestations of neurofibromatosis: café au lait spots, subcutaneous neurofibroma, or pedunculated neurofibroma. Almost all of these patients require correction and fusion. It has been the experience of many that these

curves usually progress and eventually produce the most severe deformity seen in the patient with scoliosis. Many believe that, once the diagnosis is made, correction and fusion should be performed. Their belief stems from an appreciation of the marked deformity that usually develops if correction and fusion is not done. The propensity for these patients to develop neurologic problems has been well defined by Cobb and by Curtis.[18]

In the patient with neurofibromatosis and scoliosis, one must not consider performing a laminectomy for relief of the symptoms of spinal cord pressure secondary to neurofibroma before performing a spine fusion. It has been the experience of those who have performed

Fig. 5.56D.

such a procedure, prior to stabilization of the spine, that the results are often disastrous. The neurologic deficit may increase precipitously.

Postempyema and Post-thoracoplasty Scolioses

Postempyema and post-thoracoplasty scolioses[6,7,46,71,120] are becoming less of a problem because of the decreased incidence of empyema and thoracoplasty and the successful way in which the problems associated with them are currently handled. These scolioses should always be looked for, particularly in the skeletally immature. The patient who has had either empyema or a thoracoplasty should be followed by serial x-ray films of the spine if there is any suggestion of a developing scoliosis. Correction and fusion are indicated when a significant curve develops or when definite

progression is demonstrated. It is usually in childhood that a significant scoliosis develops from either of these causes.

Muscular Dystrophy

The patients with muscular dystrophy who develop scoliosis often develop an extreme amount of deformity. The recognition of the associated disease is extremely important. These patients must not be placed in recumbency during the period of time required for correction and fusion. To do so will cause the muscular atrophy to progress to the point where walking may no longer be possible. In selected patients, we have performed correction and fusion with spinal instrumentation in an effort to improve their sitting ability and prolong their useful life (Fig. 5.70). Again, the

Fig. 5.56. (*E*) Forced lateral bend to the right demonstrates that reduction is possible of the major curve, T4 to T11, to 25°. (*F*) After the posterior window has been removed for preoperative marking, the major curve now measures 34°. The metal strips over two methylene blue intradermal marks injected into the skin overly the posterior spinous processes of the end vertebrae of the selected fusion area.

use of halo-pelvic distraction has proven to be valuable.

Postirradiation Scoliosis

This is a specific type of acquired scoliosis.[2,3,22,69,74] It is usually seen as a result of the irradiation therapy administered to infants in the course of treatment of either a Wilms' tumor or a neuroblastoma. A careful study of these patients reveals that no definite changes are seen in the irradiated segments until approximately 2 years after the therapy was administered. The changes that occur are attributable to the growth inhibition secondary to the irradiation. The vertebral bodies show irregular ossification and, in many instances,

resemble lesions seen in osteochondrodystrophy. The scarred outline of the vertebral body may be visible and appear as an os within an os. This form of structural scoliosis may progress (Fig. 5.71). Since these patients have had their insult early in life, the growth inhibition produced may be severe, and, therefore, the resulting deformity may be severe. In our series of 37 patients, all patients who have developed a postirradiation scoliosis have received more than 1,200 R tumor dose. All patients in whom the tumor or the surgery involved the spine were excluded from this study.

This type of scoliosis has the same characteristics as all other structural scolioses, i.e., wedging, rotation, and definitive curve pattern.

Fig. 5.56F.

These patients should be subjected to the same careful clinical and roentgenographic follow-up. Correction and fusion should be performed on those who show continuing progression, or who have developed a significant angular deformity. In our series only 2 patients have progressed to the degree that they required correction and fusion. Where the necessary surgery to remove the tumor included the excision of spinal elements or when the tumor itself invaded the structure of the spine of the patient, the degree of scoliosis that followed was almost without exception progressive and severe.

Summary

In summary, it would seem that intelligent management of a patient with scoliosis is dependent upon appreciation of etiology. The vast majority of patients do not require correction and fusion. When correction and fusion is indicated, it must be carefully planned and carried out. If these criteria are met, successful correction and fusion can be obtained and the results are gratifying.

It is our considered opinion that in treating scoliosis surgically, the surgeon must have an extensive understanding of the mechanics of the spine. He should handle the problem frequently and he should have available an anesthesiologist who is familiar with scoliosis and who is capable of handling the endotracheal anesthesia required.

The surgeon must realize that the opportunity to obtain correction and fusion for the rest of the patient's life normally occurs only once during that lifetime. Salvage procedures for loss of correction or for inadequate fusions are, at best, second rate. Time, therefore, is not of the

Fig. 5.56. (*G* and *H*) After instrumentation the curve now measures 25°. As indicated in the text, most of the correction should be obtained preoperatively.

essence, but adequate correction and a solid and mature fusion are.

Postlumboperitoneal Shunt Lordosis

For the past 10 years we and others[26,50] have become increasingly concerned about the effect upon the spine that lumboperitoneal shunting for communicating hydrocephalus can produce. Most often the patient develops a fixed, progressive lordosis (Fig. 5.72). Less often a significant degree of scoliosis develops.

Nonoperative treatment is ineffectual whether braces, traction, or exercises are employed.

We have found that in the patients with fixed lordosis, the posterior approach is ineffective. Therefore, our routine is to perform anterior

wedge resection and place the patient in 90-90 skeletal traction. If the wedge does not close within 10 days to 2 weeks, we perform a second stage procedure posteriorly. At that time the facets opposite the level of the anterior wedge are resected and this permits desired correction (Fig. 5.73).

The scoliosis that occurs in these patients is also a very rigid type but does respond to turnbuckle jacket correction and fusion.

Removal of the shunt has no beneficial effect upon the spinal deformity or its progression. We feel that this type of shunting procedure should be avoided because of its destructive effect upon the spine. The unanswered question to date is how extensive a posterior spine fusion, if any, should be performed following the correction of lordosis. Based on our limited

Fig. 5.56*H*.

Fig. 5.57. (A) Risser localizer jacket extending well up over the posterior aspect of the head and down over the buttock. A posterior window has been cut out for preoperative level marking and through which the surgery will be performed. (B) Anterior view showing the molded chin piece, the throat, and abdominal windows. (C) Posterior window has been removed and the operative sites for both the fusion and the left posterior iliac crest donor site can be seen.

Fig. 5.57*B*.

Fig. 5.57C.

Fig. 5.58. Halo-femoral traction. (*A*) Halo. (*B*) Traction (*C*) Halo cast. This patient was treated in traction preoperatively. Postoperatively we could not use instrumenntation. He was placed in a halo cast after primary wound healing.

Fig. 5.58C.

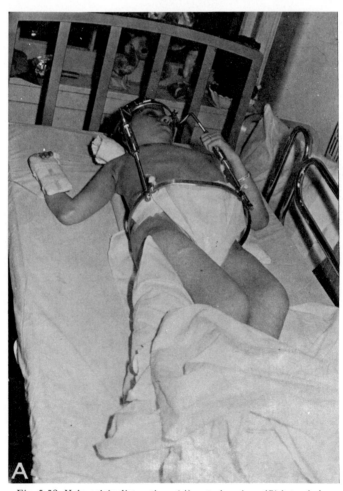

Fig. 5.59. Halo-pelvic distraction: (A) anterior view, (B) lateral view.

354

Fig. 5.59B.

Fig. 5.60 (A). C.M. The original films demonstrate a major curve, D5 to L2. After correction and fusion it was found that the fusion extended from D4 to L1.

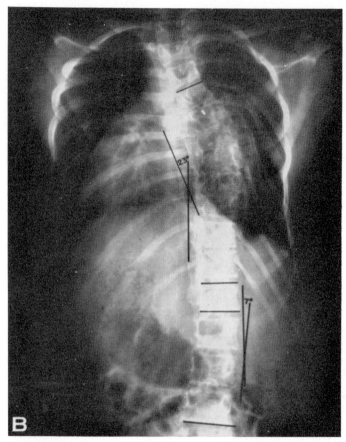

Fig. 5.60 (*B*). C.M. Ten months postoperatively. Fusion area, D4 to L1, measures 23°; L1 to L4 measures 7°.

Fig. 5.60 (*C*). C.M. Thirty-one months postoperatively. Fusion area, D4 to L1, measured 32°, and this measurement has been consistent since 12 months postoperatively. Note that there is recurrent angular deformity between L1 and L2; this deformity was originally part of the major curve and was omitted in error in the fusion area. The angular deformity between L1 and L4 is 44°.

Fig. 5.60 (*D*). C.M. The patient was placed in a turnbuckle jacket and the angular deformity was reduced 7°. Fusion was extended from L1 to L4. The patient has maintained this correction without loss.

Fig. 5.61. K.R. Idiopathic scoliosis. (*A*) Major, structural, curve extends from T6 to T12. Pedicle rotation is not neutral until L1. Therefore, fusion is extended to L1 (*B*). This excellent correction has been maintained and there has been no adding to the major curve from below.

Fig. 5.62. Solid fusion.

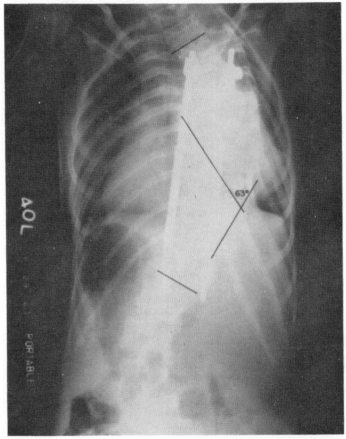

Fig. 5.63. P.S. Spine instrumentation performed as described by Harrington. This patient has shown no significant loss of correction in 1 year.

Fig. 5.64. (A) K.S. Adolescent idiopathic scoliosis. Age 12 at time of surgery. Treated in a localizer cast preoperatively. (B) Discharged 11 days postoperative; ambulatory, wearing a newly applied localizer cast. This correction has been maintained.

Fig. 5.64*B*.

Table 5.4. Follow-up of Patients with Spinal Fusion

A. Occurrence of Pseudoarthrosis

Graft	No. of Patients	Pseudoarthrosis	
		no.	*%*
Homologus	54	18	33
Autogenous	81	8	9.9

B. Number of Vertebrae in Fusion Area 4-8

Homologus	54	20	37
Autogenous	63	2	3

C. Number of Vertebrae in Fusion Area 9-14

Homologus	26	9	35
Autogenous	37	8	22

Fig. 5.65 (*A*). K.W. Postpolio scoliosis with a major curve extending from D7 to L3 and measuring 75°. This patient underwent correction and fusion.

Fig. 5.65 (*B*) K.W. One year postoperatively. Spine fusion, D7 to L4, measuring 15°.

Fig. 5.65*A* and *B*.

Fig. 5.65C and D.

Fig. 5.65 (*E*). K.W. Bending film to the concavity of the major curve, demonstrating that the opposite curves, D1 to D7, measureing 30°, and L4 to the sacrum, measuring 7°, would permit reduction of the major curve through pseudarthrosis.

Fig. 5.65 (*C*). K.W. Sixteen months postoperatively. Loss of correction is 30°. Patient has been ambulatory 6 months. Note loss of correction at apex.

Fig. 5.65 (*D*). K.W. Oblique films. *Arrows* point to pseudarthrosis.

Fig. 5.65*F* and *G*.

Fig. 5.65 (*H*). K.W. Oblique film. Arrows pointing to the area of repair of pseudarthrosis. This patient has shown no further loss in more than 3 years.

Fig. 5.65 (*F*). K.W. Bending film toward the convexity of the major curve, D7 to L4, measuring 33° as compared to 45° in the standard film. This demonstrates obvious motion at the level of pseudarthrosis.

Fig. 5.65 (*G*). K.W. Postoperative film following Risser jacket correction and repair of pseudarthrosis, D11 to D12, measuring 22°. Note the large mass of bony fusion at the level of repair.

Fig. 5.66*A* and *B*.

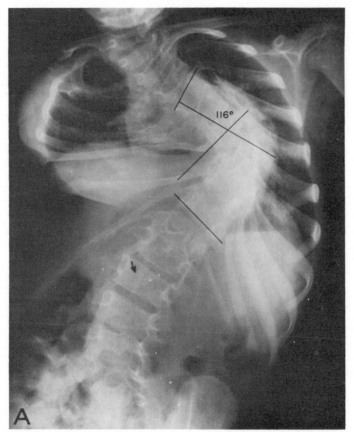

116°

A

Fig. 5.67. (A). C.W. Five-year-old female with congenital osteopathic scoliosis. Major curve, D5 to D11, 116°. Serial x-rays have not shown any progression of the angular deformity, but repeated neurologic examination revealed development of diminished sensation of L5 and S1 and progressive loss of function in the right peroneuals. On the original examination and for a year thereafter the neurologic examination of the extremity had been negative.

Fig. 5.66 (A). Postpolio scoliosis with a cervical component to the major curve.
Fig. 5.66 (B). Postoperative film following correction and fusion. When the scoliosis involves the cervical region, the serial films must include it.

Fig. 5.67 (*B*). Myelogram demonstrating diastematomyelia, level of L1. Surgical correction resulted in return of sensation and no further progression of peroneal weakness.

Fig. 5.68. G.M. Neuropathic scoliosis, von Recklinghausen. This patient had all the characteristic skin manifestations of neurofibromatosis. Notice the short, sharp, angular major curve, D4 to D8, measuring 82°. This curve pattern is typical of those seen in neuropathic scoliosis.

Fig. 5.69. M.B. Neuropathic scoliosis, von Recklinghausen. This patient has all the characteristic skin manifestations. The fifth, sixth, seventh, and eighth ribs show "neurotrophic" effect There is marked wedging of D7 out of proportion to the rest of the curve.

Fig. 5.70. Muscular dystrophy. (*A*) This patient's muscular dystrophy is advanced. He is unable to sit alone without external support. (*B*) Simple manual suspension currects most of his deformity. Patients of this category are on occasion considered for correction and fusion provided their life expectancy and general medical condition warrants. With such marked telescoping and limited extremity power, the desirability of stabilizing the spine is obvious. Since the advent of spinal instrumentation and halo-pelvic distraction, the possibilities for performing such surgery are improved.

Fig. 5.70*B*.

Fig. 5.71. (*Top, left*) Postirradiation scoliosis, 1962. Patient is white male, age 12; Wilms' tumor excised at age 4. (*Top, right*) Progressive increase over next 2 years, but none since he became skeletally mature (*bottom, left*). Lateral roentgenogram demonstrates postirradiation change, os within os. This is "the scar of the insult of the irradiation" (*bottom, right*).

Fig. 5.72. C.C. Lumboperitoneal shunt performed as an infant. His lordosis is fixed and progressive. Note the narrow disc space, L3-L4, level of the operative procedure posteriorly. Many of these patients show this particular change suggesting failure of the disc space to expand, similar to that seen when a fusion has been performed in early childhood.

Fig. 5.73. A.S., 14 years of age. Lumboperitoneal shunt was performed in infancy. Progressive lordosis was noted to have its onset at age 3 and obviously noticeable by age 8. (*A*) Preoperative roentgenogram demonstrating 125° of fixed lordosis (*B*) Following the first stage, anterior wedge resection L3-L4, the lordosis reduced only partially after 3 weeks in 90-90 traction. After second stage, the resection of the facets at L3-L4, the lordosis is corrected.

Fig. 5.73B.

experience, it would appear that in the skeletally immature patient, a spine fusion and Harrington instrumentation should be added to the posterior procedure. We have had one patient whose deformity recurred at a higher level and required secondary surgery. She was skeletally immature. The older patients have not shown this.

References

1. Albee, F. H., and Kushner, A.: Albee spine fusion operation in treatment of scoliosis, *Surg. Gynecol. Obstet., 66:* 797, 1938.
2. Arkin, A. M., Pack H. F., Ransohoff, N. S., and Simon, N.: Radiation-induced scoliosis, *J. Bone Joint Surg., 32A:* 401, 1950.
3. Arkin, A. M., and Simon, N.: Radiation scoliosis; experimental study, *J. Bone Joint Surg., 31A:* 394, 1960.
4. Balmer, G. A., and MacEwen, G. D.: The incidence and treatment of scoliosis in cerebral palsy, *J. Bone Joint Surg., 52B:* 134, 1970.
5. Barr, J. S.: Turnbuckle brace, 3 point pressure brace for correction and treatment of ambulatory care of scoliosis, *J. Bone Joint Surg., 18:* 760, 1936.
6. Bisgard, J. D.: Thoracogenic scoliosis; influence of thoracic disease and thoracic operations, *Arch. Surg., 29:* 417, 1934.
7. Bjork, V. O.: Scoliosis and herniation after osteoplastic thoracoplasty, *J. Thorac. Cardiovasc. Surg., 38:* 81, 1959.
8. Blount, W. P., and Moe, J. H.: *The Milwaukee Brace,* Baltimore: The Williams & Wilkins Co., 1973.
9. Bonnett, C., Perry, J., Brown, J. C., and Greenberg, B. J.: Halo-femoral distraction and posterior spine fusion for paralytic scoliosis, *J. Bone Joint Surg. 54A:* 202, 1972.
10. Cobb, J. R.: Treatment of scoliosis, *Conn. Med. J., 7:* 467, 1943.

11. Cobb, J. R.: Outline for study of scoliosis, *Instruct. Lect. Am. Acad. Orthop. Surg., 5:* 1948.

12. Cobb, J. R.: Technique, after-treatment and results of spine fusion for scoliosis, *Instruct. Lect. Amer. Acad. Orthop. Surg., 9:* 65, 1952.

13. Cobb, J. R.: Scoliosis, quo vadis, *J. Bone Joint Surg., 40A:* 507, 1968.

14. Cobb, J. R.: The problem of the primary curve, *J. Bone Joint Surg., 42A:* 1413, 1960.

15. Collis, D. K., and Ponseti, I. V.: Long-term follow-up patients with idiopathic scoliosis not treated surgically, *J. Bone Joint Surg., 51A:* 425, 1969.

16. Cowell, H. R., Hall, J. N., and MacEwen, G. D.: Genetic aspects of idiopathic scoliosis, *Clin. Orthop., 86:* 121, 1972.

17. Curtis, B. H.: Classification of Myelomeningocele and Congenital Spinal Defects, pp. 3-10, *Symposium on Myelomeningocele,* St. Louis: C. V. Mosby Co., 1972.

18. Curtis, B. H., Fisher, R. L., Butterfield, W. L., and Saunders, F. P.: Neurofibromatosis with paraplegia; report of 8 cases, *J. Bone Joint Surg., 51A:* 843, 1969.

19. Dewald, R. L., Mulcahey, T. M., and Schultz, A. B.: Force measurement studies with the halo-hoop apparatus in scoliosis, *Orthop. Rev., 2:* 17, 1973.

20. Dewald, R. L., and Ray, R. D.: Skeletal traction for the treatment of severe scoliosis; The University of Illinois halo-hoop apparatus, *J. Bone Joint Surg., 52A:* 233, 1970.

21. Donaldson, W. F., and Wissinger, H. A.: The results of surgical exploration of spine fusion performed for scoliosis, *West. J. Surg., 72:* 195, 1964.

22. Donaldson, W. F., and Wissinger, H. A.: Axial skeletal changes following tumor done radiation therapy, *J. Bone Joint Surg., 47A:* 1469, 1967.

23. Donaldson, W. F.: Scoliosis Associated with Spina Bifida and Myelomeningocele, pp. 40-42, *Post Graduate Course on the Management and Care of the Scoliosis Patient,* New York, 1969.

24. Donaldson, W. F.: The Problem of Pseudoarthrosis in Scoliosis Surgery, pp. 75-77, *Post Graduate Course on the Management and Care of the Scoliosis Patient,* New York, 1969.

25. Donaldson, W. F., Wissinger, H. A., and Stone, C. S.: Exploration of scoliosis spine fusions, *J. Bone Joint Surg., 51A:* 205, 1969.

26. Donaldson, W. F.: Neural Spinal Dysraphism, *Spinal Deformity in Neurological and Muscular Disorders,* St. Louis: C. V. Mosby Co., to be published.

27. Dwyer, A. F.: Anterior instrumentation in scoliosis, *J. Bone Joint Surg., 52B:* 782, 1970.

28. Dwyer, A. F.: Screw and cable correction of scoliosis, *J. Bone Joint Surg., 52B:* 193, 1970.

29. Dwyer, A. F., Newton, M. C., and Sherwood, A. A.: An anterior approach to scoliosis; preliminary report, *Clin. Orthop., 62:* 192, 1969.

30. Edmonson, A. S.: Evaluation of Milwaukee brace treatment in idiopathic scoliosis, *J. Bone*

31. Evarts, C. M., Winter, R. B., and Hall H.E.: The spinal traction syndrome—arteriomesenteric—duodenal obstruction associated with correction of spinal curvature with report of 3 illustrative cases, *J. Bone Joint Surg., 53A:* 198, 1971.

32. Ferguson, A. B.: Study and treatment of scoliosis, *South. Med. J., 23:* 116, 1930.

33. Ferguson, A. B.: Roentgen diagnosis in extremities and spine, *Instruct. Lect. Amer. Acad. Orthop. Surg., 2:* 214, 1947.

34. Ferguson, A. B.: Roentgen interpretations and decisions in scoliosis, *Instruct. Lect. Amer. Acad. Orthop. Surg., 7:* 160, 1950.

35. Ferreira, J. H., and James, J. I. P.: Progressive and resolving infantile idiopathic scoliosis; differential diagnosis, *J. Bone Joint Surg., 54B:* 648, 1972.

36. Filho, N. A., and Thompson, M. W.: Genetic studies in scoliosis, *J. Bone Joint Surg., 53A:* 199, 1971.

37. Galante, J., Schultz, A., DeWald, R. L., and Ray, R. D.: Forces acting in the Milwaukee brace on patients undergoing treatment for idiopathic scoliosis. *J. Bone Joint Surg., 52A:* 498, 1970.

38. George, K., and Reppstein, J.: A comparative study of the two popular methods of measuring scoliotic deformity of the spine, *J. Bone Joint Surg., 43A:* 809, 1961.

39. Goldstein, L. A.: Results in the treatment of scoliosis with turnbuckle plaster cast correction and fusion, *J. Bone Joint Surg., 41A:* 321, 1959.

40. Goldstein, L. A.: Surgical management of scoliosis, *J. Bone Joint Surg., 43:* 167, 1966.

41. Goldstein, L. A., and Evarts, C. M.: Follow up notes on articles previously published in the *Journal;* further experiences with the treatment of scoliosis by cast correction and spine fusion with fresh autogenous iliac-bone grafts, *J. Bone Joint Surg., 48:* 962, 1966.

42. Goldstein, L. A.: Treatment of idiopathic scoliosis by Harrington instrumentation and fusion with fresh autogenous iliac-bone grafts, *J. Bone Joint Surg., 51A:* 209, 1969.

43. Graham, J. J., Schack, J. A., and Liggett, A. S.: Cardiopulmonary function in scoliosis; preoperative and postoperative study, *J. Bone Joint Surg., 52A:* 399, 1970.

44. Gucker, T.: Experience with poliomyelitic scoliosis after fusion and correction, *J. Bone Joint Surg., 38A:* 1281, 1956.

45. Gucker, T.: Changes in vital capacity in scoliosis; primary report on effects of treatment, *J. Bone Joint Surg., 44A:* 469, 1962.

46. Gurd, F. B.: Scoliosis accompanying chronic infected open pneumothorax; its causation and correction, *Arch. Surg., 5:* 366, 1922.

47. Hall, J. E.: The management of scoliosis, *J. Bone Joint Surg., 52A:* 408, 1970.

48. Hall, J. E., Chan, D., Spira, I., and Roth, A.: Dwyer instrumentation and anterior spine fusion, unpublished data.

49. Hall, J. E., and Gillespie, R.: Idiopathic scoliosis treated by Harrington instrumentation and spine

Joint Surg., 51A: 202, 1969.

fusion, *J. Bone Joint Surg., 53A:* 198, 1971.

50. Hall, J. E., and King, J. D.: Hyperlordosis following lumbar peritoneal shunts for hydrocephalus, *J. Bone Joint Surg., 53A:* 198, 1971.

51. Hall, J. E., and Spira, I. S.: Dwyer anterior instrumentation and interbody fusion of the spine in the management of scoliosis, *J. Bone Joint Surg., 54A:* 201, 1972.

52. Hardy, J. H., Cooke, R. W., and Einbund, M.: Hyperalimintation in the treatment of "cast syndrome," *J. Bone Joint Surg., 54A:* 200, 1972.

53. Harrington, P. R.: Treatment of scoliosis, *J. Bone Joint Surg., 44A:* 591, 1962.

54. Harrington, P. R. First Progress Report: A Surgical Correction of Paralytic Scoliosis. Monograph.

55. Harrington, P. R.: Treatment of scoliosis; correction and internal fixation by spine instrumentation, *J. Bone Joint Surg., 44A:* 591, 1962.

56. Hibbs, R. A., Risser, J. D., and Ferguson, A. B.: Scoliosis treated by fusion operation, end-result study of 360 cases, *J. Bone Joint Surg., 13:* 91, 1931.

57. Hilal, S. K., and Keim, H. A.: Selective spinal angiography in adolescent scoliosis, *Radiology, 102:* 340, 1972.

58. Hodgson, A. R.: Correction of fixed spinal curves, *J. Bone Joint Surg., 44A:* 591, 1962.

59. Houtkin, S., and Levine, D. B.: The halo yoke; a simplified device for attachment of the halo to a body cast, *J. Bone Joint Surg., 54A:* 881, 1972.

60. James, J.: Idiopathic scoliosis, *J. Bone Joint Surg. 36B:* 36, 1954.

61. James, J.: Two curve patterns in idiopathic structural scoliosis, *J. Bone Joint Surg., 33B:* 399, 1951.

62. James, J.: Infantile idiopathic scoliosis, *Clin. Orthop., 21:* 106, 1961.

63. James, J.: Infantile structural scoliosis, *J. Bone Joint Surg., 41:* 719, 1959.

64. James, J.: Symposium on the treatment of organic spinal deformities; the indications for correction and fusion, *Proc. Soc. Roy. Med., 51:* 236, 1958.

65. James, J.: Paralytic scoliosis, *J. Bone Joint Surg., 38B:* 660, 1956.

66. James, J. I. P.: The etiology of scoliosis, *J. Bone Joint Surg., 52B:* 410, 1970.

67. Johnson, B. E., and Westgate, H. D.: Methods of predicting vital capacity in patients with thoracic scoliosis, *J. Bone Joint Surg., 52A:* 1433, 1970.

68. Kane, W. J., and Moe, J. H.: A scoliosis prevalence survey in Minnesota, *Clin. Orthop., 69:* 216, 1970.

69. Katzman, H., Waugh, T., and Berdon, W.: Skeletal changes following irradiation of childhood tumors, *J. Bone Joint Surg., 51A:* 825, 1969.

70. Kendrick, J.: Correction of scoliosis by use of modified turnbuckle jacket, *Cleve. Clin. Q., 4:* 16, 1937.

71. Kergin, F. G., and Dewar, F. P.: Pleural decortication in prevention and treatment of

thoacogenic scoliosis (resulting from fibrothorax), *Arch. Surg., 61:* 705, 1950.

72. Lamarre, A., Hall, J. E., Weng, T. R., Aspin, N., and Levison, H.: Pulmonary function in scoliosis 1 year after surgical correction, *J. Bone Joint Surg., 53A:* 195, 1971.

73. Leatherman, K. D.: Resection of vertebral bodies, *J. Bone Joint Surg., 51A:* 206, 1969.

74. Leatherman, K. D.: Radiation deformities of the spine, *J. Bone Joint Surg., 52A:* 405, 1970.

75. Levine, D. B., Wilson, R. L., and Doherty, J. H.: Operative management of idiopathic scoliosis; a critical analysis of 67 cases, *J. Bone Joint Surg., 52A:* 408, 1970.

76. Lowman, C. L.: Relation of abdominal muscles to paralytic scoliosis, *J. Bone Joint Surg., 14:* 763, 1932.

77. Loynes, R. D.: Scoliosis after thoracoplasty, *J. Bone Joint Surg., 54B:* 484, 1972.

78. MacEwen, G. D., and Cowell, H. R.: Familial incidence of idiopathic scoliosis and its implications in patient treatment, *J. Bone Joint Surg., 52A:* 405, 1970.

79. MacEwen, G. D., and Kirsch, P.: The structural response of the idiopathic curve to the Milwaukee brace, *J. Bone Joint Surg., 53A:* 196, 1971.

80. MacEwen, G. D., Winter, R. B., and Hardy, J. H.: Evaluation of kidney anomalies in congenital scoliosis, *J.Bone Joint Surg., 54A:* 1451, 1972.

81. Mankin, H. J., and Scheck, J.: Cardiopulmonary function in mild and moderate idiopathic scoliosis, *J. Bone Joint Surg., 46:* 53, 1964.

82. Mathews, R. S., and Stelling, F. H.: Second look spinal exploration for scoliosis, *J. Bone Joint Surg., 52A:* 409, 1970.

83. McCarroll, H. R.: Attempted treatment of scoliosis by unilateral vertebral epiphyseal arrest, *J. Bone Joint Surg., 43A:* 965, 1960.

84. McKenzie, K. G., and Dewar, F. P.: Scoliosis with paraplegia, *J. Bone Joint Surg., 31:* 162, 1919.

85. Moe, J. H.: Changing concepts of the scoliosis problem, *J. Bone Joint Surg., 43A:* 471, 1961.

86. Moe, J. H.: A critical analysis of methods of fusion for scoliosis on evaluation in 266 patients, *J. Bone Joint Surg., 40A:* 529, 1958.

87. Moe, J. H.: The management of idiopathic scoliosis, *Clin. Orthop., 9:* 169, 1957.

88. Moe, J. H.: Management of paralytic scoliosis, *South, Med. J., 50:* 67, 1957.

89. Moe, J. H., and Gustilo, R. B.: Treatment of scoliosis, results of 196 patients treated by cast correction and fusion, *J. Bone Joint Surg., 46:* 293, 1964.

90. Moe, J. H.: Presidential address, *J. Bone Joint Surg., 54A:* 1789, 1972.

91. Moe, J. H., and Kettleson, D. N.: Idiopathic scoliosis; analysis of curve patterns and the preliminary results of Milwaukee brace treatment in 169 patients, *J. Bone Joint Surg., 52A:* 1509, 1970.

92. Nachemson, A.: A long-term follow-up study of nontreated scoliosis, *J. Bone Joint Surg., 51A:* 203, 1969.

93. Nachemson, A., and Elfstrom, G.: A force-indicating distractor for the Harrington rod procedure, *J. Bone Joint Surg., 51A:* 1660, 1969.

94. Nachemson, A., and Elfstrom, G.: Intravital wireless telemetry of axial forces in Harrington distraction rods, *J. Bone Joint Surg., 53A:* 194, 1971.

95. Nachemson, A., Bake, B., Bjure, J., Grimby, G., Kaslichy, J., and Lindh, M.: Clinical follow-up and regional lung function studies in patients with nontreated idiopathic scoliosis, *J. Bone Joint Surg., 52A:* 401, 1970.

96. Nash, C. L., Jr., Brodky, J. S., and Croft, T. J.: A model for electrical monitoring of spinal cord function in scoliosis patients undergoing correction, *J. Bone Joint Surg., 54A:* 197, 1972.

97. Nash, C. L., Jr., and Moe, J. H.: A study of vertebral rotation, *J. Bone Joint Surg., 51A:* 223, 1969.

98. Nastasi, A. J., LeVine, D. B., and Veliskakis, K. P.: Pain patterns associated with adolescent idiopathic scoliosis, *J. Bone Joint Surg., 54A:* 199, 1972.

99. O'Brien, J. B.: Halo-pelvic traction in the correction of spinal deformities, *J. Bone Joint Surg., 52B:* 801, 1970.

100. O'Brien, J. P., and Yau, A. C. M. C.: Anterior and posterior correction and fusion for paralytic scoliosis, *Clin. Orthop., 86:* 151, 1972.

101. O'Brien, J. P., Yau, A. C. M. C., Smith, T. K., and Hodgson, A. R.: Halo-pelvic traction, *J. Bone Joint Surg. 53B:* 217, 1971.

102. Perry, J., Bonnett, C., and Ulin, R.: Halo-femoral traction as a method of preoperative correction of paralytic scoliosis, *J. Bone Joint Surg., 51A:* 402, 1970.

103. Ponseti, J., and Friedman, B.: Prognosis in idiopathic scoliosis, *J. Bone Joint Surg., 32A:* 381, 1950.

104. Puranik, S. R., Keiser, R. P., and Gilbert, M. G.: Arteriomesenteric duodenal compression in children, *Am. J. Surg., 124:* 334, 1972.

105. Raycroft, J. F., and Curtis, B. H.: Spinal Curvature in Myelomeningocele. Natural History and Etiology, pp. 182-201, *Symposium on Myelomeningocele,* St. Louis: C. V. Mosby Co., 1972.

106. Riseborough, E. J., and Shannon, D.: The effects of scoliosis on pulmonary function as determined by studies with xenon-133, *J. Bone Joint Surg., 52A:* 400, 1970.

107. Risser, J. C.: Scoliosis treated by fusion, preliminary report on some observations in 348 cases, *Am. J. Surg., 4:* 496, 1928.

108. Risser, J. C.: Important practical facts in treatment of scoliosis, *Instruct. Lect. Amer. Acad. Orthop. Surg., 5:* 1948.

109. Risser, J. C.: Scoliosis, prognosis, *J. Bone Joint Surg., 18:* 607, 1936.

110. Risser, J. C.: The iliac apophyses; an invaluable sign in the management of scoliosis, *Clin. Orthop., 11:* 111, 1958.

111. Risser, J. C.: Scoliosis, *Instruct. Lect. Am. Acad. Orthop. Surg., 14:* 91, 1957.

112. Risser, J. C., and Norquist, D. M.: A follow-up study of the treatment of scoliosis, *J. Bone Joint Surg., 40A:* 555, 1958.

113. Salerno, N. R., and Edeiken, J.: Vertebral scalloping in neurofibromatosis, *Radiology, 97:* 509, 1970.

114. Shannon, D. C., Riseborough, E. J., Laercio, M. V., and Kazemi, H.: The distribution of abnormal lung function in kyphoscoliosis, *J. Bone Joint Surg., 52A:* 131, 1970.

115. Silver, R. A., Nickel, V. L., Perry, J., and Bonnett, C.: The evaluation of pulmonary function in patients with scoliosis, *J. Bone Joint Surg., 52A:* 400, 1970.

116. Simmons, E. H., and Garside, H.: Biochemical and clinical study of anterior spinal instrumentation, *J. Bone Joint Surg., 52A:* 407, 1970.

117. Smith, A., Butte, F. L., and Ferguson, A. B.: Treatment of scoliosis by wedging jacket and spine fusion, *J. Bone Joint Surg., 20:* 825, 1938.

118. Sriram, K., and Bobechko, W. P.: Surgical Management of Spinal Deformities in Myelomeningocele, Proceedings, Scoliosis Research Society, 1970.

119. Sriram, K., Bobechko, W. P., and Hall, J. E.: Surgical management of spinal deformities in spina bifida, *J. Bone Joint Surg., 54B:* 666, 1972.

120. Stauffer, E. S., and Mankin, H. J.: Scoliosis after thoracoplasty; a study of 30 patients, *J. Bone Joint Surg., 48:* 339, 1966.

121. Tambornino, J. M., Armbrust, E. N., and Moe, J. H.: Harrington instrumentation in correction of scoliosis; a comparison with cast correction, *J. Bone Joint Surg., 46:* 313, 1964.

122. Urbaniak, J. R., and Stelling, F. H.: Progression of the scoliotic curve after completion of the excursion of the iliac epiphyses; a preliminary report, *J. Bone Joint Surg., 51A:* 205, 1969.

123. Vanderpool, D. W., James, J. I. P., and Wynne-Davis, R.: Scoliosis in the elderly, *J. Bone Joint Surg., 51A:* 446, 1969.

124. Van Lockum, W. H.: The surgical treatment of scoliosis, *Instruct. Lect. Am. Acad. Orthop. Surg., 5:* 1948.

125. Van Lockum, W. H.: Surgical scoliosis, *Surg. Clin. North Am.,* 1951.

126. Westgate, H. D., and Johnson, B. E.: Effects of scoliosis therapy on pulmonary function, *J. Bone Joint Surg., 52A:* 400, 1970.

127. Westgate, H. D., and Johnson, B. E.: Preoperative pulmonary evaluation and postoperative respiratory management of patients with severe thoracic scoliosis, *J. Bone Joint Surg., 53A:* 195, 1971.

128. Westgate, H. D., and Moe, J. H.: Pulmonary function in kyphoscoliosis before and after correction by the Harrington instrumentation method, *J. Bone Joint Surg., 51A:* 935, 1969.

129. Wilson, P. D., Jr., Veliskakis, K., and LeVine, D. B.: Neurofibromatosis and scoliosis; significance of the short, angular spinal curve, *J. Bone Joint Surg., 51A:* 203, 1969.

130. Winter, R. B., and Moe, J. H.: Scoliosis and the

Marfan syndrome, *J. Bone Joint Surg., 51A:* 204, 1969.

131. Winter, R. B., Moe, J. H., and Eilus, V. R.: Congenital scoliosis; a study of 234 patients treated and untreated, *J. Bone Joint Surg., 50A:* 1, 1968.

132. Winter, R. B., Moe, J. H., and Leonard, A.: The anterior approach for deformities and diseases of the spine, *J. Bone Joint Surg., 52A:* 406, 1970.

133. Wynne-Davies, R.: *Heritable Disorders in Orthopaedic Practice.* pp. 166-171, London: Blackwell Scientific Publications, 1973.

134. Yau, A., O'Brien, J. P., Smith, T., and Hodgson, A. R.: The treatment of scoliosis in Hong Kong, *J. Bone Joint Surg. 53A:* 200, 1971.

135. Young, L. W., Oestreich, A. E., and Goldstein, L. A.: Roentgenology in scoliosis; contribution to evaluation and management, *Amer. J. Roentgenol., 108:* 778, 1970.

136. Zaousses, A. L., and James, J. I.: The iliac apophyses and the evaluation of curves in scoliosis, *J. Bone Joint Surg., 40B:* 442, 1958.

CHAPTER 6

The Neck and Shoulder

CONGENITAL DEFORMITIES

Spina Bifida

Spina bifida is the term applied to the hiatus or gap due to failure of fusion of the laminae of the neural arches, through which a sac may protrude. This sac may or may not contain nerve elements, and the degree of defect determines the type of resulting deformity.

Etiology

Spina bifida occulta occurs on occasion in the neck as a congenital skeletal defect without any protrusion of the dura. Occasionally a meningocele, perhaps containing spinal fluid but no neural elements, originates from the dura and protrudes through the laminal defect.

Clinical Picture

A spina bifida occulta is suspected if superficially on the neck there is a localized overgrowth of hair of a small dimple. Very rarely is there a lump or protrusion large enough to palpate. A dimple responsible for repeated attacks of meningeal irritation may be hidden by occipital hair.

Treatment

The dimple may be a clue to a congenital dural sinus, particularly if it has a midline location. The sinus may be responsible for meningeal irritation and even for meningitis if infection arises from it. Its removal is indicated. Great care in the excision and adequate closure of the dura are essential to a successful result. Removal of the frank occipital and cervical myelomeningocele falls in the province of neurosurgery.

Klippel-Feil Syndrome

The Klippel-Feil syndrome might better be termed a congenital fusion in which two or more vertebrae become anatomically fused to each other. Such spines appear quite disorganized by roentgenogram.

Etiology

The origin of such deformities cannot be laid to the failure of ossification centers to develop because it antedates the period of their formation.

Clinical Picture

The cervical spine is limited in motion. The neck appears to be short, and, if sufficient involvement has occurred, the head may seem to be resting between the shoulders, and broad "webs" of skin and soft tissue extend out to the shoulders. Some neurologic changes may accompany this deformity owing to involvement of the cord. X-rays reveal vertebral disorganization with multiple anomalies. There is no characteristic distribution of the involved vertebrae.

Treatment

Severe though this disability may be, there is no treatment that will fully correct the deformity. Stretching by traction and passive exercises are used. Plastic improvement of the skin "webs" may be indicated.

There is a significant association of major anomalies with the Klippel-Feil syndrome. Of great significance are those involving the renal system. In our series of 20 patients, 16 were found to have absence of one kidney. Cardiac anomalies and other musculoskeletal anomalies such as congenital absence of the thumb also occur. An intravenous pyelogram is important as part of the work-up since ptosis of the other kidney and secondary involvement may also occur.

The excessive motion of those joints that are free above and below the fixed segments may lead to cord impingement in adult life.

Fig. 6.1. Multiple vertebral and rib anomalies in upper thoracic spine in patient with Klippel-Feil syndrome.

Sprengel's Deformity

A cephalad position of the scapula, which lies above its normal position and between the spines of the second to seventh dorsal vertebrae, appears to be congenital. This deformity has also been designated congenital elevation of the scapula, congenital high scapula, and undescended scapula. Sprengel made a preliminary report on the omovertebral connection in 1880 and reported 4 cases of the deformity in 1891.

Cavendish[2] has researched still earlier reports. The first description was that of Ealenberg in 1863. Willett and Walsham reported 2 cases in 1880 and 1883 and included excision of the omovertebral bone with improvement of function in their treatment.

Putti's operation entailed transplantation of the scapula to a lower level by excision of the protruding part of the scapula and its muscle attachment. Modification and various methods of holding the scapula down have been de-

Fig. 6.2. In Kleippel-Feil syndrome, the shortening of the cervical spine brings the head toward the chest. The deformed appearance is accentuated by a tendency toward webbing over either shoulder.

Fig. 6.3. Short cervical spine in Klippel-Feil syndrome.

scribed by Delchef (1922), Schrock (1926), Green (1957),[4] and Allen (1964).[1] Woodward's[9] procedure in 1961 was a radical departure from these methods. Macfarland (1950)[6] made a case for massive scapula excision, particularly of the protruding elements, leaving only the glenoid and coracoid processes as a means of improving the appearance of the patient.

The anlage of the scapula can be differentiated at the 5th week in the embryo. At this point, it lies opposite the lower four cervical and upper two thoracic vertebrae. During the 9th week of embryonic development, the descent of the scapula begins. By the 3rd month, its descent is complete. It is the rule rather than the exception to find associated anomalies of the cervical and thoracic spine as well as of the ribs. In one-third of the cases, an omovertebral bone is found. It may be osseous, fibrous, or cartilaginous. It arises from the proximal vertebral border and may be joined to processes of the lower cervical vertebrae.

Etiology

Various origins of the deformity have been suggested. Horwitz in 1908 mentioned a number of possibilities, including excessive intrauterine pressure related to an improper amount of amniotic fluid. Defective musculature or an abnormal articulation could in essence tie the scapula to its embryonic position and arrest its development.

The "bleb" theory was stated by Engel,[3] who, in 1943, postulated such an abnormal condition as failure to achieve midline union sufficiently early. Cerebral spinal fluid could, in such a case, escape from the fourth ventricle into the subcutis of the adjacent neck region. Such blebs, as they spread over the neck, would result in pressure and inflammation. A Klippel-Feil deformity could then occur in the neck and a Sprengel's deformity in the shoulder area. Engel believed that the escape of fluid from the fourth ventricle normally forms the subarachnoid space. If the bleb spreads over the upper limb, deformities of the humerus, radius, and ulna, and ultimately syndactylism and other anomalies of the fingers, could occur.

Clinical Picture

The condition is unilateral and results in an elevated shoulder and a neck that appears short. The youngster does not appear to be standing

Fig. 6.4. High scapula on the left constituting Sprengel's deformity.

both the axillary and vertebral borders are increased. There is a rotary change that cocks the upper medial angle of the scapula toward the midline and the inferior angle consequently toward the axilla.

The omovertebral connection, by its union to the lower cervical area and by its being, in substance, a complete bony union, may limit motion of the scapula markedly.

As Greenville and Coventry[5] have remarked, surgical intervention is determined by three considerations: (1) the deforming appearance, (2) the loss of a function, such as abduction of the arm, and (3) pain.

Pain is not ordinarily a factor in the childhood period. The deforming appearance is the principal presenting complaint, and the child is usually seen at approximately age 7-10. It is important to recognize that the appearance may worsen because the deformity is of the type that progresses with growth. Function may become increasingly limited, and pain may eventually result.

Treatment

From a conservative viewpoint, voluntary elevation of the opposite shoulder markedly improves the appearance. Exercises for the opposite shoulder may be helpful in this regard. Although we have tried such a program during several years with a number of children, we have not been able to procure persistent voluntary elevation of the scapula. The range of motion can occasionally be improved by stretching and by such exercises as chinning on a bar.

Operative procedures that have been developed include (1) removal of the omovertebral bone alone to improve motion, (2) extensive subperiosteal stripping of the scapula and removal of a large part of its upper portion, and (3) complete freeing of the scapula by subperiosteal dissection and anchoring of it as far as possible distally by attachment to a rib through fascia.

In any procedure, the danger of decreasing the traction of the scapula on the brachial plexus, which may result in paralysis of the arm, must be borne in mind. Such an eventuality shows up principally as deltoid and biceps weakness and must be carefully watched for. Here Robinson has added an important proce-

fully upright, and indeed some scoliosis of the upper dorsal and lower cervical region is usually present. The palpable outline of the scapula, measured from its superior to its inferior border, reveals the fact that it is smaller than the scapula of the opposite side. On the other hand, roentgenogram confirms the fact that

Fig. 6.5. Roentgenogram with congenital high scapula and accompanying lower cervical-upper dorsal scoliosis.

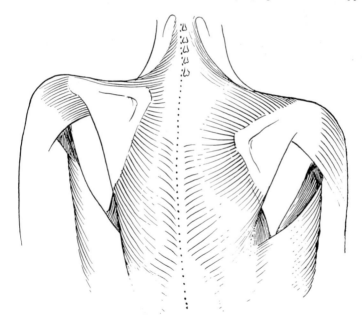

Fig. 6.6. In the operation for Sprengel's deformity reported by Woodward, the incision is made in the midline from the fourth cervical to the ninth dorsal spine. The skin is undermined to the vertebral border of the scapula. (From J. W. Woodward: Congenital elevation of the scapula, *Journal of Bone & Joint Surgery, 43A:* 219, 1961.)

dure. Its value lies in preventing this complication and thereby allowing a more radical descent of the scapula no matter which procedure is used. This increases the validity of the end results in terms of better cosmesis and function. Robinson's addition is essentially

morcellation of the middle third of the clavicle. The middle third is excised subperiosteally. It is divided into small segments and replaced in a manner to hold the periosteal cuff open. The cuff and soft tissues are then resutured.

We formerly pulled the scapula down into a

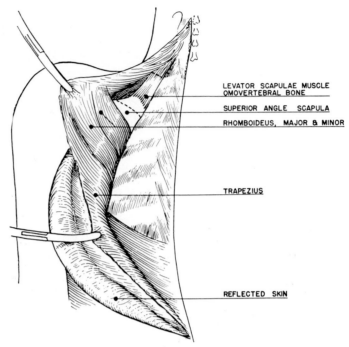

LEVATOR SCAPULAE MUSCLE
OMOVERTEBRAL BONE

SUPERIOR ANGLE SCAPULA

RHOMBOIDEUS, MAJOR & MINOR

TRAPEZIUS

REFLECTED SKIN

Fig. 6.7. Dissection of the muscle flap is begun inferiorly by detaching the origin from the spine. The omovertebral attachment is sectioned. (From J. W. Woodward: Congenital elevation of the scapula, *Journal of Bone & Joint Surgery, 43A:* 219, 1961.)

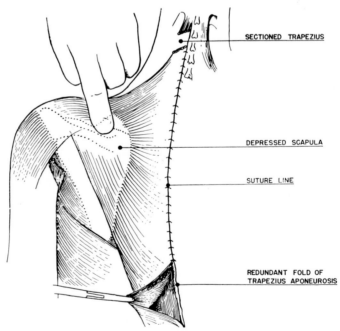

SECTIONED TRAPEZIUS

DEPRESSED SCAPULA

SUTURE LINE

REDUNDANT FOLD OF
TRAPEZIUS APONEUROSIS

Fig. 6.8. After division of the trapezius superiorly, the muscle flap is drawn down until the scapula lies approximately opposite that of the normal side. Care must be taken to avoid overstretching the spinal accessory nerve and the brachial plexus. The muscle flap is sewn into its new attachment on the spine. (From J. W. Woodward: Congenital elevation of the scapula, *Journal of Bone & Joint Surgery, 43A:* 219, 1961.)

surgical pouch by spring traction, but the procedure described by Woodward has, in our clinic, been an improvement over this procedure.

In Woodward's procedure, a midline incision is made from the fourth cervical to the ninth

Fig. 6.9. When the deformity has been repaired, a redundant portion of the trapezius is excised after the scapula has been pulled down.

dorsal spine. The skin and subcutaneous tissues are undermined to expose the vertebral border of the scapula. It is now possible to lower the scapula without moving the skin with it if the medial attachments (midline) holding it are cut.

The trapezius is identified in the lower reaches of the incision and is separated from the latissimus dorsi by blunt dissection. The origin of the trapezius is removed from the spinous processes by sharp dissection. The major and minor rhomboids are divided at their origin as dissection progresses. The rhomboids and the proximal trapezius are separated from the serratus and sacrospinalis. This continuous sheet of muscle is retracted to give access to the omovertebral bone or fibrous bands arising from the superior vertebral border. The spinal accessory nerve lying on the undersurface of the trapezius may easily be stretched and must be guarded during this phase of the operation. This is also true of the nerve to the rhomboids.

Any breaking of the supraspinatous portion of the scapula is removed by rongeurs at this stage. Subperiosteal stripping is avoided. The superior portion of the trapezius usually has to be sectioned at about the fourth cervical level. The levator scapulae muscle is releaved.

It is now possible to pull this muscle sheet distally until the spine of the scapula lies about opposite the one on the normal side. The inferior angle should not be used as a measure of correction since overpull might result.

As the aponeurosis of trapezium and rhomboids is held down, it is sewn into its new position at the midline. Because one works

Fig. 6.10. Postoperative application of spring traction to inferior angle of scapula. The scapula is freed and pulled down into a surgically created pouch if this procedure is followed. This is not necessary in Woodward's operation.

from above downward, a fold is created. It may be clipped off at the lower end, and the defect created may be sutured.

A Velpeau type dressing is worn for several weeks before active use of the shoulder is begun. In Woodward's series, 1 patient had demonstrable weakness and sensory loss which returned after a 6-month interval. Keloid formation in scars in this area is not unlikely.

Discussion

Cavendish has classified congenital elevation of the scapula into the following grades: Grade 1: very mild, the shoulder joints are level and deformity invisible when the patient is dressed; Grade 2: the shoulder joints are almost level, but there is a visible protuberance when the patient is dressed; Grade 3: moderate, the shoulder joint is elevated 2-5 cm, a very visible deformity; and Grade 4: severe, the shoulder is elevated so that the superior angle of the scapula is near the occiput with or without neck webbing.

Loss of ability to fully abduct the arm—a very definite loss of function enters into the

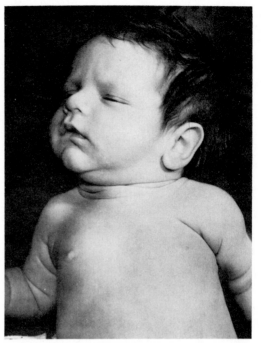

Fig. 6.12. Congenital absence of the pectoralis major muscle with the creation of an abnormal skin fold across the area normally occupied by that muscle.

Fig. 6.11. Congenital absence of the sternocleid mastoid muscle. The area normally occupied by the sternocleidmastoid muscle is retracted on inspiration and expanded on expiration.

consideration for surgery as well as cosmetic appearance.

If surgery is to be considered for correction, then because of the tendency of this lesion to be progressive, it should be done in the young age group, roughly from 4 to 7 years. One can expect improvement in function and appearance but absolute anatomic likeness to the opposite shoulder is frequently not obtained. However, the change is sufficient to justify the procedure.

An important addition to any procedure for an elevated scapula is morcellation of the middle third of the clavicle. This allows a more radical descent of the scapula to be obtained by surgical correction without an accompanying loss of function of the cords of the brachial plexus.

References

1. Allen, F. G.: The surgical treatment of Sprengel's shoulder, J. *Bone Joint Surg., 46B:* 162, 1964.
2. Cavendish, M. E.: Congenital elevation of the scapula, *J. Bone Joint Surg., 54B:* 395, 1972.
3. Engel, D.: The etiology of the undescended scapula and related syndromes, *J. Bone Joint Surg., 25:* 613, 1943.
4. Green, W. T.: The surgical correction of congenital elevation of the scapula (Sprengel's deformity), *J. Bone Joint Surg., 39A:* 1439, 1957.
5. Greenville, W., and Coventry M.: Congenital high scapula (Sprengel's) deformity, *Proc. Mayo Clin., 31:* 465, 1956.
6. McFarland, B. L.: Congenital Deformities of the Spine and Limbs, Ch. 6, p. 107, *Modern Trends in Orthopaedics,* London: Butterworth & Co., 1950.
7. Duthie, R., and Ferguson, A. B., Jr.: *Mercer's Orthopaedic Surgery,* Ed. 7, p. 148, Baltimore: The Williams & Wilkins Co., 1973.
8. Pessolano, C.: Sprengel's deformity, *Pennsylvania Med. J., 14:* 99, 1958.
9. Woodward, J. W.: Congenital elevation of the scapula, *J. Bone Joint Surg., 43A:* 219, 1961.

Absence of Muscles or Muscle Groups

Congenital absence of a muscle or muscle group may result in contracture if the function of the absent muscle is not substituted for by other muscles controlling the part.

Bracing and exercises carrying the part through a full range of motion may be indicated until the function of the absent muscle can be substituted for by transplant if necessary. Not all absences of muscle groups lead to deformity since the extent of the damage varies with the anatomic location. Thus absence of the palmaris longus is not significant, but unilateral absence of the sternocleidal mastoid may lead to deformity.

The muscle group most frequently affected is the pectoral, and the trapezius is next in order. Although any muscle may be affected, proximal or trunk muscles appear most liable to involvement. Absence of the sternocleidal mastoid is not infrequent

Familial Nuchal Rigidity

This condition is one of rigidity of the cervical spine. It is probably the direct antithesis of Ehlers-Danlos disease, which is one of hypermobility of all joints of the body.

Etiology

Enler-Danlos disease, which is associated with hyperelasticity of the skin and fragility of the skin and blood vessels, has been proved to be an inherited, dominant constitutional dyscrasia. It is thought that familial nuchal rigidity is likewise inherited by dominant transmission.

Clinical Picture

This condition is characterized by an inability to flex the neck due to relatively short ligaments and soft tissues on the posterior or dorsal aspect of the vertebral column. It is sometimes confused with ankylosing arthritis.

Treatment

Treatment is unavailing.

ACQUIRED DEFORMITIES

Deformity due to Position in Utero

Considerable interest has been aroused in recent years concerning the question of just how much fetal position determines the presence of deformities existing at birth. We do on occasion see a child born with what appears to be bilateral contractures of the sternocleidal mastoid muscles.

Etiology

Rarely this is due to a congenital loss or a stretching of the antagonistic posterior cervical muscles and ligaments. More often, however, it appears to be a positional contracture and is associated with a generalized rounded kyphosis of the entire spine similar to that of the fetal position.

Clinical Picture

There is a flexion deformity of the neck. Frequently the deformity is accompanied by an acute hip flexion deformity or by such severe flexion that the legs lie up along the abdominal wall. The head is flexed on the neck, and the whole of the spine presents a generalized, rounded dorsal and lumbar kyphosis.

Treatment

In such a case, gradual correction by traction, starting in the line of deformity with the child on a hard bed and with pads or pillows placed to conform to the deformities and then continuing with less and less padding until the spine and head is flat, brings about complete correction. If the legs are involved, the line of traction is gradually shifted. Correction is not sufficient and treatment should not cease until a normal lumbar curve has been obtained and the head can be easily hyperextended. Many minor contractures can be overcome merely by manual manipulation. Maintenance of the corrected position for a period may be necessary to allow overstretched muscles to become relatively shortened with growth of the skeleton.

Muscular Torticollis

Muscular torticollis does not appear to be a congenital anomaly but has a high association with breech births. There are many other possible reasons for a characteristic tilt and rotation of the head in childhood other than a contracture of the sternocleidomastoid muscle but this causation is most common in childhood. Osseous defects, neurogenic disturbances, ocular and middle ear pathology as well as underlying emotional disturbances have been suggested as possible causes of the deformity.

Fig. 6.13. Posterior view—muscular torticollis in older child showing tilt and elevation of shoulder on affected side.

Frederick Taylor (1875) writing in London first described the pathology of the muscle as an "induration of the sterno-mastoid muscle or sterno-mastoid tumour." He found fibrous tissue displacing the muscle fibers and interspersed among them so that the muscle was enlarged. The changes were present throughout the muscle in his particular case, a 6-week-old infant. Isacius Minnius (1685), a Dutch surgeon, had reported tenotomy of the muscle for torticollis.

Embryology of Sternocleidomastoid Muscle

Lidge, Bechtol, and Lambert[18] reviewed the evolutionary development of the sternocleidomastoid muscle. They pointed out that in mammals both the trapezius and the sternocleidomastoid is innervated by the spinal part of the accessory nerve and by branches of the anterior rami of the cervical nerves and this double innervation is unique. This muscle was apparently originally developed in the bronchial arch region. The visceral nerve supply shifted with its relocation. In lower forms this mass is supplied by the vagus nerve; in higher forms the

Fig. 6.14. Muscular torticollis becoming more evident with growth and involving primarily the clavicular portion of the sternocleidal mastoid

main nerve supply is the spinal accessory nerve. (The nucleus of this nerve is closely related to the nucleus of the vagus nerve.) In higher forms of life, the nerve supply to both the sterno-cleidomastoid and trapezius may be related to the nerve supply to the muscles of the gastrointestinal tract.

The muscles are derived from the mesoderm and arise in the lateral portion of the occipital region as a common muscle mass. As they migrate to the shoulder girdle, the accessory nerve is carried along with the muscle mass. The muscle mass first appears in the 7-mm embryo as the caudel member of the bronchial arch series. In the 11-mm embryo the trapezius portion is separate and extends to the sixth cervical nerve. The sternocleidomastoid extends virtually to the clavicle. At the 16-mm stage the muscles are separate throughout their length. The sternocleidomastoid extends from the mastoid process to the clavicle. The trapezius extends by the 20-mm stage to the occipital cartilage.

The accessory nerve supply from the cervical region is secondary—not developed directly as if the muscle came from a myotome.

The vagus complex consists of both vagus and accessory nerves, the more caudal portion of the vagus becoming a motor nerve primarily known as the spinal accessory to innervate both the sternocleidomastoid and trapezius. Additional innervation to this nerve as it is carried down the neck is obtained from the roots of the spinal cord down as far as the fourth cervical segment.

The sternocleidomastoid arises from the

Fig. 6.15. Fibroplastic process in congenital torticollis. The dark area in the upper right portion of the section represents calcium deposition (×140).

anterior end of the superomedial line and at the mastoid process anteriorly. The two distal heads are divided into an attachment to the superior border of the medial third of the clavicle—the other head crosses the sternoclavicular joint and extends by fibrous bands to the sternum.

The proximal blood supply consists of a short but major supply to the upper end and is derived from the occipital artery. The sternal head is supplied by a branch of the superior thyroid artery. The clavicular head is supplied by an artery running upward as a branch of the thyrocervical trunk or from one of the branches of this trunk, the transverse scapular artery. The venous drainage is multiple, numerous, and overlapping to all the major veins of the neck.

Etiology

The process present in the sternocleidomastoid muscle is unique and is not completely understood, making theories of causation of muscular torticollis difficult. The breech presentation incidence in this condition may be brought on by a preexisting position of the head. As early as 1670 von Roonhysen attributed the condition to the abnormal pressure on or position of the head in utero. Stromeyer in

1838 thought that the sternocleidomastoid muscle was ruptured during birth. Unfortunately, evidence for the hemorrhage when a resected muscle is examined pathologically does not exist.

In 1883 experimental hematoma was produced by Witzel by tearing muscle. No resemblance to the hyperplastic process present in this condition was found. Petersen[24] in 1886 felt that adhesions had formed between the amnion and the face of the embryo, bringing about a position of the head which interfered with development of the sternocleidomastoid muscle.

Volkman (1885) believed that the process was an infectious myositis. In 1980 Golding-Bard initiated a neurogenic theory—the deformity being secondary to a cerebral lesion occurring during intrauterine life. Anderson in 1893 believed that there was both an intrauterine type of torticollis and a birth injury type. In 1895 Mikulicz mentioned ischemia as a possible cause—a general anoxia and local trauma to the muscle. By 1906 Nove-Josserand and Viannaz developed a concept of each of the three segments of blood supply to the muscle being independent to a given segment of the muscle. In extreme rotation during labor the tensed sternocleidomastoid may compress blood vessels supplying the muscle as they pass beneath it.

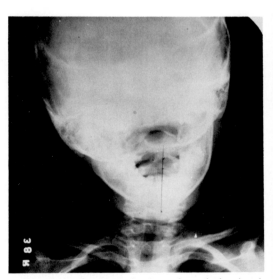

Fig. 6.16. Open-mouth view of cervical spine in patient with muscular torticollis, revealing tilt but accurate alignment of chin, spine of C2, and base of odontoid; there is no evidence of cervical subluxation.

The first recorded case of bilateral torticollis was reported by Morse in 1915. Bilaterally shortened muscles after a caesarian delivery were obviously not the product of birth trauma. Morse felt that it was due to a hyperextended position of the fetal head.

In 1923 Jones and Lovett felt that abnormal intrauterine pressure was the cause and called attention to the association of the disease with forefoot and equinovarus deformity.

Krogius (1924) called the condition a defect in the muscle blastoma itself—connective tissue formation at the expense of muscle fiber formation. And uniquely he called attention to the fact that this could be an active process continuing in the years after birth.

Middleton in 1930 stated that he was unable to demonstrate thrombosed veins in the sternocleidomastoid, and found no evidence to support the hematoma theory. He pointed out that the mass palpable in the sternocleidomastoid is from the outset firm, hard, and cartilaginous in feel. He noted also the development of the tumor several weeks after birth as being inconsistent with a hematoma. Greenstein reported a case of congenital muscular torticollis in 1950. The delivery was a caesarian section performed before the onset of labor and 2 weeks prior to the expected date of delivery.

Pathology

Taylor's original description in 1875 brought out the histologic character of the lesion. Fibrous tissue had developed between bundles of muscle fibers destroying and displacing them. The middle portion of the muscle was most densely occupied by the process with fibrous tissue alone being seen.

Numerous observations have been made of the fact that no evidence for hematoma is found including Whitman (1891) and Parker (1893). Witzel described the secondary changes in skull and face that occur with growth in this disease (1883). The affected side of the head and face becomes relatively atrophic.

In 1929 Von Lachun reported that in 3 cases that he examined the muscle was normal above and below the site of the fibrous hyperplasia. In 1 case, however, the process extended throughout the muscle rim into both clavicular and sternal heads. Muscle fibers were interspersed with the firbous tissue.

At infancy on gross examination the tumor appears to be glistening fibrous tissue resembling a soft fibroma. Microscopically there is young and cellular fibrous tissue with remnants of the original muscle fibers. Some of these fibers are vacuolated and undergoing degeneration. In the older child the process has matured there is no degenerating muscle or young fibrous tissue. There are scattered collections of muscle fibers in the fibrous tissue. The author has found calcification in this fibrous tissue.

The fibrous tissue has been observed to be continuous with the tendon at either end where it has extended that far.

Adams states that giant cells have been seen and describes them as masses of sarcolemmic nuclei possibly representing attempts at regeneration of muscle fibers.

Clinical Picture

The mass in the sternocleidomastoid muscle may be evident at birth, but most frequently it is not noticed until after approximately 10 days to 2 weeks, when it is seen as a hard, immobile, fusiform swelling in the muscle. Delivery has usually been difficult or a breech presentation. The swelling increases in size for 2-4 weeks and then gradually subsides over a 5-8-month period.

The deformity is produced by contracture of the involved muscle, the occiput being held constantly toward the involved side and the chin being rotated toward the opposite shoulder.

With persistence of the deformity, the skull becomes foreshortened, the level of the eyes changes, the side of the face on the involved side becomes flattened, and the mastoid process becomes more prominent. The clavicle and shoulder become elevated as compared to the opposite normal side. With continued growth and no treatment, a lower cervical-upper dorsal scoliosis will develop.

Treatment

When recognized early after birth, deformity can be corrected by gentle, yet even and persistent, stretching to an overcorrected position; i.e., the head is stretched over toward the shoulder opposite to the side of involvement, and the chin is rotated toward the side of involvement. Many useful tricks and artifices may be used to stimulate the child to turn the head toward the involved side. The crib may be placed so that he must turn to the desired position of overcorrection in looking for window light or for a favorite rattle. A special skull cap with an arm attachment has been used so that weight and use of the arm pull the head over. Placing sandbags along the head has been found useful.

Removal of the tumor is not necessary and has the disadvantage of deforming the outline of the neck. In the rare case that is not fully corrected after exercises, the sternal portion of the muscle can be lengthened and divided from the mastoid process at its origin. Such a procedure preserves the neck outline.

In older patients, correction of deformity can usually be obtained by lengthening of the sternal portion and detachment of the clavicular head of the sternocleidal muscle. An upper pole myotomy can also be done, if it is necessary. The overcorrected position can be maintained by a special collar.

Rotary Subluxations

An inability to rotate the head may occur as an acute episode in children who undergo some injury, even a minor one, in the course of play.

Fig. 6.17. Cervical subluxation at C1 and C2 evidenced by malalignment of axis of C2 (base of odontoid and spine of C2) in relation to chin (correlating with C1).

There is usually some history of trauma, mild or severe, after which the child suddenly develops an inability to rotate the neck to one side. A sore throat or upper respiratory infection may also precede the symptoms in some cases. The resulting "wryneck" or torticollis is characterized by spasm and tenderness on the long side of the torticollis instead of on the short side, where it is seen in such conditions as myositis. There is also limitation of motion toward the long or stretched side. Stimson and Swenson[30] stated that this acquired deformity is the result of a unilateral subluxation without associated fracture of the second or the third cervical vertebra. A. B. Ferguson, Sr., described a rotary subluxation that causes such a deformity between the atlas and axis. In a series of cases of our own, we were able to demonstrate that subluxation occurred in both places simultaneously in this deformity, there being a subluxation between C1 and C2, as well as between C2 and C3. It is the opinion of many that these subluxations occur in childhood because of the slope of the articular facets, which gradually change until the more stable adult situation is reached. The subluxation occurs in the upper three vertebrae, in which the more horizontal slope of the facets allows sufficient rotation.

Clinical Picture

Following a respiratory infection or some injury at play, or in connection with muscle spasm as the result of a cervical gland infection, the child complains of pain and inability to move the head. The head is tilted to one side and can be pushed further toward that side without pain. The rotation is limited to one side, and when the anomaly is acute, lateral tilt is also limited. Muscle spasms and tenderness are also evident on the long or stretched side. There may also be tenderness of the spines of the first and second cervical vertebrae.

Pathology

The pathology can be demonstrated by roentgenogram. An open-mouth anteroposterior view of the first and second cervical vertebrae is necessary for diagnosis. The symphysis of the mandible, the body of the second cervical, and the spine of the second cervical lie in a position of constant relationship, one to the other. If a true anteroposterior view is taken, they all lie on the same line. If the view is slightly oblique, they all are displaced in relative proportion to each other. If, however, a rotary subluxation has taken place, one of these points will be out of line in relation to the other two. The mandible is carried to one side since its position is associated with the first cervical vertebra. The body of the second cervical and its spine give a line indicating the plane of rotation, which deviated from that indicated by the mandible. In the lateral stereo view, the unilateral subluxation between the second and third cervical vertebrae can be seen, the facet of the second cervical riding upward and forward on its mate below without complete dislocation.

Treatment

Reduction may occur quite easily and quickly with the use of cervical traction, and often within 24–48 hr the neck is freely movable. A modified Thomas collar may be used for a period thereafter to prevent recurrence, usually until all tenderness and any respiratory infection have subsided.

References

1. Berkhizer, D. J., and Siedler, F.: Non-traumatic dislocations of the atlanto-axial joint, *J. A. M. A., 95:* 517, 1931.
2. Chandler, F. A.: Muscular torticollis, *J. Bone Joint Surg., 30A:* 556, 1948.
3. Chandler, F. A., and Altenberg, A.: Congenital muscular torticollis, *J. A. M. A., 125:* 476, 1944.
4. Coakley, W. A., Teplitsky, D., and Diaz, A.: Infections of head and neck, *Am. J. Surg., 77:* 469, 1949.
5. Compere, E. L.: Excision of hemivertebrae for correction of congenital scoliosis, *J. Bone Joint Surg., 14:* 555, 1932.
6. Compere, E. L.: Neck, shoulder, and arm syndrome, *New Orleans Med. Sci. J., 104:* 473, 1952.
7. Coutts, M. D.: Atlanto-epiphyseal subluxation, *Arch. Surg., 29:* 297, 1934.
8. Hartley, J. B., and Burnett, C. W. F.: Spina bifida and its associated skull defects, *Arch. Dis. Child., 18:* 173, 1943.
9. Herz, E., and Hoefer, P. F. A.: Physiologic analysis of involuntary motor activity, *Arch. Neurol. Psychiat., 61:* 129, 1949.
10. Horwitz, A. E.: Congenital elevation of scapula, *Am. J. Orthop. Surg., 6:* 260, 1908.
11. Howorth, M. B.: Spasmodic torticollis, p. 1963, *Textbook of Orthopedics*, Philadelphia: W. B. Saunders Co., 1952.
12. Jacobson, G., and Alder, Dennis, C.: Evaluation of lateral atlanto-axial displacement in injuries of the cervical spine, *Radiology, 61:* 355, 1953.
13. Jeanopolous, C. J.: Congenital elevation of the scapula, *J. Bone Joint Surg., 34A:* 883, 1952.
14. Jones, R. W.: Spontaneous hyperemic dislocations of the atlas, *Proc. Roy. Soc. Med., 25:* 1, 1931-32.
15. Kaplan, E. B.: Personal communication.
16. Keith, A.: *Human Embryology and Morphology*, Ed. 6, Baltimore: The Williams & Wilkins Co., 1933.
17. Lewis, W. H.: The development of the arm in man, *Am. J. Anat., 1:* 145, 183, 1901-1902.
18. Lidge, R. T., Bechtol, R. C., and Lambert, R. C.: Congenital muscular torticollis, *J. Bone Joint Surg., 39A:* 1165, 1957.
19. Mercer, R. D.: Atlas-asix dislocation following cervical adenitis, *Cleve. Clin. Q. 11:* 161, 1952.
20. Nelson, W. E.: Skeletal Defects, p. 1449, *Textbook of Pediatrics*, Ed. 5, Philadelphia: W. B. Saunders Co., 1950.
21. Nicholson, J. T.: Spontaneous reduction of cervical spine dislocations, *J. A. M. A., 115:* 2063, 1940.
22. Patton, E. F.: Cervical subluxation, *Ann. West. Med. Surg., 3:* 258, 1949.
23. Peters, K., et al.: *Handbuch der Anatomie des Kindes*, Vol. 2, 1938.
24. Petersen, J.: Zur Frage des Kopfricher Hamatoms bei Nengeborenen, *Zbl. Lymak, 10:* 797, 1886.
25. Pick, D. M.: Spina bifida and its associated malformations, *Wis. Med. J., 50:* 659, 1951.
26. Schrock, R. D.: Congenital elevation of scapula, *J. Bone Joint Surg., 8:* 207, 1926.
27. Shands, A. R.: Affections of neck and shoulder, p. 434, *Handbook of Orthopedic Surgery*, Ed. 2, St. Louis: C. V. Mosby Co., 1940.
28. Shoul, M. I., and Retro, M.: Manifestations of Klippel-Feil syndrome, *Am. J. Roentgenol., 68:* 369, 1952.
29. Smith, A. D.: Congenital elevation of scapula, *Arch. Surg., 42:* 529, 1941.
30. Stimson, A. B., and Swenson, P. C.: Unilateral subluxation of the cervical vertebrae without associated fracture, *J. A. M. A., 104:* 1578, 1935.
31. Sutra, C. J., and Mishkin, R. D.: Familial nuchal rigidity; form of hypomobility of vertebral column which clinically may be misdiagnosed as ankylosing arthritis (antithesis to Ehler-Danlos disease), *Bull. Hosp. Joint Dis., 13:* 155, 1952.
32. Taylor, J. C.: Breech presentation of hyperextension of the neck and intrauterine dislocation of cervical vertebrae, *Am. J. Obst. Gynec., 56:* 381, 1948.
33. Townsend, E. H., Jr., and Rowe, M. L.: Mobility of the upper cervical spine in health and disease, *J. Pediat., 10:* 567, 1952.
34. Ward, J., and Learner, H. H.: A review of the subject of congenital hemihypertrophy and a complete case report, *J. Pediat., 31:* 403, 1947.
35. Wycis, H. T., and Moore, J. R.: The surgical treatment of spasmodic torticollis, *J. Bone Joint Surg., 36A:* 119, 1954.

CHAPTER 7
The Upper Extremity

BY FRANK STELLING, M.D.

The hand of the child is fundamentally no different from the hand of the adult in its response to injury, in its healing characteristics, and in the therapeutic principles pertaining to it. Yet there are certain important differences which should be pointed out. In the adult, the major cause of disability is trauma due predominantly to industrial accidents. In the child, the major disabilities are caused by paralytic conditions and congenital abnormalities; trauma is a less frequent but a no less important cause. The same surgical principles apply to the child as to the adult; however, techniques must be varied to fit the individual problem. Some conditions, such as the spastic hand and congenital abnormalities, should be approached differently in the child than in the adult. With some problems encountered in childhood, the therapy must be a conservative one directed toward prevention of deformity until the patient has reached maturity, when definitive procedures can be performed. Occasionally, time-consuming reconstructive procedures that would not be attempted in adults because of the economic problem they would engender may be carried out in children.

There are many important differences between the hand of the child and that of the adult that affect the timing of surgical procedure; the type of suture material, dressings, skin graft, bracing, and immobilization used; the length of treatment and the type of surgical procedure performed. These differences pertain to the size and maturity of the hand; the maturity, cooperation, and adjustment of the patient; the thickness of skin and the types of scar and contracture of skin; the maturity of bone and the reaction of bone to surgery; the mobilization and immobilization of joints and the reaction of joints to injury; the maturity of tendons and the attachment of tendons to growing bones; the maturity of the nervous system and the relationship of sensory impairments to reconstructive procedures.

This chapter deals mainly with conditions common to children and with the application of sound therapeutic principles. No attempt will be made to deal with functional anatomy or the many basic fundamentals of hand surgery, all of which are most important and absolutely necessary in any attempt to carry out the procedures to be described.

CONGENITAL ANOMALIES

Congenital anomalies of all types account for about 25-30% of all the admissions to children's hospital services throughout the United States. Deformities of the hand comprise 20-30% of this group. Of the total number of patients admitted to the Shriners' Hospitals as of April 1962, the records of 100,894 cases have been reviewed, and of this number of admissions, there were 52,203 congenital anomalies of all types. Approximately 2% of this total were congenital anomalies involving the upper extremity. No single deformity can be considered common, and some are extremely rare and need not be mentioned in this section. Most of the deformities are mixed in nature, and in nearly every instance treatment must be individualized. In spite of this, certain general principles of treatment for the more common groups of anomalies will be considered here.

The etiology of congenital anomalies of the hand has not been definitely established. The theories which have been advanced will not be discussed here, but it would seem that the most acceptable theory is that of mutations which are subsequently inherited.

Radial Meromelia (Hemimelia), Complete or Incomplete

Radial meromelia, hemimelia, congenital absence of the radius, congenital clubhand, clinarthrosis, and aplasia or hypoplasia of the radius are all terms used in the literature to denote a deformity of the hand manifested by radial deviation resulting from a defect in the radius. Clubhand is a descriptive term denoting some type of deformity of the hand, but actually it means very little. Clinarthrosis, absence of the radius, and hypoplasia or aplasia of the radius are all medical terms relating to deformities of joint or of bone alone. In 1961 Frantz and O'Rahilly[3] pointed out that these deformities involve a great deal more than bone or joint and therefore suggested that everyone use the term, "radial hemimelia," which would describe the entire deformity. Recently, because of an argument based on the fact that hemimelia means half and that in many instances half is not particularly correct and that partial would be more explanatory, it has been suggested by the Committee on Prosthetics Research and Development that the term "hemimelia" be changed to "meromelia." Radial meromelia therefore can be further differentiated by describing it as "longitudinal, paraxial" when these are associated anomalies in the radial part of the hand or as "intercalary" when there is only an absence of the radius, etc., just as already written.

This condition is a manifestation of a defect in the radial elements of the limb bud. Similarly, an ulnar clubhand may occur in association with an ulnar defect. It has been found that the dividing line between radial and ulnar meromelias lies along the index finger. Quite often the thumb is absent in radial clubhands associated with a defect in the radius, whereas often the last three fingers are absent in the defects in the ulna.

Associated Anomalies

The skeletal changes which occur in the upper extremity usually involve most of the bones. The scapula is commonly reduced in size, and the clavicle may be short. The humerus is usually shorter than normal, and either end may present some deformity. The carpal bones are rarely complete in number. Most frequently absent is the navicular, which is followed by the greater multangular. Quite frequently, the first metacarpal is absent. Varying combinations occur with regard to the relationship of the first metacarpal and the thumb. If the first metacarpal is missing, the thumb usually has no function and very often is a soft-tissue appendage.

Muscular Defects

Numerous defects in the muscles accompany the condition. If the thumb and first metacarpal are present, the extensor pollicis longus and brevis and the abductor brevis are also present, and the muscles of the thenar eminence are usually normal. If the first metacarpal is absent, however, these muscles are commonly missing. The pronator teres may be missing if the radius is completely absent, or it may be underdeveloped if there is a partial defect in the radius. The flexor pollicis longus is apt to be absent unless the entire thumb and first metacarpal are present, in which case it is likely to be normal. The muscles about the shoulder and arm are frequently involved. The pectoralis major may have an abnormal insertion or its clavicular or costal portions may be absent. The pectoralis minor and the deltoid are usually present, although the latter muscle may have an abnormal insertion or it may fuse with the triceps or the brachialis. The biceps is frequently missing; however, if it is present in a patient with complete absence of the radius, it inserts into the lacertus fibrosus. The brachialis varies, but is usually present, and the triceps is usually normal. The brachioradialis is found to be missing when the radius is completely absent; however, occasionally it will be present and inserted into the ulna. The extensor carpi radialis longus and brevis may be absent, or they may be fused with the extensor digitorum communis, which is usually present and normal. The supinator is commonly absent unless the proximal radius is present.

Vascular Defects

The arterial system shows numerous abnormalities. The brachial artery may be normal, or it may divide into two branches high in the arm. The ulnar artery is usually normal, but the radial artery is frequently small or absent. The median nerve is not infrequently the most superficial structure found on the radial aspect of the forearm. For the most part, the ulnar nerve is normal and supplies the usual intrinsic muscles in the hand.

Treatment

Many different methods have been devised

Fig. 7.1. Typical bilateral clubhand with poor development of the thumbs.

Fig. 7.2. Clubhand with absence of thumb.

through the years to improve these hands. Most of the operative procedures devised for the condition have varied from producing fair improvement to being of questionable value. The general methods of treatment of this condition at the present time are: (1) conservative stretching and splinting, and the development of the use of the hand without a surgical procedure; (2) stretching and splinting followed by tenotomy and soft-tissue surgery to get the hand over the ulna, followed by fusion of the wrist or of the ulna into the carpus; and (3) conservative or surgical procedures to get the hand over the wrist, followed by some bony procedure in order to keep the hand in the new position without a definite stabilization. In general, the operative procedures that have been described in the literature have been confined to tenotomy of the contracted muscles, osteotomy of the curved ulna and addition of a stabilizing bone graft to replace the absent radius, and splitting of the ulna into radial and ulnar portions. Most of these procedures result in a fusion of the wrist joint; if such is the result, the appearance of the hand is certainly more pleasing, but sometimes it is questionable whether the functional value of the hand has been increased or not.

Conservative Treatment

Conservative treatment should be started in all cases as early as possible. In the correction of the deformity, plaster casts, splints, or braces should be used until the soft tissues have been stretched to the greatest degree that the bony deformity will allow. As soon as possible, the deformity is corrected by plaster casts. Following this, small correction braces or splints may be used on a part-time basis while stretching is carried out as a daily routine by the parents. Some authorities believe that this is the only treatment that should be used. Quite often if treatment is continued during the entire growth period, the hand remains deformed, but the child adapts to the deformity. Stretching and the movement of the parts keep the hand functionally sound, and it is amazing to see how well these children can use the hand at the termination of the growth period. The appearance of the hand is not particularly pleasing, but quite often its function is very satisfactory, and perhaps better than that of a hand with a wrist fusion alone.

Surgical Treatment

Riordan,[6] in 1955, reported in the *Journal of Bone and Joint Surgery,* a modification of the surgical method of Starr which he felt to be a more promising surgical procedure for the treatment of the radial meromelia or congenital absence of the radius, and quite a number of us undertook these surgical procedures with varying results. In actuality, the procedure functioned well for a number of years after the

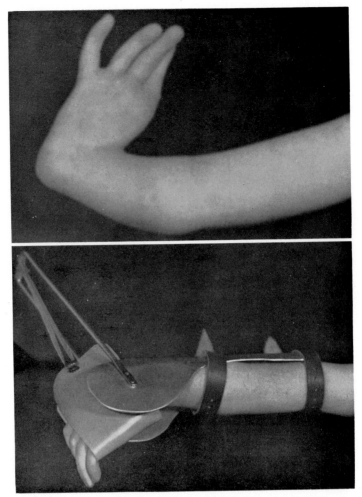

Fig. 7.3. Typical clubhand showing the use of a clubhand splint. The splint is used on a part-time basis to give active stretch in order to lessen the deformity.

procedure had been performed, and, at first, it was the thought of Riordan and quite a number of us that this transplanted fibula into the ulna would grow. In very few instances this actually occurred but the number of cases of increasing growth were so few as to not make this procedure a procedure of choice as we at one time hoped that it would be. In the previous editions of this book, this has been written up as a surgical technique of value in the treatment of this condition. However, in 1963, at the meeting of the American Orthopaedic Association at Hot Springs, Virginia, Dr. Riordan read a paper which as yet has not been published in which he reviewed all of his cases to that time and suggested a better method of treatment in that the fibula transplant had failed to grow in most instances and therefore there was a recurrence of the deformity of the hand. At that time and since, he has advocated that the hand and wrist be surgically transposed over the distal end of the ulna, leaving the ulnar epiphysis intact. He found that if this were done at a very early age, the ulnar epiphysis would expand in breadth if the wrist were held over it long enough. The expanded ulna epiphysis would act as a buttress and hold the hand over the distal ulna giving a good alignment between the forearm and the hand and also a mobile joint. So far, he has been pleased with this procedure. We have done these since 1960 and have been pleased with our results also. We have reviewed all of our cases that were performed according to

Fig. 7.4 (*Left*). X-ray of radial clubhand before surgery.

Fig. 7.5 (*Right*). X-ray of same case after correction, which involved a fibular graft to the ulna and an osteotomy of the ulna.

Riordan's first method and we, too, have had the same problems that he experienced, as have others. We have been able to correct some of the difficulties of those cases that have been performed according to his first method by performing an osteotomy of the ulna just at the junction of the bifurcation between the fibular graft and the ulna, in other words at a low point and adjusting the osteotomy so that the hand is again in proper alignment with the forearm. In some instances some of the tendons must be lengthened in order to hold this, but this has allowed us to correct the radially deviated hand and still maintain good function. In performing the new procedure of Riordan, the carpus must be exposed either through a radial incision and, as in his first procedure, one must be quite careful of the median nerve which quite often is exposed directly under the skin, with many small branches, particularly sensory branches, running out both to the dorsal and volar aspects of the radial side of the hand. The tendons are usually not lengthened, but fascial bands are resected and the carpus is exposed. Sometimes an incision must be made over the ulnar side in order to expose the ulnar epiphysis and, in certain instances, the entire procedure has been performed through just a transverse ulnar incision. Care is of utmost importance as far as the distal ulnar epiphysis is concerned in that it be allowed to grow. Therefore, nothing is done as far as the ulnar epiphysis is concerned other than its exposure. If the soft tissues are too tight, several of the carpal bones may be removed so that the hand can be placed directly over the ulnar epiphysis. Sometimes the entire proximal carpal row is removed, and, if this is not enough, some of the midcarpus in the distal row may be removed in order to allow the hand to be positioned over the ulna. All we need here is a joint with the ulna opposing the central part of the hand. This is then locked in place by the use of a longitudinal Kirschner wire and sometimes by a transverse Kirschner wire through the metacarpals, and a cast is applied with the hand in corrected position. Once this has been performed the wounds are closed. There is usually redundancy on the ulnar side, and, if there is any tension on the longitudinal incision on the radial side, this should be closed by Z-plasty in order to relieve the tension on the scar. A long-arm cast is applied with the wrist held in the neutral position and the elbow in flexion. The cast is maintained in this position and changed at intervals over a long period of time, sometimes as long as 1 year or more. Sometimes a brace is used instead of a cast. Many types of braces are used. In our experience they are not quite as useful as a well molded cast, except that the cast must be changed frequently and there is always the problem of water. It is of utmost importance, however, that the hand be maintained over the ulnar epiphysis until the ulnar epiphysis has grown and expanded so as to form a buttress to keep the hand from rotating back into a radially deviated position. Once stability has occurred by x-ray and by clinical observation, then, and only then, can all immobilization be discontinued. The procedure in our experience should not be performed after the child has attained the age of 5 years since the ulnar epiphysis will not tend to grow enough in order to allow the proper expansion and buttressing effect. Riordan[6] has indicated that this is best done in children who are quite small and has actually performed this procedure during the first month of life. The cases in which we have performed this newer Riordan procedure actually have not been followed long enough as yet for us to be perfectly certain that we will be able to maintain this in every instance as a flexible part that is motored well for functional use. Riordan has indicated that in some instances this did not occur but he was able to go ahead with wrist fusion and have still a more satisfactory extremity than if this had been left alone to develop as a clubhand.

Fig. 7.6. Thumb-clutched hand with finger deformities.

Instruct. Lect. Am. Acad. Orthop. Surg., 15: 172, 1958.

Congenital Flexion and Adduction Deformity of Thumb (Pollex Varus, Thumb-Clutched Hand, Congenital Clasped Hand)

This anomaly is a rare deformity which tends to be an inherited trait. The thumb is characteristically held adducted into the hand, and there is marked flexion of the metacarpophalangeal joint. Quite frequently there are coexistent flexion deformities of the proximal interphalangeal joints of the fingers; such deformities give rise to the term "thumb-clutched hand." The skin of the flexor surface of the fingers and thumb is usually contracted. This contraction is thought to be secondary to the true pathology. The flexion deformity of the proximal interphalangeal joints of the fingers may exist without the thumb deformity, but this is considered to be a rare occurrence. In most instances, it has been found that there is a hypoplasia or absence of the extensor pollicis brevis and a secondary adduction flexion contracture of the thumb. In the finger deformities, it is believed that there is a hypoplasia or absence of the intrinsic musculature.

Treatment

The results of treatment depend upon the stage in which therapy is started. Many of these

References

1. Albee, F. H.: Formation of radius congenitally absent; condition 7 years after implantation of bone graft, *Ann. Surg., 87:* 105, 1928.
2. Bunnell, S.: *Surgery of the Hand,* Philadelphia: J. B. Lippincott Co., 1944.
3. Frantz, C. H., and O'Rahilly, R.: Congenital skeletal limb deficiencies, *J. Bone Joint Surg., 43A:* 1202, 1961.
4. Hiekel, H. V. A.: Aplasia and hypoplasia of the radius, *Acta Orthop. Scand.,* Suppl. 39, 1959.
5. Kato, K.: Congenital absence of the radius, *J. Bone Joint Surg., 6:* 589, 1924.
6. Riordan, D. C.: Congenital absence of the radius, *J. Bone Joint Surg., 37A:* 1129, 1955.
7. Riordan, D. C.: Congenital absence of the radius; a 15 year follow-up, *J. Bone Joint Surg., 45A:* 1783, 1963.
8. Starr, D. E.: Congenital absence of the radius, a method of surgical correction, *J. Bone Joint Surg., 27:* 261, 1943.
9. Stelling, F. H.: Surgery of the hand in the child,

cases have been noted in adults with persistent disabling finger and thumb deformities. If the deformity is seen early, conservative measures should be instituted. The thumb should be mobilized out of the palm into extension and abduction and should be held in this position by some type of splint. White and Jensen[2] use a special elastic abduction splint which can be easily removed for cleaning. Wechesser[1] uses a plaster case for several months and changes the cast at 4- to 6-week intervals in order to allow for growth. Most of his cases develop good function with this conservative care. If the deformity returns following the release of the part after conservative immobilization, then it is to be expected that the tendon is either absent or nonfunctional, and tendon transplants should be done. White transplants the common extensor tendon of the index finger into the extensor surface of the metaphysis of the base of the proximal phalanx of the thumb and has shown excellent results in these cases. Sometimes the skin is tight on the flexor surface and a Z-plasty or releasing incision with a full-thickness graft should be utilized. The contracture has been limited to the skin and does not usually involve fascia and deeper structures in the small child. In the adult, contracture of all elements of the thumb web is to be expected.

References

1. Wechesser, E. C.: Congenital flexion-adduction deformity of the thumb (congenital "clasped thumb"), *J. Bone Joint Surg., 37A:* 977, 1955.

2. White, J. W., and Jensen, W. E.: The infant's persistent thumb clutched hand, *J. Bone Joint Surg., 34A:* 680, 1952.

3. Zadek, I.: Congenital absence of extensor pollicis longus of both thumbs: operation and cure, *J. Bone Joint Surg., 16:* 432, 1934.

4. Zumoff, B.: Congenital symmetrical finger contractures, *J. A. M. A., 155:* 437, 1954.

Stenosing Tenovaginitis of Thumb— "Trigger Thumb"

This condition is characterized by a flexion deformity of the interphalangeal joint of the thumb, and it occurs in adults as well as in children. In the adult, it is irritative in origin and due to repeated trauma, and in the child it is congenital. Snapping is usual in adults and rare in children. It is generally thought that the lesion is of congenital origin in infants even though in some instances it is not present until weeks or months after birth. Zadek[6] cites a case that developed in an infant with a history of minor trauma of one thumb and that was thought to have been a result of the injury; however, a few months later, the other thumb developed the same deformity with no history of trauma. The pathology was found to be the same in both thumbs.

Pathology

The gross pathologic appearance of this lesion is that of an encircling constricting fibrocartilaginous band of the sheath of the flexor pollicis longus at the level of the

Fig. 7.7. Congenital absence of the intrinsic muscles without clutched thumb.

metacarpophalangeal joint. Usually as this constriction is released, an indentation or groove in the tendon and thickening on either side of this indentation are seen. Sometimes the tendon bulges to double its normal size on either side of the groove.

Clinical Picture

The interphalangeal joint of the thumb is held in a position of fixed flexion. There is inability to extend the joint actively. Usually the thumb can be flexed actively a few degrees. In some instances the distal joint can be forcibly extended, but it locks in flexion as soon as flexion is again initiated. The joint cannot be passively extended, and any attempt to do so causes pain. As extension of the joint is attempted, the tendon becomes taut distal to the metacarpophalangeal joint, and the skin of the flexor surface of the joint blanches. There is a thickened area on the flexor surface of the thumb at the level of the metacarpophalangeal joint. This area may at times be sensitive.

Treatment

If the interphalangeal joint can be passively extended and splinted in this position for 3 weeks, the thumb sometimes resumes normal function and is permanently rid of the deformity. In most instances, however, this treatment is unsuccessful, and the deformity recurs. The treatment of choice is incision of the flexor tendon sheath, preferably by means of two incisions through each side of the annular constricting band and removal of a small

section of the sheath. The incision in the skin should be made transversely in a line with the crease at the metacarpophalangeal joint. A longitudinal incision crossing the skin crease produces a serious, painful scar which can produce a flexion deformity. Care must be taken not to injure the digital nerves. The results of this therapy are usually excellent.

References

1. Fahey, J. J., and Bollinger, J. A.: "Trigger thumb" in adults and children, *J. Bone Joint Surg., 36A:* 1200, 1954.
2. Jahss, S. A.: Trigger finger in children, *J. A. M. A., 107:* 1463, 1936.
3. Miller, J. W.: Pollex varus, a report of 2 cases, *Univ. Michigan Med. Bull., 10:* 1, 1944.
4. Sprecher, E. E.: "Trigger thumb" in infants, *J. Bone Joint Surg., 31A:* 672, 1949.
5. White, J. W., and Jensen, W. E.: "Trigger thumb" in infants, *Amer. J. Dis Child., 85:* 141, 1953.
6. Zadek, I.: Stenosing tendovaginitis of the thumb in infants, *J. Bone Joint Surg., 24:* 326, 1942.

Syndactylism

Syndactylism is the most frequent anomaly of the hand, and it occurs in all degrees of severity. The simplest involvement is an incomplete web formation between two fingers with no bone or joint deformity. Extreme involvement may take the form of severe webbing of all the fingers accompanied by incomplete segmentation of the bony parts and multiple joint deformities. Syndactylism is frequently bilateral and is sometimes seen in conjunction with webbing of the toes or other deformities of the foot. The deformity is thought most frequently to be inherited. Of the series of cases

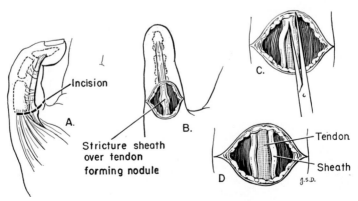

Fig. 7.8. Operation for "trigger thumb." The incision in the skin is transverse, and the incision in the tendon sheath is longitudinal.

reviewed at the Shriners' Hospital in Greenville, South Carolina, almost all of the patients have been found to originate from a single family.

In many instances syndactylism is complicated by associated deformities such as symphalangism, brachydactyly, and polydactyly. In our experience, one is more likely to find these complicating factors than not. They alter the prognosis considerably. The final prognosis in many instances of multiple congenital anomalies naturally depends upon what we have to work with. By means of a combination of basic procedures, including removal of proper parts, separation of syndactyly, and sometimes transposition of fingers, the best functional result is attained. The resulting hand is not going to be pretty or even normal in appearance, but function is always the first consideration. In these instances, the appearance should be the best that can be attained under the circumstances. Each case must be considered individually, and the surgeon himself must decide exactly what the total plan of treatment is to be and what function may finally be attained. The latter must be clearly stated, both to himself and to the family of the child.

Treatment

The results of therapy vary according to the degree of deformity, the number of fingers involved, and the amount of bony fusion. Partial webbing of the skin without bone or nail involvement can be totally corrected. The

Fig. 7.9 (*Top*). Bilateral syndactylism involving two fingers. There is no bone, joint, or nail deformity. This child is only 2 years of age, and a good operative result should be expected.

Fig. 7.10 (*Bottom*). The functional and cosmetic results following surgery are good.

Fig. 7.11. Method of surgical treatment for syndactylism. The sides of the finger are covered with split-thickness grafts; the base, by two triangular flaps that cross.

there are separate nails, no bony attachment, and only intervening soft-tissue involvement. In such cases, the prognosis is excellent.

The surgical procedure for the separation of these fingers is always performed under a tourniquet. The incision is begun by constructing pedicles in the form of V-shaped flaps on both sides of the web at the level of the metacarpholangeal joint. The points of the Vs are toward the fingers, and the flaps extend out approximately 1/2 inch. The flaps are then dissected from the finger in a manner that permits some subcutaneous tissue to remain attached to the skin. The web is then separated from both fingers, care being taken to cut in an irregular line, either waving or angulating, in order to prevent longitudinal scarring when the graft is attached. The soft tissues are separated by blunt dissection after the skin incisions have been completed. The neurovascular bundles are carefully protected. If the phalanges are fused, they are separated with a bone cutter and trimmed back smoothly. In instances of a single nail for two fingers, the nail is split and a portion of it and of its matrix on the cut side is then removed so that the skin graft may be brought around the margin of the nail. The resulting defect produced on the opposing sides of the two fingers should then be covered by a skin graft.

Two different types of skin graft may be used. In very small children, because it is almost impossible to decide what thickness a split-thickness graft would be, it may be best to use a full-thickness skin graft. In older children, we like a thick split-thickness skin graft, which can be removed from the volar aspect of the forearm on the same side as the hand to which it is to be grafted. This skin is taken with a dermatome and fashioned to cover the area so that its edges meet the wavy or angulated edges previously constructed. The two V flaps are crossed and sutured across the existing web at the palm. It is not necessary to bring the points completely across; however, if this can be done without producing tension and without discomfort to the child, it is performed. A small amount of overlap is also perfectly acceptable because the skin graft can be made to cover the defect. The sutures used are 4-0 or 5-0 interrupted catgut. These sutures do not cause any increased reaction, and they fall out at the proper time; therefore there is no necessity to

presence of bone or joint deformities invariably causes some permanent deformity, in spite of the best operative procedures. Syndactyly is so varied in its manifestations and complications that it is impossible to prescribe one method of treatment. The basic principles are the same, but the timing of the procedure, the type of immobilization, and the follow-up are all affected by the severity of the condition and the complicating factors present.

Webbing without Concurrent Discrepancy in Length. In such instances, because the discrepancy of finger lengths present is not sufficient to cause increasing joint deformities, it is thought best to defer surgery until the child is almost school age. The primary reason for this is that the skin grafts are more easily held in place by rigid immobilization at this age and that neater primary healing, less scar, and better definitive results are obtained. Secondary operative procedures are rarely necessary, even when there is some bony attachment between the distal phalanges; however, better functional and cosmetic results can always be expected if

Figure 7.12. Syndactylism involving three fingers. Note the deformity of the nails and of the longer fingers. There is also lack of segmentation of the distal phalanges. A good result can be expected here, but there will probably be some fixed joint contracture of the middle finger. The patient should have been treated surgically at a younger age for a better result.

Fig. 7.13. Brachydactylia, syndactylism, and symphalangism. The hand can be improved by separating the index and adjacent finger, but the middle finger joints will still be restricted in motion.

Fig. 7.14 (*Top*). Bilateral syndactylism of three fingers plus extra digits on the lunar side.

Fig. 7.15 (*Bottom*). Appearance after surgical release of the syndactylism and removal of the entire ray on the left and digit on the right.

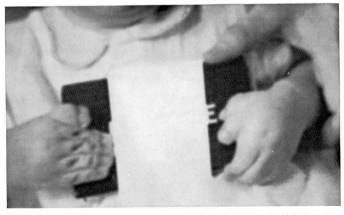

Fig. 7.16. Bilateral syndactylism of all four fingers and bifid thumbs.

struggle with the child in order to remove sutures and no danger of pulling the new skin graft off, nor is there any reason to anesthetize the child to remove the sutures. The tourniquet is always released prior to skin closure, and a dry field is attained before any part of the wound is closed. The donor site is covered with scarlet red gauze, which is allowed to remain in place until the skin underneath has reepithelized. The recipient site is covered, preferably with paraffin gauze, and the hand is placed in a skeleton splint of steel or aluminum at the end of which small holes are drilled at the level of the end of the finger. The splint is padded to protect the back of the hand, and stainless steel wire sutures are placed through the fingernail and then through the splint so that the fingers are held in full extension and also in abduction. The proximal end of the splint is then incorporated in a plaster cast extending beyond

Fig. 7.17. Same case as in Figure 7.16 after correction of the syndactylism and removal of the radial thumbs. There is some residual scarring on the flexor surface, but functional ability is excellent.

Fig. 7.18. Severe syndactylism with deformity of only the middle and ring fingers. There is a wedged phalanx in the thumb. The result here will not be excellent, but the fingers will be greatly improved.

411

Fig. 7.19. Same case as in Figure 7.18. Deformities of the feet.

Fig. 7.20. Surgical correction of bifid distal phalanx. This type of surgical correction of a bifid distal phalanx should not be performed in the growing child because of the probability that increased deformity will result from the growing epiphyses.

Fig. 7.21. This procedure, which leaves the bone and joint untouched, would be used in the case of bifid distal phalanx. If further definitive surgery should be necessary, it should be done after the patient has reached maturity.

the elbow, which is at 90° in the older age group. In very young children 1 or 2 years old, this cast is extended over the shoulder and chest in order to give more secure immobilization. The cast is left in place for a period of about 2 weeks, and then the dressing is removed. Most of the sutures come out at that time. The wounds are redressed, and splints are left in place for another week. At the end of that time, the strenuous immobilization is removed, and small splints are applied to keep the fingers in extension and abduction for at least 3 more weeks. During this period of time, it has been found, even in the older children, that the joints do not stiffen, and there is no permanent joint damage due to the immobilization. In no instance should work be done on both sides of any one finger. This may jeopardize circulation and cause loss of the finger.

Syndactyly with Discrepancy in Length of Adjacent Parts. When the little finger is attached to the ring finger or the thumb to the index finger (which is rare), or when the entire group of fingers is involved in a mitten of skin, surgery should be performed much earlier. It should be done sometime after 1 year of age and before 2 years; otherwise increasing joint deformities in the longer finger will occur. In these cases, surgery is performed with the full knowledge that immobilization is difficult and almost impossible. If immobilization is not perfectly secure, motion occurs and causes many degrees of scarring and subsequent "scarring in" because of partial or total loss of the graft. This produces skin contracture usually of the flexion type, which is not as severe as lateral or rotary deformity. Later, Z-plasty or skin graft inlays after section of the cicatrix are necessary. Skin contracture need not always result. We should try our best to achieve perfect immobilization in order to avoid secondary scarring and secondary surgical procedures, but the parents should be told that these procedures may be necessary. The surgical procedure in very young children is same as that described above, except that immobilization may be obtained, if the finger is perfectly straight, by means of a small Kirschner wire inserted centrally through the phalanges. The wire may be left in place for a period of 3 weeks and then exchanged for a plastic or metal splint. Care must be taken that the wire be

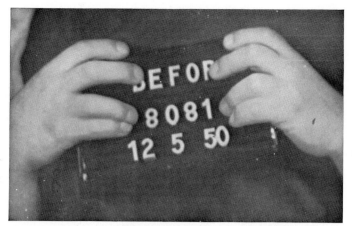

Fig. 7.22. Bilateral syndactylism of two fingers with no bone or nail deformity. The child is young, and excellent cosmetic and functional results should be anticipated with proper surgery.

Fig. 7.23. Same case as seen in Figure 7.22. Postoperative appearance showing a good functional result.

Fig. 7.24. Bilateral syndactylism of two fingers. There is some nail and joint deformity.

Fig. 7.25. Same case as seen in Figure 7.24. Surgery was performed early enough to correct the joint deformity.

centrally located. The procedure of immobilization described above is then added to this, the plaster being extended above the shoulder in all instances. If there is doubt in these very young children as to the thickness of skin, it is best to use a full-thickness skin graft taken from the flexor crease of the elbow of the same side.

Polydactylism

Polydactylism is inherited and often accompanies syndactylism, brachydactylism, and other congenital anomalies. It is probably the most common congenital anomaly, but because some of the small finger appendages attached by a fine skin pedicle are tied off with a suture in the nursery by the obstetrician or pediatrician, they are lost in statistical analyses.

The anomaly occurs in three main types: (1) an extra soft-tissue mass not adherent to the skeleton and frequently without bone joints or tendons; (2) a duplicate digit containing all elements and attached to a large metacarpal head or to a bifurcated metacarpal; and (3) a complete extra digit with a full metacarpal.

Treatment

Cases of the first type which show a very small pedicle at birth can be easily treated by tying off the pedicle with a piece of silk. The result is usually a normal-appearing hand without deformity. Sometimes the soft-tissue attachment is too thick for this type of treatment, and, in such cases, it is best to wait until the child is older (4-5 years) before carrying out a surgical resection. Extra digits do not cause functional difficulty in the early years of life. In some instances, it is difficult to decide which digit should be sacrificed, and careful study and observation for a considerable period of time become necessary before the decision to operate can be made. If there is any doubt whatsoever in cases of polydactyly as to which finger should be sacrificed, it is best to wait until one can be definitely certain of the function of the various parts before deciding which part should be retained and which deleted. Structures should also have developed enough to be identified with certainty. In many cases of polydactyly, there are split tendons or a central tendon with a Y-split to the two segments. Such variations should be checked at the time of surgery, and the functional structures should be left in the remaining part. In cases of double thumb in which there is one metacarpal or a partially segmented metacarpal, the dissection must be very careful. Too often when the radial thumb is removed, the abductor attachment is taken down and lost. This attachment should be searched out anatomically and reattached in proper relationship to the part remaining. When a part is removed, one must be sure that the part remaining can function properly. Occasionally, the tendons of an accessory digit may be transferred to provide function in the remaining digit.

Injury of the epiphysis, either traumatic or surgical, may produce deformities. For this reason certain surgical procedures that are of a definitive nature and involve the bone structure itself often must be delayed. In the treatment of a congenital duplication of the distal phalanx of the thumb, it has been suggested that central segments of the bone be removed, the remaining parts fitted together to form one bone, and the soft tissues closed over, in order to form one distal thumb segment. If this procedure is performed in a growing child, it is nearly certain that deformity will occur from the damage to the epiphysis. It is believed far better in the young child to produce a syndactylism surgically, to leave the bone alone except for pulling the two bone segments toward each other, and to leave a broad distal thumb with two bones and nails covered with one envelope of skin. A split nail will be produced, but this should cause little difficulty, and if definitive reconstruction is necessary, it can be performed at or after maturity.

Cleft Hand

This is a rare deformity with many variations and often concomitant with other types of congenital malformations, such as syndactylism, brachydactylism, and symphalangism. The usual deformity is a central cleft dividing the hand in two parts. The digits in each part may be webbed partially or completely, or they may be free. Most frequently, one or more rays are missing. In some cases, there may be a radial and ulnar ray with no digits between them. In others, the hand may be normal except that it lacks a central digit. In nearly all instances, the patient uses the hand almost like a claw, opposing one part to the other for grasping.

Treatment

The treatment must be individualized to the type of deformity present. In instances in which only two functioning units are present and there is no webbing, the hand is best left untreated.

Webbing should be released as described in the section on syndactylism, and the cleft should be eliminated by closure of the palm and hand defect. If a central digit or digits are missing but their metacarpals are present, the metacarpal should be excised and the two parts of the hand closed.

Megalodactylism

Hypertrophy of one or more digits or of the entire hand is a rare anomaly. These hypertrophies may be the result of true anomalies of development, but there is definite evidence that a large number of them have neurofibromatosis as the underlying pathology. McCarroll,[9] Moore,[11] and Brooks[2] have shown cases of increase in length as well as breadth or of soft tissues and bone due to neurofibromatous changes in the digit. The neurofibroma itself is usually unobtrusive, and the associated hypertrophy is the most notable condition.

Treatment

A good deal of the enlargement may consist entirely of soft-tissue hypertrophy in which large tortuous nerves and nodular tumor masses are located. When this is the case, resection of the soft-tissue masses, the grossly enlarged tortuous nerves, and the redundant skin may produce a nearly normal finger, although sensation may be somewhat diminished. It is advisable to perform this procedure in stages to avoid circulatory damage to the entire part. If the digital nerve is uninvolved, it should be preserved, and excess tissues should be removed from its periphery. In some instances, the length of the finger and of the associated bony deformity is too great, and parts of the finger

Fig. 7.26. Congenital anomalous development of a joint in the fingers. There is a large double first metacarpal of the middle finger and marked joint contracture.

Fig. 7.27. Same case as seen in Figure 7.26 after complete ray excision and narrowing of the hand. The child has very good function.

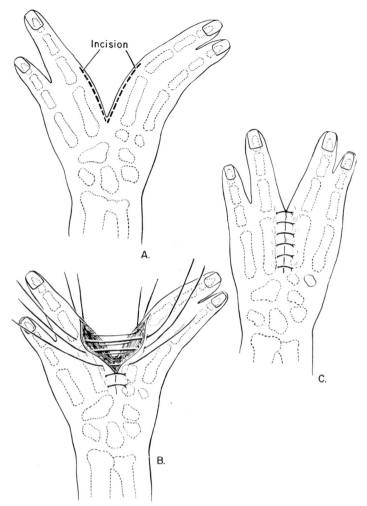

Fig. 7.28. Narrowing of the hand to improve its cosmetic appearance. Function should always be the main consideration, however.

Fig. 7.29. Extra ulnar digits.

417

Fig. 7.30. Same case as seen in Figure 7.29, showing the final result after surgical excision.

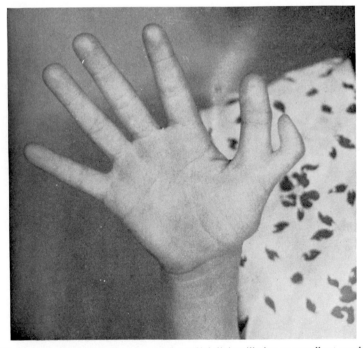

Fig. 7.31. Bifid thumb. Excision of the radial digit will give an excellent result.

Fig. 7.32. Lobster claw hand. No treatment is prescribed for this type of case.

Fig. 7.33. Congenital hypertrophy or megalodactylia.

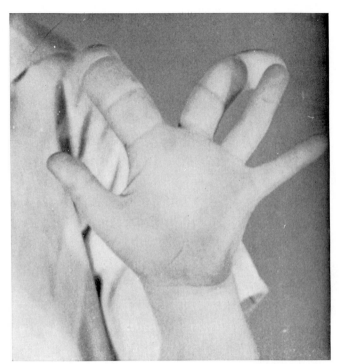

Fig. 7.34. Congenital hypertrophy or megalodactylia.

Fig. 7.35. Congenital grooves and bands with amputations associated with partial syndactylism. Some improvement cosmetically and functionally can be obtained by deepening the webs.

Fig. 7.36. Typical Streeter's dysplasia (congential amputation and annular grooves).

may have to be sacrified. If the finger is severely deformed and enlarged so that it is a poorly functioning unit in an otherwise normally functioning hand, it is probably best to sacrifice it. A ray amputation in these cases produces a result that is excellent functionally and cosmetically.

Annular Grooves and Congenital Amputations

These ringlike bands appear circumferentially about the arm, forearm, leg, fingers, and toes. The exact etiology is unknown; however, they are not due to amniotic bands. The grooves may be shallow, involving only skin and subcutaneous tissue, or they may extend through the fascia to any depth. The deeper ones often interfere with lymphatic and venous return and cause distal edema. At times, the portion of the extremity that is distal to the groove is lost. This definitely occurs in utero, and amputations are then present in the newborn. Single or multiple amputations of fingers or of the hand frequently accompany these annular grooves.

Treatment

When the grooving is superficial, no treatment is necessary and the groove should be left alone. Deep grooves, particularly those interfering with lymphatic drainage, should be corrected. The groove is excised by means of incisions that go beneath it until normal structures are encountered and that zigzag in a manner approximating the subcutaneous tissue and skin so that a constricting scar is avoided. The excision should not be accomplished in one procedure, but rather in stages, one-half to one-third of the groove being released at a sitting, in order to avoid circulatory embarrassment.

Brachydactylism

Interference with embryonic development may cause shortening of one or more digits. The phalanges may be decreased in number of length, or the metacarpal may be shortened. Various combinations may occur simultaneously. It is not uncommon for this condition to occur concomitantly with syndactylism or polydactylism.

Treatment

There is really no treatment for brachydactylia. The fingers may be almost normally formed, and they may function quite satisfactorily. The accompanying deformities of syn-

Fig. 7.37. Correction of annular groove by surgical excision. This is best done in stages one-third to one-half of the circumference being released at one sitting.

dactylism or polydactylism should be corrected as described above.

Agenesis and Incomplete Development

Absence or incomplete development of parts may involve an entire extremity or parts of one. This section deals with such deformities as amelia, or complete absence of an upper limb; hemimelia, or absence of the forearm and hand; acheiria, or absence of the hand; adactylia, or absence, complete or incomplete, of the digits, including the metacarpals and phalanges; aphalangia, or absence of phalanges, complete or incomplete; and phocomelia, including complete phocomelia—or absence of an entire arm except the hand and fingers, proximal phocomelia—or complete absence of only the proximal segment of an arm, and distal phocomelia—or complete absence of only the forearm. In some instances, the involvement may be quite extensive, even to the point of producing a quadruple amputee. It may be so mild, however, as to produce a perfectly normal skeleton except for the absence of a phalanx or even a part of one phalanx. Sometimes the stump of a part is smooth and has no external

evidence of a part distal to it; however, by x-ray there are at times evidences of incomplete development of the distal limb bud. In other instances, there is a fairly well developed arm but a poorly developed forearm and a limb bud for the hand. Usually these small processes are valueless from a functional standpoint and are in the way as far as the fitting of prostheses is concerned.

A deformity of the fingers may be manifested in many ways. There may be complete absence of a finger or an entire ray, or of the entire radial or ulnar side of the hand. The fingers may be present but incompletely developed, and there may be other associated anomalies such as partial or complete syndactylism, symphalangism, or any group of such associated deformities.

Treatment

Unfortunately, when a part is absent, there is no way to add or replace it. Usually one must accept deformity, particularly if there is incomplete loss of a part such as a forearm, arm, or hand. In cases of amelia, and of hemimelia and phocomelia in which no definitive procedures

Fig. 7.38. Severe partial brachydactylia and syndactylism. This child was very much upset by the deformity. Excision of the middle and ring fingers and moving the middle ray ulnarward would render the deformity much less noticeable.

Fig. 7.39. Congenital absence of both forearms and of left lower leg with flexion contracture of both knees. The flexion contractures were corrected by posterior surgical release and skeletal traction. The right leg was then braced, and a prosthesis was fitted on the left. The patient now walks with crutches at the age of 3 years.

can be accomplished to give satisfactory terminal usefulness to the part, prostheses should be used. Numerous factors have been shown to

Fig. 7.40. Congenital absence of the first metacarpal with poorly developed phalanges. There is some function in the long flexor and the extensor (adactylia, partial, intercalary) (floating thumb).

determine whether the prosthesis will be functionally useful or a failure. Two of the most important are (1) the age at which the prosthesis is fitted and (2) the attitude of the family. Aitken and Frantz[1a] have pointed out that when the child with an amputation is presented for care, it is imperative first to establish enough rapport with the family to convince them that the prosthesis is desirable and necessary. The family must exercise its authority to promote acceptance of the prosthesis, repetitive wearing, and practice until functional gain makes wearing the prosthesis seem desirable. This will not be done unless the family is first convinced that prosthetic restoration is a sound principle.

For years it was thought unnecessary to fit children who had limb deficiencies until they were old enough to decide for themselves whether they needed a prosthesis or not. In recent years, fitting was begun just before school age at about 4-4½ years, but now most authorities who work constantly with this problem believe that the best final results are obtained when the prosthesis is fitted as early as possible. Prosthetic tolerance and functional use are now obtained in children only 6 months of age. As soon as the child can sit well and balance, it is well to fit these congenital limb deficiencies with a passive type of mitten that

Fig. 7.41. Same case as seen in Figure 7.40 after transfer of index finger to thumb position.

Fig. 7.42. (*Left*) Congenital absence of the hand. A prothesis should be fitted at an early age (about four years).

Fig. 7.43. (*Right*) Congenital absence of the forearm and hand. This patient should have a prosthesis with an elbow joint at the age of about 4 years.

Fig. 7.44. Rudimentary bud of forearm and hand. Improved function and appearance may be attained by sacrificing the bud and fitting the remaining arm stump with a prosthesis.

offers some cosmetic restoration and also permits palmar prehension. At the age of approximately 2½ years, the two-pronged, voluntary-opening, terminal device should be fitted. When these prostheses are fitted early, the children are found to adapt to them quite nicely; the prosthesis actually becomes a part of the child.

Small, useless appendages, if present, should be sacrificed in order to gain an accurate fitting of the prosthesis. When there is an abnormal appendage that may have some functional use in stabilizing a prosthesis or in helping to control some of the movable parts, it should be left intact, regardless of how small or unsightly it may be, and the prosthesis itself should be altered to fit and utilize this valuable part.

Children do well with quite short arm and forearm stumps. It is amazing to watch the function of a multiplying action joint with a short stump. People usually count stumps but rarely count fingers. Any useless part should be sacrificed. The appearance is always improved by such procedures, and quite often function is also improved. When children have been born without certain functions, they tend to adapt to the deficiency without great difficulty, to become quite agile, and to substitute very nicely for the missing parts. Such substitution should certainly be encouraged. If phalanges are absent but metacarpals are present, the webs

Fig. 7.45. Congenital absence of the thumb with excellent function of fingers.

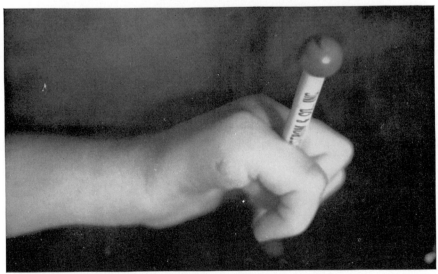

Fig. 7.46. Same case as seen in Figure 7.45. Use of pencil showing substitution pattern. Surgery should not be considered unless the deformity is bilateral, in which case the index finger might be transposed for the thumb on one side.

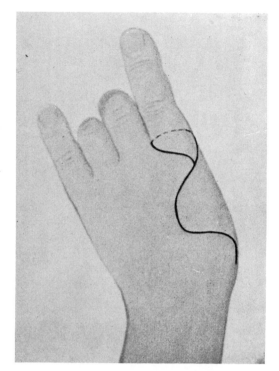

Fig. 7.47. Plan of incision used in first stage of transfer of index finger to thumb position.

Fig. 7.48. Congenital maldevelopment. The right hand can be improved cosmetically by removal of the poorly developed radial and ulnar digits.

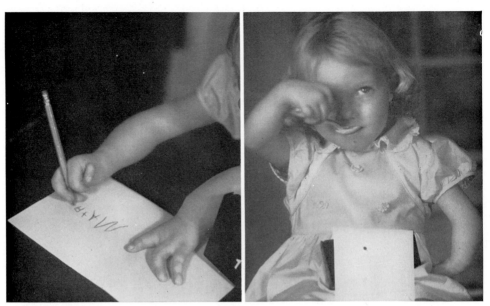

Fig. 7.49. Same case as seen in Figure 7.48 showing adaptability at an early age. Function will improve in this case with use and time.

Fig. 7.50. Same case as seen in Figures 7.48 and 7.49 after transfer of index finger to thumb position.

Fig. 7.51. Hand of child with multiple congenital anomalies.

Fig. 7.52. X-ray of same hand as seen in Figure 7.51 showing absence of thumb phalanges, partial absence of finger phalanges, and syndactyly.

Fig. 7.53. Hand shown in Figure 7.51 after syndactyly separation of index finger and transfer of entire index ray to first metacarpal. A usable thumb with good sensation has been constructed.

Fig. 7.54. Multiple congenital skeletal anomalies. The child has adapted well to the use of one finger on the right. He can lace shoes and tie bows as quickly as anyone.

Fig. 7.55. (*Top*) Congenital absence of digit with webbing of the first metacarpal space. The child has congenital deafness and congenital anomalies of the ears in addition.

Fig. 7.56. (*Bottom*) The result after Z-plasty deepening of the thumb web.

may be deepened so that the metacarpals may be used for grasping. The first metacarpal is particularly valuable for such an adaptation.

Absence of Thumb. If the entire thumb ray is absent bilaterally, a pollicization may be performed on one side. It is better to perform this type of surgery in late childhood when the structures have some maturity and are relatively easy to work with and when the child is at an age of cooperativeness and understanding. The procedures we have been most pleased with have been done between the ages of 7 and 10.

We have been very happy in recent years with the results of the one-stage procedure of transfer of the index finger to the thumb position on a neurovascular pedicle, as described by Littler and Cooley,[8a] for both congenital and traumatic absence of the thumb. It is generally thought that, if there is a unilateral absence of the thumb, the procedure

is not necessary, but if the absence is bilateral, the mobile thumb ought to be developed.

Many procedures for dealing with the so-called floating thumb have been described. These procedures attempt to utilize the existing hypoplastic thumb as a post and, in some instances, to obtain a post plus a little mobility if any tendon structures are present in the hypoplastic thumb. Some of the procedures have been successful, but they always leave the thumb in a poor position. It is always a post, and its appearance and function are never as good as one desires. It is not nearly as functional as an index finger that has been properly moved to the thumb position.

Depending upon what structures are present, many modifications of the procedure may be necessary. In some instances, an existing first metacarpal allows a relatively simple procedure. In other instances, there may be no

Fig. 7.57. Widening the adductor web by Z-plasty to procure additional function of thumb.

Fig. 7.58. Symphalangism in mother and daughter. X-rays of the child's feet show incomplete segmentation of calcis, cuboid, talus, and navicular.

thumb tendons, either extrinsic or intrinsic, and no carpal bones. In such cases, the procedure is somewhat more diffcult but certainly possible, and it gives, in our experience, excellent results. Usually when the entire digit, including all musculature, has been removed, we have found that a sublimis type of opponens transfer gives better stability and even more function of the moved finger. The procedure, which has been well described by Littler, involves making a flap on the radial side of the hand. A racket type of incision is made about the base of the index finger; it comes down radialward and dorsalward and then swings back from the dorsal surface of the hand to the level of the "take-off" position of the thumb. The entire wound, which circumscribes the index finger, is opened up; then, the surgeon working from the dorsal surface, the dorsal aponeurosis is sectioned between the second and third metacarpals, along with the deep transverse metacarpal ligament and any interdigitating fibers between the extensor tendons of the index and middle fingers. The vessels are demonstrated at this point, and the artery and vein to the radial side of the middle finger are identified, ligated, and servered in order that the vessels to the index finger may remain intact and that the entire finger may be mobilized. The nerve is usually separate at this level. If it is not, it can be mobilized by sharp dissection about as far back as one desires so that the nerve fibers are left running out to the middle finger and index finger separately. If the entire finger is moved, the interossei are detached and the metacarpal is exposed. The metacarpal may then be sectioned at the base and also at the neck so that its shaft is completely removed. We have utilized the head of the second metacarpal more or less as a carpal bone. In one instance, we attached this bone to its own base at an angle of almost 90°. It united and, in spite of our wishes to the contrary, has continued to grow and to add length to the finger. In 2 other cases since that one, we left the head of the metacarpal in the position of the carpus and attached it to the base of the second metacarpal bone very insecurely so that bony union

Fig. 7.59. (*Top*) Triphalangeal thumb bilateral, the middle phalanx being wedge-shaped.
Fig. 7.60. (*Bottom*) Hands are shown after removal of middle phalanx. Excellent functional and cosmetic results.

would not occur; in both instances, the head has remained as we desired it, so that it has been used as a carpal bone, and has not increased in length, the metaphysis being constantly absorbed. We therefore have a fibrous union at this level and the proximal phalanx is utilized as the first metacarpal. The flexor and extensor tendons motivate the finger, and if after a year of use there is not enough take-up in these tendons, they can be shortened above the wrist. In our experience to date, we have not had to perform this second procedure.

A transfer of the index finger should be done any time after the child has reached a cooperative age. We have not thought it necesarry to do this very early but like to get it done about the age of 5 or 6 years. After the procedure has been performed, the skin is sutured with interrupted 4-0 sutures or 51-0 chromic catgut, and a pressure dressing and a cast that holds the thumb in a position of opposition are applied. To date we have had no difficulties with arterial insufficiency. Venous stasis has at times presented a small problem, but not yet enough difficulty to warrant treatment other than observation. We have been very careful to observe Littler's original suggestion that as many venous structures as possible be saved in the skin so that there is little interference with venous return. This is very important.

Symphalangism

This condition results in failure of the interphalangeal joints to develop and occurs most frequently as a loss of the distal interphalangeal joint. The condition is frequently hereditary. There is no treatment, and, as a rule, the patient does not realize the presence of the deformity and usually adapts well from a functional standpoint.

Triphalangeal Thumb

Sometimes a thumb develops the appearance of a finger. This may occur with failure of development of the thenar muscles and lack of a wide intermetacarpal space between the first and second metacarpals, along with the existence of three phalanges in the ray. Another variation is a more or less normally developed thumb with three full phalanges. This thumb is more satisfactory in that the function is more normal and treatment is usually unnecessary. On occasion, one of the three phalanges may be deformed or wedge-shaped. In such instances, the deformed phalanx, which is fortunately most often the middle one, can be removed surgically so that the two normal phalanges will approximate each other They will form a good joint. The ligaments should be sutured, and most often the thumb will have very good function and appearance.

References

1a. Aitken, G. T., and Frantz, C. H.: The juvenile amputee, *J. Bone Joint Surg., 46A:* 1376, 1964.
1. Barsky, A. J.: Congenital anomalies of the hand, *J. Bone Joint Surg., 33A:* 35, 1951.
2. Brooks, B., and Lehman, E. P.: The bone changes in Recklinghausen's neurofibromatosis, *Surg. Gynecol. Obstet, 38:* 587, 1924.
3. Bunnell, S.: Contractures of the hand from infections and injuries, *J. Bone Joint Surg., 14:* 27, 1932.
4. Bunnell, S.: *Surgery of the Hand,* Philadelphia: J. B. Lippincott Co., 1944.
5. Colonna, P. C.: Some common congenital deformities and their orthopedic treatment, *New York J. Med., 28:* 713, 1928.
6. Frantz, C. H., and O'Rahilly, R.: Congenital skeletal limb deficiencies, *J. Bone Joint Surg., 43A:* 1202, 1961.
7. Johnson, H. M.: Congenital cicatrizing bands, report of a case with etiologic observations, *Am. J. Surg., 52:* 498, 1941.
8. Kanavel, A. B.: Congenital malformations of the hand, *Arch. Surg., 25:* 1932.
8a. Littler, J. W., and Cooley, S. G. E.: Congenital dysplasia of the thumb, *J. Bone Joint Surg., 46A:* 912, 1964.
9. McCarroll, H. R.: Clinical manifestations of congenital neurofibromatosis, *J. Bone Joint Surg., 32A:* 601, 1950.
10. MacCollum, D. W.: Webbed fingers, *Surg. Gynecol. Obstet., 71:* 782, 1940.
11. Moore, B. H.: Some orthopedic relationships of neruofibromatosis, *J. Bone Joint Surg., 23:* 109, 1941.
12. Sachs, M. D.: Familial brachyphalangiae, *Radiology, 35:* 622, 1940.
13. Stelling, F. H.: Surgery of the hand in the child, *J. Bone Joint Surg., 45A:* 623, 1963.

CEREBRAL PALSY

Reconstruction of the hand disabled by cerebral palsy is one of the most difficult tasks confronting the surgeon who treats hand conditions. The results are frequently disheartening, and in general, treatment should be conservative. There are very few cases in which surgical intervention is advisable or beneficial. Many factors serve to complicate the treatment of these hands. One of the first and most important steps is the careful classification of these cases into one of the basic types, *i. e.,* true spastics, athetoids, tension athetoids, ataxias, or rigidities. Therapy which may prove valuable in one of these groups can well be completely ineffective or contraindicated in another. Because the classification may at times be difficult, careful observation and repeated examinations are necessary before a definite therapeutic plan can be developed.

A second major factor which plays an important part in determining treatment is the mentality of the child. Many of these children are retarded and lack the cooperativeness necessary to hand surgery. Another factor that contributes greatly to the difficulties of treatment is that even in specific groups there are great variations in the severity of involvement. In certain cases, spasticity and poor coordination may seem to play the greatest part in dysfunction; however, there may also be a definite weakness of the opposing muscle. In

Fig. 7.61. These figures show typical attempt of the spastic to grasp. Active flexion of the wrist is performed in order to release the spastic finger flexion. The fingers are incoordinately flexed, and final grasp is achieved through extension of the wrist, which enhances the use of the spastic finger flexors. The child with this pattern can be trained, and surgery can often be avoided.

the very young cerebral palsied child, major emphasis should be placed on preventing a fixed position. The fingers, thumb, wrist, and forearm should be stretched passively several times daily. Frequently, children affected unilaterally do not recognize the effective hand as such and make no attempt to use it as a hand. Early recognition of the hand should be taught by means of toys, colored beads, and blocks to stimulate interest. Occasionally, the doctor or parent attempts to restrict the good hand in order to force the child to use the affected one. This procedure is condemned as it has been definitely shown that restricting a dominant

hand may lead to serious psychologic difficulties such as stuttering, loss or lack of speech, and behavior problems. Occasionally, after the child has discovered the dominant hand, restriction of the other may cure a psychologic complex.

Splinting and Physical Therapy

Following a period of observation, some of these children may be helped by the use of a small cock-up splint, or a splint with an outrigger to hold the thumb in extension may be necessary. Occasionally, rigid splints or

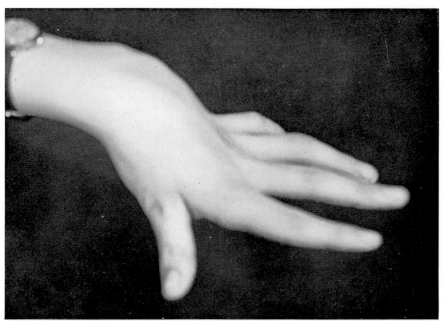

Fig. 7.62. Cerebral palsy, spastic type, showing reach and poor ability to get the thumb away from the palm.

Fig. 7.63. Same case as seen in Figure 7.62. Patient with wrist immobilized passively in extension and ulnar deviation, showing active ability now to get the thumb away from the palm for better function. Ability to extend the fingers is not quite as good, but it would still be quite effective for reach. This patient would profit from a wrist fusion.

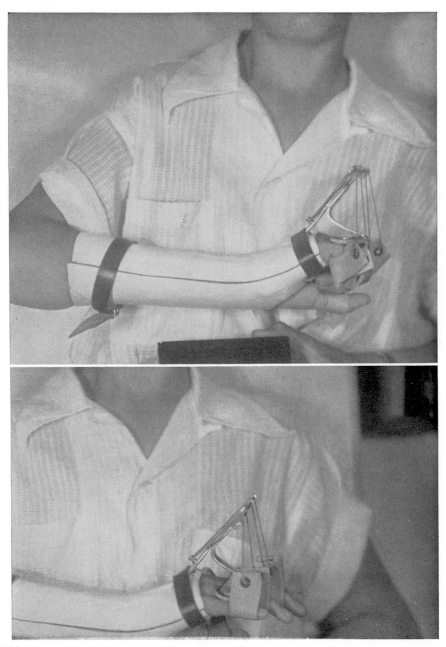

Fig. 7.64. Removable plastic splint with active rubber band traction outriggers for finger and thumb extension. The bar prevents hyperextension of the metacarpophalangeal joint. This splint is used on a part time basis in order to attempt to teach proper patterns.

Fig. 7.65. Cerebral palsy showing attempt to extend the fingers and wrist.

Fig. 7.66. Same case as seen in Figure 7.65 after transplantation of the flexor ulnaris to the common extensors and the flexor radialis to the extensor pollicis brevis. The patient has a good grip, but now hyperextends the wrist and is unable to extend the fingers away from the palm. The condition would be improved now by a wrist fusion in a neutral position. This pattern sometimes occurs after transplantation of wrist flexors into finger extensors owing to a resulting active insufficiency of wrist flexion.

Fig. 7.67. True spastic cerebral palsy showing patient's attempt to extend the fingers and wrist (*top*) and to grasp (*bottom*).

plaster bivalves may be used at night or on a part-time basis during the day in order to hold the forearm in a supinated position and to aid in passive stretching exercises. Later, as the child begins to develop and becomes more cooperative, active exercises can be added to the treatment program. Physical therapists are helpful in teaching the child and parents specific exercises outlined by the doctor. Major functions to be stressed are those of reaching, releasing the fingers, stabilizing the wrist in extension, grasping, and releasing the fingers.

Patients with true spasticity usually tend to flex the wrist as the fingers are extended incoordinately. They also have difficulty extending the thumb out of the palm. As grasp is attempted, varying degrees of wrist flexion hinder active grasping function of the fingers. Frequently, the thumb is in a position of adduction prior to finger flexion, and this position interferes severely with pick-up and attempted pinch. In most of these cases, if one extends the wrist in order to aid the strength of grasp, the patient may be unable to extend the fingers effectively

Fig. 7.68. Same case as seen in Figure 7.67, showing reach and grasp after wrist fusion in a neutral position.

for function. Treatment must be carried out many times daily, and parental cooperation and understanding are essential.

The preceding conservative program is used in all types of cases and should be the only type of treatment for ataxias, athetoids, and tension athetoids. with athetoids, one of the prime initial efforts should be to teach the patient active relaxation. Time is a great factor here, but again understanding on the part of the family and helpfulness of those charged with the care of the patient may make a great difference. It is amazing to see one of these patient attempt to write or to use a typewriter

Fig. 7.69. Reach and grasp following transplantation of the flexor ulnaris to the common extensors and the flexor radialis to the extensor pollicis brevis. Prior to surgery, the thumb was held flexed, the fingers were clenched, and the wrist was markedly flexed. Now the patient has better reach and grasp, but the thumb hyperextends. This has since been improved by an arthrodesis of the metacarpophalangeal joint.

while fighting the marked overflow. Surgery in some of these cases produces much poorer function, and in very few instances does it produce the desired effect.

Surgical Treatment

Occasionally, surgical intervention definitely improves the function in these hands. At the North Carolina Cerebral Palsy Hospital, Goldner,[3] taking into consideration physical status and mental condition, found only 12 patients acceptable for hand surgery out of 300 selected as eligible for general treatment.

Prior to selecting a case for surgery, it is advisable that the surgeon follow the patient for a long period to make sure that the proposed procedure has at least a reasonable chance of improving function. The use of casts or splints may be extremely helpful in making a decision. The brace or cast may be placed on the extremity so as to hold it in the position that might be attained by surgery. The use of the hand in the cast or splint is observed over a period of time before a decision is made. Before a definitive surgical procedure is attempted a detailed examination of the muscles must be made. Phelps[8] has emphasized that in addition to the charting and evaluation of spastic muscles, the power of other associated muscles must be evaluated and their degree of control noted. The importance of evaluating the power of nonspastic muscles is emphasized because certain antagonistic muscles may show a great weakness and at times may be completely flaccid. This is particularly true in the muscles controlling the wrist and fingers. If there is a flaccid paralysis in the antagonistic muscles, relieving the spasticity will not solve the problem.

Surgery should be used only as an adjunct to the general treatment of the hand in cerebral palsy. Many of the operative procedures have been devised for other types of neurologic involvement, and it should be emphasized that, when these procedures are used on the cerebral palsied child, the final results are never as satisfactory. The procedures used in cerebral palsy for improvement of the spastic hand should be those which stabilize the wrist in order to permit better finger function, get the thumb away from the palm to allow the hand to be opened and closed effectively, and improve supination. Certain minor procedures may be helpful, and occasionally, an excellent result may be obtained. Intricate procedures which are often used for polio should be left to the surgeon who is well versed in hand surgery.

Arthrodesis of the wrist is performed in order to improve the function of the digits and correct deformity of the wrist. The flexor carpi ulnaris is often a strong spastic muscle capable of producing considerably deformity. Steindler described a procedure in that the spastic flexor carpi ulnaris was released from its insertion, brought subcutaneously through a channel

Fig. 7.70. These figures show a hand of a child with cerebral palsy, true spastic type, following a wrist fusion in ulnar deviation with the wrist in a neutral position regarding flexion and extension. The patient is able to extend the fingers and to get the thumb away from the palm for grasping. Prior to surgery, the patient clenched the fingers and thumb into the palm and had difficulty attempting to get them away from the palm.

from the ulnar side across the dorsal aspect of the forearm, and transferred into an osseous opening in the distal radius in the radial styloid. This removed the deforming force of the ulnaris as a strong ulnar deviator and flexor, and aided in active supination of the forearm. Green[4] later modified this procedure by transferring the flexor carpi ulnaris into the extensor carpi radialis longus. This actually is a better procedure since it adds a powerful active dorsiflexion which improves wrist and finger control and also, because of the position of the transfer, will add some supinatory effect. It is less desirable than the Green transfer, which removes the deforming force of ulnar deviation and flexion and provides the active force of promoting dorsiflexion of the wrist in supination, however. In 1962 Green and Banks[5] reported an end result study of 39 cases and rated 24 in the excellent to good group, 15 in the fair group, and only 2 as poor results. They felt that surgical procedure was the single best way to improve function of the hand and fingers in cerebral palsy. They also noted that they had not had to perform a wrist arthrodesis in the past 20 years. They emphasized the importance of proper evaluation of cases before utilizing this procedure. In every instance the transfer should not be performed until the soft tissues causing fixed deformity were corrected, such as release of flexion of the wrist or fixed pronation of the forearm. They felt it was very important to utilize proper follow-up care in the use of proper splinting and utilization of physical therapy in the form of active assistive exercises until the patients were able to actively function to the best possible ability before discontinuing all protection and functional training. In his discussion of the paper by Drs. Green and Banks, Goldner[3] indicated that he did not believe that arthrodesis should be abandoned. There are definitely some cases that previous procedures have failed or others in which stability can only be obtained by arthrodesis. Hands requiring stability of the wrist are helped considerably by arthrodesis just past the neutral position in extension. This position allows more effective and efficient use of the fingers. Not infrequently this positioning of the wrist causes the fingers to be tightly clenched in the palm and unable to extend. This condition should be known prior to surgery, and a first procedure would be to transplant one of the strong wrist flexors into the finger extensors. Occasionally, this procedure is all that is necessary; however, a wrist fusion is usually needed to provide for adequate stability.

The thumb-in-palm deformity is one of the most disabling encountered in the spastic hand. If the deformity is mild, ulnar deviation of the hand at the wrist increases the tension of the extensor and abductor mechanism of the thumb and thus pulls the thumb phalanges and the first metacarpal toward the radial side. This was first emphasized by Cooper,[2] and it is wise, in arthrodeses of the wrist, to place the hand in moderate ulnar deviation in order that this mechanism may become effective in pulling the thumb up out of the palm. It should be remembered that if the flexor pollicis longus is spastic or contracted and the thumb web is tight, no amount of ulnar deviation of the hand produces an effective result in getting the thumb out of the palm. A hypermobile metacarpophalangeal joint often results in the deformity that pulls the thumb into the palm, and weakness of the intrinsic musculature of the thumb may lead to the thumb-in-palm position.

Spasticity or contracture of the thumb web may be treated by sectioning the web fascia and stripping the dorsal interosseous muscle from the first metacarpal, as well as tenotomizing the adductor pollicis. These procedures are often done in conjunction with fusion of the metacaropohalangeal joint. If the extensor mechanism is inactive or weak, transplantation of an active wrist or finger flexor to the extensor pollicis longus should be carried out. Sometimes this leads to an imbalance with hyperextension of the metacaropohalangeal joint and, when it does, a fusion of this joint should be added.

References

1. Burman, M. S.: The spastic hand, *J. Bone Joint Surg., 20:* 133, 1938.
2. Cooper, W.: Surgery of the upper extremity in spastic paralysis, *Q. Rev. Pediatr., 7:* 64, 1951.
3. Goldner, J. L.: Reconstructive surgery of the hand in cerebral palsy and spastic paralysis resulting from injury to the spinal cord, *J. Bone Joint Surg., 37A:* 1141, 1955.
4. Green, W. T.: Transplantation of flexor carpi ulnaris for pronation-flexion deformity of the wrist, *Surg. Gynecol. Obstet., 75:* 337, 1942.
5. Green, W. T., and Banks, H.: Flexor carpi ulnaris

transplant and its use in cerebral palsy, *J. Bone Joint Surg., 44A:* 1343, 1962.

6. Green, W. T., and McDermott, L. J.: Operative treatment of cerebral palsy of spastic type, *J. A. M. A., 118:* 434, 1942.

7. McCarroll, H. R.: Surgical treatment of spastic paralysis, *Instruct. Lect. Am. Acad. Orthrop. Surg., 6:* 134, 1949.

8. Phelps, W.: Prevention of acquired dislocation of the hip in cerebral palsy, *J. Bone Joint Surg., 41A:* 440, 1959.

POLIOMYELITIS

Poliomyelitis frequently involves the upper extremity and results in residual weakness and a poorly functioning hand. In some instances, the hand is so severely involved that very little functional value is maintained; however, by certain operative procedures, the value can be increased. The aim of these procedures is to reroute tendons, in order to prevent or correct deformities caused by strong musculature and to increase the efficiency of poorly functioning muscle. Occasionally, a completely paralyzed muscle can be replaced by tendon transplantation. In other instances, substitution patterns are developed, or can be developed with help, so that a fairly valuable hand is obtained. Occasionally these substitution patterns may be strengthened or enhanced by surgical procedures.

From the very onset of the acute disease, function should be the final goal of the care and treatment of the hand. The joints should be kept mobile, and secondary contractures and deformities should be prevented by proper utilization of active and passive exercises and by splinting the hand in the position of function. During the sensitive stages of the disease, passive splints may be used to rest the parts and thus to prevent stretching of painful, weakened muscles. Later, as sensitivity and muscle spasm disappear and muscle power begins to return, certain active splints are used. These splints are devised to afford helpful stabilization of the wrist action in some 10 or 15° of dorsiflexion. They are made of spring type metal to afford support and yet maintain flexibility. Outriggers are used to help finger extension or flexion, or both, with spring metal or elastic bands. Opponens splints are usually rigid or semirigid in order to keep the thumb in the opposed, functioning position. They may be made of plastic or metal.

In the younger age groups (up to 10 years) it is best to utilize functional splinting for a period of years even though certain operative procedures might be available to improve function and thus to replace the splint. There are several reasons for this recommendation: (1) operative procedures are technically more difficult in the young child; (2) the refined hand movements that are necessary for taking over tendon transplants are lacking because of incomplete development of the nervous system; (3) the best results are attained with full cooperation, which is often lacking in the younger age group; and (4) bone growth should be complete, or nearly complete, to prevent disproportion between the bony framework and the tendon transplantation.

In some exceptional cases, waiting should definitely be avoided. These cases are mainly those in which the tendon to be transplanted is producing bone or joint deformity in spite of splinting and exercises.

Certain conditions that are present in polio are not always present in traumatic hands and are favorable to both the patient and the surgeon. On the other hand, other conditions exist which make rehabilitation more difficult and uncertain.

Unfavorable conditions:
1. Disseminated muscle weakness.
2. Substitution patterns.
3. Involvement of the trunk and other extremities.

Favorable conditions:
1. Good skin and subcutaneous tissue.
2. Normal sensation.
3. Good mobility of joints.

The procedures devised to improve hand function surgically may be divided into three groups: (1) arthrodeses, (2) tendon transfers, and (3) tenodeses. Of these three groups, the tendon transfers are the most valuable and produce a better functioning hand.

Arthrodeses

Arthrodeses should be used only as a last resort. Occasionally, an arthrodesis is indicated to free tendons for other usage, but, in polio, the loss of joint motion in the upper extremity may be disabling. All other methods of improving function should be carefully considered before such a procedure as fusing the wrist is undertaken. This procedure should be regarded as a last resort, and the relationship of a stiff wrist to the total function of the patient's extremity must be determined. Occasionally, it may be seen that the finger and thumb function could undoubtedly be improved by utilizing the wrist tendons following stabilization; however, after careful consideration, it may be found that wrist motion will be much more useful than an improved finger and thumb function. Fusion of the wrist in the wheelchair patient may cause loss of ability to use the chair, and may thus disable him completely if the chair is his only means of locomotion. Other patients need a flexible wrist in order to shift the body weight. A fusion of the wrist here might well prevent the patient from moving about. It is important in all instances to consider the affected hand in relation to body function as a whole before permanently stabilizing a joint. Arthrodesis of the metacarpophalangeal joint is certainly of value and sometimes necessary to correct deformity and to increase the usefulness of the fingers; however, it should not be done if it can possibly be avoided. The avoidance of this procedure is especially necessary in a severely handicapped person who requires a flat hand in order to push himself about. It has also been found that arthrodesis weakens the grasp and thus makes the use of crutches extremely difficult. It is wise, when arthrodesis is considered, to defer the procedure as long as possible, preferably until maturity. The reason for this is that the person should be allowed to try a vocation first. The relationship of the hand to his vocation is extremely important, and he may be greatly handicapped by such a permanent procedure as an arthrodesis.

The bone block procedure may be helpful in improving the function of the hand, but it should be remembered that it is a poor procedure if the patient is a crutch walker.

Arthrodesis of the interphalangeal joint of the thumb is valuable if other means of stabilization are found impossible.

Tendon Transplantation

It has been found that tendon transplants are by far the best procedures for increasing the function of the hand. Occasionally, active motors are not available, and it has been found best to perform passive or active tenodeses,

Fig. 7.71. A hand in which all wrist flexors have been transplanted into finger and thumb extensors. The stabilizing effect of the wrist flexors has been lost; the wrist cocks back and the fingers do not extend in the metacarpophalangeal joints.

Fig. 7.72. Same case as seen in Figure 7.71. If the wrist is stabilized toward flexion, the fingers then extend beautifully. It is always best to leave at least one wrist flexor intact when transferring a tendon, whether it be for cerebral palsy, polio, or brachial palsy.

which will be discussed later. A tendon must never be moved without careful consideration and an accurate muscle evaluation. It is frequently necessary to retest the muscles several times in order to get an accurate picture of the muscle power, and it is often difficult in the young child to obtain an accurate muscle test. It is to be remembered that occasionally two muscles acting together may produce a functioning unit, even though each muscle has only 50% of normal power. A muscle used for transplantation should have at least 85% of normal power.

It should be remembered that transplanting a tendon should not excessively weaken the portion of the hand from which it is taken. For example, a strong wrist extensor should not be transplanted in order to gain finger flexion or opposition when the remaining wrist flexors are weak. The procedure would result in loss of the stabilizing function of wrist extension and would thereby defeat the purpose of the original transplant, which was to strengthen the grip. If there is any doubt regarding the power of a muscle, an incision should be made over the belly, and the color and texture of the muscle should be inspected.

In adults, it has been found advisable to wait for a period of 2 years before attempting a tendon transplantation. In children up to the age of 12, it is best to wait for even longer periods. With proper splinting, substitution patterns which will make surgery entirely unnecessary may evolve. In children, it is better to err on the side of waiting too long than to perform surgical procedures without careful consideration.

Opposition. Paralysis of opposition is a major disability. The transplant of choice for restroing opponens function is based on use of the sublimis tendon of the ring finger as a motor. The prerequisties for this procedure are: (1) a profundus of the ring finger that is adequate for flexion of the digit without the sublimis, (2) a strong flexor pollicis longus, (3) a strong extensor pollicis longus and abductor pollicis longus, (4) a good or normal flexor digitorum sublimis, (5) absence of bone, joint, or soft-tissue deformity of the thumb, (6) a strong flexor carpi ulnaris, and (7) functional strength of the fingers and the palmar arch.

If these conditions do not exist, the pro-fundus of the ring finger may be reinforced with an adjacent profundus or sublimis. The flexor longus, the abductor, or the extensor of the thumb may be strengthened by another transplant. The most suitable tendon for such strengthening is the long extensor of the wrist. The indicis proprius can often be used to great advantage for strengthening the extensor pol-licis longus. The flexor carpi ulnaris may be reinforced by the extensor carpi ulnaris. These procedures will be described in detail later. If there is deformity or contraction of the thumb, it should be corrected prior to any attempts at tendon reconstruction. Sometimes a tenotomy

Fig. 7.73. Loss of opponens and atrophy of thenar eminence.

Fig. 7.74. Same case as seen in Figure 7.73, after opponens transplantation of the sublimis of the ring finger to the base of the proximal phalanx of the thumb, with the flexor carpi ulnaris used as a pulley.

of the adductor of the thumb is necessary to release soft-tissue contracture of the web space. Parmanent tightness of the joints may be relieved by a rotation osteotomy of the first metacarpal. Occasionally, in a thumb with a strong flexor pollicis brevis and no disability other than a weakened or absent opponens, an osteotomy of the first metacarpal may produce a satisfactorily functioning result that obviates the necessity of an opponens transplant.

The opponens transfer should pull from the region of the pisiform for best mechanical efficiency. When the sublimis is used, this is accomplished best by bringing the tendon beneath and around the ulnar side of the flexor carpi ulnaris at its insertion as a pulley. The tendon should be attached to the thumb on the ulnar side of the proximal phalanx. The transplanted tendon should pass across the base of the palm subcutaneously from the pisiform to the metacarpophalangeal joint of the thumb. Proper tension is of utmost importance and is gained only by experience with the procedure. If the tendon is inserted too loosely, it will lack sufficient strength to oppose properly. If it is inserted too tightly, it may migrate over the metacarpophalangeal joint and cause a hyper-extension contracture. Following transfer, the hand should be immobilized in a plaster splint that holds the wrist in approximately 30° of flexion and 15° of ulnar deviation. Immobilization should be continued for a period of 3 weeks. Active exercises should follow, but an opponens splint should be used for protection between exercise periods. If the sublimis of the ring finger is not sufficiently strong, the sublimis of the middle finger may be used satisfactorily. Occasionally, it may be necessary to reinforce a transplanted weaker sublimis. This can be done by suturing an additional tendon into the musculotendinous junction of the sublimis tendon. In the absence of sublimi,

Fig. 7.76. Same case as seen in Figure 7.75, showing the support given by an opponens splint.

the extensor carpis ulnaris may be used, if its length is prolonged with a free tendon graft. It is passed around the ulnar border of the wrist proximal to the dorsal carpal ligament so that no pulleys are required.

Rerouting of Extensor Pollicis Longus. Frequently, the thumb drifts into ulnar deviation at the metacarpophalangeal joint. This position often cannot be corrected by opponens transfer. The condition may be alleviated and the opponens transfer made more effective, however, by rerouting the extensor pollicis longus tendon.

In this procedure, the dorsal carpal ligament is sectioned, and the extensor pollicis longus is removed from its groove and brought volarward in the subcataneous tissue. Its position is maintained by a subcutaneous suture that holds the tendon in direct line with the thumb ray. The dorsal carpal ligament is then resutured.

Reinforcement of Pulley for Opponens Transfers. At times the opponens transfer migrates toward the radial border of the wrist, and thus reduces the power and effectiveness of the transplant. The usual reason for this migration is weakness of the flexor carpi ulnaris. It can be corrected by suturing the extensor carpi ulnaris into the tendon of the flexor carpi ulnaris, according to the following procedure.

A hockey stick incision is made over the volar ulnar border of the wrist. The flexor carpi ulnaris is then freed, and the forearm is pronated. The extensor carpi ulnaris is isolated and sutured through a slit in the flexor carpi ulnaris. Fixation is maintained by interrupted

Fig. 7.75. Typical pinch of opponens loss plus a weak first interosseous.

Fig. 7.77. Effect of imbalance of the long flexors, intrinsics, and long extensors due to weak wrist extensors. Thenar muscles are absent, except for the long thumb flexor and extensor and the long abductor.

silk sutures. The anastomosis is performed just proximal to the route of the opponens transfer around the flexor carpi ulnaris tendon.

The index finger stands next to the thumb in functional importance. Loss of intrinsic power of this finger along with weak or absent opposition of the thumb is more commonly seen than weakness in all the remaining extrinsic muscles of the hand in poliomyelitis. Absence of the intrinsic power of the index finger prevents extension of the distal two phalanges and abduction of the finger into a position opposite the opposed thumb in the formation of the pinching mechanism. Strong extrinsic flexors and extensors of the index finger do not replace the dorsal and volar interossei and lumbricale muscles in the pinching mechanism. The clinical picture is usually that of cocking or hyperextension of the metacarpophalangeal joint when pinching is attempted. It is due to a loss of stability in flexion of the metacarpophalangeal joint.

If restoration of the intrinsic factor, particularly with regard to stability in flexion of the metacarpophalangeal joint, is attempted, transfers must insert into the lateral band, and function is better mechanically when the insertion is from the volar aspect of the hand. Many procedures for the restitution of this function have been described. Probably the most popular is that of sublimis transfer into the lateral band, as described by Bunnell.[1] Even in the absence of actively functioning musculature, tenodeses according to the methods of Fowler and of Riordan[12] are sometimes performed to stabilize these joints. These procedures will be discussed to some extent below. Frequently, the indicis proprius is transferred into the lateral band tendon to afford good abduction of the index finger. This transplant restores abduction and extension, but does not stabilize the metacarpophalangeal joint in flexion. Irwin and Eyler[10] have described a procedure which is excellent for the restoration of the abduction element in flexion and extension and also the stabilizing effect of intrinsic power on the metacarpophalangeal joint. This is the split sublimis procedure.

In this procedure, a long finger sublimis is severed at the proximal joint of the finger and withdrawn at the musculotendinous junction. The tendon is split into two tails. One tail is introduced through the lumbricale canal and inserted into the lateral band past the lubricale insertion. The other is inserted into the volar and dorsal interosseous tendons of the first dorsal interosseous. The wrist is kept in neutral position, the metacarpophalangeal joints are flexed 80°, and the interphalangeal joints are fully extended. The hand is immobilized for a period of 3 weeks, after which active exercises are begun.

Fig. 7.78. This opponens transplant functions well, but there is practically no abductor brevis or flexor pollicis longus to give stability.

Finger Flexion. Irwin[9] stated that weakened profundi may be successfully reinforced by being placed in continuity with other strong profundi or sublimi. When this procedure is performed properly, excellent results are obtained. It is accomplished by splicing the strong tendons into the weakened ones proximal to the volar carpal ligament. The wrist extensors work more or less synergistically with the long flexors of the fingers, and it has been found that wrist extensors work well in restoring finger flexion. The extensor carpi radialis longus has a good excursion and works well when it is woven into the profundus tendons at the musculotendinous junction. The anastomosis should be made under considerable tension; the little finger should be under the greatest tension, and each adjacent finger under progressively less tension. It should be made with the fingers in a position of relaxed flexion. A plaster splint is applied for about 3 weeks, and active motion follows its removal. Prior to utilization of an extensor of the wrist as a transplant, particularly to the flexor side, the ability to extend the wrist in the absence of this tendon must be assured. The remaining wrist extensor muscles should be inspected directly. If a strong extensor carpi radialis tendon is not available, transfer of the extensor carpi ulnaris into the flexor digitorun profundus tendons may give good restoration of finger flexion. The excursion of the flexor carpi ulnaris is not great enough to give satisfactory finger function. The brachioradialis works moderately well, but its excursion is less than that of the long extensor of the wrist. Restoration of common extensor action restores the ability to extend the metacarpophalangeal joints and stabilizes these joints, but it does not extend the interphalangeal joints in the absence of good intrinsics. The extensor carpi radialis also works very well in a restoration of common extensor function. It is transferred to the finger extensors more easily and with less concern than to the flexors, inasmuch as it can work as a stabilizer of the wrist when it is anastomosed into the extensors.

In this procedure, the extensor of the wrist is sectioned at its insertion into the base of the metacarpal, freed up in a retrograde fashion from under the carpal ligament, and then redirected along the dorsal surface of the forearm subcutaneously and anastomosed into the extensor tendons at their musculotendinous junctions. The anastomosis must be made with the extensors in considerable tension and with the metacarpophalangeal joints in extension.

Fig. 7.79. As strength is added, the grip is lost and the thumb flexes. This functional anomaly can be avoided by inserting one slip of the sublimis into the metacarpal and one into the phalanx so that the metacarpal is brought into opposition equally with the rest of the thumb.

Relative differences in tension are accomplished by suturing the little finger tighter than the adjacent ring finger, the ring finger slightly tighter than the middle finger, and so on. The extensor carpi radialis brevis can also be used to replace extensor communis function. The extensor carpi ulnaris is of fair usefulness, and the brachioradialis has been found to be an excellent motor, for this purpose. The wrist flexors, being synergistic with finger extension, may be used quite satisfactorily as replacements for common extensor function. The flexor carpi radialis and ulnaris can be used successfully; however, they are not as satisfactory as the radial extensors of the wrist.

Restoration of Finger Function by Tenodesis

As has been previously established, an arthrodesis in the hand paralyzed by polio is rarely indicated. The procedure might be considered in order to free valuable tendons for transplantation to weakened fingers and thumb; however, in evaluating the activity of the patient, one might find loss of flexibility of the wrist to be a great handicap. Irwin[9] and his associates at Warm Springs have found instances of patients who could be aided considerably be a tenodesis. Wrist motion can be retained, and in instances in which conventional transfers cannot be performed because of insufficient musculature, the tenodesis action can be utilized with quite effective results.

Grasp with the wrist extended is the result of two types of muscle action, namely, a primary flexion of the fingers caused by contraction of the flexor muscle mass and a secondary flexion of the fingers due to the increased distance, with the wrist extended, between the origin and the insertion of the long flexors. Conversely, flexion of the wrist may extend the fingers as a result of increasing the distance from the origin to the insertion of the long extensors. In the presence of weakness or loss of the long extensors or flexors of the fingers, grasp may be enhanced greatly by tenodesis of the afflicted motors. The fixation can be accomplished by implanting the common tendon mass into bone, which creates a tenodesis, or by transferring an actively contracting muscle into the tendon mass to form a dynamic tenodesis. Irwin emphasized that the distinction between a dynamic tenodesis and a standard transfer is a difficult one. A dynamic tenodesis is a transfer which, when the tendon is inserted into a common tendon group, such as the flexors of the fingers, relies mainly on wrist action for its function and only secondarily on the transplanted active muscle. Tenodeses should be reserved for patients who lack sufficient motors for conventional transfers. The patient must possess a mobile wrist that he can manipulate into flexion and extension, mobile fingers, and a functional elbow. An active wrist extensor greatly enhances the value of a flexor tenodesis; however, in the absence of active wrist extension, the wrist may be made to fall into the extended position by gravity when the forearm is supinated and the elbow flexed. The grasp that results is necessarily very slight, but an effective hook that the patient may utilize to considerable advantage is created. Active wrist flexion is less important than wrist extension to the grasp. In the absence of active motors, the wrist normally falls into a position of pronation and flexion when the elbow is flexed. The status of the intrinsics of the fingers plays an important role in the final result. Extensor tenodesis will not fully extend the fingers unless active intrinsics are present. Interestingly enough, finger extension may improve with flexor tenodesis if the lumbricales are functional. Lumbricale efficiency is increased when the profundi are stabilized.

According to the technique described by Irwin, flexor tenodesis is performed through a semilunar incision overlying the volar surface of the wrist. The median nerve is identified and carefully retracted from the field. The profundus tendons are identified by applying manual traction to each tendon and observing for flexion of the distal phalanges. The position of the fingers is adjusted to correspond to that assumed by the normal hand lying at rest on a flat surface with the wrist supinated. If the tenodesis is to be of the passive type, a small window is made in the distal end of the radius, and the profundus tendons are inserted into the bone with the aid of a single wire suture. Should a dynamic tenodesis be indicated, the position of the fingers is fixed by anastomosing any available transfer into the common tendon mass. Anastomosis is secured with the aid of twisted steel wire sutures. The technique for insertion of the extensor tenodesis is the same. The common extensors are isolated through a semilunar incision from the dorsum of the wrist to the ulnar side of the tubercle of Lister. Anastomosis is accomplished while the hand is in a position of rest. Active transfers are inserted under moderate tension. Immediate postoperative immobilization is secured with dorsal and volar plaster splints. Flexor tenodeses are immobilized with the wrist in full flexion and the fingers extended, and extensor tenodeses with the wrist in full extension and the fingers extended. Three weeks postoperatively, the splints are removed, and mobilization of the hand and wrist is initiated.

References

1. Bunnell, S.: Surgery of the intrinsic muscles of the hand other than those producing opposition of the thumb, *J. Bone Joint Surg., 24:* 1942.
2. Bunnell, S.: Active splinting of the hand, *J. Bone Joint Surg., 28:* 732, 1946.
3. Bunnell, S., and Howard, L. D.: Additional elastic hand splints, *J. Bone Joint Surg., 32A:* 226, 1950.
4. Coonrad, R., Eyler, D., and Irwin, C. E.: Splint sublimis transfer for paralysis of the intrinsic muscles of the index finger; Correspondence Club Letter, Duke Training Program, 1951.
5. Eyler, D. L., and Markee, J. E.: The anatomy and function of the intrinsic musculature of the fingers, *J. Bone Joint Surg., 36A:* 1, 1954.
6. Foerster, O., Fusion of metacarpals of thumb and index finger, *Acta Chir. Scand., 67:* 350, 1931.
7. Goldner, J. L., and Irwin, C. E.: An analysis of paralytic thumb deformities, *J. Bone Joint Surg., 32A:* 627, 1950.
8. Irwin, C. E.: Apparatus for the upper extremity disabled by poliomyelitis, *Instruct. Lect. Am. Acad. Orthop. Surg., 9:* 208, 1952.
9. Irwin, C. E.: Dynamic tenodesis, presented at the American Academy of Orthopaedic Surgeons, January 1956.
10. Irwin, C. E., and Eyler, D. L.: Surgical rehabilitation of the hand and forearm disabled by poliomyelitis, *J. Bone Joint Surg., 33A:* 825, 1951.
11. Kirklin, J. W., and Thomas, C. G.: Opponens transplant; an analysis of methods employed and results obtained, *Surg. Gynecol. Obstet., 86:* 213, 1948.
12. Riordan, D. C.: Tendon transplantation in median nerve and ulnar nerve paralysis, *J. Bone Joint Surg., 35A:* 312, 1953.
13. Royle, N. D.: An operation for paralysis of the intrinsic muscles of the thumb, *J.A.M.A., 111:* 612, 1938.
14. Thompson, C. F.: Fusion of metacarpals of thumb and index finger to maintain functional position of the thumb, *J. Bone Joint Surg., 24:* 907, 1942.

RHEUMATOID ARTHRITIS

Rheumatoid arthritis is a generalized systemic disease affecting both children and adults. In children, the disease may vary considerably in its mode of onset. Frequently, it begins in one joint and subsequently spreads to involve all joints. When it remains localized to one or two joints, as it occasionally does, it becomes a problem in diagnosis. It may be manifested by generalized joint involvement with marked toxicity, anemia, weight loss, splenomegaly, and fever.

When the hands are involved, marked deformity causing severe permanent dysfunction and disability frequently results. Primary joint involvement is not the only deforming factor. Secondary muscle spasm and eventual myostatic contracture contribute to the hand deformity. The muscles are in spasm because of irritation of the synovial reaction, but later they become fibrosed and permanently shortened. Microscopically, the muscles, tendons, and ligaments show multiple foci of inflammation and later fibrotic contracture. Some ligaments actually degenerate and thus permit subluxation of the joints. Some of the tendons may degenerate and rupture at focal spots of granulation. The joint changes and the ligamentous and tendinous involvement all play a part in the deformity, but the position of the deformity is largely due to a muscle imbalance among the long flexors, the long extensors, and the intrinsics. Because of this disturbance of the normal equilibrium in these three groups of muscles, all of the clinical forms of arthritis involving the hands and fingers result in two types of deformity, namely, the clawhand and the pillroller hand. In the clawhand, the metacarpophalangeal joints are pulled into hyperextension by the long extensors and thus overcome the resistance of the intrinsic muscles. The fingers flex in the middle joints and extend in the distal joints. The more usual of the two deformities is the pillroller hand, in which there is flexion of the metacarpophalangeal joints due to the intrinsic contracture. The middle and distal joints are thus pulled straight by the lateral bands, or at times the middle joint may be hyperextended and the distal joints may flex. The position of the wrist seems to play a great part in the effect of the deformity on the hands and fingers in both of these conditions. In the clawhand, the wrist is in flexion; therefore, the passive tension on the extensors leads to hyperextension in the metacarpophalangeal joints. In the pillroller hand, the wrist remains in extension and the finger extensors are relaxed. The spastic contracture of the intrinsic muscles, which are not being opposed by the relaxed finger extensors, causes the metacarpophalangeal joints to become markedly flexed. The interphalangeal articula-

tions assume a position of hyperextension because of the contracture and tightness of the intrinsic musculature. The thumb is usually drawn into flexion and adduction. The imbalance between the short flexors and adductors and the abductor group usually results in adduction and flexion of the carpometacarpal joint. The metacarpophalangeal joint is overflexed and thus causes hyperextension of the distal joint because of the pull of the long extensor. Deformity of the thumb is more often noted in the pillroller type of hand.

Treatment

Because of the systemic nature of rheumatoid arthritis, treatment of it must first be generalized; however, great attention should also be given to the local involvement and the prevention or correction of deformity. It is rare to see a patient who has in any way been neglected from a general standpoint. It is not unusual, however, to find that the general treatment has been carried out but that there has been very little effort locally to prevent crippling contractures. With the advent of newer remedies for rheumatoid arthritis and the improvement in general care and treatment, conservative local measures should become much more efficient and promising in the prevention and correction of deformities such as those that occur in the hand. In cases that are seen early—prior to the development of contracture—the treatment to prevent the deformity should start early and proceed actively under careful observation. The development of deformity is insidious, and frequently the doctor and family procrastinate until a serious deformity results. The family physician or pediatrician should handle the general medical care of the patient, but the orthopaedist should see the child early during the stage of irritation and painful swelling, before the occurrence of permanent contracture and deformity. If the development of deformity due to the imbalance of musculature is anticipated, proper splinting may be instituted, and the occurence of serious disability may be completely avoided. Dunnell[1] and Steindler[5] have emphasized that the muscles are contracted from irritation and are in a state of spasm. It is only later that they become structurally changed by progressive fibrosis.

Fig. 7.80. Rheumatoid arthritis prior to therapy showing the range of extension and flexion.

Steindler stated that a spastic muscle is an extensible one which has retained its elasticity, whereas a fibrosed muscle has lost its elasticity. The arthritic muscle remains in a reflex spastic state for a considerable period. The correction of this reversible condition by mechanical means and the restoration of balance by muscle reeducation offer a wide therapeutic opportunity for the acute and subacute case of rheumatoid arthritis. These factors greatly improve the prognosis for the arthritic hand in children who are seen prior to the development of fixed contracture and bone deformity. Even

when a definite contracture has developed, it is usually still in the stage of reflex spasm rather than of fixed myostatic contracture. Physical therapy in the form of heat, splinting, paraffin baths, and active exercises should be utilized to the fullest. Surgery is rarely indicated. In the early stages of swelling, pain, and muscle spasm, paraffin and whirlpool baths are more effective. Early development of flexion contracture of the wrist can be prevented by passive splinting with a cock-up splint. Active use of the hand should be encouraged, and fixed immobilization is to be avoided. Splints should be retention ones, which are designed only to maintain position, and should not be applied for corrective effect.

Active splinting is quite effective. The active splint should perform one purpose only; however, several splints, each exerting a different type of effect, may be used in the same case at different periods. Active splints using mild elastic traction or spring effect may be made by the bracemaker. If there are not available, simple plaster splints using spring wire or elastic

traction can be fashioned inexpensively. By utilizing the active splints part time to help overcome muscle spasm and imbalance, fixed deformities can be prevented.

Active exercises for the fingers, wrist, and forearm are essential in the treatment and should be combined and properly balanced with gentle passive stretching of tight joints. Emphasis is placed on gentle stretching and manipulative treatment, which must be undertaken with great care never to approach the

Fig. 7.81. Same child as seen in Figure 7.80, 10 months later, after use of paraffin baths, whirlpool and active exercises, and active splinting.

Fig. 7.82. Active splints made of plaster with rubber band traction; they can be removed for use of the limb and for physical therapy.

Fig. 7.83. Hands with rheumatoid arthritis showing advanced stage of deformity: flexed wrist, hyperextended proximal finger joints, flexed middle joints. and extended distal joints.

456

Fig. 7.84. Metal active splint to hold wrist in dorsiflexion and bar to prevent metacarpophalangeal extension during active stretch on the proximal interphalangeal joints. This splint is worn part time while gentle passive stretching and active exercises are used and, at other times, during active use of the hand in general daily activity.

point of tearing capsular tissues. The treatment program is attended by some increase in pain, which may be allayed by the administration of salicylates. Children usually tolerate treatment better than adults and are quite cooperative.

Utilization of the foregoing measures, accompanied by proper education of the family regarding the chronicity of the treatment, usually produces gratifying results. Only after a period of from two to ten years usually does the disease become completely burned out, and some residual deformities may be expected at the end of this period; however, major crippling can usually be minimized, and in many instances it can be completely prevented.

References

1. Bunnell, S.: Surgery of the rheumatic hand, *J. Bone Joint Surg., 37A:* 759, 1955.
2. Bunnell, S., and Howard, L. D.: Additional elastic hand splints, *J. Bone Joint Surg., 32A:* 226, 1950.
3. Bunnell, S.: Active splinting of the hand, *J. Bone Joint Surg., 28:* 732, 1947.
4. Peacock, E., Jr.: Dynamic splinting for prevention of deformities and correction of hand deformities, *J. Bone Joint Surg., 34A:* 789, 1952.
5. Steindler, A.: Arthritic deformities of the wrist and fingers, *J. Bone Joint Surg., 33A:* 849, 1951.

TRAUMA

Trauma in its many varieties, and particularly that due to the increased mechanization of the modern age, accounts for a vast number of hand disabilities and deformities. Children are susceptible to many of the same types of trauma as adults, and their reaction to injury, in spite of minor variations, is practically the same. Most of the variations have to do with skin thickness, growth and healing ability of bone, and joint mobility. Some of these variations from the adult tend to be helpful in treatment, but others make the treatment more difficult. Children have surprising powers of adaptation and are able to accomodate well to the loss of a part. They are able to substitute functions and to accept their disabilities and deformities better than one might at first suppose. Sometimes it is best to defer large reconstructive procedures until the child is older. Delay may result in sufficient accommodation to the difficulty to make treatment unnecessary. It is advisable also in that young children do not cooperate well, and because their small extremities are hard to immobilize, the postoperative care is difficult and sometimes unsuccessful.

The basic principles of treatment of traumatic deformities in children are the same as those in adults; therefore, the entire field is not covered here. Certain injuries which are common in children are discussed in detail, and variations in basic treatment of other types of trauma are given.

Volkmann's Ischemic Contracture

Volkmann's ischemic contracture is one of the most serious deformities of the hand and forearm, and the most dreaded complication of injuries about the elbow and forearm, particularly in children. Steindler[33] stated that from a purely pathologic viewpoint, ischemic contracture is a fibrous reaction of the muscles of the forearm, particularly those of the flexor group. The contracture may involve the muscles in toto or in part, and cases have been reported in which muscles of the hand alone were involved. In one instance, all of the muscles, except one sublimis muscle, escaped involvement.

The fully developed ischemic contracture actually is a combination of deformities. The characteristic picture is that of pronation of the forearm, flexion of the wrist and interphalangeal joints, and hyperextension of the metacarpophalangeal joints. The hyperextension of the metacarpophalangeal joints is largely a result of passive insufficiency of the extensors and is not necessarily indicative of intrinsic loss. Although this picture is the one most frequently seen, variations of it may be encountered. Common variations are the absence of hyperextension of the metacarpophalangeal joints and a flexion contracture of the wrist similar to that seen in radial nerve palsy. The thumb is frequently involved; an adduction contracture and the inability to oppose may place it in a plane with the involved fingers.

Etiology

Since Volkmann's original description,[34] numerous investigators have tried to solve the problem of pathogenesis of this lesion, and excellent papers, from both clinical and experimental standpoints, have been written on the subject. Each of these papers conveys the impression that the investigator has proved his premise to be the correct one. Bardenheuer[1] originated the venous obstruction theory, and his work has been adequately substantiated by other authorities in the field. Brooks and his associates[3] have done some excellent experimental studies that prove quite conclusively that the lesion can be produced experimentally by complete venous obstruction. Volkmann's original arterial deficit theory has been substantiated by numerous investigators and by much experimentation.

Griffiths[11, 12] has produced an excellent work giving convincing proof that the lesion is due to arterial occlusion and muscle infarction. Others hold that the lesion is merely an unusual variety of contracture due to nerve injury. In many instances, it is undoubtedly true that there is peripheral nerve damage in addition to the contractures, but there has been no definite proof that direct injury to the nerve is the primary cause of ischemic contracture. There can be little doubt, however, that constriction lasting for a long enough period of time to close large vessels does exert pressure over the median and ulnar nerves and leads to neuritis and degeneration. Leriche and his workers attributed great significance to irritation of the sympathetic nerve supply that results in peripheral vasoconstriction.

In view of these conflicting clinical and experimental impressions, the etiology of Volkmann's contracture could be either arterial or venous obstruction. It is also not illogical to assume that in certain cases all of the previously postulated factors might well play a part.

Because of the popularity of circulatory obstruction as the etiology of Volkmann's ischemic contracture, constricting casts, bandages, and dressings have long been associated with the condition. There are cases on record, however, in which no dressing or cast was used, and yet the condition developed. In spite of this, casts or bandages can be very definite contributing causes, and for this reason, careful supervision and vigilance are essential features in the treatment of all injuries about the elbow and forearm.

Pathology

In the initial stages, the subcutaneous tissues become cyanotic and infiltrated with blood. The superficial veins engorge, and there is swelling of the extremity. Deep fascia and muscle envelopes are tight, and when cut, they tend to gap and retract markedly and to show a very pale, yellowish-gray musculature. In later stages, the muscles may become gray and may have shortened muscle fibers and evident fibrous cords. Within 48 hr after the onset, polymorphonuclear leukocytes accumulating about the fibers produce a typical inflammatory appearance. Organization of the exudate begins within 4 or 5 days and is usually well established within 10 days. Destruction of muscle fibers varies directly with the severity of the case. All gradations of involvement can occur; in mild cases almost all of the muscle fibers function normally, whereas in severe cases all of the muscle substance may be replaced by connective tissue.

Histologically, the connective tissue forms in bundles which ramify throughout the muscle bellies and replace necrotic muscle fibers. The fibrous tissue has a fibrillar aspect and forms a meshwork in which isolated areas are of viable muscle tissue.

Clinical Picture

Following the treatment of an acute injury such as a fracture or dislocation, there is usually a period of relative comfort to the patient. The earliest signs and symptoms of Volkmann's contracture usually appear within 4-6 hr, but they may develop as late as 48 hr after treatment. Cases are recorded in which the symptoms have developed as late as a week after the initial injury. Following the period of initial comfort, there is usually a sudden onset of severe pain in the arm and in the volar aspect of the forearm. The fingers become cold, cyanotic, and swollen. The pain increases in intensity and is often incompletely relieved by narcotics. Paresthesias develop, and even though the fingers may feel numb, they are often hypersensitive to touch. As the condition progresses, voluntary motion is lost, and the fingers assume a flexed position. Passive extension of the fingers causes severe pain. The radial pulse is usually absent. The pain disappears after about 48 hr, contracture of the flexor group of muscles occurs, and a clawhand subsequently develops. Clinically, the presence of coldness, swelling of the fingers, cyanosis, and absence of the radial pulse are most important early signs; however, it must be noted that pallor, rather than cyanosis, is sometimes present and is equally important. Pain in the forearm accompanied by fixed flexion of the fingers and increased pain in the forearm on passive extension of the fingers are serious signs; if preventive treatment is to be attempted with any hope of success, earlier signs must be sought.

Treatment

The treatment of Volkmann's contracture is prophylaxis. The condition is easily missed in its earliest stages, and recognition is essential if successful preventive measures are to be initiated. As a result of the injury the patient is expected to have some pain and some swelling and tenderness of the fingers. Procrastination during this important stage is an easy matter, and differentiation between normal discomfort and an impending Volkmann's contracture may be difficult. It should be remembered that, following proper therapy of injuries such as fractures and dislocations, the pain should rapidly subside. Cases of undue and prolonged pain should be watched with suspicion. All injuries about the elbow and forearm in children must be meticulously watched and preventive measures vigilantly initiated as soon as increased swelling, cyanosis, coldness, and pain appear. The time to treat Volkmann's contracture is at its very beginning. Once there has been degeneration and fibrosis with contracture of the muscle, no power can restore the muscle to normal. From then on, we must think in terms of improvement but never of cure.

Early Phase. As soon as the signs and symptoms of impending Volkmann's contracture appear, one must first remove all dressings, bandages, and splints and relieve the acute flexion of the elbow. One of the best methods of maintaining immobilization of the supracondylar fracture without acute flixion and without bandages or external splints is traction by means of a Kirschner wire in the olecranon. The use of repeated stellate ganglion blocks frequently improves circulation. Should notable improvement—evidenced by pink, warm fingers and the return of a radial pulse—appear with these measures, the case may be watched. If this happy state does not appear within 3 or 4 hr, surgical intervention is mandatory. Surgery is performed with the intent of relieving obstruction. The incision is made lengthwise over the flexor surface of the forearm, and it joggs across the antecubital space to avoid crossing the flexion crease of the elbow. The skin usually gaps as it is cut, and the deep fascia is found to be very tight as it is incised. The brachial, radial, and ulnar arteries are freed, and

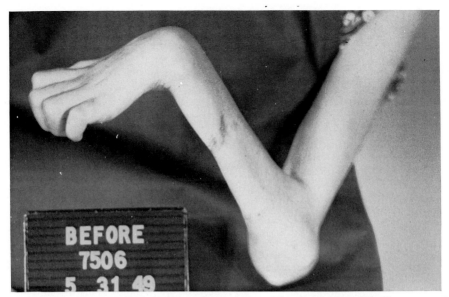

Fig. 7.85. Typical deformity seen in Volkmann's contracture. There is atrophy of the forearm, acutely flexed wrist and interphalangeal joints, and hyperextended metacarpophalangeal joints.

the muscle groups of the forearm are separated. In making incisions through the deep fascia, one must remember that the forearm consists of a series of deep fascial compartments. The release of one compartment when another is involved is not the solution to the problem. It is important to relieve the tension in each compartment. Closure is confined to the skin, and if it cannot be accomplished without tension, a split-thickness skin graft should be utilized.

Neurolysis of the ulnar and median nerves has been advocated and should be considered when primary involvement of the nerve appears to be present. At surgery, a few constricting bands or dense adhesions causing complete strangulation of the nerve may be discovered. The nerve, in this case, should be carefully freed by sharp dissection and saline neurolysis.

Late Phase. Treatment of the established contracture is as varied as the theories of pathogenesis. The reason for this is that the established contracture is not always the same. Various combinations and degrees of muscle involvement with or without nerve damage present many types of contractures. Initial treatment during this stage should be conservative. In early cases, gradual stretching according to the method of Sir Robert Jones[18] is excellent treatment. By means of a rigid splint

hinged at the wrist, first the interphalangeal joints are gradually extended, then the metacarpophalangeal joints are extended, and finally the wrist is brought into extension. The splint should be removed several times daily so that the hand may be actively and passively exercised and treated with heat and massage. Rapid or forceful correction of the deformity produces overstretching, laceration, and hemorrhage and invites recurrence. There are many other methods of gaining gradual correction of the deformity by the use of bivalve casts, semirigid splints, elastic traction splints, glove traction splints, and other pieces of apparatus. The general principle of gentle but persistent stretching of the deformity remains applicable to every method.

In cases in which there is sufficient viable muscle to provide for practical function and muscle balance of the hand, passive stretching exercises and splinting may be the only treatment necessary. In some instances, it may be found that certain structures are not stretching and are more deforming than valuable. These structures should be sacrificed. Steindler[33] states that the contracture resistance of muscle varies with the number of joints the muscle motivates. The short-fibered, uniarticular muscles of the wrist joint are very much more resistant in contracture than are the muscles of the fingers, which have a wider contractile range because of the greater length of their muscle fibers. The flexor carpi ulnaris offers the most resistance, and lengthening or even sectioning of this tendon should be performed when necessary. The same principle holds true for the flexor carpi radialis and the flexor pollicis longus.

Reconstruction

A thorough knowledge of the mechanics and function of the hand and an ability to assess the deformity with utmost care are prerequisites to attempting surgical reconstruction of the deformity caused by Volkmann's ischemic contracture. Surgical procedures must be meticulously designed to salvage as much as possible from a serious deformity. Excellent results are rarely obtained because of extensive damage to the functional mechanism of the hand. These hands have a poor appearance; however, some function which will greatly decrease the handicap of the patient can frequently be obtained. Occasionally, nothing can be done to improve function, and the surgeon must be satisfied to accept this fact and to improve the hand cosmetically if possible. The end results are innumerable, and because each case presents an entirely different problem, many operative procedures have been advocated for a single condition. A procedure which is suitable for one problem may be quite unsatisfactory for another. The general groups of procedures which are at present in common usage are: (1) sliding of the flexor muscle origin distalward; (2) lengthening of tendons; (3) shortening of static structures, including carpectomy and shortening of the radius and ulna; and (4)

Fig. 7.86. Severe Volkmann's contracture upon attempted flexion in an 8-year-old girl. Pedicle graft over the volar aspect of the lower forearm has been performed at the site of a skin slough.

Fig. 7.87. Attempted extension in patient seen in Figure 7.86. Below the elbow, only the wrist extensors, common extensors, and thumb extensors are functioning. These muscles are greatly inhibited due to the flexion contractures.

Fig. 7.88 (*A-E*). Same case as seen in Figure 7.86 after multiple tendon transfers. The figures show the function of the hand on active flexion (*A*) and extension (*B*) of fingers, opposition (*C*), writing (*D*), and grasping a glass (*E*). The procedures were the following: (1) the extensor radialis longus and brevis were transplanted to the profundus and sublimis tendons after all of the flexor tendons had been released, (2) the brachioradialis was transplanted into the flexor pollicis longus, (3) the extensor carpi ulnaris was elongated by means of grafts from the long toe extensors and was then transplanted through the intermetacarpal spaces to the lateral bands, and (4) the extensor pollicis brevis was elongated by means of the palmaris longus tendon and was rerouted around the ulna to replace the opponens function. (The last procedure gave only a fair result and is not a good procedure owing to the weakness of the extensor pollicis brevis. Function is enhanced by use of an opponens splint.)

Fig. 7.88 (E)

tendon transposition with or without carpal arthrodesis.

The first procedure releases flexion contractures of the wrist, but detachment is possible for only a short distance because of the restriction of the median nerve branches. Lengthening of the wrist flexors, combined with stretching and other operative procedures, is often helpful. Lengthening of the finger flexors is rarely of benefit. This procedure may allow the finger to be extended, but usually, when the length is increased, the active contractile power of flexion is diminished or lost in the functional range. Shortening of the long bones has decreased in popularity, and it is now thought that, if actual shortening of the static parts will aid function, carpectomy is the

Fig. 7.89. Volkmann's contracture of less severity. This patient had some function of the flexor profundus and sublimis, but these muscles were weak and had contractures. Wrist flexors were strong, but the extensors were poor.

Fig. 7.90. Same case as seen in Figure 7.89 showing extension.

procedure of choice. In well selected cases, this procedure provides good functional results and frequently improves the appearance of the hand. Tendon transplantations following a careful muscle evaluation frequently aid the functional improvement of the hand. This is especially true of the transplantation of extensors to the flexor muscles. Capsulectomies of the metacarpophalangeal joints are often indicated; but, not infrequently, the contracture is so severe that the resection of the metacarpal

Fig. 7.91. Same case as seen in Figures 7.89 and 7.90, showing flexion following mobilization by physical therapy and transfer of the flexor carpi ulnaris to the base of the third metacarpal. The result

of these procedures was a dynamic tenodesis function whereby extending the wrist with the transfer allowed the tight finger flexors to grasp more or less passively.

Fig. 7.92. Function attained in a case of moderately severe Volkmanns' contracture after carpectomy.

heads or metacarpophalangeal arthroplasty is necessary.

The end results of treating established cases of Volkmann's ischemic contracture are by no means excellent in anyone's hands. The recovery of some degree of function in these cases is often more appreciated by the patient than a brilliant correction of a mild deformity in another condition. The rehabilitation of these hands presents a great challenge and offers great possibilities is a meticulous therapeutic plan is carried out.

References

1. Bardenheuer, E.: *Deutsch. Z. Chir., 108:* 44, 1911.
2. Brooks, B.: Experimental study of Volkmann's paralysis, *Arch. Surg., 5:* 188, 1922.
3. Brooks, B. Johnson, G. S., and Kirtley, J. A., Jr.: Simultaneous vein ligation, *Surg. Gynecol. Obstet., 59:* 496, 1934.
4. Bruce, J. R.: Localized Volkmann contracture, *J. Bone Joint Surg., 22:* 738, 1940.
5. Burman, M. S., and Suturo, C. J.: Brief communications; esperimental ischemic contracture, *Ann. Surg., 100:* 559, 1934.
6. Cohen, H. H.: Adjustable volar-flexion splint for Volkmann's contracture, *J. Bone Joint Surg., 24:* 189, 1942.
7. Fleming, C. W.: Case of impending Volkmann's ischemic contracture treated by incision of deep *fascia*, Lancet, 2: 293, 1931.
8. Foisie, P. S.: Volkmann's ischemic contracture. *N. Engl. J. Med., 226:* 671, 1942.
9. Garber, J. N.: Volkmann's contracture as complication of fractures of forearm and elbow, *J. Bone Joint Surg., 21:* 154, 1939.
10. Glen, F. W.: Vascular injuries complicating supracondylar fractures of humerus in children, with case report, *Bull. Jackson Mem. Hosp., 3:* 29, 1941.
11. Griffiths, D. L.: Volkmann's ischemic contracture, *Lancet, 2:* 1339, 1938.
12. Griffiths, D. L.: Volkmann's ischemic contracture, *Br. J. Surg., 28:* 239, 1940.
13. d'Harcourt, J., and d'Harcourt, M.: A contribution to the study of Volkmann's ischemic contracture, *Madrid Med., 6:* 237, 1935.
14. Harris, C., and Riordan, D. C.: Intrinsic contracture in the hand and its surgical treatment, *J. Bone Joint Surg., 36A:* 10, 1954.
15. Horwitz, T.: Significance of venous circulation about elbow in patho-mechanics of Volkmann's contracture, *Surg. Gynecol. Obstet. 74:* 871, 1942.
16. Jepson, P. N.: Ischemic contracture, *Ann. Surg., 84:* 785, 1926.
17. Jones, E. B.: Volkmann's ischemia; observations at open operation. *Br. Med. J., 1:* 1053, 1940.
18. Jones, R.: Address on Volkmann's ischemic contracture with special reference to treatment, *Br. Med. J., 2:* 639, 1928.
19. Jones, S. G.: Volkmann's contracture, *Am. J. Surg., 43:* 325, 1939.
20. Laigle, L.: Evolution of ideas concerning Volkmann's syndrome, *Medicine, 19:* 893, 1938.
21. Massart, R.: Volkmann's disease, ischemic contraction of the flexor muscles of the fingers: pathogenesis and treatment, *Presse Med., 43:* 1695, 1935.
22. Meyerding, H. W.: Volkmann's ischemic contracture, *J. A. M. A., 94:* 394, 8, 1930.
23. Meyerding, H. W.: Volkmann's ischemic contracture, *Surg. Clin. North Am. 10:* 49, 1930.
24. Meyerding, H. W.: Fracture of elbow and Volkmann's ischemic contracture, *Minn. Med., 22:* 100, 1939.
25. Meyerding, H. W., and Krusen, F. H.: Treatment of Volkmann's ischemic contracture, *Ann. Surg., 100:* 417, 1939.
26. Middleton, D. S.: Discussion of Volkmann's ischemic contracture, *Lancet, 2:* 299, 1928.
27. Murphy, J. B.: Myositis, *J. A. M. A., 63:* 1949, 1914.
28. de Nuce: Ischemic contracture. *Rev. Orthop., 20:* 97, 1909.
29. Plewes, L. W.: Occlusion of brachial artery and Volkmann's ischemic contracture, *Br. Med. J., 1:* 1054, 1940.
30. Powers, C. A.: The ischemic paralysis and contracture of Volkmann, *J. A. M. A., 48:* 759, 1907.
31. Pusitz, M. E.: Abortive treatment of Volkmann's ischemia, *J. Kans. Med. Soc., 35:* 448, 1934.
32. Rowlands: *Lancet, 2:* 1168, 1904.
33. Steindler, A.: Ischemic contracture, *Surg. Gynecol. Obstet., 62:* 358, 1936.
34. Volkmann, Pithia, and Bilrath: *Handbuch der Chirurgie, 2:* 846, 1882.
35. White, J. W., and Stubbins, S. G.: Carpectomy for intractable flexion deformities of the wrist, *J. Bone Joint Surg., 29:* 131, 1944.

Wringer Arm

"Wringer arm" is a descriptive term applied to an upper extremity that has been caught between two rollers. The injury occurs most frequently in childhood and is usually caused by a power-driven washing machine. Hardin and Robinson[3] reported 35 cases of which 30 were children under the age of 6 years.

Pathogenesis and Pathology

The compressive force and friction produced by the rollers cause damage primarily to the skin and soft tissues of the hand, the forearm, and the elbow region. The severity of the

Fig. 7.93. Wringer injury. Besides deep slough shown here, the child has paralysis of the radial, ulnar, and median nerves.

damage depends upon the length of time the extremity has been between the rollers, the rapidity of revolution, the width of approximation, and the tension of the rollers. The prognosis is much better in the younger age groups because of the elasticity and flexibility of the bones, joints, and ligaments.

In these injuries, the hand usually enters the roller first with the fingers in the extended position. The rollers are usually elastic enough to allow the hand and the distal portion of the forearm to pass through them without great damage. As the forearm proceeds through the roller, however, tension usually builds up because of the increasing width of the upper arm and elbow, and the elbow usually bears the brunt of the avulsing action of the rollers.

Bones are rarely damaged, but muscles, tendons, and nerves may be crushed, torn, or avulsed without a break in the skin. The most common damage is that of separation of the skin from its subcutaneous attachments by the mechanical action of the moving rollers. A collection of blood and serum beneath such a full-thickness skin area delays the reestablishment of good blood supply. If this condition goes unrecognized and untreated, the overlying skin remains separated and sloughs. Venous thrombosis and lymphatic obstruction occur frequently. The arteries in the affected zone are less easily injured than the veins; they continue

to circulate blood into the damaged area and thus cause engorgement and subsequently necrosis. Occasionally, flaps of skin are completely separated and expose contused or macerated muscle. At times, tendon ends are completely stripped from their muscle attachments.

Clinical Examination

Immediate evaluation should include the determination of nerve and tendon function distal to the site of the injury and roentgenographic examination for possible bone or joint damage. In cases seen immediately after injury, the swelling and ecchymosis may be mild to moderate, and may mislead the physician who is inexperienced in treating these conditions. Occasionally, the damage may be limited to abrasion, contusion, and edema of the skin. In many instances, however, extravasation of blood and serum separate the skin as a flap from the forearm or arm, and severe sloughs occur. The extent of damage cannot always be determined early, and the prognosis should always be guarded.

Treatment

Regardless of the initial appearance of the injury, the patient should be hospitalized and observed for at least 48 hr. Conservative treatment, making use of viable skin to cover the damaged area, should be employed. Pressure dressings and elevation of the extremity minimize the edema of the damaged limb. The area should be cleansed with soap, preferably Phisoderm with hexachlorophene, and water and dressed with sterile dressings. The use of pressure dressings applied as one dresses a new skin graft often prevents separation of the skin from the underlying tissues. The dressing should be changed after 48 hr and, if a hematoma has lifted the skin, aspiration should be performed and the pressure dressing reapplied. In late cases with severe extravasation, the collection of blood should be aspirated or released by multiple small incisions, and the wound should then be dressed with pressure dressings and subsequently elevated and observed.

Definitive reconstructive surgery should be deferred until all inflammatory induration has subsided and the degree of soft-tissue destruction can be ascertained. The surface should be well covered in all cases before tendon and bone reconstruction is attempted. If the injury has produced a flap, resuture will usually be unsuccessful. Farmer[2] has successfully excised the fat and subcutaneous tissues to convert the flap into a full-thickness graft. The depth of injury limits this type of treatment, which requires a suitable underlying bed. A split-thickness graft should be used in cases of permanent loss of skin, but because this graft usually results in shrinkage, secondary coverage should be carried out. If bone, tendon, joint, or nerve is exposed, an immediate pedicle graft is imperative. Rotation or sliding flaps are usually unsuccessful because of tissue damage and circulatory impairment to the immediately surrounding tissues.

The thoracicoabdominal area is a convenient source of skin for covering these severely damaged areas according to the method of Hardin and Robinson.[3] The flaps are developed conventionally; they have a superior base and should be one-third larger than the defect to allow for shrinkage. The length should not exceed the base by more than two times. The flap is carried to the external oblique fascia and is transferred without any removal of fat. The abdominal defect may be closed by undermin-

ing, or if it is too large for undermining, coverage may be completed with a split-thickness graft. The graft is dressed with moderate pressure, and the joint is immobilized to relieve any motion or tension on the graft base. Detachment and revision is carried out in approximately 3 weeks. If tendon repairs or grafts are necessary, all joints should be thoroughly mobilized possively prior to surgery. The skin should be well healed and induration should have subsided before definitive work is attempted; otherwise summation of scarring is likely.

References

1. Dupertius, S. M.: An evaluation of skin grafts for hand coverage, *J. Bone Joint Surg., 34A:* 811, 1952.
2. Farmer, A. W.: Treatment of avulsed skin flaps, *Ann. Surg., 110:* 951, 1939.
3. Hardin, C. A., and Robinson, D. W.: Coverage problems in treatment of wringer injuries, *J. Bone Joint Surg., 36A:* 392, 1954.
4. MacCollum, D. W.: Wringer arm, a report of twenty-six cases, *N. Engl. J. Med., 218:* 549, 1938.
5. MacCollum, D. W., Bernhard, W. F., and Banner, R. L.: The treatment of wringer arm injuries, *N. Engl. J. Med., 247:* 750, 1952.
6. Posch, J. L., and Weller, C. N.: Mangle and severe wringer injuries of the hand in children, *J. Bone Joint Surg., 36A:* 57, 1954.

Lacerations of Hand and Fingers

Damaged tendons may occur as a result of lacerations, burns, crushing injuries, friction wounds, or combinations of traumata such as those seen in wringer or mangle injuries, which are discussed above. Most lacerations are of the fingers and are due to grasping sharp cutting surfaces. The treatment of these wounds in children varies in no way from the treatment in adults. Boyes[4] has grafted tendons in 2-year-old children with excellent results. The tendons grow in length and continue to function well with growth. Because of the smallness of the parts, the difficulty of immobilization, and the poor cooperation of the very young, it is thought best to wait until the child is at least two years of age before performing tendon grafts. Joints should be kept mobile by passive exercise until surgery can be performed. No tendon surgery should be done until good skin coverage has been attained and all scars have

Fig. 7.94. Attempted flexion after severance of the flexor sublimis and profundus in an 11-year-old boy.

Fig. 7.95. Same case as seen in Figure 7.94. Range of flexion after removal of the sublimis and profundus tendons and graft of the palmaris longus to the profundus in the palm. The graft was extended to the base of the distal phalanx.

been released. The bony parts should be intact, and all joints of the involved digits should be passively mobilized before tendon surgery.

If the profundus tendon has been cut distal to the sublimis attachment, the distal end of the cut profundus can be advanced to a bony attachment at the base of the distal phalanx. The distal piece of the cut tendon is then

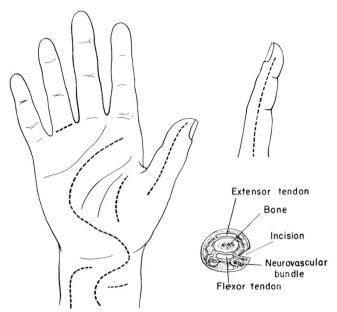

Fig. 7.96. Incisions useful in hand operations.

Fig. 7.97. Severed profundus tendon in the right little finger between the proximal and middle creases of the finger. One slip of the sublimis had also been severed, and there was deep scarring and destruction of this pulley.

removed. The suture is made by means of a stainless steel, pullout wire suture attached into the bone at the base of the distal phalanx. The tendon soon accommodates to its new length, and a satisfactory functional result is obtained. If one or both tendons are cut in the area on the volar surface between the sublimis insertion and the distal palmar crease, both tendons should be removed. A graft should be placed from the profundus tendon in the palm out through the finger to a bony attachment into the proximal end of the distal phalanx. This is done according to the method of Bunnell, 12-14 with No. 34 stainless steel wire sutures. If pulleys have been destroyed, they are replaced by means of tendons wrapped about the phalanges or metacarpal necks and passing subcutaenously on the dorsal surface outside the extensor apparatus. The suture line in the pulley should be fixed in an area not in contact with the tendon graft. The hands are immobilized routinely in plaster splints to relieve

Fig. 7.98. Same case as seen in Figure 7.97, showing flexion and extension after a tendon graft. The sublimis and profundus tendons were removed. The palmaris longus was grafted from the profundus in the palm through the finger to the base of the distal phalanx. The proximal pulley was reconstructed from a part of the removed sublimis tendon.

Fig. 7.99. Same case as seen in Figures 7.97 and 7.98, showing the definite function of the profundus and its strength after the profundus graft.

tension on the graft for a period of 3 weeks. Following removal of the cast, active exercises and physical therapy are begun. If a tendon seems to be tied down, a tendolysis may be necessary, but such a procedure should not be premature in a child, inasmuch as adhesions, if they occur, often stretch out after several months of active and passive exercises. In the majority of instances, the tendon begins to function well within the first weeks after removal of the casts or splints.

Lacerations occurring the flexor aspects of the fingers are best treated by débridement, cleansing, and skin suture; the graft should be an elective procedure and should be deferred to a later time. In lacerations involving the

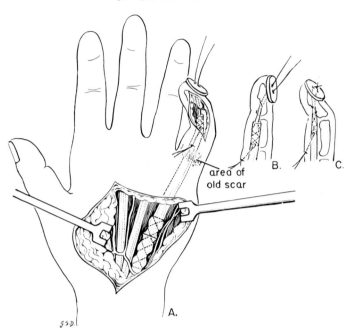

Fig. 7.100. Free tendon graft after removal of profundus and sublimis and attachment of graft to distal phalanx according to the Bunnel technique.

extensor aspects of the hand and fingers, the extensor tendons should be sutured primarily.

Children are not infrequently seen with deformities of the hand and fingers that are due to unrecognized lacerations of the peripheral nerves higher in the arm or forearm. Many of these lacerations have been treated as simple, small cuts, without due recognition of the nerve damage. Fixed contractures that have occurred should be corrected if the injuries are seen late, and the nerves should then be explored just as in the adult patient, the ends being sutured carefully with No. 6-0 silk on an atraumatic needle. If this procedure is carefully performed, a great number of these children regain full function. Satisfactory results may be expected as late as 2 years after the injury for return of motor function and even later for the return of sensation. Digital nerves damaged in the hand and fingers should be sutured, according to a meticulous technique, with No. 6-0 silk on an atraumatic needle at the time of débridement.

If motor function does not return, any of various reconstructive transplants can be performed with good results. In the case of a radial nerve loss, good results are usually obtained by transplanting the wrist flexors into the finger and thumb extensors. The most common procedure is to move the flexor ulnaris into the common extensors, the palmaris longus into the abductor and extensor brevis of the thumb, and the flexor carpi radialis into the extensor pollicis longus. There are other methods of utilizing these same muscles just as effectively, but their use depends upon individual variations.

In ulnar and median paralyses, the main loss is that of intrinsics, and the consequent loss of finger extension and thumb opposition is quite disabling. The many different kinds of transplants that may be used to restore these functions will not be enumerated. Deformities can be overcome completely or partially by appropriate tendon transfers and arthrodeses designed to restore muscle balance and to bring the thumb and fingers to functional positions. Often there is a dearth of transferable tendons, so that only the most important intrinsic function can be restored. In children, it is best to avoid arthrodeses if possible. Irwin's dynamic tenodesis may give adequate function by utilizing a few tendons and retaining joint motions. Occasionally, injury makes it necessary to sacrifice digits or a portion of the hand.

Fig. 7.101. Application of Bunnel technique (Fig. 7.100), showing function of hand following transplantation of flexor carpi radialis to extensor pollicis brevis and abductor pollicis longus, palmaris longus to extensor pollicis longus, and flexor carpi lunaris to common finger extensors.

Fig. 7.102. Radial nerve palsy due to trauma.

Fig. 7.103. Ulnar nerve palsy due to laceration over the flexor surface of the ulnar side of the elbow. This palsy is only 5 months old, and the wound is well healed. No finger contractures are present. The nerve should be explored and sutured at this time.

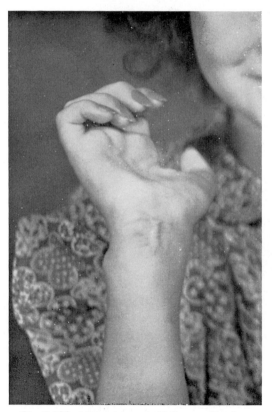

Fig. 7.104. Attempt to extend fingers after laceration at the ulnar surface of the wrist. The ulnar nerve was severed at that level, and the intrinsic function was consequently lost.

Such a loss is always disabling; however, the axiom that the thumb should be preserved or restored at all costs should always be kept in mind by the surgeon.

Sometimes parts of fingers or entire fingers must be sacrificed. The loss of a finger is disabling, but not nearly as disabling as the loss of a thumb. In instances of loss of the terminal part of the thumb, the simple procedure of deepening the web space by a Z-plasty may greatly improve the function. Sometimes when both phalanges are lost and the first metacarpal, along with its musculature, is retained, certain procedures may increase the length and usefulness of the thumb. Lewin[21] has described an advancement procedure that uses a bone graft into the metacarpal and a skin graft onto a nonopposing surface, lifts the intact skin up over the bone graft, and inlays the skin below the surface. This procedure may add to the length and give sensation on the opposing surface to serve greatly for the previous loss. Littler,[22] who has gone even further, uses almost the same principle, except that when the thumb is retained and all of the fingers, including the metacarpals, have been lost, he elevates the skin flap and inserts a bone graft from the ilium underneath it, opposes normal skin from hand, with its sensation, against the thumb, and then fills the part that is not to be opposed with a skin flap from the abdomen. This procedure improves the function of the hand by providing an effective post for the intact thumb to work against; this post had good sensation in the part that opposes the thumb.

A tube pedicle may be constructed and a bone equal to the length of the missing thumb may be moved into the pedicle and grafted into the first metacarpal. The motor function of such a reconstructed part is usually excellent

Fig. 7.105. Same case as seen in Figure 7.104, showing the result 2 years after ulnar nerve suture. The patient has completely recovered intrinsic function and sensation in the hand.

Fig. 7.106. Loss of hand except for the thumb due to trauma. This patient would benefit greatly by Littler's procedure, which gives a post for the thumb to work against.

Fig. 7.107. Loss of phalanges of the thumb and of the index and middle fingers due to trauma.

Fig. 7.108. Same hand as seen in Figure 7.107 after bone grafting of the second metacarpal into the first metacarpal through a pedicle graft, release of the pedicle, and closure. Good functional and cosmetic improvement.

but because its sensation is poor, its usefulness is inadequate. This inadequacy may now be circumvented, however, by transferring skin from a less valuable finger, such as the little or ring finger. The skin is taken from the flexor surface at the tip and, with its neurovascular bundle, is transferred according to the method of Littler to the opposing end of the thumb. This addition should make for much better functional results, but great care is necessary in performing this type of surgery.

References

1. Abbott, L. C., Saunders, J. B., and Bost, F. C.: Arthrodesis of the wrist with the use of grafts of cancellous bone, *J. Bone Joint Surg., 24:* 883, 1942.
2. Boyd, H. B., and Stone, M. M.: Resection of the distal end of the ulna, *J. Bone Joint Surg., 26:* 313, 1944.
3. Boyes, J. H.: Repair of motor branch of the ulnar nerve in the palm, *J. Bone Joint Surg., 37A:* 920, 1955.
4. Boyes, J. H.: Flexor tendon grafts in fingers and thumb, *J. Bone Joint Surg., 32A:* 489, 1950.
5. Bruner, J. M.: Problems of postoperative position and motion in surgery of the hand, *J. Bone Joint Surg., 35A:* 355, 1953.
6. Bunnell, S.: Active splinting of the hand, *J. Bone Joint Surg., 28:* 732, 1946.
7. Bunnell, S.: Digit transfer by neurovascular pedicle, *J. Bone Joint Surg., 34:* 772, 1952.
8. Bunnell, S.: Physiological reconstruction of the thumb after total loss, *Surg. Gynecol. Obstet., 52:* 245, 1931.
9. Bunnell, S.: Primary and secondary repair of flexor tendons of hand, *Plast. Reconstructr. Surg., 12:* 65 1953.
10. Bunnell, S.: Repair of tendons in the fingers and description of two new instruments, *Surg. Gynecol. Obstet., 26:* 103, 1918.
11. Bunnell, S.: Surgery of the intrinsic muscles of the hand other than those producing opposition of the thumb, *J. Bone Joint Surg., 24:* 1, 1942.
12. Bunnell, S.: Suturing tendons, *Instruct. Lect. Am. Acad. Orthop. Surge.,* Lect. 1-5, 1943.
13. Bunnell, S.: Treatment of tendons of the hand, *J. Bone Joint Surg., 23:* 240 1941.
14. Bunnell, S.: *Surgery of the Hand,* Philadelphia: J. B. Lippincott Co., 1944.
15. Dial, D.: Reconstruction of the thumb after traumatic amputation, *J. Bone Joint Surg., 21:* 98: 1939.
16. Dunlop, J.: The use of the index finger for the thumb: some interesting points in hand surgery, *J. Bone Joint Surg., 5:* 99, 1923.
17. Goldner, J. L.: Deformities of hand incidental to pathological changes of the extensor and intrinsic muscle mechanisms, *J. Bone Joint Surg., 35A:* 115, 1953.
18. Graham, W. C.: Flexor tendon grafts to the fingers and thumb, *J. Bone Joint Surg., 29,* 553, 1947.
19. Joyce, J. L.: Results of new operation for

substitution of the thumb, *Brit. J. Surg., 16:* 362, 1929.

20. Koch, S. L., and Kanavel, A. B.: Purposeful splinting following injuries of the hand, *Surg., Gynecol. Obstet., 68:* 1, 1939.

21. Lewin, M.: Partial reconstruction of the thumb in a one stage operation, *J. Bone Joint Surg., 35A:* 573, 1953.

22. Littler, J. W.: Architectural principles of reconstructive hand surgery, *Surg. Clin. North Am., 31:* 463, 1951.

23. Littler, J. W.: Free tendon grafts in secondary flexor tendon repair *Am. J. Surg., 74:* 315, 1947.

24. Littler, J. W.: Tendon transfers and arthrodeses in combined median and ulnar nerve paralysis, *J. Bone Joint Surg., 31A:* 225, 1949.

25. Littler, J. W.: The neurovascular pedicle method of digital transposition for reconstruction of the thumb, *Plast. Reconstructr. Surg., 12:* 303, 1953.

26. Littler, J. W.: Transfer of free skin graft with neurovascular pedicle presented at the American Society of Surgery of the Hand, 1956.

27. Riordan, D. C.: Tendon transplantation in median nerve and ulnar nerve paralysis, *J. Bone Joint Surg., 35A:* 312, 1953.

28. Siler, V. E.: Primary tenorrhaphy of the flexor tendons in the hand, *J. Bone Joint Surg., 32A:* 218, 1950.

Burns

Burns involving the hands are unfortunately common injuries in children. Involvement of other parts of the body, which is very frequent, greatly complicates the overall treatment program. The burn usually involves only the skin and spares the tendons, bones, and joints; however, if it is treated improperly in the early stages, secondary involvement of these structures may cause severe crippling disability of the hand. The deformity produced may take almost any form and is often quite grotesque. The most common deformity is that of flexion of the wrist and hyperextension of the metacarpophalangeal joints combined with flexion of the interphalangeal joints or with flexion of the proximal interphalangeal joints and extension of the distal joints. This type of deformity tends to be most frequent since pain and muscle spasm cause overpull of the wrist flexors and stretching of the common extensors. This causes a hyperextension of the proximal finger joints, which often results in lateral slipping of the lateral bands to produce severe finger deformities. These burns are sometimes severe enough to cause loss of major deep structures, particularly of ligaments and tendons. Occasionally, fingers or parts of fingers or practically

Fig. 7.109. Burn healed by granulating in without any skin coverage. There is a severe cicatrix contracture.

the entire hand is lost. If the wounds are allowed to become septic or if there is an accumulation of necrosis after poor débridement, joints and tendons become fixed rapidly and often permanently. Because the skin of children and infants is relatively thin, deeper involvement may occur initially than would have been the case in an adult with a similar burn. Fortuantely, the joints of a child do not stiffen quite as rapidly as those of an adult. On the other hand, children do not tolerate burns in general very well during the initial phases.

Treatment

The systemic treatment of burns in children does not differ from the therapy indicated in adults. The general care of toxemia, shock, and sepsis, all of which are of great importance, will not be discussed here. An attempt will be made to outline and cover only the more important aspects of the local care of the hand. It is essential that all efforts should be made to allay pain, prevent sepsis, débride early, and cover as soon as possible with skin grafts. Splinting in the postion of function is extremely important to prevention of deformity.

Early. Methods of early treatment are con-

Fig. 7.110. Same case as seen in Figure 7.109, after excision of scar and replacement by full-thickness skin graft from the abdomen.

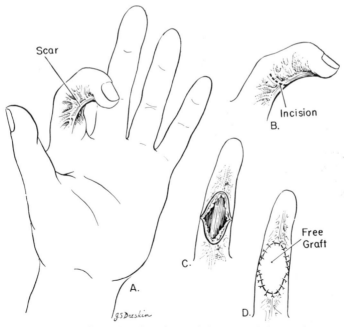

Fig. 7.111. Procedure for release of cicatrix with free graft.

Fig. 7.112. Longitudinal cicatrization after burn. The contracture may be released by a Z-plastic procedure with an excellent result.

troversial, but the majority of authorities are of the opinion that open surgical drainage is the treatment of choice. Hand burns seen in the first 12 hr, or even those seen after sepsis has occurred should be treated in the following manner with the general idea of gaining skin coverage as soon as possible. This goal can be attained by early débridement, daily cleansing, and use of wet dressings. As soon as the general condition permits, the entire hand should be cleansed gently and thoroughly by means of large gauze sponges with hexachlorophene and Phisoderm in water. The blisters should be opened and necrotized, and charred tissue should be removed. This procedure should be exacting and meticulous. Several layers of fine mesh gauze should be wrapped around the part. Each finger should be dressed separately and placed in the position of function. The wrist should be dorsiflexed, the fingers in semi-flexion, and the thumb slightly flexed and in opposition. Sterile mechanic's waste may then be applied to hold these positions, and the entire bulky dressing should be kept wet with normal saline solution. Metal or plastic splints may also be included, if they are necessary, but usually the bulky mechanic's waste dressing holds the position satisfactorily. The dressings are changed under water, and the patient is encouraged to move his fingers actively as much as possible. Necrotic tissue in trimmed away as it is encountered. Most burned hands can be prepared in this manner for split-thickness

coverage within 2-4 weeks. In most instances involving the dorsal aspect of the hand and fingers, split-thickness skin will serve permanently. On the palmar aspect of the hand and fingers, the split graft is used only for temporary coverage. It is later replaced with full-thickness skin grafts.

Late. Unfortunately, many burned hands are seen only after severe scarring and contractures have occurred. No burn wound should be allowed to "granulate and heal in." Every burn should be covered as soon as possible.

When scarring of the dorsal surface of the fingers occurs, the scar can be dissected completely free, and the fingers flexed and immobilized on an aluminum splint. The area can be covered with a split-thickness skin graft. The aluminum splint can be prepared and cut to the proper shape prior to surgery and then sterilized and molded into the position desired in the operating room. Pressure dressings are applied over the graft, and the entire part is dressed with bulky pressure dressings that incorporate the splint. The dressings are changed in about 10 days, and immobilization is continued for approximately 1 month; then mobilization is begun by means of physical therapy in the form of active exercises and whirlpool treatment. The splint is used on a part-time basis until the end of the 6th week. Scars involving the palm should be removed, and the hand should be splinted with the fingers in extension after a full-thickness graft has been applied. The graft is obtained from an area on the abdomen containing as little hair as possible.

The graft is outlined according to a pattern, and the dissection, which is carried out with the graft under tension, follows a plane in the fine white fibers that attach the skin to the subcutaneous tissue. No fat is removed with the skin. The graft is cut slightly larger than the wound to allow for shrinkage. It is sutured accurately into the bed, which should be perfectly dry in order to prevent formation of

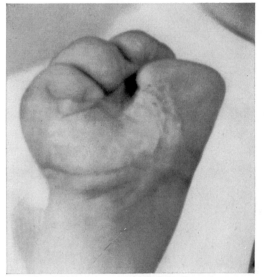

Fig. 7.113. Severe scarring following a burn.

Fig. 7.114. Same case as seen in Figure 7.113, after freeing of scar and application of a full-thickness graft to release the thumb alone and the fingers en masse from the palm.

Fig. 7.115. Same case as seen in Figures 7.113 and 7.114, after the webs between the fingers had been released as in syndactylism.

Fig. 7.116. (*Left*) Flexor cicatrix due to an old burn. (*Right*) After release of scar and coverage by diamond inlay of free, full-thickness skin from the abdomen.

Fig. 7.117. The result of poor early handling of a burn. There was no splinting. Healing has occurred by granulating in, which has produced heavy cicatrization and inexcusable deformity due to contracture.

Fig. 7.118. Soon after burn due to friction. This child grasped a belt of a rapidly rotating motor.

hematomas. A central holding stitch or two is often used to prevent slippage.

The donor site can usually be closed by excising the subcutaneous fat undermining the defect and closing. If the defect is very large, a split-thickness graft may be needed to cover it without tension. In most instances, it is necessary to immobilize the elbow in flexion and to attach the part of the cast that covers the elbow to the splint to keep it from slipping. Longitudinal scares involving the flexor surfaces of the finger and web spaces are not uncommon in burns of the hand. They may be released by Z-plasty or multiple Z-plasties or by cutting the longitudinal scar transversely to allow the finger to extend and then inserting a diamond-shaped full-thickness graft. The release of tension by

Fig. 7.119. Free full-thickness grafts used in the palm to replace cicatrices.

Fig. 7.120. Severe burn of hand and wrists mainly on the dorsal surfaces with fixed hypertension contractures of the metacarpophalangeal joints, flexion contracture of the proximal interphalangeal joints, and hyperextension of most of the distal interphalangeal joints.

Fig. 7.121. Same case as seen in Figure 7.120. Active splinting is used to help relieve some of the contractures.

Fig. 7.122. Same case as seen in Figures 7.120 and 7.121, after removal of the dorsal scar of the wrist, hand, and fingers to the proximal interphalangeal joints and coverage with split-thickness grafts. Release of the distal extensors of the lateral bands may improve the fingers by releasing the extension contracture of the distal joint and the flexion of the proximal interphalangeal joint, which have occurred through buttonholing of the lateral hands.

these methods results in the gradual disappearance of the scar and the contracture.

Dry fields are essential. Immobilization as described above is mandatory. When final coverage for hands and fingers has been secured and mobilization has been attained, fixed deformities due to tendon, bone, or joint damage may remain. If the middle extensor slip of the extensor apparatus scars down, the lateral bands slip laterally, causing flexion of the middle joint and extension of the distal joints. The middle slip should be freed and the lateral bands sectioned. This procedure allows the distal phalanx to flex into the mallet finger position but allows for better function in the proximal and middle joints. In severe cases the joint surfaces may be extensively damaged and the tendons and ligaments scarred beyond repair. Arthrodesis in a functional position may be the treatment of choice. Occasionally, an amputation may be most desirable. The decision depends upon the individual case. If flexor tendons have been lost, they may be replaced by grafting as in other traumatic flexor tendon injuries (see "Lacerations of Hand and Fingers"). Frequently the results are rather discouraging because of other involvement, such as joint tightness and trauma to the capsule, caused by the burn itself. Tendon grafts should not be undertaken until good skin coverage has been secured in the area of transplantation. It is also imperative that a

Fig. 7.123. (*Left*) Flexion contractures in volar skin of all fingers. (*Right*) After a diamond-shaped, free, full-thickness graft.

Fig. 7.124. Flexion contracture of the ring and middle finger is due to a burn. The skin only was involved on the ring finger. The tendons and the proximal interphalangeal joint were scarred in the middle finger. Both fingers were released and covered with a free, full-thickness skin graft. Later, the middle finger was covered by a pedicle flap from the abdomen, and a free tendon graft was inserted. The tendon used was the palmaris longus tendon from the profundus tendon in the palm, and it was attached to bone at the base of the distal phalanx.

Fig. 7.125. Same case as seen in Figure 7.124. Result 4 years after treatment. (In an adult, amputation of the middle finger would have been the procedure of choice.)

Fig. 7.126. Result after release of a severe cicatrix in the palm due to burns. There is still flexion tightness of the skin in the fingers. The fingers will be released and the defect filled by a free, full-thickness graft, just as in the palm.

Fig. 7.127. (*Left*) Severe burn with contracture of the middle finger and loss of the ring and little fingers in a girl of 7 years. (*Right*) Release of the scar and removal of the fourth and fifth rays; some of the skin from the fillet was used to cover the scarred areas.

Fig. 7.128. Severe deformity of the hand due to cicatrix of the skin involving mainly the dorsal aspect.

Fig. 7.129. Same case as seen in Figure 7.128 after release of scar and application of free, full-thickness grafts from the abdomen.

Fig. 7.130. Severe burn with loss of all fingers. The first metacarpal remained, and its intrinsic muscle attachment is intact.

range of passive motion of maximal function be attained in the involved joint before the tendon work is started. In many instances, only partial restoration is possible; however, because of the serious disability which occurs as a result of severe burns to the hand, reconstruction should always be attempted in order to gain at least some functional, and possibly cosmetic, improvement.

References

1. Barsky, A. J.: Surgical repair of unusual dermatological conditions, *Surg. Clin. North Am., 19:* 459, 1939.
2. Blair, V. P., and Brown, J. B.: Use and uses of large split grafts of intermediate thickness, *Surg. Gynecol. Obstet., 49:* 82, 1929.
3. Brown, J. B.: Surface defects of the hand, *Am. J. Surg., 46:* 690, 1939.
4. Brown, J. B., and McDowell, F.: Persistence of function of thin grafts through long periods of growth, *Surg. Gynecol. Obstet., 72:* 848, 1941.
5. Brown, J. B., and McDowell, F.: *Skin Grafting of Burns,* Philadelphia: J. B. Lippincott Co., 1943.
6. Bunnell, S.: Contractures of the hand from infection and injuries, *J. Bone Joint Surg., 14:* 27, 1932.
7. Bunnell, S., and Howard, L. D.: Additional elastic hand splints, *J. Bone Joint Surg., 32A:* 226, 1950.
8. Cohen, H. H.: An adjustable volar flexion splint, *J. Bone Joint Surg., 24:* 189, 1942.
9. Conway, H.: Whole thickness grafts in correction of contractures due to burn scar, *Ann. Surg., 109:* 286, 1939.
10. Davis, J. S.: Use of small deep grafts in repair of surface defects, *Am. J. Surg., 47:* 280, 1940.
11. Dupertius, S. M.: An evaluation of skin grafts for hand coverage, *J. Bone Joint Surg., 34A:* 811, 1952.
12. Gillies, H.: Experience with tubed pedicle flaps, *Surg. Gynecol. Obstet., 60:* 291, 1935.
13. Goldner, J. L.: Deformities of the hand incidental to pathological changes of the extensor and

Fig. 7.131. Same hand as seen in Figure 7.130, after a Z-plastic procedure and deepening of the web between the first and second metacarpals. The function of the hand is now much improved.

intrinsic muscle mechanism, *J. Bone Joint Surg.*, *35A:* 115, 1952.

14. Harris, C., and Riordan, D. C.: Intrinsic contracture of the hand and its surgical treatment, *J. Bone Joint Surg., 36A:* 10, 1954.
15. Hovens, F. Z.: Preoperative and postoperative care in skin grafting, *Surg. Clin. North Am., 20:* 1087, 1940.
16. Howard, L. D., Jr.: Contracture of the thumb web, *J. Bone Joint Surg., 32A:* 267, 1950.
17. Jones, R., Jr.: Management of old contractures of upper extremity resulting from third degree burns, *South. Med. J., 4:* 789, 1941.
18. Koch, S. L.: Complicated contractures of the hand, *Ann. Surg., 98:* 546, 1933.
19. Koch, S L., and Kanavel, A. B.: Purposeful splinting following injuries of the hand, *Surg. Gynecol. Obstet., 68:* 1939.
20. Mason, M. L.: Plastic surgery of hands, *Surg. Clin. North Am., 19:* 227, 1939.
21. Padgett, E. C.: Free full thickness skin graft in correction of soft tissue deformities, *J. A. M. A., 98:* 18, 1932.
22. Padgett, E. C.: Skin grafting in severe burns, *Am. J. Surg., 43:* 626, 1939.
23. Padgett, E. C.: Skin grafting and three-quarter thickness skin graft for prevention and correction of cicatricial formation, *Ann. Surg., 113:* 1034, 1941.
24. Padgett, E. C.: *Skin Grafting,* Springfield, Ill.: Charles C Thomas, 1942.
25. Sheehan, J. E.: Use of free full thickness skin grafts, *J. A. M. A., 112:* 27, 1939.
26. Tanzer, R. C.: Prevention of postoperative hematoma in surgery of the hand: use of compression suture, *J. Bone Joint Surg., 34A:* 797, 1952.

BRACHIAL PALSY—BIRTH TYPE

A paralysis due to injury of the roots of the brachial plexus at birth became a more common clinical entity as fetal and maternal mortality associated with difficult deliveries was reduced. Still further refinement of obstetric technique has reduced the incidence in recent times.

Smellie mentioned this complication of delivery in 1764. The mechanism of the paralysis was described by Duchenne in 1872 and by Erb in 1874. The predominant upper arm lesion bears their names. Klumpke described the lower arm type in 1885.

Etiology

Fixation of the shoulder or head followed by traction and lateral flexion of the neck by means of either the trunk, an arm, or the head, acting as a lever, has been thought to be the mechanism of injury.

Pathology

In 36 of 54 patients reviewed by Wickstrom[8] and others, the involvement centered about the fifth and sixth cervical roots. In these cases of principally upper arm involvement, damage was most commonly minimal. It was represented at the root by edema and mild intraneural hemorrhage and by some tearing of fibers although the root remained intact. Recovery sometimes occurred in only a few days, but more commonly complete return was evidenced in 3-6 months.

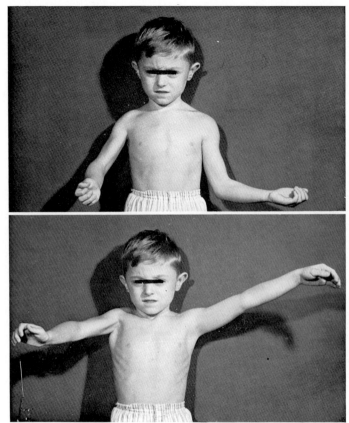

Fig. 7.132. (*Top*) Limited external rotation due to contracture in brachial palsy. (*Bottom*) Limitation of abduction and elevation despite good deltoid power following birth type of brachial palsy.

There were 14 patients in whom all roots were involved and 4 in whom paralysis was evidenced as involving primarily the eighth cervical and first thoracic roots.

In these there was disruption of the nerve fibers, including avulsion of the roots from the spinal cord, at multiple points. Complete laceration of the roots, multiple neuromata, and gross lesions of the cord have been observed on exploration.

There were three cases of Horner's syndrome and four of sensory as well as motor loss in Wickstrom's series.

Clinical Picture

Early

Although no signs may be noted other than the loss of the Moro reflex when the infant is startled, more frequently the stricken limb is observed to remain lifeless at the side with the elbow extended. In some infants, a traumatic neuritis persists, and the infant cries when the arm is moved. Pronation of the forearm and wrist, placing the limb in the attitude of receiving a "hidden tip," is a typical finding. There may be swelling in the supraclavicular fossa due to hemorrhage or inflammation. Occasionally a fractured clavicle or humerus is seen in concert with the paralysis. Signs consistent with Horner's syndrome may be found if the thoracic root has been injured.

The upper arm, or Erbe-Duchenne, type of paralysis is most frequent; it is at least four times as common as other types. Here, damage to the fifth and sixth cervical roots result in paralysis of the deltoid supraspinatus, infraspinatus biceps, coraco brachialis, and supinator brevis.

In Klumpke's type, which involves the lower arm and the eighth cervical and first thoracic nerve roots, there is loss of the intrinsic muscalature of the hand, the flexors of the wrist, and the long flexors of the fingers. Along with involvement of the sympathetic fibers, there is dropped eyelid (ptosis), narrowing of the palpebral fissure, and constriction of the pupil on the involved side.

Sensation is ordinarily intact.

In Sever's series, [6] the right side was involved in 64% of cases. In 63 of the 1,100 cases analyzed by Sever, the involvement was bilateral.

The paralysis characteristically leads to internal rotation at the shoulder, pronation of the forearm, and flexion of the wrist.

Late

The signs of this injury in the older child are those of residual deformity. The most marked imbalance of musculature involves the shoulder, in which the internal rotators are strong and the external rotators are paralyzed.

The internal rotation contracture causes the child to hold the elbow away from the side in partial abduction in order to clear the arm from the trunk. The resulting deformity enables one to diagnose this condition on the street. Humeral scapular rhythm is lost, and there is limited abduction, most of which is really scapular elevation.

The humerus is frequently shortened out of all proportion to the muscular atrophy. The acromion may be hooked downward and elongated on x-ray examination. Posterior subluxation or dislocation of the humeral head may occasionally be present.

Pronation or supination deformities, depending on the kind of muscle imbalance, may be present in the forearm.

Fig. 7.133. Involvement of the whole arm in brachial palsy. There are forearm, hand, and wrist contractures.

Fig. 7.134. Involvement of the upper arm in brachial palsy. Note shortening, tendency to hold elbow away from trunk because of internal rotation contracture, flexed elbow but good hand.

The most common muscle weakness by far is that of the deltoid, biceps, and external rotators at the shoulder. However, it is not unusual on examining a late case to find that the muscle power is good but inhibited from maximal function by contracture.

Treatment

Treatment cannot be based on the use of a position to prevent deformity 24 hr a day. Such therapy results in contracture in abduction and internal rotation. Periodic change into the corrective position is the guiding principle of treatment. Neurologic exploration and repair of the injury have not been justified, the proximal nature of the lesion and the lack of suitable nerve sheath in young infants being major handicaps.

The arm may be pinned in abduction and external rotation by means of a diaper while the infant is recumbent. This position should be maintained for periods of 2-3 hr only, and there should be alternate periods during which the arm is free. In addition, at each diaper change the arm is passively abducted, the elbow flexed, the forearm supinated, and the wrist dorsiflexed so that a full range of motion of all joints, including those of the fingers, is gently carried out.

More efficient corrective immobilization is carried out by a so-called "Statue of Liberty" splint, which maintains abduction and external rotation and in addition controls the forearm and hand in a manner that mere splinting cannot equal. The splint is not worn continuously. It is alternated with periods during which the arm is entirely free and with periods of active and passive exercise. The splint is usually needed for the first 6 months intermittently through day and night and perhaps for an additional 6 months at night only. The child must be followed frequently enough so that the earliest opportunity to reestablish scapulohumeral rhythm through active use of the area is not missed. About one-half of the upper arm paralyses respond to this regime with satisfactory shoulder function, but function is completely normal in only 10%.

In late deformity the splint does not solve the clinical problem.

The usual problem in late cases is to increase the range of external rotation and abduction. If there is no bony deformity, this may be accomplished in part by tenotomy of the subcapularis and pectoralis major muscles, as described by Sever. If active external rotation power is not present, it may be established by the muscle transplant described by L'Episcopo.[4] In this procedure, the teres major and often the latissimus dorsi are removed from their insertions and sutured under an osteoperiosteal flap on the posterior aspect of the humerus at the same level. They are thereby converted from internal to external rotators. Abduction as well is frequently improved by this procedure.

In the presence of functioning musculature, but fixed contracture, osteotomy of the humerus above the insertion of the deltoid and rotation of the distal fragment externally inside the periosteum may be indicated.

Improvement in appearance as well as in function can be expected from a correctly done operation that has been carefully selected for the particular case.

References

1. Clark, L. P., Taylor, A. S., and Prout, T.: A study of brachial birth Palsy, *Am. J. Med. Sci., 130:* 670, 1905.
2. Fairbank, H. A. T.: Birth palsy: subluxation of the shoulder joint in infants and young children, *Lancet, 1:* 1217, 1913.
3. L'Episcopo, J. B.: Tendon transplantation in obstetrical paralysis, *Am. J. Surg., 25:* 122, 1934.
4. L'Episcopo, J. B.: Restoration of muscle balance in the treatment of obstetrical paralysis, *New York J. Med., 39:* 357, 1939.
5. Sever, J. W.: Obstetrics paralysis; its etiology, pathology, clinical aspects and treatment with a report of four hundred and seventy cases, *Am. J. Dis. Child., 12:* 541, 1916.
6. Sever, J. W.: The results of a new operation for obstetrical paralysis, *Am. J. Orthop. Surg., 16:* 248, 1918.
7. Taylor, E. S.: Brachial birth palsy and injuries of similar type in adults, *Surg. Gynecol. Obstet., 30:* 494, 1920.
8. Wickstrom, J., Haslam, E. T., and Hutchison, R.: The surgical management of residual deformities of the shoulder following birth injuries of the brachial plexus, *J. Bone Joint Surg., 37A:* 27, 1955.

CHAPTER 8

Defective Formation of Bone

Chondrodysplasia and chondrodystrophy are terms which are often used loosely without exact definition. In this chapter they are interpreted as follows: *chondrodysplasia* is defective formation of bone from cartilage resulting in relatively permanent defects in the bone structure; *chondrodystrophy* is defective formation of bone from cartilage altering the size or contour of the bone but not resulting in permanent defects in the bone structure.

These definitions exclude transformation in formed bone—osteitis fibrosa of parathyroidism, benign giant cell tumor, and benign aneurysmal bone cyst—and complete or partial absence of cartilage—hemivertebra, incomplete segmentation of vertebrae (congenital fusion), and cleidocranial dysostosis. Also excluded are effects on formed bone and on growth rate of affections of tissues about bone, as osteopsathyrosis, myelomuscular disturbances, and neurofibromatosis, and conditions resulting from stress developed by resistance of soft tissues to elongation by the growing bones, as in developmental or "congenital" coxa vara, developmental genu valgum, and developmental genu varum (Blount's disease, the Blount-Barber syndrome, or osteochondrosis deformans tibiae).

CHONDRODYSTROPHIES

Chondrodystrophia Fetalis (Achondroplastic Dwarfism)

Chondrodystrophia fetalis (achondroplastic dwarfism) begins in fetal life and is often demonstrably familial. Diminished production of growth cartilage and relatively prompt conversion of cartilage to bone cause the growth discs to be grossly and roentgenographically thin. The tubular bones are short, and often somewhat distorted, but adequately wide. The face is flat and the nose small and saddle-shaped, but the vault of the skull is voluminous. The trunk is long relative to the short extremities; this is an obvious difference from Morquio's disease, in which the trunk is short. There is no effective treatment for the systemic condition. Orthopaedic treatment is rarely necessary but, if osteotomy is contemplated for correction of deformity, union of bone fragments follows the pattern for normal bones.

Morquio's disease is a systemic disease in which chondrodystrophy is a feature. It is mentioned here to point out that the dystrophy affects chiefly the formation of bone from vertebral and articular cartilage. Because metaphyseal bone formation is less disturbed, the limbs are relatively long and the trunk relatively short. In spite of these characteristics, an exact pattern of roentgenographic bone changes is not to be expected because the degree of chondrodystrophic change varies greatly from case to case and the dysfunctioning cartilage may also produce permanent defects in bone structure (chondrodysplasia), usually central type defects, in the epiphyses and metaphyses.

Local Chondrodystrophies

Chondrodystrophy may occur locally in a restricted area or in a single bone. Some examples follow.

In developmental dorsolumbar round back, a vertebra near the dorsolumbar junction, usually the twelfth dorsal or first lumbar, may be deficient in development at its anterior superior quadrant and its anterior surface. This deficiency may occur as an incidental feature in a systemic chondrodystrophy such as Morquio's disease, but it is not infrequent as an isolated lesion. In the latter case, deformity begins in infancy or shortly thereafter with development of rounded dorsolumbar kyphos greater than the normal postural dorsolumbar round back of infancy. The deficiency of the vertebra is clearly evident and characteristic in the lateral

Fig. 8.1. Short and broad bones with abnormal outline in chondrodystrophy.

Fig. 8.2. Hip joints such as these in chondro-dystrophic patient may later become the site of degenerative arthritis. The tendency to appear as a femoral head duplication is evident.

roentgenogram. Two adjacent vertebrae may be affected. The deformity tends to progress for a few years and then to decrease and improve. Reversion toward normal development may be aided by encouraging the prone and restricting the erect posture. When deformity is great, recumbency in a posterior plaster shell or other apparatus maintaining moderate extension relative to the kyphos should be used to assure earlier and adequate recovery from the developmental deficiency.

Developmental valgus (or varus) of a phalanx is characterized by moderate shortness of the phalanx and angulation of its distal articular plane transversely relative to its proximal articular plane. The middle phalanx of a finger is the usual site of the deformity, but other phalanges, and more than one phalanx, may be

Fig. 8.3. Forearm and hand with deformity, broadening of distal radius, and shortened metacarpals.

rapidity and converted to bone at a relatively normal rate, to result in abnormally long bones and roentgenographically normal growth discs, and that, in cretinism, the production of cartilage and its conversion to bone are equally slowed so that the bones maintain a normal roentgenographic appearance but take an abnormally long time to reach a given stage of development. These chondrodystrophic features of the diseases cause no noteworthy orthopaedic problems.

Premature union of an epiphysis may cause shortness of one or more metacarpal or metatarsal bones in pseudohypoparathyroidism, clubfoot, spina bifida, and paralysis of the lower extremity occurring before the fourth birthday. This condition is a form of local chondrodystrophy secondary to abnormality of adjacent soft tissues. In some instances it may be an inherited trait. The shortness is seldom recognized before the eighth birthday. The adjacent phalanx may also be affected. Treatment to correct the shortness is not necessary. Partial premature union of an epiphysis following destruction of cartilage by injury or inflammation is not chondrodystrophy.

affected. The condition is often demonstrably familial and gene-controlled. In at least one family it is regarded as evidence of relationship. It may be detectable at birth but usually is not recognized until bone development is well advanced. The deformity does not reverse itself in the later stages of growth, but the writer has not yet seen a case in which any treatment seemed advisable.

Delayed conversion of cartilage to bone is a descriptive phrase applicable to those rare cases in which the rate of formation of cartilage is normal but its conversion to bone is delayed. The result is an unusual depth of the growth disc; the writer has seen, for example, cases in which the apophyseal disc of each ulna measured 1 inch in the axial diameter. The condition has been observed only as a local chondrodystrophy, and the cases are too few to demonstrate familial occurrence. Because no symptoms or deformities develop, the anomaly is disclosed only incidentally by roentgenogram. No treatment is necessary.

It should be noted here that, in pituitary gigantism, cartilage is produced with increased

CHONDRODYSPLASIAS

The important factors in the production of permanent defects of bone structure by defective conversion of cartilage to bone during growth are as follows.

1. One or more of the many possible predisposing factors or exciting causes of such defective formation of bone must have been present. Among these are:
   a. Normal probability that not all cell divisions will have a normal result.
   b. Increased probability of conversion defects when cartilage is older, when it grows more rapidly, or when it approaches completion of ossification. These factors make conversion defects rarer in infancy and more common in adolescence; some are not fully developed until after the pediatric age period. These factors also do much to account for the facts that conversion defects are most common at the distal metaphysis of the femur, which is the most rapidly growing metaphysis, that

Fig. 8.4. The hand in chondrodystrophy. Note irregularity in metaphyseal area adjacent to the epiphyseal line and short, broad phalanges.

epiphyseal bone formed more slowly from articular cartilage is less subject to defects, and that the portion of a long bone formed from fetal cartilage, which is young and which grows little after it begins its conversion to bone, is seldom the site of conversion defects.

c. Tension at the attachment of fibrous tissue to cartilage resulting from growth of the bone, especially rapid growth.

d. Hemorrhage or faulty development of vascular buds at the area of conversion of cartilage to bone.

e. Either hemorrhage or blebs adjacent to the conversion area.

f. Localized injury of the conversion area.

g. Familial tendencies or gene-controlled factors affecting development, as in multiple enchondromas of the hands or in diaphyseal aclasia.

h. Endocrine disturbances affecting development as in cretinism, parathyroidism, polyglandular dystrophy, or Albright's disease.

i. Affections of neighboring tissues which alter the nutrition of bone and cartilage, as in Morquio's disease, gargoylism, and generalized neurofibromatosis.

j. Any other condition which disturbs the nutrition or functioning of cartilage or adjacent bone.

2. Material which is not bone is formed at the affected area. The material may be calcareous without bone structure, or it may be cartilage or fibrous tissue. Fibrous tissue may contain giant cells or cystic

Fig. 8.5. Achondroplastic dwarf with extremities that are short relative to the trunk.

areas; it may form one large cyst. The defect may contain a mixture of the materials mentioned. For most types of defect, there is no constant relation between the predisposing or causative factor and the character of the material in the defect.

3. The defective material is left behind in situ as the bone grows in length. The axial length of the defect is thus determined by the time during which defective conversion of cartilage to bone continues and the rate of growth in that time. A defect which still extends to the cartilage at the time of examination is a continuous defect, whereas one which has become separated from the cartilage by reversion to normal bone formation is an intermittent defect.

4. The defective material is not altered by the normal remodeling process in the shaft of a long bone, nor is it subject to Wolff's law. The extent to which the defect interferes with these processes depends chiefly upon whether the defect occupies or approaches the periphery of the bone and, to a lesser degree, upon the breadth and length of the defect and the number of defects.

5. The defective material does not tend to exhibit autonomous growth. A cyst may accumulate more fluid and become larger and more rounded with resorption of adjacent bone. A sufficiently broad defect may increase slightly in breadth owing to compression in the axial diameter by soft tissues that resist elongation by the growing bone. A cartilaginous defect may retain some of its physiologic capacity to produce cartilage and bone and may express that capacity if it is stimulated by repeated motion or trauma. These are not autonomous growths. Conversion defects practically never exhibit autonomous tumorous growth except in the few cases which develop secondary malignancy or the rare cases which develop large osteochondromata.

6. Since conversion defects are often symptomless, they may attract notice only incidentally by roentgenographic examination late in life, but they are formed during the growth period and are detectable in increasing frequency up to the end of adolescence.

7. The great number of differences in appearance and character of conversion defects which may result from different combinations of the factors that have been mentioned is further augmented by variation in the number and distribution of the defects and by combinations of different defects. The possibilities seem infinite.

A few of these defects which are seen sufficiently often to appear to represent types are discussed below. They are classified as peripheral, submarginal, or central defects at articular, metaphyseal, or fetal cartilage.

Peripheral Conversion Defects

Single Peripheral Metaphyseal Chondrodysplasia

In single peripheral metaphyseal chondrodysplasia (exostosis, osteoma, osteochondroma), a portion of cartilage derived from the epiphyseal disc becomes separated at the periosteal attachment. The separated portion remains in situ in the periosteum, and its radial distance from the center of the bone remains constant as it is left behind by growth at the metaphysis. If the separation begins sufficiently early in life, the eventual site of the cartilage defect may be several inches from the metaphysis. The defect preserves the underlying bone while adjacent bone is remodeled, so that it soon appears as though there were a

Fig. 8.6. Upper extremities in chondrodystrophia fetalis (achondroplastic dwarf). Note that the trunk is relatively unaffected.

Fig. 8.7. Chondrodystrophia multiplex congenita with multiple ossification centers in the epiphyses.

Fig. 8.8. The spine in chondrodystrophy with increased anteroposterior diameter of the vertebrae and bony deformity.

projection of bone with cartilage at its crest. The projection is directed away from the near metaphysis because resorption on the far surface of the exostosis is accelerated owing to traction on the periosteum created by metaphyseal growth. The projection has the usual pencil type appearance in cases in which the defect became intermittent shortly after it began, but a broader table type projection is developed when the duration of formation of the defect was longer. The radial projection of the exostosis may be increased slightly by physiologic activity of the cartilage cap, which produces some cartilage and bone. In cases in which such activity causes the mass to be bulbous, it may be called an osteoma if it is practically entirely bony, an osteochondroma if bone and cartilage are obviously present. These distinctions and the diagnosis are usually made roentgenographically.

No autonomous tumorous growth has been mentioned in the preceding description. Usually there is none. Occasionally, the radial projection of the mass beyond its metaphyseal site is great enough to justify the suspicion that some autonomous growth has occurred, and in rare instances an osteochondromatous mass

several inches in diameter may eventually develop.

These defects are innocuous and require no treatment except that a mass in an exposed position, where it is subject to repeated irritation or traumatism from external sources or by movement of tissues over it, may be removed by surgical excision at its base for the purpose of relieving discomfort or annoyance and as prophylaxis against secondary malignancy, which eventually occurs with some frequency in such irritated lesions. This treatment is definitely advisable when an exostosis on a rib is subject to friction by an adjacent rib in breathing.

Multiple Peripheral Metaphyseal Chondrodysplasia (Diaphyseal Aclasia)

Multiple peripheral metaphyseal chondrodysplasia (diaphyseal aclasia, multiple cartilaginous exostoses, hereditary deforming chondrodysplasia, Ehrenfried's disease) is a roughly symmetric, bilateral production of metaphyseal exostoses. The long bones and ribs are principally involved, but other bones may also be affected. Each exostosis develops and may be treated as described above for single exostosis. The condition is demonstrably familial, and it affects male more often than female patients. Central metaphyseal defects of various types may be detectable in some cases.

Selected cases exhibit various degrees of relative prominence of peripheral, as opposed to central, defects and of bilateral, as opposed to unilateral, distribution. They make it impossible to define exactly the limits of diaphyseal aclasia as compared to Ollier's disease.

Unilateral Multiple Peripheral and Central Metaphyseal Chondrodysplasia (Ollier's Disease)

Unilateral multiple peripheral and central metaphyseal chondrodysplasia (unilateral dyschondroplasia, Ollier's disease) is characterized by extensive unilateral involvement of metaphyses by an assortment of narrow and broad central and submarginal continuous defects (see below); the defects are mostly cartilaginous, but some are fibrous, and sometimes they are peripheral. In the older portion of the affected area, which is formed before the metaphysis becomes completely involved, axial striae representing thin lines of relatively normal ossification between defective areas may be seen. The long bones of the lower extremity and the ilium are most commonly affected. Occasionally both sides of the body are affected, and cases intermediate between Ollier's disease and diaphyseal aclasia are encountered. Cartilage in defects within the bone may undergo nodular calcification as life advances, and in Ollier's disease this calcification may begin to appear early, even in childhood, and may falsely suggest a relationship to some form of calcinosis. When the metaphysis is completely involved throughout its breadth, the defective tissues are unable to overcome completely the resistance of soft tissues to elongation by the growing bone, and growth in length becomes deficient. This axial compression results in some lateral bulging of the defective tissue at the metaphysis; the epiphyseal disc develops over the bulged tissue, and the metaphysis thus becomes abnormally wide. The same process may result in angular deformity when involvement is less complete toward one aspect of the metaphysis. The defective formation of bone cannot be controlled. Correction of angular deformity by osteotomy may be expected to result in normal union of bone fragments. Shortness of one leg may be compensated for partially by stapling at epiphyseal disc in the opposite leg at an appropriate time, or later a bone in the opposite leg may be shortened surgically by removal of a section.

Peripheral Epiphyseal Chondrodysplasia

Pheripheral epiphyseal chondrodysplasia produces separation of a cartilaginous conversion defect from articular cartilage at the site of attachment of fibrous tissue near the epiphyseal disc, and the plaque of cartilage becomes increasingly separated from its area of origin by growth of both epiphyses at the joint until its

Fig. 8.9. The single exostosis–cartilage capped, remodeled at the base. The lesion and the bone supporting it are not remodeled, a characteristic of chondrodysplasia.

Fig. 8.10. Traumatic chondrodysplasia—linear defect in the bone laid down from the epiphyseal line arose at the site of insertion of a Kirschner wire.

position is nearly opposite the center of articulation. Motion at the joint producing friction and stress at the cartilage defect stimulate its physiologic capacity to grow, and a mass 1 or 2 cm in diameter may result. Such cartilage is slow to ossify, but it eventually does ossify centrally and cartilage usually persists at its surface.

The intermittent peripheral epiphyseal defect (sesamoidoma, benign bone-forming tumor) thus forms a cartilaginous or bony mass in fibrous tissue at a joint and suggests an unusual sesamoid bone. The mass is rarely recognized before it ossifies. As many as four or five such masses may be present at a joint, most commonly at the knee or ankle. The condition is innocuous and may be ignored unless mechanical interference with motion makes surgical removal advisable.

The continuous peripheral epiphyseal defect maintains continuity of cartilage between the defect and the epiphysis as the defect gradually becomes more displaced by growth of the two epiphyses. The asymmetric condylar mass thus formed distorts the joint in angular deformity, which increases as the mass increases. Because of such deformity, the patient is apt to be seen early, before the cartilage at the defect ossifies. Roentgenogram then suggests the presence of a space-occupying mass in the peripheral portion of the joint with corresponding angulation at the joint and underdevelopment of the adjacent aspects of the epiphyses to conform to the mass. No reactive phenomena are visible in adjacent bone or soft tissues. The knee is most commonly affected. When the patient is seen in this stage, osteotomy through the shaft of the bone for correction of the angular deformity is

Fig. 8.11. Failure to remodel in defective formation of bone from cartilage. Note persistent boxlike metaphysis on left compared with remodeled metaphysis on right.

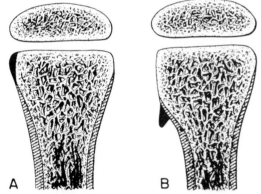

Fig. 8.12. Diagram of the formation of exostosis, which, with its cartilage cap, is not subjected to remodeling as is the uninvolved bone around it.

not advisable because it does not restore normal conformation at the joint or prevent further development of deformity. On the other hand, surgical treatment by paring off the adventitious cartilage sufficiently to approach normal conformation at the joint is feasible, and it has proved satisfactory in the 2 cases thus treated under the writer's observation; the joint remained stable, deformity did not increase appreciably, and there was no stimulation of tumorous growth of the remaining cartilage. Later in life, when physiologic ossification has developed in the cartilage mass, treatment is less satisfactory. At that time, reshaping the distorted epiphysis is not feasible because a

cartilaginous surface cannot be maintained, and the condition may not justify such radical procedures as insertion of an internal prosthesis or fusion in corrected alignment; restoration of alignment by osteotomy through the shaft of one of the bones is, therefore, the only treatment commonly justifiable, and it leaves a distorted joint operating in an abnormal plane. Obviously, it is important to recognize and treat these patients early, when the best results may be obtained.

Submarginal Conversion Defects

Submarginal metaphyseal chondrodysplasia is defective formation of bone from cartilage situated within the bone but sufficiently near the periphery to be brought to the surface eventually as the defect is left behing by the growing metaphysis and the remodeling process causes the bone to become narrower. The defect may be recognized early, when it is still entirely within the bone at the metaphyseal area, or late, when it is entirely at the surface of the remodeled narrow portion of the shaft, but it is most characteristic in the intermediate stage, when it is partly within the bone and partly at the surface and the perforation of the cortex is parallel to the long axis of the bone but oblique to the flared portion of the cortex, which it perforates. Submarginal defects may be broad enough to involve the peripheral or

Fig. 8.13. Patient with multiple cartilaginous exostoses involving the metaphyseal areas of the long bones.

The writer has not yet seen a case in which there was histologic or roentgenographic evidence that the lesion was the site of autonomous tumor growth or a case in which continued observation without surgical inter-

Fig. 8.14. Multiple cartilaginous exostoses with short ulna and fibula and bowing of the radius.

Fig. 8.15. Multiple cartilaginous exostoses with short ulna and fibula and bowing of the radius.

central areas, or they may be accompanied by other defects in those areas. A thin line of cortex visible roentgenographically may be preserved over the defect by inhibition of remodeling, and a thin calcareous wall may be formed about the defect by processes of accommodation in the adjacent bone structure. The diameter of the defect varies with the breadth of the defective formation at different times during the period of continuity so that the sides of the defect may appear wavy or even scalloped.

Benign Nonosteogenic Fibroma

Benign nonosteogenic fibroma is typically submarginal metaphyseal chondrodysplasia.

ference demonstrated increase in size of the lesion except by continued formation of defective material at the metaphysis. The material at the defect is spindle cell fibrous tissue; giant cells and foam cells may be present. The condition is innocuous, is usually discovered incidentally by roentgenogram, and requires no treatment although biopsy and more extensive surgery are often done. If symptoms are present, they can safely be assumed to be due to some other condition, such as injury at the neighboring joint.

Calcareous submarginal chondrodysplasia is present when the contents of a submarginal defect are calcareous. The calcific material does not have trabeculated or cortical bone structure, and it appears amorphous in the roentgenogram, in which it is readily visible because of its great density. Such defects of moderate length are frequently observable in adolescence and later, especially in bones of the feet and in the fibula. They may widen the cortical area peripherally or narrow the medullary canal endosteally, or both, depending upon their breadth and situation relative to the radius of the bone and the remodeled area of the bone. They are innocuous and symptomless, and they require no treatment.

Melorrheostosis

Melorrheostosis is calcareous submarginal chondrodysplasia that has developed in the metaphyseal and fetal areas along one aspect of a bone or succession of bones in a limb and that tends to correspond with a somatic segment. It has been identified in childhood but usually does not attract attention until later, when pain appears, motion becomes limited, and calcification may develop in soft tissues about the joints. The periosteum tends to adhere to the calcific mass, and pain is probably the result of stress exerted by tissues attaching to the periosteum. The pain is relieved by rest. No other treatment is necessary. Prognosis is good in that the condition is self-limited and symptoms do not become marked.

Cartilaginous submarginal (and central) chondrodysplasia is characterized by the presence of cartilage throughout most or all of the defect. This character of the material is often not identifiable until the tissue is examined, but it is suggested roentgenographically when the

Fig. 8.16. Ollier's dyschondroplasia with unilateral deformity.

defect is eccentrically situated in the bone, irregularly rounded, and not elongated axially, and it is indicated in the adult when characteristic nodular calcification has developed in the cartilage of the defect. These defects are innocuous and symptomless unless they are in exposed situations where contusion or periosteal stress can excite physiologic activity of the cartilage.

A small cartilaginous defect situated centrally in the medullary tissue where it does not deprive the bone of an appreciable amount of trabeculation is not detectable in the child but

Fig. 8.17. Ollier's disease: unilateral chondrodysplasia. Note defects in structure of bone that is laid down.

Fig. 8.18. Roentgenogram of upper extremity in unilateral chondrodysplasia with involvement of long bones and metacarpals.

Fig. 8.19. Epiphyseal osteochondroma involving medial condyle of the femur.

becomes recognizable in the adult, usually after age 30, when nodular calcification occurs within it.

A cartilaginous defect in the submarginal area brought to the surface of the cortex beneath the periosteum by the remodeling process may be too small to be detectable but may exhibit physiologic activity of the cartilage and formation of subperiosteal chondroma in adolescence or later.

A small cartilaginous conversion defect in fetal cartilage or early in metaphyseal growth is the probable source of the rare benign myxoma of bone of infancy.

The broad central cartilaginous defect (benign central chondroma) may be encountered in childhood but usually does not attract attention until later. A bone of the hands, feet, or ribs is commonly affected. The lesion is usually eccentric, and the thin cortical line at its surface may undulate instead of presenting a smooth fusiform outline. Its treatment is the same as that for other broad central defects (q.v.), and it may not be distinguished from them until tissue is examined.

Multiple Enchondromas

Multiple enchondromas of the hands constitute submarginal and central chondrodysplasia, which is apparently gene controlled. The feet may also be affected. The defects are mostly submarginal and cartilaginous, but tiny peripheral exostoses may be seen and some central fibrous or cystic defects may appear on tissue examination. The conversion defects are visible roentgenographically early in life (some may form from fetal cartilage), and they continue to

Fig. 8.20. Submarginal metaphyseal chondrodysplasia (benign nonosteogenic fibroma) in the proximal femur bilaterally.

Fig. 8.21. Fibrous tissue removed at biopsy from area of submarginal metaphyseal chondrodysplasia.

form or to be added to throughout most of the period of metaphyseal growth of the bones of the hands. Physiologic activity of the cartilage persists, probably because of the more or less constant use of the hands, and the cartilage masses tend to enlarge and may become quite big in relation to the size of the bones of origin. Individual masses which interfere with function or become tender owing to repeated pressures may be removed surgically, and the resulting cavity in the bone, if any, may be filled with bone chips. Incomplete removal of a particular mass should be avoided if possible.

Central Conversion Defects

Central chondrodysplasia develops conversion defects in the area of the bone which is not brought to the surface by the remodeling process. The defects may be single or multiple, broad or narrow, long or short, calcareous, noncalcareous, or mixed. When the breadth of the bone occupied by a defect or by a number of defects is sufficient, the operation of Wolff's law preserves enough bone about the defect to meet stresses normally applied to it and thus inhibits remodeling and presents the appearance of "expansion" of the cortex. The cortex over such an area seen roentgenographically is thin and smoothly fusiform in shape except that rigid material (cartilage or calcareous material) in the defect may cause the outline to be wavy. Such "expansion" is the hallmark of the large central defect.

Pyle's disease presents roentgenographic evidence of "expansion" toward the ends of the long bones (dumbbell bones) owing to multiple noncalcareous defects which are individually too small to be visible. A similar condition may affect a single metaphyseal area symmetrically or eccentrically. The condition is symptomless and innocuous, and it requires no treatment.

Single, broad, central noncalcareous defects in metaphyseal chondrodysplasia (osteitis fibrosa circumscripta, bone cyst, central chondroma) present roentgenographically a conspicuous area of deficient bone structure usually oval in shape but with a transverse limit toward the epiphyseal cartilage if they are continuous or only recently intermittent. "Expansion" of the cortex is present to the degree necessitated by the size and position of the lesion. The position of the lesion in the long axis of the bone depends upon the length of the bone at the time the lesion began to form. It takes more than a year of defective bone formation to form a sizable lesion, and years may pass before the lesion attracts attention. The condition is therefore rarely encountered before the age of 4, and its frequency increases thereafter. The material in the defect is not positively identifiable before tissue examination, but the roentgenogram suggests cartilage when the lesion is eccentric or its outline undulant and fibrous tissue if the lesion is well separated from the metaphysis and symmetric—the cyst tends to fracture before much separation from the metaphysis is achieved.

Broad central defects may be of mixed type and may contain some structureless calcareous material. They may also present a great variety of bizarre appearances on roentgenographic examination.

A variation of the broad central defect occurs in cases in which the defect becomes intermittent shortly after its onset. This kind of development produces only a thin plane of defective material, which is left behind by the growing metaphysis. The thin defect is not visible roentgenographically until remodeling narrows the cortex to the diameter of the defect, and then a thin transverse break in the continuity of the cortex is visible. Transverse fracture occurs spontaneously at such a defect, and if the defect does not extend completely across the bone, it may be completed by trivial injury. The writer believes that this type of defect is the commonest cause of "spontaneous" fracture precisely in the transverse plane in childhood and early adolescence.

Broad, central calcareous defects in metaphyseal chondrodysplasia (marble bones, osteopetrosis) exhibit roentgenographically a transverse dense area of structureless calcareous material toward the ends of the shafts. When the axial extent of the defects is not great, the condition is symptomless and requires no treatment. When the condition begins early in life (Albers-Schönberg disease), the abnormal bone formation is generalized and may involve bone derived from fetal as well as from metaphyseal cartilage. Little room remains for medullary tissue, and anemia and activity of accessory hematopoietic organs develop. Blindness and deafness may result from faulty development of the skull. Predisposition to the disease is probably due to a gene-controlled Mendelian recessive character. Blood chemistry and bone chemistry are essentially normal. Patients exhibiting the condition in infancy usually die young, but those with later onset and sufficient medullary tissue in the bones have a good prognosis. The bones are subject to fracture, which may be treated as similar fractures in normal bone. No other treatment is useful except medical supportive treatment to combat anemia.

Multiple, small, central calcareous conversion defects of chondrodysplasia (osteopoikilosis) are usually systemically distributed in the epiphyses and, toward the end of the growth period, in the metaphyses. The defects are irregularly rounded and rarely over five millimeters in diameter. They are symptomless and

Fig. 8.22. The forearm and hand in Pyle's disease.

require no treatment. The prognosis is excellent although the defects are permanent.

Single, small, central calcareous conversion defects form single dense nodules, visible roentgenographically, which have often been described as bone whorls and as osteosclerosis. The calcaneus, talus, and proximal femur are common sites. The lesions are innocuous and should be ignored.

Small, noncalcareous, central metaphyseal conversion defects, which have been mentioned in association with other defects (Ollier's disease, Pyle's disease, etc.), may not deprive the bone of enough structure to be visible individually in the roentgenogram. They may be visible individually, however, if adjacent bone forms a calcareous limiting wall about them. Such a defect is indicated when a small circular area of deficient bone structure is outlined roentgenographically by a thin circular calcareous wall and there is no reaction in adjacent tissue. The defect is common in the

femoral neck. It requires no treatment but should be observed over a period of time, rather than subjected to immediate biopsy, in order to confirm its innocuous character.

Defective bone formation may occur along the surface of epiphyses in Morquio's disease and in association with chondrodystrophy, spina bifida, and other conditions, but articular cartilage does not form noncalcareous defects (visible within the epiphysis) as often as does metaphyseal cartilage. Because it grows more slowly, the epiphysis is less subject to defective formation, and for the same reason, the defect must continue for a longer time in order to achieve a size which is recognizable unless it is outlined by a calcareous ring as described above. Other single noncalcareous epiphyseal defects, if visible, are apt to occupy a considerable portion of the epiphysis and to produce a bizarre effect. Lack of symptoms, lack of reaction in adjacent tissues, and a tendency of the sides of the defect to be straight and parallel to the direction of growth identify the defect in the roentgenogram. No treatment is necessary.

The vertebrae are subject to noncalcareous conversion defects at their upper and lower surfaces (commonly called Schmorl's nodes). They may be detected by roentgenogram in midchildhood as an early defect producing a shallow indentation of the ossified surface of the vertebra. If such a defect is followed through the growth period, it will be observed to increase in depth exactly as bone is added to

Fig. 8.23. Central chondrodysplasia calcified in the adult. (From A. B. Ferguson, Jr.: Calcified medullary defects in bone, *Journal of Bone & Joint Surgery, 29:* 598 1947.)

the vertebral surface by growth, the sides of the defect remaining perpendicular and the base parallel to the surface until late adolescence or later, when the defect may become somewhat rounded by adjustment of adjacent bone to it. One or more such defects can be found in most spines in adolescence and later. They are ordinarily symptomless and can be ignored, but occasionally the developmental disturbance affects the cartilage more extensively and the underdeveloped disc may be thin owing to deficiency of cartilage and nucleus pulposus. In the lumbar area, where normal motion is considerable, such a lesion may produce local ache following activity because of the poor mechanical action of the joint.

GARGOYLISM

Gargoylism (Hurler-Pfaundler syndrome, dysostosis multiplex, lipochondrodystrophy) is a disease of uncertain etiology which is sometimes familial. It begins to become apparent in the first year of life, or soon thereafter, when there is evidence of mental retardation, infantilism, and dwarfism. The skin becomes coarse and thick, and the corneas may be cloudy. Potbelly, hepatomegaly, and splenomegaly develop. Hydrocephalus is frequent. The neck is usually short, dorsolumbar round back is present, and mobility of the joints is

Fig. 8.24. Calcified cartilage matrix removed from specimen taken from patient shown in Figure 8.23. (From A. B. Ferguson, Jr.: Calcified medullary defects in bone, *Journal of Bone & Joint Surgery, 29:* 598, 1947.)

Fig. 8.25. Transverse defects laid down in the metaphyseal area adjacent to the epiphyseal line.

Fig. 8.26. Transverse "stress" type fracture in the tibia.

impaired, especially in the spine and hands. Lipoid deposits are found in some cases (but not in all) in the liver, spleen, lymph nodes, cornea, brain, and pituitary gland, and the sella turcica is enlarged. The central portion of the long bones, especially in the hands, tends to be bulbous; roentgenographically this suggests disturbance of accretion and resorption in formed bone rather than defective formation of bone cartilage. In the presence of such widespread disease, chondrodystrophic changes appear relatively minor and incidental. They are of the type seen roentgenographically in Morquio's disease but are less marked. They consist of developmental dorsolumbar round back, shortness of long bones, distorted metaphyses, and underdeveloped epiphyses. The changes in the long bones are most evident in the distal portion of the upper extremity. There is no effective treatment for the condition, and no orthopaedic treatment is advisable except the use of an extension frame or similar apparatus for inhibition or improvement of the round back.

ACHONDROGENESIS

Achondrogenesis is a lethal variety of short-limbed dwarfism that may be mistaken for neonatal achondroplasia. Most are stillborn or die shortly after birth due to respiratory insufficiency. Crown-rump length may be only mildly reduced, but limb shortening is severe. The femur may be little more than an inch in length.

The roentgenographic findings include a normal skull, retarded rib development, absent sternal ossification, severely retarded cervicothoracic spine ossification with retarded to absent ossification of the lumbosacral spine (in contrast to congenital absence of the lumbosacral spine, cartilage precursors are present), increased interpedicular distances, and marked retardation of long bone formation with metaphyseal flaring (Fig. 8.29A).

Of most significance are the alterations in

Fig. 8.27. Developing Schmorl's node, a form of chondrodysplasia. (See Fig. 8.28 for the progressive development of the lesion with growth.)

Fig. 8.28. Same patient as shown in Figure 8.27, 2 years later. Note that the edges are straight and the bottom flat and that the node has increased in depth and become well marked in the vertebra. A similar defect is beginning in the vertebra just above.

normal epiphyseal/endochondral bone formation. The integrity of the articular cartilage is lost. There is extensive periosteal erosion of the peripheral chondroepiphysis. There is excessive vascularization of the chondroepiphysis with loss of normal cartilage canal patterns. In the growth plate there are focal areas of more orderly patterns of ossification juxtaposed to much larger sections of immature and disorganized growth plate (Fig. 8.29B).

This disorder is probably an inherited biochemical abnormality affecting matrix production or elaboration (one report described a twin pregnancy, one normal child and one with achondrogenesis). It is interesting that thiourea-induced hypothyroidism and thallium adminis-

tration in chick embryos produce a similar histologic picture (Fig. 8.29C). It is postulated that thyroxin normally maintains chondroepiphyseal integrity by controlling the rate of erosion and resorption of cartilage and playing a role in synthesis or deposition of acid-mucopolysaccharide-protein complexes into the matrix.

BY JOHN OGDEN, M.D.

HUMERUS VARUS

Humerus varus is an infrequent deformity that may be found in association with hypothyroidism, mucopolysaccharidosis, rickets, and

Fig. 8.29 (*a*). Roentgenogram of still-born with achondrogenesis. Note normal skull and clavicle development, but severe retardation of the axial skeleton and significant shortening and metaphyseal flaring of the appendicular skeleton.

osteomyelitis. It is being recognized more frequently in children with thalassemia. However, the majority of cases probably occur as a result of birth trauma (usually breech delivery, with the involved arm caught over the head) or a shoulder injury in a very young child.

The major clinical problem is shortening of the arm. The forearm and hand are usually normal. Unfortunately, the length discrepancy is often not appreciated until early adolescence, when a significant deformity is already present. The difficulty of recognition until early adolescence makes close follow-up in the young, birth injured child imperative. The average shortening is 7 cm. Abduction is generally restricted, but other glenohumeral motions are usually retained.

The diagnosis is characteristic by roentgenographic examination (Fig. 8.30). The head is in marked varus and is usually flattened. The greater tuberosity may be higher than the articular portion of the humeral head. The epiphysis is parallel to the longitudinal axis of the humerus, rather than transverse or oblique. Premature fusion may occur. The medial (inferior) portion of the growth plate has a sclerotic region of bone bridging epiphysis and metaphysis. The medial cortex of the metaphysis appears to have a large defect.

Fig. 8.29 (*b*). Transverse section of distal femur with achondrogenesis. Ossification is proceeding relatively normally, but the structures of the growth plate and chondroepiphysis are severely disrupted. (*c*) Thiourea-treated proximal tibial from a chick showing increased vascular invasion of the epiphysis.

Fig. 8.30. Anteroposterior roentgenogram of the left shoulder in a 12-year-old boy with humerus varus complicating a fracture during birth. Note particularly the proximal/medial direction of the greater tuberosity (*) and the apparent metaphyseal defect(**). The growth plate above this "defect" is crossed by a bony bridge.

The mechanism of injury in most cases is damage to the medial side of the growth plate, severely limiting its capacity for normal longitudinal growth, while the lateral portion continues to grow at a relatively normal rate. Trueta produced a similar deformity in rabbits by damaging the perichondrium. As the humeral head is progressively tilted into varus, sections of the articular cartilage begin to appose metaphyseal bone. Articular cartilage, during much of longitudinal bone development, is not capable of ossification and thus will present a block to a significant bony bridge between epiphysis and metaphysis. The "defect" in Figure 8.30 is thus filled with articular cartilage "overgrown" by the widening metaphysis. With closure of the growth plate, the articular cartilage undergoes biochemical changes that allow closure of the "defect."

Treatment should be offered only to the symptomatic individual. Epiphyseodesis will lessen the risk of fracture of the long metaphyseal fragment. Realignment osteotomy may improve motion, but only at the expense of some degree of further shortening of the arm. Most cases do not require treatment.

BY JOHN OGDEN, M.D.

Reference
1. Trueta, J.: Role of the vessels in osteogenesis. *J. Bone Joint Surg., 45B:* 402, 1963.

CHAPTER 9

Epiphyseal, Metaphyseal, and Diaphyseal Affections

EPIPHYSEAL AFFECTIONS

Dysplasia Epiphysialis Hemimelica

This entity was described in 1950 by Trevor,[3] who named it "tarsoepiphyseal aclasis." It is not limited to the tarsus, nor is the tarsus constantly involved. It is an epiphyseal disease that, in a sense, represents an osteochondroma of the epiphysis. Involvement of the astragalus is striking, and the tarsal bones represent the most common site.

Clinical Picture

In reported cases, this disease is most common in the male. It is usually recognized in childhood.

A swelling at either the medial or the lateral side of the ankle or knee is the most common presenting complaint. Such a swelling is bony and hard, and because of the abnormal growth of the epiphysis on one side, deformity of the part distal to it, as, for instance, genu valgus or varus, may be apparent. There may be limitation of motion of the affected joint, and symptoms of internal derangement of the joint may arise as the growth progresses. Ligaments and tendons have to slide over these prominences and may lock on one side.

The medial side of the epiphysis is the usual site of involvement. The distal femoral epiphysis and the talus are most commonly subject to this abnormal growth. Progression is most severe in the early years of life, but it may continue through the growth period. It tends to cease as the epiphyseal lines close.

The x-ray appearance is that of an abnormal mass and an eccentric epiphyseal enlargement. There appear to be multiple centers of ossification irregularly and disorderly distributed in the involved area of the epiphysis. Diagnosis by the roentgenogram requires primarily knowledge of this condition, since epiphyseal diseases are few and none have the eccentric disorderly appearance of bone-forming elements and distortion of epiphyseal shape present here.

Pathology

The mass, when visualized at operation, has a smooth, glistening, bluish cartilage surface. Its irregularly convoluted surface joins the area of normal epiphyseal cartilage in a manner that permits no clear-cut distinction. It becomes a matter of judgement as to where the epiphysis ends. Examined by microscope, the cartilage is more hyperplastic than normal and active enchondral ossification is taking place at multiple centers within it. The appearance is very similar to that of an osteochondroma. All the elements taken by themselves are parts of normal growth; only the pattern and the organization have become disorderly.

Treatment

It is noteworthy that experience generally indicates that these epiphyses can be attacked surgically to remove the excess mass and to shape the epiphysis into something regarded as normal for a given location and a given child. There has been no particular tendency for the growth to recur, and functional improvement has been good. It is not a question of removing the lesion entirely but of reshaping the epiphysis into a functioning part. Judgement has to be used in preserving other elements of the joint.

References

1. Donaldson, J. S., Sankey, H. H., Girdany, B. R., and Donaldson, W. F.: Osteochondroma of the

Fig. 9.1. Epiphyseal osteochondroma of the medial condyle of the femur. Such a lesion belongs to the condition known as dysplasia epiphysialis hemimelica. It produces marked deformity and may be surgically remodeled to the expected anatomic shape of the bone. To permit the lesion to produce secondary deformity increases the disaster stemming from overgrowth of the lesion.

distal femoral epiphysis, *J. Pediatr., 43:* 212, 1953.
2. Fairbank, T. J.: Dysplasia epiphysialis hemimelica, *J. Bone Joint Surg., 38B:* 237, 1956.
3. Trevor, D.: Tarso epiphyseal aclasis: a congenital error of epiphyseal development, *J. Bone Joint Surg., 32B:* 204, 1950.

Epiphyseal Chondroblastoma

This lesion appears to be a distinct entity which occurs in the epiphyses of adolescents. It arises from proliferation of the chondroblast and produces foci of chondroid matrix. For a long time after Codman[1] in 1931 described 9 cases that occurred in the proximal end of the humerus, it was known as Codman's tumor. One suspects that this tumor is not yet completely understood. It has certain similarities to giant cell tumor in that it occurs in the epiphysis, but it differs in that it begins to develop before the epiphyseal line closes from the chondroblast. Giant cell tumor occurs only after the epiphysis is ossified.

Ewing[2] first noted this tumor in 1928, and he considered it a variant of the giant cell tumor. Jaffe and Lichtenstein[3] in 1942 described the lesion in further detail and renamed it a benign chondroblastoma of bone.

It is a rare tumor arising principally at the ends of long bones.

Clinical Picture

The lesion produces pain. The child is usually adolescent, the tumor rarely having been noted before the age of 10. In the series of Kunkel, Dahlin, and Young,[4] one patient was age 8. Tumors noted just after the epiphyseal lines have closed, when the patient is in the early 20s, are suspected of having originated just prior to closure of the epiphyseal line, when the chondroblast was still active. The usual duration of symptoms before the patient is seen is 1-2 years. Limitation of motion of the adjacent joint, and occasionally swelling, may be seen. A mass may be palpated if the tumor has been present for considerable time.

Pathology

The gross appearance is not very helpful, the principle feature being the epiphyseal location. With increasing duration, the lesion may extend into the metaphysis and break through the cortex, but it is usually overlain by subperiosteal bone if it does so. It may erode the articular surface. The material feels gritty when it is cut. Microscopically, the diagnosis depends on recognition of the chondroblast as the basic proliferating cell. This cell is larger than normal and has a well defined cytoplasmic membrane. Areas filled with sheets of these cells are found to be quite uniform in nature. The cellular areas lie in a matrix of hyalin, of myxoid material, and of collagenized connective tissue. Deposits of amorphous calcium lie in this matrix. Giant cells are present. Mitotic figures are rare.

Roentgen Picture

Location in an epiphysis is characteristic. The calcium in the matrix of the tumor may

Fig. 9.2. (*A*) Epiphyseal osteochondroma involving the talus and navicular with irregular ossific masses. The normal foot is shown beneath for contrast. (*B*) Exposure of cartilage-capped enlargement coming from both talus and navicular and in line with the medial ray of the foot, consistent with dysplasia epiphysialis hemimelica described by Trevor.

give it a hazy appearance, or definite foci of increased density may be seen within the radiolucent area occupied by the lesion. The lesion may be very small, occupying but a small portion of the epiphysis, or it may occupy most of the epiphysis and extend into the metaphysis. When it does so, subperiosteal new bone may wall off the lesion. The edge of the lesion in contact with bone is rather well defined and may be walled off sclerotically.

Treatment

The features of this tumor are quite charac-

Fig. 9.3. Epiphyseal chondroblastoma (so-called Codman's tumor). The tumor involves the proximal humeral epiphysis and extends into the metaphysis.

teristic, and the course is benign. Biopsy, however, is indicated. Surgical excision appears to be a satisfactory means of ablating the lesion. It may be necessary to fill the resulting defect with bone grafts. Recurrences are rare and respond to second excisions. It is generally thought that radiation therapy should be avoided.

References

1. Codman, E. A.: Ephiphyseal chondromatous giant cell tumors of the upper end of the humerus, *Surg. Gynecol Obstet., 52:* 543, 1931.
2. Ewing, J.: The classification and treatment of bone sarcoma, 365-376, *Report of the International Conference on Cancer,* Bristol: John Wright & Sons, Ltd., 1928.
3. Jaffe, H. L., and Lichtenstein, L.: Benign chondroblastoma of bone; reinterpretation of the so-called calcifying or chondromatous giant cell tumor, *Am. J. Pathol., 18:* 969, 1942.
4. Kunkel, M. G., Dahlin, D. C., and Young, H. H.: Benign chondroblastoma, *J. Bone Joint Surg., 38A:* 817, 1956.
5. Valls, J., O'Holeghi, C. E., and Schajowicz, F.: Epiphyseal chondroblastoma of bone, *J. Bone Joint Surg., 33A:* 997, 1951.

Chondrodystrophia Calcificans Congenita (Stippled Epiphyses, Fairbank's Disease)

This condition cannot be recognized from the roentgen film alone. It is associated with flexion contractures and congenital cataracts.

Several types of roentgen findings may be confused with the more serious classic form of the disease. A child with clinically normal extremities may be noted to have multiple ossification centers, for the epiphyses of coalescence may be seen. The epiphyseal centers appear none the worse for this method of ossification as growth progresses, and the child goes on to normal growth and development both clinically and roentgenographically as the centers fully coalesce.

Very rarely, areas of calcification in the articular cartilage are seen in infancy. These areas are amorphous. The child goes on to normal development. There is no apparent relation to calcinosis and no detectable disturbance of calcium metabolism.

The irregular ossification of the epiphyses that is clinically serious is associated with flexion contractures of the knees, hips, elbows, wrist, and fingers. The involved limb is short and readily detectable when unilateral congenital cataracts are noted. The skull is normal. The child is hypotonic and remains in the lower growth percentiles.

Roentgen Features

The epiphyses of the distal femur and proximal tibia are most commonly involved. Multiple ossification centers give a stippled appearance. The upper extremity often shows changes around the elbow joint. The ossification centers may be distributed like a necklace of pearls through the epiphysis. Irregular outlines of the bones of the tarsus may be visible. Where growth is affected the bones are short and thick.

Prognosis

A number of these infants appear to have little resistance to infection and die before 1 year of age.

Little is known of the underlying abnormality. The cartilage of the epiphysis may contain fibrous areas in which normal cartilage structure is lost and degenerative changes occur. There is extreme vascular invasion of the cartilage. Occasional areas of mucoid degeneration may calcify.

Spondyloepiphyseal Dysplasia (Pseudoachondroplasia)

There is shortening of the long bones in this disease. It becomes evident after the second year of extrauterine growth, but is usually not apparent before this age group. It is transmitted as a Mendelian dominant.

Clinical Picture

The child is short or dwarfed when seen at age 4 and over, but is not apparently dwarfed at birth. The skull is not involved and the facies consequently normal. Painful hips and a gluteus medius limp is the clinical feature that brings the patient to medical attention. The disease is compatible with a normal life expectancy.

Roentgen Picture

The long bones show many features of chondrodystrophy. Such bone as is formed has normal texture and microscopically is undistinguishable from normal bone. The bones are short and broad and tend to be widened in the metaphyseal area to accommodate the irregular epiphyses.

The gross irregularity in shape of the formed epiphyses is the distinguishing characteristic. Particularly evident are the hips with irregu-

Fig. 9.4. Shortening of the long bones, flaring of the epiphyseal metaphyseal area, and irregular shape of the small bones of the hands and feet are all features of chondrodystrophic bone formation with multiple joint involvement due to deformity.

Fig. 9.5. Spondyloepiphyseal dysplasia in (A) mother age 40, (B) daughter age 15, and (C) son age 14. The gross irregularity of the proximal femoral epiphyses can be expected to lead to the arthritis present at age 40. (D) The spine shows progressive diminution of height of the proximal lumbar vertebra and irregular notching of the anterior angles of the vertebral bodies.

larity so gross that it leads to secondary arthritic changes. The knees may also be affected.

The vertebrae are similarly involved with diminished height and irregular shape and widening. There is hypoplasia of the upper lumbar vertebrae and deficient ossification at the anterior angle of the vertebrae.

The pelvis is normal except for the hip joints and tends to be broad.

Fig. 9.5 C and D.

Treatment

The gross joint irregularities are unfortunately already the seat of extensive pathology when seen. There is no known prevention for the specific abnormality in growth of the epiphyses and vertebrae.

The joints can be aided by orthopaedic measures appropriate to the individual case and respond to these measures including replacement in a normal way.

Ellis-Van Creveld Syndrome

For those who like to consider generalized disturbance of bone formation from cartilage which has a particular distribution as a syndrome, this entity appears fairly clear-cut.

The youngster shows a shortening of the extremities that is most pronounced distally. The teeth and nails are underdeveloped (ectodermal dysplasia). There is bilateral polydactyly with fused or duplicated metacarpals. Delayed maturation of the primary ossification center of the phalanges, deformity of the proximal end of the tibial epiphysis, and possible association with congenital heart disease complete the picture.

The child looks somewhat like an achondroplastic dwarf though his deformity is not so severe. The skull is normal, and there is no nasal deformity. The trunk is normal in length for the child's age, but the limbs are disproportionately short. The polydactyly is evident, and other minor anomalies or variations may be associated with this malformation. The denti-

Fig. 9.6. Shortening and irregular shape of the distal long bones, a feature of Ellis-Van Creveld syndrome and diastrophic dwarfism.

tion is retarded. Intelligence is normal; at least, retarded intelligence is not part of the syndrome.

The acetabuli may be slightly hypoplastic. The shortening of the long bones, which is most marked in the lower leg and the lower arm, is evident. The anomalies of the metacarpals are varieties of duplication or fusion and polydactylism. The depression of the lateral proximal tibial epiphysis has appeared in cases reviewed by the author to be due to an epiphyseal osteochondroma of the lateral condyle of the femur.

Osteochondromas and other forms of chondrodysplasia arising from the metaphyseal side of the epiphyseal line are not present.

Treatment

Recognition of this youngster as having a form of achondroplastic dwarfism with other anomalies is the first step. Explanation to the parents and care of the psychologic hazards of this situation for both the parents and the child are important. The youngster should be followed to full maturity in order too obtain maximal function.

Pleonosteosis

This is a rare congenital and hereditary syndrome which principally involves the skeletal system. André Leri,[2] who described the anomaly in 1921, used the prefix "pleon-" to signify the superabundance of the changes.

There is enlargement of the epiphyses and precocious and excessive ossification of bones arising from cartilage, which give rise to limitation of the joints of the body. Watson-Jones[3] noted an increase in the collagenous tissue of major ligaments and the presence of fibrocartilage and mucinous material. There was a marked absence of elastic fibers.

Clinical Picture

The hands are short and spadelike, the stature is short, and mongoloid facies may be present. The digits have flexion contractures; the thumb is broad, and the first metacarpal is in a valgus position. There may be such skin changes as accentuated skin creases, thickened hollow palms, and a condition resembling scleroderma in the hands and forearms. The

knees may be in valgus and may have a hyperextension deformity.

The disease is apparent early in life and becomes more obvious with growth. The pathogenesis of the syndrome is not known. The hereditary transmission appears to occur by means of a dominant autosomal gene.

Treatment

The individual deformity has to be evaluated along orthopaedic lines as at the knees and in the hands. In general no treatment is indicated except in cases in which a noticeable deformity can be improved in appearance and function.

References

1. Leri, A.: Une maladie congenitale et hereditaire de l'ossification: la pleonosteosis familiale, *Bull. Mém. Soc. Méd. Hôp. Paris, 75:* 1228, 1921.
2. Rukavina, J. S., Falls, H. F., Holt, J. F., and Block, W. D.: Leri's pleonosteosis, *J. Bone Joint Surg., 41A:* 397, 1959.
3. Watson-Jones, R.: Leri's pleonosteosis, carpal tunnel compression of the median nerve and Morton's metatarsalgia, *J. Bone Joint Surg., 3B:* 560, 1949.

Diastrophic Dwarfism

It is possible to separate out from the entities of Morquio's chondrodystrophy, achondroplasia, multiple epiphyseal dysplasia, and arthrogryposis, an entity which results in considerable deformity and dwarfism below 5 feet in height.

A typical diastrophic dwarf would present as an infant with finger deformities, short finger and broad palm, hypermobile thumb, bilateral clubfeet, and dysplastic or dislocated hip. In addition, there would be thickened and protruding external ears.

The condition affects both sexes equally and is quite rare. It is transmitted by a single autosomal gene and has a distribution in the offspring of a particular union typical of this type of transmission. This separates if from achondroplastic dwarfism which is a mutant condition from normal parents or arthrogryposis which is not transmitted by hereditary patterns.

The condition was described by Jackson[1] in 1951, Lamy and Marateaux[2] in 1960, and in a clear-cut description by Stover, Hayes, and Holt in 1963.[3]

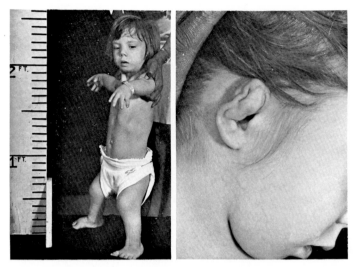

Fig. 9.7 (*Left*). Diastrophic dwarfism with short extremities and enlargements around epiphyseal areas.
Fig. 9.8 (*Right*). Deformed ear in diastrophic dwarfism.

Clinical Picture

The interphalangeal joints of the fingers may be fixed in a hyperextension contracture and they are short. The thumb, by contrast, is held away from the palms but has loose capsular structure and is hypermobile. The ears are thickened, protruding, and irregular shaped. Cleft palate has been reported as an occasional associated anomaly. The club feet and limited abduction at the hips with trochanters above Nélaton's line are evident in most, but not all, cases.

Roentgen Features

The femurs reveal delay in appearance of the epiphyses. Where the distal bony epiphysis does appear, it tends to be medially displaced, and, as development of both the femoral and tibial epiphyses progresses, they are flattened with flaring metaphyses and somewhat irregular in outline. At the hips there may be a coxa vara rather than dislocated epiphysis made difficult to recognize by the late development of the bony center. Occasionally both ulna and fibula are short with bowing of the radius and flaring of the distal metaphysis. The first metacarpal is typically rudimentary and very short. The phalanges ossify in an irregular manner.

A structural scoliosis appears early and progresses in severity toward adulthood.

Treatment

All adults reported have been well under 5 feet, varying from 3 feet to 4 feet, 6 inches. There is some muscle involvement as shown by abnormal electromyographic motion units and occasional denervation fibrillations. An elevated serum glutamic oxaloacetic transaminase has been reported.

All of this is to emphasize that the equinovarus feet are difficult to correct, with muscle imbalance frequently an accompaniment which must result in early tendon transplant. The hips are difficult to correct due to the epiphyseal deformity. The treatment follows the standard attacks on the various deformities with phychiatric support for both parent and child afflicted with dwarfism.

References

1. Jackson, W. P. M.: Irregular familial chondro-osseous defect, *J. Bone Joint Surg., 33B:* 420, 1951.
2. Lamy, M., and Marateaux, P.: L'anisme diastrophique, *Presse méd., 68:* 1977, 1960.
3. Stover, C., Hayes, J. Y., and Holt, J. F.: Diastrophic dwarfism, *Am. J. Roentgenol., 89:* 914, 1963.

METAPHYSEAL AFFECTIONS

Morquio's Disease

The entity called Morquio's disease was first

Fig. 9.9 (*Top, left*). In the upper extremity the roentgenogram reveals the thumb held away from the palm, the short broad metacarpals and phalanges, and the bowed radius with flaring metaphysis, a picture that is consistent with diastrophic dwarfism.

Fig. 9.10 (*Bottom*). The hip joints exhibit gross malformation with widening of the proximal femoral metaphysis and lateral displacement of the femoral shaft. The acetabulum mirrors the incongruity of the proximal femur. The ossification center for the proximal femoral epiphysis is delayed in its appearance.

Fig. 9.11 (*Right*). The distal femoral epiphysis has a displacement of its ossification center. The shortened tibia and flared metaphysis are also evident.

described by Morquio[3] in 1929 as a "form of familial osseous dystrophy." Chondrodystrophy is characterized by an altered rate in the formation of bone from cartilage.

The characteristics of this disease include dwarflike stature, a marked kyphos usually centering at the dorsolumbar junction, and involvement of the hips and other major joints in the changes of chondrodystrophy. These are noted clinically as enlargements and deformity. The bones of the skull and face are not involved, and the intelligence is normal.

In infancy there is little to raise the suspicion of Morquio's disease. The short trunk relative to the extremities gradually becomes evident with growth. There is often ligamentous laxity and lack of coordination resulting in a delayed walking age. Corneal opacities and dental abnormalities develop with maturity.

The disease has been recorded slightly more frequently in male patients, but both sexes are affected. According to Fairbanks, more than one member of a family is involved in about one-third of the cases.

Etiology

There is apparently an autosomal recessive mode of inheritance. Keratosulfate is found in the urine in childhood, gradually ceasing past puberty. The nature of the disturbances producing widespread disturbances of bone structure and shape, ligamentous laxity, and corneal opacities is still unknown.

Clinical Picture

The presence of Morquio's disease is ordinarily not recognized until after the child begins to walk. The disease is symptomless until the patient is older and secondary changes have developed in joints. The standing posture is characteristic. The spine is in flexion, and there is an accentuated kyphos at the midspine area. The knees tend to be flexed and the feet pronated. Valgus at the knee is quite common. As the age of the patient progresses, these deformities tend to become more severe. The gait tends to be a bilateral Trendelenburg type that results in waddling owing to the varus deformity at the hips.

The head may appear enlarged in relation to the short trunk and extremities, but usually it is normal in size and shape for the chronologic age. The kyphos and round back result in a lordotic curve through the lumbar area; the curve is usually quite short and accentuated. The shortening of the spine is out of proportion to that of the extremities. The hands may reach the knee level. There is limited extension of the spine, and in older patients there may be some lateral elevation resulting in mild scoliosis.

In achondroplastic dwarfs the proximal portion of the extremities may be excessively short, but this is not true in chondrodystrophy. In the lower extremities in particular, the ends of the bones in the epiphyseal and metaphyseal areas may be enlarged. Such enlargements are more readily noted at the knee than elsewhere.

Motion at the hip joint, which is usually involved in the disease, is often limited, and flexion contractures of mild degree are frequently present. There may be an inability to extend the knee completely. However, cases of excessive ligamentous laxity about the joints have been described. Enlargement of the interphalangeal joints is not common, but it may occur. The hand is broad and has broad and blunt fingers.

Narrowing of the chest anteriorly and protrusion of the sternum is common. The chin may be prominent and a short, flat nose is characteristic. The corneal opacities seen by slit lamp examination appear early. The shoulders and elbows may be limited in terms of full extension (elbow) or abduction (shoulder.)

Keratosulfate is found in the urine. Life expectancy is limited with cardiopulmonary involvement resulting in demise prior to age 40.

Roentgen Findings

Although the rate of formation of bone from cartilage may be altered, there is no area of persistent failure of ossification as there is in chondrodysplasia. Delayed growth of cartilage and failure of remodeling produces short, broad bones.

In the vertebrae, the transverse and anteroposterior diameters are increased. The upper and lower surfaces are irregular and poorly defined. The anterior border may be much smaller than the posterior, so that the vertebra may be wedge-shaped. The wedging may appear to be more at the expense of either the upper or lower half rather than symmetric, however.

At an area of kyphosis, one vertebra, usually the first lumbar, may appear smaller and more irregularly wedged than the others, and it may be displaced posteriorly. The epiphyseal lines of the long bones are widened, deepened, and irregular. The metaphyseal areas are broad and out of proportion to the diaphyses. Not all epiphyses are necessarily involved.

The ribs are more horizontal than usual and may present an expansion at either end. The hips are involved, the changes becoming more evident with increasing age. The femoral heads show marked epiphyseal irregularity and flattening. The femoral necks are shortened and broad, and they tend toward a varus deformity. According to Fairbanks, these changes are markedly progressive; the child may appear normal early in life only to develop changes later. Other joints may or may not be involved.

The metacarpals and phalanges are short and

Fig. 9.12. The spine in Morquio's disease with abnormal shape, flattening, and increased anteroposterior diameter of the vertebrae.

expanded at their extremities. Ossification in the bones of the hand may be delayed and may be irregular in outline when it does appear.

Differential Diagnosis

Achondroplasia is differentiated clinically and roentgenographically. The spine is of normal height; the prominent buttocks and lumbar lordosis with a round back or kyphos are characteristic. The shortening of the limbs occurs principally in the proximal segments. Joint degenerative changes are not seen, and genu valgum is not a feature. The bone is affected by failure to form in some areas rather than by slowness and irregularity of the rate of formation.

In "dysostosis multiplex" or gargoylism the patient is mentally deficient, the facial features coarsened and heavy, the liver and spleen enlarged, and the cornea cloudy.

Tuberculosis and other causes of dorsal vertebral collapses and subsequent kyphos are readily distinguished clinically. It should be remembered that chondrodystrophy of Morquio's type is a generalized disease and that roentgenograms reveal the generalized involvement.

Fig. 9.13. Involvement of epiphyseal and articular cartilage at the hip in Morquio's disease. The tendency toward a flat acetabular roof is apparent.

Treatment

There may be frequent respiratory tract infections requiring treatment. Hernias, loss of hearing, visual problems, and ear infections all complicate the disease. The teeth may be of poor quality requiring attention.

The use of the Milwaukee brace may be necessary to stabilize progressive kyphosis. The prominent genu valgum may complicate the walking disability to the point of requiring elective correction. The ligamentous laxity at the knee makes correction difficult and soft tissue reefing and subsequent bracing is often required.

References

1. Gordenich, I. F., and Lenzi, L. Morquio-Ullrich disease; new mucopolysaccharidosis, *J. Bone Joint Surg., 46A:* 743, 1964.

2. Langer, L. O., Jr., and Carey, L. S.: The roentgenographic features of the k.s. mucopolysaccharidosis of Morquio, *Am. J. Roentgenol., 97:* 1, 1966.
3. Morquio, L.: Sur une forme de dystrophie osseuse familiale, *Bul. Soc. Pediatr. Paris, 27:* 145, 1929.
4. Schenk, F. A., and Haggerty, J.: Morquio's disease; radiologic and morphologic study, *Pediatrics, 34:* 839, 1964.

Familial Metaphyseal Dysplasia

A rare bone disease, familial metaphyseal dysplasia was described in 1931 by Edwin Pyle.[2] Its outstanding feature is a failure to remodel bone laid down by growth from the epiphyseal line. The cases previously described in the literature have had a familial incidence. The distribution is symmetric and the metaphyseal areas of long bones are involved. The wide, flask-shaped metaphyses may result in confusion with Gaucher's disease. Phalanges, metacarpals, and metatarsals may also be involved.

Fig. 9.14. Familial metaphyseal dysplasia with failure of bone laid down by the epiphyses to remodel. This disease indicates nicely the amount of growth from one epiphysis as compared to another.

By roentgen examination, the lack of involvement of bone originating from fetal or membranous material is striking; therefore, the pictures show beautifully the relative percentages of growth from either end of a long bone. The area laid down by any one epiphyseal line has not been subject to remodeling. With the increased width there is a lack of normal development of bone cortex. The vertebrae may have an increased anteroposterior diameter. The pubis and ischii may be markedly widened. Skull changes, particularly a decrease in the transverse diameter at the base, may be noted.

The clinical picture is not striking. The osseous lesions ordinarily are found incidentally on a routine x-ray examination. Valgus at the knee has resulted in discovery of the anomaly in some children. Osteotomy may be necessary

if the deformity justifies it. Treatment is ordinarily not otherwise indicated.

References

1. Feld, H., Switzer, R. A., Dexter, M. W., and Langer, E. M.: Familial metaphyseal dysplasia, *Radiology, 65:* 206, 1955.
2. Pyle, E.: Case of unusual bone development, *J. Bone Joint Surg., 13:* 874, 1931.

Solitary Bone Cyst

A solitary bone cyst is usually brought to the attention of the orthopaedic surgeon by pathologic fracture. Rarely it may be incidentally found on roentgen examination. Although found in the adult, this lesion is peculiarly a disease of children and young adults. It has been termed osteitis fibrosa, but is not associ-

Fig. 9.15. Note small area of original fetal bone compared with unremodeled areas above and below in both tibia and fibula (familial metaphyseal dysplasia).

normal bone may be visualized distal to the epiphyseal line. The walls of the cyst are never wider than the width of the epiphyseal line in solitary bone cyst.

The second theory notes that the mechanism of production may be an exaggeration of the resorptive phase, during which calcified cartilage is replaced by bone. This phase, which is characterized by a proliferation of vessels and giant cells, according to Geschickter and Copeland,[4] may produce a loss of structure when it is exaggerated and may thus result in the cyst.

The location is conspicuously that of areas of high rates of growth and extensive remodeling. What part trauma plays in the picture is still unknown.

Clinical Picture

Pain, swelling, and mild deformity may be complaints that caused the patient to seek

ated with the generalized skeletal changes found in hyperparathyroidism, which is followed by polycystic lesions in the bones and bone atrophy.

Silver[5] reviewed the so-called "benign cyst of the bones" in 1912. In 97 cases, only 18 were past the age of 20 years. The usual age group in which bone cysts are discovered is that from 6 to 15 years. In addition to the long bones, the calcaneus is sometimes affected. The vast majority of cysts occur in the humerus or femur, however. There is a tendency for the lesion to predominate in males.

Etiology

The underlying prime factor that causes the area immediately adjacent to an epiphyseal line to become productive of cyst tissue rather than of bone is unknown. Trauma and hemorrhage have been suggested, but there are two opposing theories of the mechanism. The first assumes that the epiphyseal line in difficulty gives rise, not to normal bone, but to cyst tissue. This process may already have eased when the patient is first seen, and an area of

Fig. 9.16. Diagram of distribution of solitary bone cyst. Solid black areas are most frequently affected. (From C. T. Geschickter and M. M. Copeland: *Tumors of Bone*, J. B. Lippincott Co., Philadelphia, 1949.)

Fig. 9.17. Fracture in solitary bone cyst. The fracture will not result in healing of the cyst.

medical attention. The pain is quite low grade except in instances of acute fracture, and, as a result, it may have existed for considerable time before the patient is seen. There may have been no preceding symptoms. When the cyst occurs in areas such as the femoral neck, hemorrhage into the joint may initially result in confusion with entities that may cause pain and spasm at the hips.

The site of these complaints is characteristic. The most common area involved is the proximal femur. It is usually apparent on viewing the x-ray film that either the trochanteric epiphysis or the capital femoral epiphyseal line is more closely related to the cyst. The second most common site is the proximal tibia. Other long bone sites may occasionally be involved. The older the patient and the longer the duration of symptoms, the further removed from the epiphyseal line the cyst may reasonably be found.

So-called acute bone cysts may have a duration of but a few months and are regarded by Geschickter and Copeland as giant cell variants which may be related to giant cell tumor. These cysts have not progressed down the shaft with growth but are situated close to the epiphyseal line. Garceau and Gregory,[3] in tabulating the incidence of healing of the cyst in those cases with fracture, found that it was fifteen per cent both in their own cases and in those in the literature.

Roentgen Findings

This lesion is not actually expansile, although superficially it may appear so. There is an area of loss of normal bone structure which is contained within thinned cortex. The actual width of the cyst is never greater than the width of the epiphyseal line. The cyst area has not been subject to remodeling, but this process has taken place distal to it. When the cyst is removed from the epiphyseal line, it is seen that remodeling has also taken place proximal to it. The remodeling of the normal bone results in the expanded appearance of the cyst by contrast. When the width of the lesion is greater than that of the epiphyseal line from which it may have arisen, serious doubt of the diagnosis

Fig. 9.18. Fibrous lining membrane from wall of simple bone cyst.

Fig. 9.19 (*Left*). So called "immature state" of solitary bone cyst with epiphyseal lines still directly adjacent to the cyst. (*Right*) Postoperative view after bone grafting. (Courtesy of Elmer King, M.D.)

of solitary bone cyst should arise. Lesions such as syphilitic gumma and giant cell tumor should be considered.

The juncture of the cyst with the normal cortex is a symmetric one; that is, the normal cortex thins on both its exterior and its interior surfaces to the width of the cortex overlying the lesion.

Pathology

The cyst wall on examination at operation may be greatly thinned and may fracture on slight pressure. There may be little or no lining, but some areas of fibrous tissue are usually found. The cyst contents usually consist of fluid either yellow or reddened by recent hemorrhage. Except in the region of recent fracture, there is no indication that new bone formation is going on exteriorly.

In the areas of fibrous tissue lining the wall there is no evidence of fibrous tissue proliferation, but there are occasionally osteoblasts and new bone. The more central fibrous tissue, if present, is quite loose and myxomatous.

Evidence of old hemorrhages is sometimes noted. In the areas of fresh hemorrhage a giant cell reaction may be present. Bone formation from cartilage is not seen; and when there is osteoblastic activity, it takes place in fibrous tissue.

The so-called giant cell variant of the solitary bone cyst may tend more to be subcortical and most frequently is found in the region of the greater trochanter of the femur. The tissue is featured by numerous giant cell areas close to the epiphyseal line in a stroma of considerable intercellular tissue and fibroblasts.

Treatment

The solitary bone cyst lends itself well to carefully performed surgery. A belief has arisen that fracture heals cysts of this type, but this belief is not borne out by experience. When the cyst is small, i.e., when its long axis is ½ inch or less, the healing reaction about a fracture line extending approximately ¼ inch on either side of it may indeed ablate the cyst or render it of little consequence. In larger cysts, such a reaction is not expected.

If the cyst has suffered a recent fracture, its healing reaction may be utilized by surgery performed during the phase of callus proliferation. Not all cysts must have surgery, however.

The optimal time for operation in a case of cyst which has rendered the bone mechanically inadequate arises when a centimeter or more of normal bone has been laid down between the epiphyseal line and the cyst itself. Attempts to ablate the cyst when there is no evidence that normal bone is being developed from the epiphyseal line may be followed by recurrence. Garceau and Gregory have emphasized the high recurrence rate in patients operated on below the age of 10.

The operation has two aims: (1) to remove the contents of the cyst and (2) to stimulate a repair reaction which will cause bone to be laid down in the cyst area. At surgery, the area involved is usually wider than the expected width of bone subject to remodeling and has a bluish cast. Normal-bleeding bone should be visualized at both proximal and distal ends of the cyst cavity after curettement. There is occasionally a small quantity of fibrous tissue that can be obtained by curetting. It is helpful to displace the wall segment removed in order to visualize the cyst to the far side so that it abuts against the remaining wall, thereby obliterating the cyst cavity. Bone grafts are used to fill the cavity remaining.

Bone grafts are inserted so that contact with the parent bone is made at both ends of the cyst. If chips are used, large cystic spaces which the bone would have difficulty in bridging, are avoided, and the cavity is not packed so tightly that development of the repair reaction is impeded. Autogenous bone is preferable but may be impractical in the presence of large cystic areas. Where bone bank bone is used, match stick grafts derived from ribs are inserted into the cyst cavity so that they run longitudinally and have good contact in normal cancellous bone areas.

Carefully performed operative procedures in a patient in whom the cyst area is removed from the epiphyseal line by normal cancellous bone one centimeter or more in depth, and in the older child, may be expected to yield good results.

References

1. Alldrédge, R. H.: Localized fibrocystic disease of bone: results of treatment in 152 cases, *J. Bone Joint Surg., 24:* 795, 1942.

2. Elinslic, R. C.: Fibrocystic diseases of the bone, *Br. J. Surg., 2:* 17, 1914.
3. Garceau, G. J., and Gregory, C. F.: Solitary unicameral bone cyst, *J. Bone Joint Surg., 36A:* 267, 1954.
4. Geschickter, C. T., and Copeland, M. M.: *Tumors of Bone,* Ed. 3, Philadelphia: J. B. Lippincott Co., 1949.
5. Silver, D.: The so-called benign cyst of the bones, *Am. J. Orthop. Surg., 9:* 563, 1912.
6. Stewart, M. J., and Hamel, H. A.: Solitary bone cyst, *South. Med. J., 43:* 927, 1950.

Aneurysmal Bone Cyst

This lesion of bone once was classified within a group of conditions known as "atypical giant cell tumor." Jaffe and Lichtenstein[3] in 1942 reclassified it as an individual entity. It appears to be confined to the young, the youngest reported patient being 2 years and 3 months and the majority under the age of 30 years.

Aneurysmal bone cyst is a benign lesion occurring in the metaphyses of long bones and occasionally in the spine and flat bones. It produces local pain and symptoms secondary to its pressure on adjacent structures. It destroys bone and thus gives rise to the characteristic described as a "blow out."

Etiology

The cause is unknown. Aberrant vessel formation has been suggested by Donaldson.[2] Jaffe[3] suggests that the lesion is engrafted onto some preexisting lesion in bone, such as a nonossifying fibroma or fibrous dysplasia. Trauma appears to draw attention to the lesion but is not a primary cause.

There are characteristics in the pathology which have led some observers to the belief that the lesion is essentially a hemangioma in bone. In one of Donaldson's cases reported in 1962, roentgenograms of the involved bone had been made in connection with a femoral fracture. A metaphysis that appeared normal upon roentgen examination was shown distal to the fracture at that time; 1½ years after healing of the fracture, the area involved was the site of an aneurysmal bone cyst.

Clinical Picture

The patient is usually under 30 years of age. Pain at the site of involvement is the most frequent presenting complaint. In patients with spine lesions, paraplegia as well as back pain may be the presenting complaint. The involved area may have collapsed with trauma or manipulation.

Swelling and tenderness are present over the involved area. There is an equal incidence in male and female.

Roentgen Picture

In the long bones, the aneurysmal bone cyst is located in the metaphysis. It is ovoid in shape

A. ANEURYSMAL BONE CYST   B. IMMATURE SIMPLE BONE CYST   C. MATURE SIMPLE BONE CYST   D. GIANT CELL TUMOR

Fig. 9.20. *Dotted line* represents the width of the adjacent epiphyseal plate and its metaphysis. The *shaded areas* represent the typical sites of involvement in a long bone with various types of cystlike lesions of bone. The aneurysmal bone cyst is frequently eccentric. The immature bone cyst is metaphyseal; it abuts directly on the epiphyseal line and usually extends entirely across the metaphysis. The mature simple cyst is not remodeled, as the normal bone around it is, and the result is an apparent expansion of the lesion as the epiphysis starts laying down normal bone. The giant cell tumor involves the epiphyseal area in an older age group after the epiphyseal line has closed. (From W. A. Donaldson: *Journal of Bone & Joint Surgery, 44A:* 25, 1962.)

and usually eccentrically located. The cortex overlying it has been destroyed, and the lesion is not bounded by a thin shell of new bone. The edge is benign in character rather than actively destructive. In the spine, it is usually found in the posterior elements, such as the spinous processes and lunimae, rather than in the body of the vertebra, although it may advance into the posterior portion of the vertebra. The lesion may produce a mass that balloons out from its original site.

Pathology

Although the metaphyses of long bones and spine are the most frequent site, it has been found in the calcaneous, clavicle, scapula, ilium, occiput metacarpals, and metatarsals. When exposed surgically, the lesion is covered by a thin layer of subperiosteal bone. Beneath this lies a bloody, red tissue which is soft. Occasionally, the area may be filled with fluid, but there is a well marked lining. Microscopically, the lesion contains numerous blood-filled spaces contained by fibrous tissue septa with osteoid. There are giant cells of the foreign body type that vary greatly in density from area to area. In the septa, in addition to active fibroblasts and osteoid, some areas of immature bone may be seen.

Treatment

Aneurysmal bone cyst is a benign lesion apparently capable of increasing to great size if untreated. Its secondary effects, such as paraplegia, are most serious.

The lesion responds to curettement, which is apparently, however, not always sufficient. In one of the author's cases, a previous procedure consisting of curettement and replacement with bone chips had failed to cure the conditions. In this case, the area was resected en bloc and cure resulted. In contrast to simple bone cysts, these cysts appear to respond beneficially to x-ray therapy in doses varying between 600 and 2,000 R.

Th surgical approach, especially in children,

Fig. 9.21. Aneurysmal bone cyst in a 19-year-old girl. The eccentric position of the lesion is well demonstrated. The cortex has been destroyed, and the lesion is covered by a thin shell of new bone.

appears preferable, however, because growth areas may be affected. Roentgen therapy may be necessary in surgically inaccessible areas.

References

1. Coley, B. L., and Miller, L. B.: Atypical giant cell tumor, *Am. J. Roentgenol., 47:* 541, 1942.
2. Donaldson, W. F.: Aneurysmal bone cyst, *J. Bone Joint Surg., 44A:* 25, 1962.
3. Jaffe, H. L., and Lichtenstein, L.: Solitary unicameral bone cyst with emphasis on the roentgen picture, pathologic appearance, and pathogenesis, *Arch. Surg., 44:* 1004, 1942.
4. Lichtenstein, L.: Aneurysmal bone cyst: a pathologic entity commonly mistaken for giant cell tumor and occasionally for hemangioma and osteogenic sarcoma, *Cancer, 3:* 279, 1950.

Tibia Vara

Three forms of tibia vara are encountered in childhood. By far the commonest of these is tibia vara or bowlegs associated with growth stress. Such a condition is commonly seen in orthopaedic and pediatric practice. This form of tibia vara is associated with internal tibial torsion and is of mild degree. It is present at birth—apparently a remnant of intrauterine position—and persists with sleeping on the stomach.

Deformity due to asymmetric growth of the proximal tibial epiphyseal line with apparent osteochondritis (or Blount's disease) is occasionally seen and must be particularly considered in unilateral tibia vara. Varus deformity of the tibia due to various forms of rickets and other growth disturbances of the epiphyseal line, such as chondrodystrophy, is not quite rare. When tibia vara is associated with generalized disease, such as osteogenesis imperfecta, it is usually an incidental part of a generalized deformity.

Clinical Picture

Complaint of the deformity is not ordinarily made until the child begins to walk and the

Fig. 9.22 (*Left*). Patient with tibia vara. Note the change of angle in the proximal tibial area and secondary pronation of feet.
Fig. 9.23 (*Right*). Posterior view.

Fig. 9.24. Weight-bearing roentgenogram in tibia vara due to growth stress. Note the medial facing of the distal tibial surface and secondary pronation of feet.

rolling gait, the wide-spaced knees, and the secondary pronation of the foot become evident. Infants are seen usually because the associated internal tibial torsion has resulted in turning inward of the foot to a sufficient degree to alarm the parents.

Infants with tibia vara due to growth stress are most often quite stocky and unusually active. Those with Blount's disease do not exhibit evidence of generalized disease. However, in instances of rachitic and other growth disturbances of the epiphyseal line, there is usually a generalized diminished rate of growth as well.

Roentgen Findings

The findings on the x-ray film are most helpful in differentiating among the various causes of tibia vara.

Growth Stress. Here the angulation takes place in the proximal tibia. The epiphyseal line is normal. There is a characteristic increase in width of the medial cortex that is most prominent at the junction of the proximal and middle thirds. The plane of knee ankle joint faces slightly medialward instead of lying parallel to that of the knee. The deformity is equal in both legs.

Blount's Disease. The height of the proximal tibial epiphysis is diminished on its medial aspect, and the epiphyseal line is narrowed and irregular on this side. The metaphysis immediately below this area is irregularly ossified, and there is breaking medially. The diminished growth in this area causes angulation to take place proximally. The deformity is often unilateral.

Rickets. The irregularity and widening of the epiphyseal line are evident at once. The fraying of the metaphysis, its cuplike deformity, and generalized osteoporosis are later changes. The angulation of the tibia, in contradistinction to that due to growth stress, takes place at the junction of the mid and distal thirds, and there is maximal thickening of the medial cortex in this area. A similar angulation of the distal femur helps to contribute to the deformity.

Prognosis

Growth Stress. The deformity has a tendency to improve with weight-bearing and growth. Eventually, at approximately age 3-4 years, it actually tends to pass over to genu valgum.

Blount's Disease. The condition tends to subside spontaneously after a 3-4-year period, and there is reconstitution of the epiphyseal line and filling in of the irregularly calcified medial metaphysis.

Rickets. The response to antirachitic therapy is dependent on the type of rickets involved and is discussed elsewhere.

Treatment

Tibia vara results in medial facing of the ankle joint and secondary pronation of the foot to get it flat on the floor. In order to avoid this foot position, the foot must be supported by a longitudinal arch pad. A 1/8-inch inner heel wedge is added to support the pad and to stimulate medial growth. After adequate alignment of the foot with the leg, the child is followed, as growth itself tends to straighten

Fig. 9.25. Prominent breaking of medial metaphysis of both femora and tibiae. (*Left*) The tendency toward irregular ossification at the proximal tibia is no longer present. (*Right*) One year later the deformity still appears severe, but one may expect these legs to straighten through growth with appropriate foot support.

the leg is the deformity is due to growth stress. Osteotomy of the tibia is not necessary.

In Blount's disease the foot is similarly supported. The activity of the disease is followed by roentgenogram; and when the disease is quiescent and growth restored to normal, surgical correction by osteotomy may be considered if the deformity is of sufficient degree. Braces which are built with partial correction of the malalignment are sometimes used in an endeavor to prevent the development of severe deformity.

The rachitic bowleg with deformity in the distal third of the tibia does not have the tendency toward spontaneous correction that exists in angulation of the upper third. It is obviously poor judgment to attempt correction in the presence of active disease; but once the disease is controlled, osteotomy may be considered. This may involve correction of the femur as well, in order to get knee and ankle aligned in the same plane.

Osteopoikilosis (Osteopathia Condensus Disseminata)

This condition is characterized by dense calcific densities irregularly spotted about the ends of the long bone of the extremities. They are found in the small bones of the hands and feet as well.

The appearance was described by Stredi in 1905. It is of importance only to avoid confusion with clinical entities of more serious import. The opacities are of gross size, giving a bizarre appearance of the roentgenogram of the skeleton, but not affecting the external form or function of the skeleton. It is a familial condition and may be accompanied by hereditary multiple exostoses. The opacities articulate with the normal trabeculae about them, but are flat expanses of unvarying density. The nodules tend to be spherical and occasionally elongated. Microscopic examination reveals that they are composed of dense lamellated bone, similar to cortical bone.

Reference

1. Hinson, A.: Familial osteopoikilosis, *Am. J. Surg.*, *45:* 566, 1939.

DIAPHYSEAL AFFECTIONS

Marfan Syndrome (Arachnodactyly)

Marfan's syndrome, also known as arachnodactyly, is a relatively rare familial disorder of

Fig. 9.26. Blount's disease. (*Top*) Irregular ossification and diminished height of metaphysis and epiphysis medially on right. (*Bottom*) Healing in previously affected area.

unknown etiology in which there are widespread abnormalities of the skeletal, cardiovascular, and ocular systems. In 1896, Marfan[9] made the first report of the syndrome which now bears his name and described the long extremities and long, spidery fingers, the hallmark of the skeletal abnormalities. In 1902, Achard coined the name arachnodactyly to describe the spider-like fingers seen in the classical case of Marfan's syndrome and this term and the eponym have been used interchangeably to describe the syndrome ever since. Since then, it has been estimated that between 350 and 400 cases have been reported in the literature, including detailed pathologic studies of over 70 cases.

McKusick[10] suggests the term "Marfan syndrome" for this generalized disease involving mesodermal tissue and producing an undefined defect. Although the disease is known as arachnodactyly in orthopaedic circles because the skeletal abnormalities it causes often bring the patient to medical attention, Marfan syndrome is probably a better term since not all patients exhibit skeletal manifestations. "Arachnodactyly" refers to the long "spider-like" fingers. Marfan suggested "dolichostenomelia" which emphasized long extremities.

Marfan's syndrome is characterized by excessive length of the long bones, loose joints and ligaments, ectopia lentis, dilation of the aorta, and defects such as inguinal hernia.

Fig. 9.27. Dense sclerotic areas articulating with the normal bone stria are observed tending to a metaphyseal location in the proximal femur (osteopoikilosis, see page 540).

The disease effects approximately 1.5 per 100,000 population. According to McKusick, at least 85% of the cases actually can be shown to have been inherited as autosomal dominants when appropriate genetic studies are conducted, with the remaining 15% being spontaneous mutations. It has also been shown the incidence is the same in both sexes and in both whites and Negroes.

Etiology

That the disease is transmitted as a dominant trait was brought to medical attention by Weve[17] of Utrecht in 1931, who designated the disease "dystrophia—mesodermalis congenita—typus Marfans."

In 1958, Tjio and Puck first reported variability in size of human satellited chromosomes. At first no significance was ascribed to the variation in satellite size, but in 1960, Tjio, Puck, and Robinson[16] described the results of chromosome studies in 2 patients with Marfan's syndrome and noted that one of the patients possessed a tremendously enlarged satellite on one member of pair 21 while the other patient had a similarly greatly enlarged satellite on one member of pair 13. Handmaker[5] presented evidence in 1963 that there was no correlation between enlarged satellites and Marfan's syndrome. He found that in chromosome studies of 8 patients with Marfan's syndrome, none of them possessed a chromosome satellite enlarged any greater than those observed in any of their unaffected relatives.

In an experiment performed in 1961, Prockop[12] reported an increase in urinary bound hydroxyproline excretion in patients with Marfan's syndrome. His values demonstrated that while normal subjects excreted less than 34 mg of hydroxyproline per day, those with Marfan's syndrome excreted between 38 and 90 mg per day. Jones et al.[6, 7] confirmed this in 1964 when they compared urinary hydroxyproline excretion in Marfan's syndrome

Fig. 9.28. In the tibia the tendency of the opacities to occupy a metaphyseal location in osteopoikilosis is evident (see page 540).

Fig. 9.29 (*Left*) and Fig. 9.30 (*Right*). Diagnosis: arachnodactyly. Note long extremities and digits, scoliosis, and eye defect.

with age matched controls. They found that preadolescent and adult patients with Marfan's syndrome consistently excreted greater amounts of hydroxyproline than did the controls. The vast majority of the urinary hydroxyproline in both of these studies was excreted bound to peptides and the amount of free hydroxyproline was consistently insignificant. Stetten[15] found that exogenous ^{15}N-labeled hydroxyproline was not incorporated into collagen but rather remains as free hydroxyproline and is excreted as such in the urine. From this it was inferred that, without significant hydroxyproline in the exogenous form, most of the hydroxyproline in the body and in the urine must be derived from the breakdown of collagen. Prokop therefore suggested that the increased hydroxyproline excretion in the urine of subjects with Marfan's syndrome must indicate a more rapid than normal rate of collagen breakdown in this condition.

An association between the abnormalities produced in experimental animals fed *Lathyrus odoratus* (sweet pea) seeds and the abnormali-

ties of Marfan's syndrome has also been postulated. Ponseti and Shepard found that white rats fed a diet containing 50% *Lathyrus odoratus* seeds all developed kyphoscoliosis—apparently the result of osteoporosis and collapse of several vertebrae. Aneurysms of the thoracic aorta in 6 of 16 rats were also found and histopathologic studies on these demonstrated marked medial necrosis. They concluded that the sweet pea seeds contained a toxic factor which had its primary effect on the development of mesodermal structures. In 1954 these same investigators[11] found that rats fed *Lathyrus odoratus* developed epiphyseal plates containing a cartilage matrix that appeared to lose cohesion, and the same diets produced loosening and detachments of the tendinous and ligamentous insertions with defects such as recurrent shoulder dislocations.

Subsequently, the toxic agent of the sweet pea seed has been identified as being β-aminopropionitrile (BAPN). Rats fed BAPN have been found to have an increased amount of soluble collagen that could be extracted in neutral salts and also a comparable increase in urinary hydroxyproline peptides Jasin and Ziff concluded that the increased amounts of bound hydroxyproline in the urine represented an increase in this soluble collagen fraction. In 1963, Gross[4] found that guinea pigs fed 0.5-1.0 mg of BAPN/kg/day showed an increase in the amount of collagen that was extractable in neutral salts and that this soluble collagen would not reprecipitate with prolonged incubation as would normal soluble collagen. He proposed that previously formed intramolecular bonds and intermolecular bonds in the normal collagen molecule had been disrupted by the BAPN.

Macek et al.[8] stated in 1967 that the fibroblasts form a basic molecule of the tropocollagen which consists of three polypeptide chains. In the youngest developmental forms the individual chains are not cross-linked so that this form of collagen which is called α-collagen is very labile and degradates easily. During fibrillogenesis, the three fundamental chains of tropocollagen are cross-linked together to a higher degree and further tropocollagen units aggregate. This is how β-collagen, and, from this, gradually insoluble collagen forms are formed.

In summary, these studies have shown that there is an increase in urinary hydroxyproline excretion in Marfan's syndrome, and this is thought to represent collagen breakdown, that lathyrism results in many Marfan-like abnormalities, and the lathyrism produces an increased urinary hydroxyproline excretion due to a block in collagen cross-linking.

The problem that arises with any hypothesis as to the basic defect in Marfan's syndrome is that it must explain the wide variety of clinical manifestations involving the skeletal, cardiovascular, and ocular systems.

Pathologic studies have shown that aortic aneurysms in patients with Marfan's disease show a form of medial necrosis in which there is marked disarrangement of the normal orientation of the elastic lamellae with whorls of elastic fibers, increased vascularization and large areas of cystic degeneration. However, if it is remembered that there is a large component of collagen in the wall of the aorta, an explanation of the histologic findings might go as follows: the collagen may actually act to hold the elastic fibers in their normal lamellar orientation and thus a defective collagenous element may result in disorganization of the elastic fibers in the wall of the aorta. The increased vascularity observed may result from dilitation of the vasa vasorum. Ectopia lentis and myopia could also readily be explained by a possible defect in collagen since both of these (i.e., the suspensory ligament of the lens and the sclera of the eye) are largely collagenous structures.

Clinical Picture

The dislocated lens that accompanies the development of pigeon chest deformity or scoliosis may bring the patient to medical attention. Later in life, back pain, joint pain, and effusion may occur. Cardiac symptoms may occur at an early age, but usually begin in the late teen-age group. Once left-sided failure has occurred, the prognosis, as in syphilitic aortitis, is very grave, the patient seldom living more than 2 years.

The orthopaedist is often consulted because of deformity, which may consist of pronated feet, scoliosis, or round back deformity. Some patients have subluxated elbows. The patient is usually thin and notes generalized weakness. There is no evidence that the muscles are involved, however, and there is a normal creative coefficient.

The edge of the dislocated lens may be visualized on dilating the pupil. Retinal detachment is not uncommon. The sclerae may be blue, and the patient may be myopic.

An increase in pubis-sole height over that of pubis to vertex is a common abnormality, although the total height is not necessarily increased. Some patients are unusually tall.

Some diagnostic ratios have been given. A hand-to-height ratio greater than 11% or a foot-to-height ratio greater than 15% are thought to be diagnostic. A middle finger that is one and a half times greater than the metacarpal is easily ascertained. Elasticity of the tissues is often noted by a high-riding patella due to stretching out of the patellar tendon.

In 1960, Sinclair, Kitchin, and Turner[14] suggested a new measurement which they found useful in making the diagnosis of arachnodactyly. They averaged the ratios of the length to the width of the second through fifth metacarpals and found that 80% of normal

Fig. 9.31. Elongated metacarpals and phalanges result in long, graceful hands in Marfan's syndrome.

Fig. 9.32. Excess laxity of the ligaments permits excess mobility of the joints in arachnodactyly.

Fig. 9.33. Femora in arachnodactyly.

subjects had values between 7.0 and 8.0, with the other 20% having values below 7. In patients with Marfan's syndrome, they found that over 90% had values between 8 1/2 and 10. Another useful measure for the diagnosis of Marfan's syndrome is the ratio of the distance from the vertex to the pubis and the distance from the pubis to the sole. In normal whites this ratio varies with a mean of 1.08 to 0.94 between the ages of 4 and 14, respectively; in Marfan's syndrome the ratio is much lower with an average of approximately 0.85 at 14 years of age. The reason for the reduction in this ratio in Marfan's syndrome is not difficult to appreciate when one considers the fact that not only are the extremities longer but also the frequently found kyphoscoliosis reduces the numerator of the ratio.

Kyphoscoliosis is not ordinarily noted before 10 years of age, but may become quite severe as growth progresses. The pigeon breast deformity is often present anteriorly. Most of the spine deformity is in the thoracic spine.

The aortic dilation begins at the aortic ring and involves the ascending aorta; the patient may develop a dissecting aneurysm.

The two most outstanding features of the cardiovascular system in Marfan's syndrome are: (1) dilatation of the aortic ring with resultant aortic insufficiency and (2) dissecting aneurysm of the ascending aorta. However, the many other cardiovascular complications associated with Marfan's syndrome include abdominal aortic aneurysms, mitral regurgitation secondary to redundant chordae tendinae, artial septal defects, tetrology of Fallot, coarctation of the aorta, and even one reported case of patent ductus arteriosus.

The joints hyperextend, and the limbs are flail-like.

The ocular manifestations of Marfan's syndrome are numerous but the most important include: (1) ectopia lentis—usually bilateral—in which the suspensory ligaments of the lens are relaxed or fragmemted with the lower ligaments most frequently being the most defective so that the lens is displaced upward, (2) myopia—secondary to the excessive length of the eyeball which is again thought to be due to a defect in the connective tissue elements of the sclera, (3) spontaneous retinal detachment, (4) coloboma of the iris or lens, and (5) associated blue sclera.

Other manifestations of the disease include: (1) congenital cystic lung disease which may result in spontaneous pneumothorax, (2) small skin papules that occur most often over the neck and are composed of what histologically looks like whorls of elastic fibers in continuity with the dermis (these occur rarely in Marfan's syndrome but, when they do, they are also virtually pathognomonic of the syndrome and have been given the name Meischer's elastoma),

and (3) striae of the skin over the pectoral region are also frequent.

Mental retardation is not a conspicuous component of the syndrome.

Roentgen Picture

The excessive length of the bone compared to its width is apparent. The long bones tend to be especially long distally. The increased length of the finger as compared to the metacarpal is apparent on a film of the hand. Skeletal maturation is normal.

Treatment

The various systems that can be involved in this desease demand highly specialized care in each area. Both cardiac and ocular systems must be thoroughly evaluated initially to determine the need for referral.

The orthopaedic complaints can be individually dealt with although the total condition affecting the patient still remains unsolvable in terms of remedy for the fundamental metabolic defect.

Generalized weakness demands a resistive

Fig. 9.34. Roentgenogram of a patient with arachnodactyly. There is unusual length of long bones and phalanges and a mild scoliosis.

exercise program. The training effect from these exercises in these patients is less than normal, but sufficient help is apparent to the patient that a carefully graded program is indicated.

Since the scoliosis can be expected to be progressive early bracing (Milwaukee-Blount brace) is indicated with regular visits for evaluation of progression and consideration of fusion when indicated.

The long feet may lead to symptoms with arch supports an early necessity. Eventually triple arthrodesis may be indicated.

References

1. Aegerter E., and Kirkpatrick, J. A.: *Orthopedic Diseases*, p. 123, Philadelphia: W. B. Saunders Co., 1958.
2. Bacchus, H.: A quantitative abnormality in serum mucoproteins in the Marfan syndrome, *Am. J. Med., 25:* 744, 1958.
3. Goodman, R. M.: Thoughts on various genetic disorders of connective tissue, *Med. Times, 94:* 1361, 1966.
4. Gross, J.: An intermolecular defect of collagen in experimental lathyrism, *Biochim. Biophys. Acta, 71:* 250, 1963.
5. Handmaker, S. D.: The satellited chromosomes of man with reference to the Marfan's syndrome, *Am. J. Hum. Genet., 15:* 11, 1963.
6. Jones, C. R., et al.: Urinary hydroxyproline excretion in normal children and adolescents, *Proc. Soc. Exp. Biol. Med., 115:* 85, 1964.
7. Jones, C. R., et al.: Urinary hydroxyproline excretion in Marfan's syndrome as compared with age matched controls, *Proc. Soc. Exp. Biol. Med., 116:* 931, 1964.
8. Macek, J., Hurych, J., Chvapil, M., and Kadecova, V.: Study on Fibroblasts in Marfan's syndrome, *Hum. Genet. 3:* 87, 1967.
9. Marfan, A. B.: Une corde déformation congenitale des quatre membres plus prononcée aux extrémités characterisée par l'allongement des os avec un certain degré d'amincissement, *Bull. Mêm. Soc. Méd. Hôp. Paris, 13:* 220, 1896.
10. McKusick, V. A.: *Heritable Disorders of Connective Tissues*, Ed. 2, St. Louis: C. V. Mosby Co., 1960.
11. Ponseti, I. V., and Shepard, R. S.: Lesions of the skeletal and of other mesodermal tissues in rats fed sweet pea seeds, *J. Bone Joint Surg., 36A:* 1031, 1954.
12. Procop, D. J.: Significance of urinary hydroxyproline in man, *J. Clin. Invest., 40:* 843, 1961.
13. Sinclair, R. J. G.: The Marfan syndrome, *Bull. Rheum. Dis., 8:* 153, 1958.
14. Sinclair, R. J., Kitchin, A. H., and Turner, R. W.: The Marfan syndrome, *Q. J. Med., 29:* 19, 1960.
15. Stetten, M. R.: Dietary N^{15}-hydroxyproline, *J. Biol. Chem., 181:* 31, 1949.
16. Tijo, J. H., Puck, T. T., and Robinson, A.: The human satellited chromosomes in normal patients and in two patients with Marfan's syndrome, *Proc. Nat. Acad. Sci., 46:* 532, 1960.
17. Weve, H.: Neben Arachnodaktylie, *Arch. Angenh., 104:* 1, 1931.

Progressive Diaphyseal Dysplasia

The rare disease, progressive diaphyseal dysplasia, is characterized by muscular wasting, progressive laying down of subperiosteal new bone in the diaphyseal areas of long bones, and mild neuromuscular disturbances. The syndrome has also been termed Englemann's disease.

Etiology

The cause is unknown. Some observers have likened the anomaly to muscular dystrophy because of the progressive muscular weakness and familial incidence. Instances of the disease have been found in relatives of the patient who were unaware of any disorder.

Clinical Picture

Males appear to be more commonly affected. The disease is usually discovered in the 4-10-year age group. Easy fatigue or a gait abnormality usually bring the patient for examination. The latter may consist of waddling, difficulty in going up or down stairs, or limp. The patients are frequently underweight and show general growth disturbance. Pain is not a feature.

The legs are thinned, the reflexes may be hyperactive, and there may be swelling and prominence of the diaphyseal areas of long bones. Tenderness is not prominent. The complete blood count, serum, calcium, phosphorous, and alkaline phosphatase have not been noted to be remarkable.

Roentgen Features

Neuhauser[1] has emphasized the symmetric skeletal distribution of the diaphyses of the long bones and the thickening of the cortex from both the periosteal and the endosteal sides. The epiphyses and metaphyses are normal, and there is an abrupt termination of the lesion in extremities which are relatively long for the individual.

Fig. 9.35. Progressive diaphyseal dysplasia. The diaphysis is widened and the cortex is widened from both periosteal and endosteal sides.

Pathology

Thickening of the periosteum accompanied by alteration of the cortex by bone resorption and accretion results in a change to bone of the cancellous type. The marrow frequently is fibrous and has mononuclear and hematopoietic foci. There is no evidence of the effect of an inflammatory agent. Cartilage formation at the epiphyseal line and conversion to bone in the metaphysis are apparently normal.

Treatment

Some individuals noted to have the disease are able to live full lives without disabling muscular weakness. Some follow a progressive, downhill course. Muscle exercises, including resistive ones to strengthen available musculature, have been of some value. No medication has been proved to alter the course of the disease.

References

1. Neuhauser, E. B. D., Schwachman, H., Wittenborg, M., and Cohen, J.: Progressive diaphyseal dysplasia, *Radiology, 51:* 11, 1948.
2. Riley, C. M., and Schwachman, H.: Unusual osseous disease with neurologic changes, *Am. J. Dis. Child., 66:* 150, 1943.

Infantile Cortical Hyperostosis

This is an infantile disease in which the diaphysis of long bones, the mandible, and the

Fig. 9.36. Involvement of diaphysis of the tibiae and fibulae in progressive diaphyseal dysplasia. Note the symmetry of involvement.

Fig. 9.37. Same case as in Figure 9.36. Three years later the cortex is beginning to have a mottled appearance.

Fig. 9.38. Involvement of mandible in infantile cortical hyperostosis, lateral view.

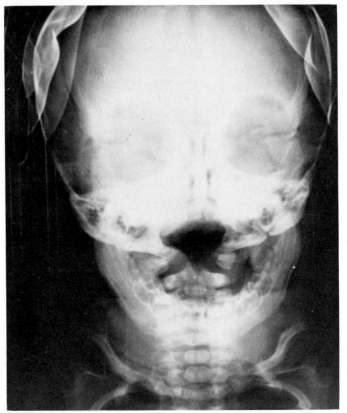

Fig. 9.39. Anterior view of patient seen in Figure 9.38. Clinically, swelling due to this bony reaction may be mistaken for osteomyelitis.

scapula are characteristically involved by the deposition of subperiosteal new bone. It was first reported in the German literature by Roske in 1930, but was brought to American attention principally by Caffey (1939), whose name is sometimes given to this disease. The mandibular swelling, a principal sign, has led to an erroneous diagnosis of osteomyelitis in many cases. The disease occurs in the first 6 months of life and is more common in the male.

Clinical Picture

Swelling about the jaw without heat or redness leads to a suspicion of the diagnosis. Swelling over the scapula is also especially characteristic, but not as frequent. The infant is usually irritable and may have a low grade fever which runs a chronic course. Leukocytosis usually accompanies the fever.

Thw swelling is often tender and asymmetric. The tibia, humerus, and clavicle are often involved in conjunction with the mandible and scapula. The small bones of the hands and feet, along with the vertebrae, are exempt.

Roentgen Picture

Subperiosteal swelling occurs along the diaphysis, usually starting centrally and then spreading throughout the length. It may appear more marked on one side than on the other. The edges of this new subperiosteal bone are smooth; it is laid upon the cortex in layers and separated from it by a thin dark line. In later stages, the subperiosteal new bone and the old

Fig. 9.40. Early involvement of the tibia in Caffey's disease.

Fig. 9.41. Severe involvement with obliteration of bony architecture by bony reaction in Caffey's disease.

cortex are not well delineated from each other. the area of new bone tending to become confluent. The new bone laid down in the scapular region is more masslike and is sometimes confused with tumor. The lesion may be differentiated from osteomyelitis by the fact that the accompanying deep soft-tissue swelling is diaphyseal rather than metaphyseal.

Pathology

Biopsies have revealed the areas of subperiosteal bone formation but have not shown signs of active inflammation. The marrow is often vascular and exhibits fibrosis and activity of cells in the form of osteoclasts. Cultures of these lesions have been sterile.

Treatment

The disease is self-limited; it runs for 10 or 11 months at the longest. It is not affected by antibiotics. The swelling subsides, and the bones appear normal eventually by roentgenogram. The disease is more widespread than osteomyelitis and does not exhibit bone destruction. Scurvy is inappropriate to the age group in which this disease arises. When the bone heals, it does so by widening the medullary cavity so that the cortex lies in the area of bony thickening. As the bone increases in width and length, the developing bone catches up with the increased width created by the disease, so that with sufficient growth the bone is reconstructed.

Reference

1. Caffey, J., and Silverman, W. A.: Infantile cortical hyperostoses, *Am. J. Roentgenol., 54:* 1, 1945.

Osteoid Osteoma

Recognition of the osteoid osteoma lesion followed the publication in 1935 of a paper by Jaffe[1] which revealed its clinical and pathologic characteristics. It is seen as a cause of chronic bone pain in children, adolescents, and young adults. The nature of the lesion is still in doubt. Opinion supports a benign neoplasm, chronic infection, and unusual bone repair. Due to its unusual pathology and difficulty in classification, it has occupied the attention of many

Fig. 9.42. Healing in which the widened shape is maintained and results in a widened medullary cavity. Eventually growth in length and width at the metaphysis will obliterate this evidence of disease. This represents the expected result following Caffey's disease.

writers. Notable reviews were published by Jaffe[2] in 1945 and by Sherman[3] in 1947.

Clinical Picture

The entity is more common in males, and the majority of cases occur in the age group between 6 and 12 years. It is rare in Negroes. The two most common areas of involvement are the tibia and the femoral neck. Involvement of a vertebra is not unusual. Other bones may be involved.

The usual patient is seen because of pain that began insidiously but has lasted for many months. The pain is accentuated at night, is localized, and may be relieved by aspirin. It characteristically has gradually increased in severity until medical advice is sought.

If the osteoma is in the lower extremity, examination frequently reveals an antalgic limp.

Fig. 9.43. Subperiosteal and endosteal ossification in diaphysis of tibia in osteoid osteoma. The area of the nidus is well delineated.

There is usually quite severe atrophy of the soft tissues. A location close to a joint may cause limitation of motion. Superficial locations cause muscle spasm, limitation of motion, and tenderness on palpation of the spine of the involved vertebra. There is no fever and no abnormality of routine blood studies.

Roentgen Examination

The characteristic picture is that of a radiolucent nidus surrounded by sclerosis. There may be a central calcified area within the nidus. Demonstration of the radiolucent center may be quite difficult in the presence of excessive sclerosis. With a cortical location, the periosteum is often raised, and there may be considerable thickening of the bone. Lesions in an early stage of development and causing minimal bony reaction may easily be missed.

Pathology

There is a vascular fibrous tissue stroma which may be quite cellular. Occasional giant cells may be found. Most characteristic is an irregular deposition of osteoid tissue throughout the nidus. Some of the osteoid trabeculae may become bone. Surrounding the nidus are areas of hypertrophic bone, often with intervening fibrous tissue rather than marrow between the layers. There is no evidence of acute or chronic inflammation.

Etiology

Aside from occasional cultured organisms from the group that commonly are thought of as contaminants, there is no evidence that osteoid osteoma is an infection. There is no clinical response to infection and no pathologic evidence of it. Jaffe supports the theory that these are benign neoplasms, but there is no evidence that this "tumor" grows. The nidus is always small.

The lesion may represent repair following trauma which for some reason cannot be carried to its full conclusion. This inhibition excites the outpouring of further bony calcifi-

Fig. 9.44. Osteoid formation from osteoid osteoma.

cation to wall off the defect. The repair under difficulty may be caused by a vascular lesion.

Treatment

The course of mature osteoid osteoma appears to be chronic persistence of the lesion. Some authors have reported cases in which after a period of years the nidus and pain cleared although bony sclerosis was still evident.

The response to surgical removal of the nidus is dramatic and satisfactory. It is appropriate to ensure removal of the essential part of the lesion—the nidus. This is done by inserting drills above and below the area presumed to contain the lesion. An x-ray is then taken in the operating room. When the nidus is demonstrated to lie between the drills, it is removed en bloc.

References

1. Jaffe, H. L.: Osteoid osteoma; a benign osteoblastic tumor composed of osteoid and atypical bone, *Arch. Surg., 31:* 709, 1935.
2. Jaffe, H. L.: Osteoid-osteoma of bone, *Radiology, 45:* 319, 1945.
3. Sherman, M. S.: Osteoid-osteoma (review of the literature and report of 30 cases), *J. Bone Joint Surg., 29:* 918, 1947.
4. Wallace, G. T.: Some surgical aspects of osteoid-osteoma, *J. Bone Joint Surg., 29:* 777, 1947.

Pseudarthroses in Childhood

Pseudarthroses in childhood have various backgrounds. The congenital type is rare by

Fig. 9.45. Congenital anterior angulation of the tibia possibly preliminary to pseudarthrosis.

Fig. 9.46. Diagram of delayed osteotomy used in correcting angulation when bone healing is suspect. (*Left and center*) Initial operation dividing one-half of the involved bone and leaving the mass of bone chips. (*Right*) Second operation dividing the second half of the bone when callus has formed at the first area.

Fig. 9.47. Pseudarthrosis of tibia and fibula with narrowing of bone progressively toward the involved area.

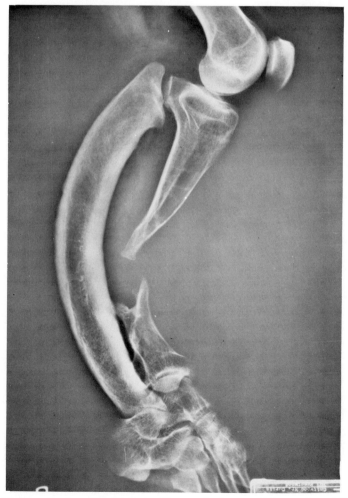

Fig. 9.48. Hypertrophy of the fibula in old unresolved congenital nonunion of the tibia.

Fig. 9.49. (*A*) Anterior angulation of the tibia with beginning narrowing of the medullary canal. (*B*) Implantation of fibula into distal portion of bowed tibia. (*C*) Straightening of the tibia 4 years later. (*D*) Remaining lateral bow of the tibia with nonunion of the fibula.

comparison with other anomalies. They are noted at birth or shortly thereafter and are most frequent in the mid or distal third of the tibia or fibula. Thay have also been found in the femur, clavicle, humerus, ulna, and first rib.

Strangely, some pseudarthroses appear to develop with gradual narrowing of the bone. The medullary cavity becomes sclerosed, and a fracture, either spontaneous or induced, occurs. The end result of both types appears the same. The area of the pseudarthrosis consists of the meeting place of two narrowed bony structures, both of which have lost their medullary cavity. Green and Rudo[4] reported the finding of neurofibroma at the site of the pseudarthrosis, and others have confirmed their finding. How-

Fig. 9.51. Double onlay grafts for pseudarthrosis with double fixation of both proximal and distal end bone chips filling in the area of bone narrowing. (Modified from H. B. Boyd: Congenital pseudarthrosis, *Journal of Bone & Joint Surgery, 30A:* 274, 1948, and J. R. Moore: Autogenous bone graft in the delayed treatment of congenital pseudarthrosis, *Journal of Bone & Joint Surgery, 31A:* 23, 1949.)

Fig. 9.50. Diagram of by-pass cortical graft of McFarland. Bone chips may also be used to fill in the interval between the graft and the parent bone.

ever, in some cases little is noted other than a binding structure of dense connective tissue about the pseudarthrosis.

The area of pseudarthrosis is sometimes bound by a bulbous mass consisting of irregularly distributed cartilage and fibrous tissue. When this is the case, there is no marked narrowing of the bone, but there may be adjacent cystic changes in the bone.

Fig. 9.52. Amputation occasionally may be necessary for failure to achieve union of congenital tibial lesion. Use of the heel as above achieves good end bearing stump without problem of the bone growing through the soft tissues.

Boyd and Sage[2] reported 15 cases of congenital pseudarthrosis of the tibia and noted that 2 presented the microscopic picture of fibrous dysplasia in the tissue between the bone ends. Moore[6] noted that of 178 cases reported from the Shrine Hospitals of North America, 17 were recorded as revealing neurofibromatosis at the site of the pseudarthrosis. Aegerter[1] has suggested that neurofibromatosis, fibrous dysplasia, and congenital pseudarthrosis are in some way related. Fibrous dysplasia here may represent an inability to produce normal bone in one or more areas and a metaplasia into primitive bone. The hamartomatous proliferation of fibrous tissue may lead to a mistaken diagnosis of neurofibroma. Aegerter believes that the fibroblastic masses seen in all three conditions have a common cause, namely, an alteration of the nerve pathways to the areas in which they occur. The alteration may be a neurofibromatous mass or masses in the nerves supplying the area, but the definitive presence of neurofibroma in the bone has not yet been adequately delinated.

The author has seen tibiae, that appeared normal by roentgenogram, go on, after a simple childhood fracture, to develop this lesion. In some, the development of cystlike lesions appears clearly to be a part of the disease; such lesions either inhibit union or threaten union after it is obtained. In these cases, the microscopic picture most closely resembles that of fibrous dysplasia. On the other hand, fractures in children with previously diagnosed fibrous dysplasia have gone on to heal without difficulty.

Treatment

If operation is delayed, considerable overlapping often occurs. In some cases, the bone at the pseudarthrosis narrows, and considerable atrophy of the distal fragment makes reconstruction still more difficult. The author believes, as Boyd does, that operation should be performed as soon as the general condition of the patient is at the optimum. The parents should clearly understand that operative procedures may have to be repeated, and, if union is obtained and cystic changes or narrowing of the bone begin to threaten that union, regrafting should not be delayed.

The history of treatment includes many well thought out and noble attempts to secure union, but many of these attempts have been quite discouraging.

J. R. Moore[7] has described a procedure in which each of the united fragments of the tibia is held by two transfixing pins and placed in an Abbott leg-lengthening apparatus. An os novum type of graft is raised on the opposite tibia and, along with a smaller fibular graft, is used 18 days later to bridge the defect. The pertinent points in technique, as detailed by Moore, are that (1) the bone grafts must overlap the fragments by 2 inches or more, (2) fixation with four pins is essential, (3) the graft is held in position until a well defined medullary cavity has appeared, and (4) the graft should not be delayed more than 18 days.

MacFarland[5] has used two procedures. One is a double onlay graft that was later described again by Boyd. The second is a by-pass graft technique in which a tibial cortical and cancellous graft from the opposite leg is inserted into the proximal and distal tibial fragments. The graft is posterior and does not directly attack the pseudarthrosis. It is so placed that the stress of use is transmitted through it and causes hypertrophy.

MacFarland has favored the by-pass technique rather than the double onlay graft, as he believes the former is more certain to produce a good result.

Charnley[3] has successfully used intramedullary fixation, including tibia and os calcis, along with grafting but without lengthening.

Whatever method is used, the chances of success are slim unless the greatest care is taken to ensure that no fundamental principle in the treatment of nonunion is neglected. Such principles include elimination of infection,

adequate fixation, good soft-tissue coverage, wide bone contact, good general health of the patient, and placement so that the graft will be functional. Once union is secured, regrafting should not be delayed if the bone shows a tendency to narrow in any portion. Gradually increased and protected weight bearing helps to develop the bone.

References

1. Aegerter, E. E.: The possible relationship of neurofibromatosis, congenital pseudarthrosis, and fibrous dysplasia, *J. Bone Joint Surg., 32A:* 618, 1950.
2. Boyd, H. B., and Sage, F. P.: Congenital pseudarthrosis of the tibia, *J. Bone Joint Surg., 40A:* 1245, 1958.
3. Charnley, J.: Congenital pseudarthrosis of the tibia treated by the intramedullary nail, *J. Bone Joint Surg., 38A:* 283, 1956.
4. Green, W. T., and Rudo, W.: Pseudarthrosis and neurofibromatosis, *Arch. Surg., 46:* 639, 1940.
5. MacFarland, B.: Pseudarthrosis of the tibia in childhood, *J. Bone Joint Surg., 33B:* 36, 1951.
6. Moore, B. H.: Peripheral nerve changes associated with congenital deformities, *J. Bone Joint Surg., 26:* 282, 1944.
7. Moore, J. R.: Delayed autogenous bone graft in treatment of congenital pseudarthrosis, *J. Bone Joint Surg., 31A:* 23, 1949.

CHAPTER 10

Metabolic and Generalized Orthopaedic Conditions

HISTIOCYTOSIS X

A solitary eosinophilic granuloma or multiple granulomas in bone and soft tissue, comprising Hand-Schüller-Christian disease and Letterer-Siwe disease, have been considered different manifestations of the same disease process by Tauber (1941) Malloy (1942), and Lichtenstein[6] (1953). Lichtenstein used the term histiocytosis X.

Clinical Features

Cheyne estimated the incidence of this condition as 1:2,000,000 per year. It is most common in the first 4 years of life and equally distributed between the sexes. Approximately one-half the patients will clearly recover. Of those who die, the course is rapidly progressive within 4 years and the vast majority of these come from the infantile group. The age of onset carries a prognostic significance.

Just under 10% will have no detectable bony lesions. Lymph node involvement alone is entirely compatible with survival, but with involvement of the liver one-half of the patients have died. Progressive anemia leads to a poor prognosis. Petechiae and hemorrhage internally appear to play a part in this anemia. Massive marrow replacement is also seen. The lungs may be involved leading to fibrosis and cysts. About 25% of the patients will have a rash not unlike seborrheic dermatitis.

The skull, femur, and spine are the most common sites of skeletal involvement.

Roentgen Features

The spine lesion is one of the causes of vertebral plana or "Calvé's disease." The involvement tends to be in the posterior portion of the vertebrae but progresses to occupy most of the body and, as it does, the body is compressed, loses height, and can become wafer thin.

When a lesion is in a bone it can occupy the metaphysis or diaphysis and only rarely the epiphysis. It is totally lucent within the area it occupies, through destroyed cortex it becomes radiologically visible. The edge is smooth rather than grossly destructive.

The amount of reaction about the lesion is variable from slight to moderate. A considerable amount of periosteal reaction can occur.

Histologic Features

The histiocyte containing eosinophilic cytoplasm is the characteristic cell, with a variable infiltration of eosinophilic leukocytes in addition. These are contained in a granuloma with blood vessels running into the lesion from the periphery.

In Letterer-Siwe disease, the histiocytes are smaller with paler cytoplasm and tend to resemble reticulum cells.

The histocytes accumulate in a cellular lipid. The cholesterol content of the tissues is only raised in the region of these cells, representing a change in cellular metabolism. In Hand-Schüller- Christian disease, the cells are markedly swollen.

When the histocytes are proliferating and accumulating cholesterol, the eosinophils and blood vessels may be less prominent.

References

1. Abt, A. F., and Denenholz, E. J.: Letterer-Siwe's disease: splenohepatomegaly associated with widespread hyperplasia of nonlipoid-storing macrophages; discussion of the so-called reticulo-endothelioses, *Am. J. Dis. Child., 51:* 499, 1936.
2. Avery, M. E., McAfee, J. G., and Guild, H. G.: The course and prognosis of reticuloendotheliosis of bone, *Am. J. Med., 22:* 636, 1957.

3. Christian, H. A.: Defects in membranous bones, exophthalmos, and diabetes insipidus; an unusual syndrome of dyspituitarism, *Med. Clin. North Am., 3:* 849, 1920.
4. Green, and Farber, S.: Eosinophilic or "solitary granuloma" of bone, *J. Bone Joint Surg., 24:* 499, 1942.
5. Lichtenstein, L.: Eosinophilic granuloma of bone, *Arch. Pathol., 37:* 99, 1944.
6. Lichtenstein, L.: Histocytosis X, *Arch. Pathol., 56:* 84, 1953.
7. Lichtenstein, L., and Jaffe, H. L.: Eosinophilic granuloma of bone, *Am. J. Pathol., 16:* 595, 1940.
8. Oberman, H. A.: Idiopathic histiocytosis, *Pediatrics, 28:* 307, 1961.
9. Thanhauser, S. J., *Lipoidoses,* Ed. 3, New York: Grune & Stratton, 1958.

GAUCHER'S DISEASE

Gaucher's disease[3] has been known since its description in 1882. It was thought originally to be a neoplasm. Cushing and Stout[1] in 1926 reported a case involving the hip and causing a marked collapse of the proximal femur and acetabulum. With this case in a woman of 33, the disease was first recognized to involve the bone. It represents a rare familial disorder of lipoid metabolism in which kerosin is deposited in the reticulum cells of the reticuloendothelial system. These cells, which have a typical appearance, are called Gaucher cells, and they may appear in the spleen, liver, lymph nodes, and bone marrow. The disease is most common in Jewish patients. Symptoms are usually noted in childhood and adolescence, but the disease is chronic and only slowly progressive.

The most common area of bone involvement is the lower femur, which is involved in about two-thirds of the cases, and the hip is second in frequency.

According to Schein and Arkin,[5] the skeletal changes are due to infiltration and replacement of the bone trabeculae by kerosin-containing reticulum cells. This infiltration results in linear radiolucent areas that give the bone a characteristic mottled appearance. The cortex tends to become thinned, and the bone to be slightly but not markedly expanded in the metaphyseal area. The expansion is fusiform rather than lobular. Secondary changes may occur, particularly at the hip, where the femoral head may collapse or undergo aseptic necrosis. Pathologic fracture of the femoral neck and a tendency to coxa vara, as well as vertebral involvement and collapse, also occur.

These bone changes in a patient with splenomegaly, hepatomegaly, secondary anemia, hemorrhages, and brown pigmentation of the skin result in the diagnosis of Gaucher's disease. The suspicion can be confirmed by bone marrow biopsy.

Treatment

The care of these skeletal lesions consists of measures to relieve pain and to prevent deformity. Bed rest is indicated during periods of acute symptoms. The hip joint and femoral neck lesions must frequently be kept from the hazards of weight bearing and subsequent

Fig. 10.1. The femoral neck can be weakened to such an extent that a coxa vara deformity gradually develops in Gaucher's disease.

Fig. 10.2. Aseptic necrosis of the femoral head as a complication in Gaucher's disease.

deformity by non-weight bearing splints or, when indicated, by plaster spicas. In the carefully followed case, regeneration of the femoral head and development of more normal bone structure has been observed. Aseptic necrosis of the femoral head has apparently been caused by infiltration of the femoral neck.

References

1. Cushing, E. H., and Stout, A. P.: Gaucher's disease, with report of a case showing bone disintegration and joint involvement, *Arch. Surg., 12:* 639, 1926.
2. Davies, F. W. T.: Gaucher's disease in bone, *J. Bone Joint Surg., 34B:* 454, 1952.
3. Gaucher, P. C. E.: De l'epithelioma primitif de la rate, hypertrophie de la rate sans leucémie, These de Paris, 1882.
4. Milch, H., and Pomeranz, W.: Bone changes in Gaucher's splenomegaly, *Arch. Int. Med., 61:* 793, 1938.
5. Schein, A. J., and Arkin, A. M.: Hip joint involvement in Gaucher's disease, *J. Bone Joint Surg., 24:* 396, 1942.
6. Vaughan-Jackson, O. J.: Gaucher's disease with involvement of both hip joints (case report), *J Bone Joint Surg., 34B:* 460, 1952.
7. Wood, H.: Gaucher's disease with pseudocoxalgia, *J. Bone Joint Surg., 34B:* 462, 1952.

MUCOPOLYSACCHARIDOSES

McKusick has divided the mucopolysaccharidoses into five recognizable states growing out of the cases that have previously been grouped together as Hurler's syndrome. In addition to the urinary mucopolysaccharidoses, metachromatic granules may be found in circulating lymphocytes stained with toluidine blue.

MPS Type I (Hurler's Syndrome)

Type I is inherited as an autosomal recessive disease, with death ocurring at less than 10 years from respiratory infection or cardiac failure. It is marked by progressive mental deterioration, lumbar gibbus, stiff joints, chest deformity, rhinitis, clouding of the cornea, enlarged liver, "gargoyle face," short neck, broad hands with stubby fingers, and splenomegaly.

Roentgen Findings

The findings are those of various aspects of osteochondrodystrophy. In the hands the fifth metacarpal shows this most severe involvement with a hypoplastic terminal phalanx. The proximal phalanges are broadened as are the metacarpal. and both are short.

The vertebrae tend to irregularity—some with beaking. In the dorsolumbar region, a kyphos may be present with a deficiency of the anterosuperior corner of the supporting vertebrae. The intervertebral spaces may be widened.

The diaphysis of the long bones is thickened, possibly WAVY, and with the metaphyseal ends slanted to accommodate coxa valga and genu valgum.

Laboratory Findings

Evidence of chondroitin sulfate B (dermatan sulfate) in the urine is the major finding. Heparitin sulfate is increased, but less so. An acid-albumin turbidimetric test is a suitable scanning device.

MPS Type II (Hunter's Syndrome)

Type II is thought to occur through an X-linked recessive inheritance. The clinical picture is similar to that of Type I, but less severe. Mental deterioration is slower and lumbar gibbus does not occur. Clouding of the cornea is not clinically evident. Patients often live to the 30s, with precocious osteoarthritis of the head of the femur, pes cavus, congestive heart failure, thickened coronary arteries, or pulmonary hypertension. The skin may be grooved, ridged, or nodular. It occurs in 1:200,000 births. X-ray and pathologic features are as for Type I; urinary dermatan sulfate and heparitin sulfate are critical laboratory findings.

MPS Type III (Sanfilippo's Syndrome)

Type III is inherited as an autosomal recessive disease of severe mental retardation but relatively less severe somatic changes. The intellect deteriorates so that by school age

Fig. 10.3. Involvement of the distal femur in Gaucher's disease.

retardation is evident; by the teens it is marked. Clouding of the cornea does not occur. Hepatosplenomegaly is only slight or moderate. Stiffness of the joints is less severe than in Types I or II. Patients may live to the 4th decade. X-rays show minor changes, as in the anterior part of the lumbar vertebrae. The incidence is 1:200,000. An increase in urinary heparitin sulfate is the fundamental metabolic defect.

MPS Type IV (Morquio's Disease)

Type IV is inherited as an autosomal recessive disease. Patients show strikingly dwarfed (truncal) stature, knock-knees, enlarged wrists, misshapen hands, pigeon breast (sternal kyphos), short neck, semicrouching stance, broad mouth, and frequent hernias. Neurologic symptoms may occur from spinal cord and medullary compression; spastic paraplegia is frequent, with respiratory paralysis occurring in late stages. Intelligence may be normal or mildly impaired. All patients, should they reach sufficient age, show corneal opacities and cardiac manifestations such as aortic regurgitation.

Early x-rays of the spine resemble those seen in Type I mucopolysaccharidosis. Later, flattened vertebrae plus osteoporosis can be seen. Late films also show changes in femoral heads and characteristic skeletal lesions. It occurs in 1:40,000 births. Increased keratosulfate in the urine is the fundamental defect.

MPS Type V (Scheie's Syndrome)

In this autosomal recessive inherited disease, the intellect is impaired little or not at all. Stiff joints, clawhands, excessive body hair, retinitis pigmentosa, and corneal clouding may be seen. Stature is normal or low normal, the carpal tunnel syndrome with increased collagenous tissue is frequent, as is aortic regurgitation. Psychosis is seen. X-ray features are unremarkable, but skin, cornea, and conjunctiva show the same histologic changes as observed in Type I mucopolysaccharidosis. The rate of occurrence is unknown. There is increased urinary dermatan sulfate.

MPS VI (Maroteaux-Lamy Syndrome; Polydystrophic Dwarfism)

Occurring through autosomal recessive inheritance, this type shows the chief abnormal-ity of growth retardation, noted at age 2-3 years. Stunting of both the trunk and the limbs is usually present, as well as genu valgum, lumbar kyphosis, and anterior sternal protrusion. There is face abnormality, hepatosplenomegaly is usual, and bony abnormalities are severe. Corneal opacities develop fairly early. Cardiac manifestations are not seen.

X-ray features show long bones with irregular metaphysis and epiphysis slightly deformed, particularly the head of the femur, which may be fragmented, and the upper end of the humerus, which is hatchet-shaped. The distal end of the radius and ulna is oblique, the carpal and tarsal ossification centers are hypoplastic. The vertebral bodies have reduced height. The first lumbar and last dorsal vertebrae are wedge-shaped and posteriorly displaced. Pathology, prevalence, and metabolic defect are as for Type V mucopolysaccharidosis.

References

1. Dorfman, A., and Matalin, R.: The Hurler and Hunter syndromes, *Am. J. Med., 47:* 691, 1969.
2. Fratantoni, J. C., Hall, C. W., and Neufeld, E. F.: Defect of Hurler's and Hunter's syndromes. II. Faulty degradation of mucopolysaccharides, *Proc. Nat. Acad. Sci. U.S.A., 60:* 699, 1968.
3. McKusick, V. A.: The nosology of the mucopolysaccharidoses, *Am. J. Med., 47:* 730, 1969.
4. McKusick, V. A., Kaplan, D., Wise, D., Hanley, W., Suddarth, S., Sevick, M., and Maumanee, A.: The genetic mucopolysaccharidoses, *Medicine, 44:* 445, 1965.
5. Muir, H.: The structure and metabolism of mucopolysaccharides (glycosaminoglycans), and the problem of mucopolysaccharidoses, *Am. J. Med., 47:* 673, 1969.
6. Rubin, P.: *Dynamic Classification of Bone Dysplasias,* Chicago: Year Book Medical Publications, Inc., 1964.

EOSINOPHILIC GRANULOMA

One of the considered diagnosis of a cystlike lesion of bone is eosinophilic granuloma. Such a lesion totally destroys the central area that it occupies. It is most common in the skull but is often seen as an isolated lesion of the long bones. It may be a forerunner of similar lesions of the skeleton, which may be combined with visceral lesions to form the entity known as Hand-Schüller-Christian syndrome. It is much more common in children than in adults.

Pathology

Farber has studied this disease extensively and has concluded that the so-called eosinophilic granuloma represents one variant of a more basic disease process grouped under the general heading of xanthoma. The lesion is a granuloma which appears gelatinous and reddish-yellow on gross examination. Microscopically there are numerous large mononuclear phagocytes with granular to finely vacuolated cytoplasm. Numerous eosinophils are a prominent feature. They may form evident clumps, or they may be scattered diffusely. The more mature granulomas have large, vacuolated mononuclear cells rather than eosinophils.

Roentgen Findings

The contour of the individual lesions is variable in outline but tends to be either oval or round. They are totally destructive; that is, no bone remnants are contained within the area outlined by the lesion. The cortex is not expanded, but it may be destroyed. The edge of the lesion usually appears well outlined and benign; but in some lesions, particularly those in the skull, it is minutely spiculated. The reaction in bone surrounding the lesion consists of minimal increased deposition of bone rather than marked sclerosis.

The lesions are most common in the skull and ribs. Flat bones are predominantly involved. When the bones of an extremity are involved, the area closest to the trunk is the most frequent site. Involvement of the distal

Fig. 10.5. The same patient as in Figure 10.4, 4 weeks following roentgen therapy of the granuloma.

end of the extremities is virtually unknown. There is no particularly predominant site within the long bones.

Clinical Picture

In some reported series, the lesion has been more common in males. The symptoms relate to the area of involvement. Minimal pain and swelling prominent enough to be readily seen are features that bring the patient to the physician. When an area of the skull is involved, swelling is present, often with pain. The swelling is soft and not particularly tender to palpation. Unilateral exophthalmos or periorbital swelling may result from lesions in this area. Long bone involvement is more likely to cause pain.

There is little evidence of generalized illness when the patient is first seen. Loss of weight and anorexia follow multiple severe areas of involvement. The laboratory findings are not remarkable. Lichtenstein and Jaffe noted an eosinophilia in from 4 to 10% of their cases. There may be a mild leukocytosis. The calcium, phosphorus, phospatase, total protein, and blood cholesterol are usually normal.

Differential Diagnosis

Cystic lesions of the bone must be considered. These include solitary bone cyst, giant cell tumor, and benign growth defects. Solitary bone cyst is associated with the epiphyseal line, appears to be derived from it, and is not subject to remodeling. Giant cell tumor occurs in the

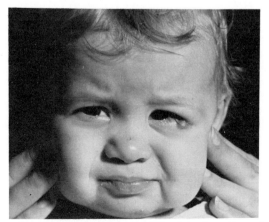

Fig. 10.4. Granuloma involving lateral portion of lower eyelid (eosinophilic granuloma).

Fig. 10.6. Eosinophilic granuloma of the tibia revealing cystlike appearance and total destruction.

tiple myeloma is an adult disease. The differentiation from solitary bone cyst may be impossible except by biopsy.

Treatment

The initial or most accessible lesion is biopsied and diagnosis follows correlation of the patient's examination, laboratory data, history, and gross and microscopic findings. The rapidity with which lesions can appear, and also disappear with treatment, is impressive.

Once the diagnosis is established, the choice between curettage and roentgen therapy depends upon the location of the lesion. Both methods are very efficacious in removing the individual lesions. In areas where other structures, such as epiphyseal lines and ovaries may be affected by roentgen therapy, currettage is favored. The accessibility of the lesions and the gravity of the procedure involved are other considerations.

The course of the patient cannot be predicted at the outset. New lesions may appear while the original lesions are being treated. As long as the entity is confined to bone, the prognosis is good. The ever present possibility of Hand-Schüller-Christian disease should, however, prompt a guarded outlook

early adult age group. Growth defects are usually linear rather than rounded and are not associated with bone reaction.

Osteomyelitis, tuberculosis, and syphilis should be borne in mind. Osteomyelitis is accompanied by clinical and laboratory evidence of infection. When eosinophilic granuloma involves a vertebra, to differentiate it from tuberculosis by roentgenogram may be quite difficult since the abscess shadow associated with tuberculosis may be duplicated by this lesion. Compere has pointed out that eosinophilic granulomas produce the picture of Calvé's disease in the vertebra.

Lesions such as Ewing's tumor and leukemia are ordinarily characterized by an infiltrating type of destruction rather than by the total destruction of an eosinophilic granuloma. Mul-

RESISTANT RICKETS AND OTHER DISORDERS OF CALCIUM AND PHOSPHATE METABOLISM

BY ROBERT KLEIN, M.D.

Patients with resistant or refractory rickets constitute a problem which is so common that all orthopaedic surgeons dealing with children should be conversant with the disease and its manifestations. Indeed, in most pediatric clinics, cases of ordinary vitamin D deficiency rickets constitute only about one-half of the total number of cases of rickets. Unless patients with refractory rickets are discovered early, they become severe orthopaedic problems. In a 5-year span, 6 cases of renal rickets and 3 cases of hepatic rickets were seen. At the same time, there were 20 cases of vitamin D deficiency rickets. There is no point in applying orthopaedic treatment to patients with resistant or other forms of rickets until the metabolic disease is brought under complete control.

Fig. 10.7. Eosinophilic granuloma of the skull with minimal bony reaction.

Fig. 10.8. Eosinophilic granuloma with dark-staining eosinophils distributed over the background of the pale-staining histiocytes.

Therefore, before refractory rickets is discussed as a clinical entity, it is important that the metabolic changes in this and related diseases be considered. No mention of the x-ray changes or the appearance on histologic section of the various forms of rickets will be considered in this chapter, since it is in general correct to state that neither gives sufficient evidence to determine etiology. "Rickets is rickets" when studied by these methods. In patients with vitamin D deficiency rickets, rickets associated with total renal failure, rickets associated with renal tubular disease, and hepatic rickets, therefore, the metabolic and clinical changes must be understood so that the proper diagnosis can be made and adequate therapy carried out.

Some Metabolic Changes in Rickets

The growing infant deprived of any extra-dietary source of vitamin D and kept from sufficient sunlight to manufacture his own vitamin D develops rickets as evidenced by x-ray, clinical, and histologic changes. His serum phosphate is low, and his serum calcium is usually normal or only slightly depressed. Serum phosphatase is very high. Actually his bone phosphatase is also high, but this is not of diagnostic importance. He absorbs calcium and phosphate poorly from the intestinal tract and excretes excessive amounts of phosphate in the urine in the face of low serum phosphate values. When the diagnosis is made and he is in a steady state, the magnitude of his phosphate excretion is not absolutely large. The excretion is, however, relatively great in view of his low serum phosphate level. His tubular reabsorption of phosphate per 100 ml of glomerular filtrate is low. He has an increased aminoaciduria, a decreased citric aciduria, and a depressed citric acid level in his blood. When he is given vitamin D in therapeutic doses, usually less than 5,000 units per day, the first response is increased tubular reabsorption of phosphate. This, coupled with the increased absorption from the gut of calcium and phosphate, leads to an elevated serum phosphate level. The administration of vitamin D also returns the aminoaciduria to normal and elevates the blood citric acid level and the citric acid excretion.

Action of Vitamin D and Parathyroid Hormone

It has been suggested recently that vitamin D acts in this instance by inhibiting directly or indirectly the secretion of parthyroid hormone. This theory explains most of the known facts, but not all of them; it requires ancillary postulations for whose validity there is no evidence at the present time. In any event, when extremely large doses of vitamin D are given to normal subjects or to patients with hypoparathroidism, the vitamin seems also to have a direct renal effect. It increases the renal excretion of phosphate. This action causes a lowering of serum phosphate and, coupled presumably with increased absorption from the gut, leads to an elevation of the serum calcium both in patients with hypoparathyroidism and in normal persons intoxicated with vitamin D. Thus, vitamin D has two different actions at different dosage levels. In ordinary therapeutic doses, the vitamin increases the tubular reabsorption of phosphate and lessens its excretion. In high doses, of the order of magnitude of 100,000 units or more per day, it increases the

renal excretion of phosphate. In addition, the administration of vitamin D at both dosage levels leads to an increased absorption of calcium from the gut.

Parathyroid hormone may elevate serum calcium by directly causing its release from bones. Vitamin D may act in a similar manner, although it has not been proved to do so. Agents lowering serum phosphate tend to raise serum calcium. The lowering of serum phosphates lowers the product of calcium and phosphate ions, and more calcium (and phosphate) are released from the bone until the point of saturation is once more reached. This is an oversimplified theory that has value chiefly as a didactic device. In any event, both parathyroid hormone and massive doses of vitamin D lower serum phosphate by increasing phosphate excretion, and they raise serum calcium. Both of these agents, in excessive amounts, lead to hypercalcemia and intoxication. The clinical aspects of vitamin D intoxication will be discussed subsequently.

Action of Vitamin D in Refractory Rickets

There is no evidence, at present, to show whether the patient with vitamin D refractory rickets has any other defects in metabolism beyond a quantitative inability to respond normally to the usually required doses of vitamin D. On the other hand, there is no proof that he responds to a large dose of vitamin D in the same fashion as a normal patient responds to small doses of vitamin D. The one bit of evidence against this latter possibility is the response of the patient with vitamin D refractory rickets when he is given a sufficient amount of vitamin D. His rickets heal, but his serum phosphate still remains lower than normal although it does rise above the pretreatment level. This response might be explained by postulating a dissociation between the two mechanisms of vitamin D action in the patient with resistant rickets. The patient with vitamin D refractory rickets may require a much larger dose of vitamin D to benefit from the ordinary antirachitic action. At the same time, however, he may require no more than the normal subject to obtain the direct renal effect of the vitamin, which is the phosphate-losing action. Therefore, with the large doses used to heal his rickets, the effect upon calcium absorption goes on normally, but the increased phosphate reabsorption, which would ordinarily take place, is partially counteracted by the directed renal phosphate-losing action of vitamin D in massive doses.

Renal Phosphate-Losing Rickets

Other diseases that have some of the same metabolic features as refractory rickets include the deToni-Fanconi syndrome, in which there is hyperphosphaturia, hyperaminoaciduria, glycosuria, and albuminuria. This is basically a disease of the renal tubules that, like other related syndromes, causes an acidosis often accompanied by the secretion of an alkaline urine. The other renal tubular diseases are difficult to separate from each other and from the deToni-Fanconi syndrome. There is a considerable argument about whether the syndrome of cystinosis is a universal concomitant of the deToni-Fanconi syndrome, occurs as part of it sometimes, or is an entirely separate syndrome. The relationship of the deToni-Fanconi syndrome to the other renal tubular diseases producing rickets is vague. These other diseases have been characterized by Gardner as having renal base-losing lesions produced by a defect either in the reabsorption of bicarbonate or in the ammonia-forming mechanism. These syndromes sometimes are associated with loss of much fixed base including calcium in the urine. They are characterized by a depressed serum pH and the secretion of an alkaline urine. Patients with these syndromes vary greatly in the number of symptoms had and the combinations in which these symptoms occur. They may show all the signs of the deToni-Fanconi syndrome, including the acidosis, phosphaturia, aminoaciduria, albuminuria, glycosuria, polyuria, and often the inability to reabsorb bicarbonate or the failure to manufacture ammonia, or they may show any combination of these symptoms and be classified under various eponyms.

The aminoaciduria in these diseases, and the changes in citric acid metabolism, also tend to disappear with the administration of vitamin D. Vitamin D decreases the phosphaturia, but complete healing of the rickets frequently occurs only after large amounts of fixed base have also been given to reduce the acidosis. In general, the rickets in these patients is not so

severe as to require orthopaedic care. Perhaps this is because many of the patients die early with uremia. It is more likely, however, that the rickets is mild because the children grow very poorly and very slowly; rickets does not often become apparent in the child who does not grow. However, these children do suffer from osteomalacia, as does the nongrowing adult who is on a diet poor in calcium and is deprived of vitamin D and sunlight over a long period of time. Milkman's syndrome may occur in the later stages of these diseases, but it occurs more frequently in patients with the syndrome to be described next.

Renal Phosphate-Retaining Rickets

Patients with a diagnosis of "renal rickets" contrast with those whose rickets is associated with a tubular defect. This group of patients is made up of individuals with chronic renal failure of diverse etiology. They present all the classic signs of chronic renal failure. They have the continuing acidosis and a retention of nitrogenous products marked by a high blood urea nitrogen or nonprotein nitrogen. In addition, they have a high serum phosphate due to

Fig. 10.9. Siblings with bowing of the tibia in resistant rickets.

depressed glomerular filtration. This is frequently accompanied by a lowered serum calcium. This situation stimulates a relative or secondary hyperparathyroidism, and in a certain number of these patients, the calcium is maintained at normal levels. Coincident with this, these patients develop signs of rickets. The excess parathyroid hormone apparently causes the release of calcium and phosphate from the bones, which leads to a failure to calcify osteoid and prevents the orderly change of growing cartilage to bone. This failure is characteristic of rickets. The acidosis contributes to the leaching of calcium from bone. Furthermore, there may be an excessive loss of fixed base, including calcium, in this condition, which also contributes to the development of the rickets.

Rickets associated with renal tubular defects, such as the deToni-Fanconi syndrome, frequently progresses to chronic renal failure. It is then impossible to distinguish from members of the group usually characterized as "renal rickets'." The nomenclature is difficult and at times confusing. However, a diagnosis of "renal rickets" usually implies rickets associated with chronic renal failure and signs of uremia in greater or lesser degrees. On the other hand, patients with specific tubular defects have no elevation of nonprotein nitrogen or of blood urea nitrogen and do not exhibit the signs of renal failure until late. The syndromes should perhaps be regrouped as renal phosphate-losing rickets and renal phosphate-retaining rickets or according to some similar classification. Admittedly there would be an overlap between the groups due to the phosphate-losing patients who develop uremia.

Fig. 10.10. Rachitic changes of the distal femoral epiphyseal line. This area, which is subject to most active growth, may be the only one to show changes and the last to regress.

Hypercalcemia

Nearly all of the changes of vitamin D intoxication are duplicated by hyperparathyroidism. The latter seems to present a higher incidence of gross renal calculi and bone rarefaction, but this may merely be a question of chronicity. When large doses of vitamin D are given by error, or for their pharmacologic action on the kidney, and there is an overdose, the first sign associated with hypercalcemia is usually anorexia followed by constipation. Polyuria, accompanied by polydipsia, occurs very early. The specific gravity of the urine is low, and if the child is very small or for some reason fluid cannot be ingested, dehydration may supervene. Nausea occurs early. As the toxic symptoms progress, there are vomiting and signs of nervous system change, accompanied by irritability, lethargy, and extreme flaccidity of the muscles. Apparently, there is actual relaxation of the ligaments because these children frequently have hyperextendable joints in addition to flaccidity. As the disease progresses, metastatic calcification may occur. Further signs of renal damage are produced, which may result from calcification of the kidney parenchyma, although presumably the earlier renal changes are merely a further manifestation of the pharmacologic, or direct toxic, action of the high doses of vitamin D upon the kidney. The renal damage may be manifested by an elevated blood nonprotein nitrogen, but this elevation, in part, may be due to the dehydration that occurs. The skin becomes sallow and pale and mottles readily. At times it is dry and coarse. Metastatic calcification occurs elsewhere throughout the body. It is apparently easily found just beneath the conjunctival tissues by slit-lamp examination.

Hypercalcemia may also be produced by immobilization of even the normal child or adult. The child, of course, is less likely to be immobilized unless he is actually in a cast or some other restraining device. However, even the comparative immobility of enforced bed rest will lead to a release of calcium and phosphate from the bones of the normal individual. This may at times be great enough to produce a hypercalcemia sufficiently severe to cause symptoms. Renal stones may be produced by the attendant hypercalcemia.

Refractory Rickets

Refractory rickets is an inherited disease. In the clinic of Children's Hospital at Pittsburgh, three generations of several families are being followed. The disease can be traced back in these and other families for several more generations. This kind of incidence is common in all such clinics. There are, of course, instances in which no previous manifestations of refractory rickets can be found. If the disease is not recognized in the parent, the children are often considered to have rickets of the usual variety, and indeed, when first seen, they are not distinguishable in any way from patients with vitamin D deficiency rickets. When they are then treated for this condition with the usual dose of vitamin D, however, no response is obtained and the rickets progresses to severe deformity.

It is important to arrest the disease in female patients before deformities of the pelvis are so great as to make delivery impossible except by cesarean section. In the older generations, the usual story is that the mother who was affected has had several cesarean sections. If the disease is not recognized, osteotomies are frequently performed for the correction of the deformity of the legs, but vitamin D is not administered except in small doses. The osteotomies heal well and the immediate results are good, but unless the rickets is controlled, the deformities recur as severely as before. It is imperative that the diagnosis be made early so that deformities can be prevented. If deformities have already occured, the disease must be brought under control before reparative surgery is performed.

If, when the patient is first seen, he is about 1 year of age, there is no way to distinguish refractory from vitamin D deficiency rickets. The physical findings in both conditions are the same, as are the chemical findings of a normal or slightly low serum calcium, a low phosphate, and an elevated phosphatase. One is suspicious of the refractory disease when the patient with rickets is several or more years of age. Suspicion is confirmed when the patient fails to respond to the ordinary therapeutic dose of vitamin D. At this time it is necessary to consider the various types of rickets that do not respond to the usual treatment. These are genetic refractory rickets and the rickets of the various renal diseases. (Chronic hepatic disease and spruelike syndromes can also cause rickets, but the etiology should be apparent whenever the rickets occurs and will not be considered here.)

Renal function should be investigated first. Simple urinalysis is exceptionally helpful in these diseases. The patient with the deToni-Fanconi syndrome has albuminuria and glycosuria, although the latter is not constantly present and repeated specimens must be analyzed. The specific gravity of urine in all these diseases tends to be low and somewhat fixed. Since the normal obligatory urinary solute excretion, coupled with the low specific gravity, characteristically produces polyuria, an accurate measurement of urinary output is helpful. Where this is not possible, measurement of fluid intake is useful. At times, the polyuria and polydipsia are enough to cause these patients to be diagnosed as suffering from diabetes insipidus. The excretion of alkaline or nearly neutral urine in the presence of systemic acidosis in practically pathognomonic of one of these renal tubular diseases, even if more sophisticated measurements, such as estimations of the ability to form ammonia or of bicarbonate reabsorption, cannot be done. Therapeutic responsiveness is of no help in distinguishing between the various renal tubular diseases and genetic refractory rickets. Both will respond to high doses of vitamin D, although the renal disease may require the additional administration of various alkalies.

When the diagnosis of genetic refractory rickets has been made, the treatment should be carried out with large doses of vitamin D given by mouth, although it can be administered intramuscularly. Unless there is some failure or difficulty in gastrointestinal absorption such as occurs in the celial syndrome, there is no reason why vitamin D should not be given by mouth. Since the required dose of vitamin D may be anywhere between 50,000 and 1,000,000 units per day, the initial dose is chosen arbitrarily. A dose near the lowest end of the therapeutic range should be used, of course. It has been our custom to start with either 50,000 or 100,000 units a day, depending upon the size of the child. If there is no response as evidenced by rising serum phosphate or falling serum phosphatase, or later by roentgen evidence of healing of the rickets, the dose is raised. We check the serum calcium, phosphate, and phosphatase values at least once a month and at the same time do a routine urinalysis plus a Sulkowitch test on the urine. An increasing Sulkowitch response should be a warning of hypercalcemia and is a help in avoiding serious signs of vitamin D intoxication. Healing occurs in the absence of a normal serum phosphate. Usually the serum phosphate is maintained just over 3 g per 100 ml. This is higher than in the untreated patient but lower than in the normal growing child. Apparently, this level of serum phosphate represents a balance between the pharmacologic effect of vitamin D in huge doses—that is, phosphate excretion—and the more physiologic effect of small doses of vitamin D in the normal child—that is, the increased tubular reabsorption of phosphate. When rickets is controlled, the serum calcium value rises to normal, if it has been slightly low, and the serum phosphatase falls within the normal range. It is difficult, at times, to maintain healing of the rickets without permitting a small amount of hypercalcemia. The patient with controlled refractory rickets usually has a higher serum calcium than he had before treatment; frequently it is at the top of the normal range or just above.

The goal in the treatment of refractory rickets is to find a dose of vitamin D that is large enough to maintain healing of the rickets and yet does not produce enough hypercalcemia to cause symptoms. In our clinic the average well controlled patient with refractory rickets has a normal serum phosphatase but a calcium that averages 11 g, and a phosphorus just slightly more than 3 g, per 100 ml. The slight hypercalcemia which he may occasionally have gives no symptoms. He eats well, gains weight, and in general looks much healthier than before. His color is improved. Although these patients begin to grow more rapidly after they are treated, even the treated patient tends to grow less rapidly than the normal, and as adults they tend to be short. However, they are not as dwarfed as the grotesque untreated patient with this disease. The excessive lordosis and potbelly of rickets disappear with treatment and, as growth continues, the visible and reparable stigmata of rickets disappear.

If treatment is carried out late, when the child is in a period of slow growth, not all of the bony deformities disappear under vitamin therapy. Patients who are not seen during the period of rapid growth, then, are the ones who require osteotomy and other surgical care. One statement that must be taken with a grain of salt is that these patients can never grow to a normal height. In this clinic, all of the patients were diagnosed after some deformity was visible, and they had already lived beyond the rapid phase of growth of the first 2 years of life; yet the possibility remains that their eventual height will be normal if they were treated early enough.

When these patients are brought in for osteotomy, the vitamin D therapy should be stopped; if it is not, immobilization tends to give them hypercalcemia, which may produce serious kidney damage. After the osteotomy, the patient should be mobilized as soon as possible. Exercises, or as much motion as possible, should be carried out even when the child is in bed in a cast. Renal stones in these patients are avoidable.

After such a patient has been controlled for a period of time, the dosage required usually is fairly stable. Fluctuations occur, however, with changes in the rate of growth, with changes in diet, and perhaps with variations in the amount of sunlight that the patient is exposed to. Until the dosage is well stabilized, these patients should be seen at least once a month for at least 1 year. The interval between visits may then be steadily increased until they are seen only once or twice a year, if good rapport is maintained with the family and if the family can be relied upon to report any changes early. After growth is stopped, the administration of vitamin D may be cut, probably entirely, without any real harm. Further bony deformities will not develop, although some degree of osteomalacia will exist. However, it has been our habit to give a large but reduced dosage of vitamin D to our adult patients. We have no evidence of the value of this treatment.

SCURVY

BY ROBERT KLEIN, M.D.

The incidence of scurvy in pediatric practice, like that of congenital syphilis, has become minimal. The very rarity of these diseases in some ways makes them important to the pediatric orthopaedic surgeon. Just as undiagnosed cases of congenital lues are referred to

him because of the pseudoparalysis that the disease induces, so the patient with scurvy may be erroneously considered to have primary bone or joint disease because of his refusal to sit or stand and because of the attending bony tenderness. When these diseases were more common they were less likely to be misdiagnosed and referred to orthopaedic care. With the widespread use of orange juice and ascorbic acid pills or drops, the few cases of scurvy seen are the result of ignorance or neglect.

The most common cause of scurvy in our experience has been the boiling of orange juice; the second most common cause has been iatrogenic. The doctor has, usually mistakenly, supposed that the baby's eczema is due to the orange juice ingested. The mother is told not to give the orange juice, but adequate provision for its replacement by ascorbic acid is not made. Breast milk ordinarily contains an adequate amount of ascorbic acid unless the mother has been on a deficient diet herself. Cow's milk contains approximately one-fourth as much vitamin C as human milk, and after pasteurization the content falls even lower.

The disease occurs most often in children between the ages of 6 months and 1 year. Scurvy should be considered by the orthopaedic surgeon when he is asked to see an infant in the latter half of the first year of life who refuses to stand or perhaps to sit, evidences tenderness in his legs, or keeps his legs drawn up in a frog leg position. As the disease progresses, the areas of tenderness may be swollen. These areas usually are the ends of the long bones. The specific symptoms are caused by the subperiosteal hemorrhages that these infants have much more often than hemorrhage elsewhere. Typical petechiae may be seen on the skin. Orbital hemorrhage occurs on rare occasions. Very rarely is there any bleeding from the gums, probably because of the paucity of teeth at this age. The gums are said to be swollen at times and sore, but we have not observed this condition. The symptoms of bone pain are also produced by the infractions that occur around the epiphyses. As the disease progresses, the patients develop beading at the costochondral junctions, which is very difficult to distinguish from the beading of rickets. In the best defined and well advanced cases, the beading is much sharper and firmer, and frequently it is tender.

Fig. 10.11. Massive ossifying subperiosteal hemorrhage in scurvy. Halo-like epiphyses are seen.

Once the diagnosis is considered, there usually is no trouble in establishing it. On close questioning a history of the lack of intake of vitamin C is usually obtainable, even though the mother may have thought that she was giving it. The differential diagnosis from trauma must be made although everday trauma probably is the cause of the infractions and some of the hemorrhages that children with scurvy have. However, in the patient with scurvy, these changes are produced by a much less severe trauma than that needed to produce the same

changes in a normal child. Moreover, the normal child who has undergone trauma usually does not have symmetric lesions.

The pseudoparalysis that some of these patients have suggests poliomyelitis, but its true nature is usually easily ascertained. The painful swellings about the joints may suggest osteomyelitis, suppurative arthritis, or even some rheumatoid process. However, these patients are much younger than patients with a rheumatoid disease usually are. The symmetric diffuse distribution of the scorbutic lesions helps rule

Fig. 10.12. Healing 1 year later of the same femur seen in Figure 10.11.

out most of these processes. Scurvy is frequently accompanied by elevation of temperature, which also might suggest infection. However, leukocytosis does not usually occur in uncomplicated scurvy. The pseudoparalysis seen in congenital·lues usually occurs at a younger age and is accompanied by other manifestations of syphilis. The distribution of the lesion in infantile cortical hyperostosis is unlike that of scurvy; the former lesion involves the mandible, clavicle, and ulna chiefly. There is no hemorrhage, and the x-ray is diagnostic of this syndrome.

Finally the roentgen appearance of the bones should confirm the diagnosis of scurvy. The most dramatic changes on x-ray are those of early healing when new bone begins to form beneath the elevated periosteum. The periosteum itself is, of course, invisible on x-ray. At times the new bone has suggested bony tumor. More important for clinical diagnosis is the ground glass appearance of the long bones due to the atrophy of the trabeculae. The cortex is thin, and the zone of provisional calcification shows increased density beneath which is a zone of rarefaction. Infractions occur at the epiphyseal line, and actual displacement of the epiphyses is occasionally seen. Calcification is seen in the form of spurs that extend out from the epiphyseal line where the periosteum is attached.

There are various tests that prove the diagnosis of ascorbic acid deficiency. Perhaps the best of these is the measurement of ascorbic acid content of the buffy coat of centrifuged blood.

Treatment of the disease, which is simple, requires the administration of ascorbic acid. Very rarely is any local treatment of the extremities needed. The normal contours of the bones may not be seen by x-ray for many months, or even for a year, if the subperiosteal bone formation has been great. The subsidence of symptoms with treatment is very rapid and very dramatic.

HEMOPHILIA

BY RONALD HILLEGASS, M.D.

History and Incidence

Although the inherited condition which we recognize as hemophilia was described in the

Talmud, the term hemophilia was first used in 1828 by Hopff, a student of Johann Schönlein of Wurzburg. He used this term to describe an inherited condition which resulted in prolonged bleeding following an injury. Hemophilia has since been specifically identified to result from a specific disorder in the clotting mechanism of blood. The most frequent disorder is a deficiency in Factor VIII (AHF) which occurs in approximately 85% of hemophiliacs. This is also called Type A hemophilia. Type B hemophilia occurs in approximately 15% of patients and results from a deficiency of Factor IX (PTC) of the clotting mechanism. This is also called Christmas disease. Both Type A and Type B hemophilia are sex-linked recessives. In addition, some people feel that Factor XI

Fig. 10.13. Knee flexion contractures in patient with hemophilia.

Fig. 10.14. Pseudotumor formation in hemophilia.

(PTA) deficiency is also a type of hemophilia, or Type C. This may occur in either males or females. Von Willibrand disease also has a deficiency Factor VIII. This disorder has an increased bleeding time, a decreased platelet efficiency, and is present in both males and females. The male has the defect in the clotting mechanism in Factor VIII and Factor IX deficiency. The female serves as the carrier for this sex-linked recessive condition. Cases have been reported in a female who has inherited the recessive trait from both her parents.

The incidence of hemophilia is approximately 8:10,000 live births, or 1:3,000-4,000 live male births. It is estimated that there are between 5,000 and 7,000 severe hemophiliacs in the United States. The importance of this is apparent when clinical evidence of arthritis is present in 89% of hemophiliacs by the age of 10.

Etiology

The patient has a genetic inability to manufacture the appropriate clotting protein, a β-globulin. Bennet and Huehns[3] had described three types of deficiency. The first is no biologic activity and no Factor VIII-type protein. The second condition is no biologic

activity but normal amounts of a Factor VIII-like protein. The third mechanism is a low level of Factor VIII activity with a normal amount of a Factor VIII-type protein. Absence of a significant level of the protein clotting factor results in a hemophiliac condition.

Clinical Picture

The patient with hemophilia usually presents with prolonged bleeding from either a relatively minor injury or a surgical procedure, or has spontaneous bleeding. This may be overt bleeding or may be a hemarthrosis or bleeding into the soft tissue. Prolonged and frequent bleeding into the joint may result in changes similar to those seen with degenerative arthritis. The involved joint may be painful and have a limited range of motion. The joints most frequently affected are the knees, the elbows, and the ankles. Pseudotumors may occur from bleeding around the periosteum and neurologic deficit may occur following pressure on a nerve from soft-tissue bleeding. The severity of bleeding is dependent on the amount of clotting factor present in plasma. If this is less than 1% of the normal level, the patient has severe hemophilia which is manifested by frequent spontaneous bleeding into the joints and soft tissues. With a level of 1-5%, moderate hemophilia is present with less bleeding and fewer chronic articular changes. When the level reaches 5-30%, the hemophilia is mild and spontaneous hemorrhages are rare.

Diagnosis

The diagnosis is suspected when there is a history of spontaneous or traumatic inappropriately excessive bleeding. If this is accompanied by a family history of hemophilia and the patient is a male, the diagnosis is more likely. Laboratory investigation must be conducted by someone who is familiar with the clotting mechanism. Only in the most severe cases is the blood clotting time prolonged and abnormal. It may be normal with a very small percentage of clotting factor. The kaolin-cephalin clotting time is a more sensitive test for Factor VIII or Factor IX deficiency. It is positive for moderate and severe deficiencies of Factors I, V, VIII, IX, X, XI, and XII. In routine coagulation studies, a thromboplastin generation test (one-stage pro-

Fig. 10.15. Changes in knee of 9-year-old boy with hemophilia. (*A*) Note marked synovial hypertrophy. (*B*) Anteroposterior view shows early enlarged epiphysis of left femur, hyperemia with increased radiolucency of epiphysis, irregularity of subchondral bone, and early cyst formation of left lateral femoral condyle. Note widened intracondylar notch. (*C*) Lateral view of left knee showing bony fusion 3 years later. Contour of epiphyses still visible. (*D*) Anteroposterior view of left knee at age 15. Well organized bony fusion. (*E*) Lateral view of left knee at age 15 demonstrating bony fusion. Note absence of "squared" patella. (*C-E* are on p. 582.)

thrombin time) may be the best method to diagnose hemophilia. This may be present with a deficiency of Factor V and with a thrombocytopenia. The most refined test is the identification of the percentage of the plasma level of a specific factor. This can be readily done for both Factors VIII and IX.

Diagnosis by radiologic methods is nonspe-

Fig. 10.5*C-E*

582

Fig. 10.16. Lateral view of knee in 13-year-old hemophiliac. Note the "square" appearance of the lower pole of the patella.

cific for hemophilia. Boldero and Kemp[4] in 1966 emphasized this. They listed three different types of x-ray changes which may be present. The first type occurs as a result of hemorrhage into the joint cavity. The second type occurs as a result of immobilization and from the reactive hyperemia which may follow hemorrhage. The third type are changes that occur in specific areas. Hemorrhage may result in a distention of the joint cavity. When this becomes more chronic, synovial thickening may be present. Subarticular erosions, reduction of the cartilage space, and collapse of the subchondral bone may be noted. Cystic changes and osteophytes will ultimately occur.

With loss of mobility and hyperemia, muscle wasting and bone atrophy occur. The trabecula pattern becomes lattice-like. Osteoporosis develops and frequently Harris lines are present. Enlargement of the epiphysis develops as a result of hyperemia.

Certain anatomical areas have demonstrated changes that are considered characteristic of hemophilia. The two most frequently noted are squaring of the lower pole of the patella and widening of the intracondylar notch of the distal femur. However, both of these may occur with other conditions, especially juvenile rheumatoid arthritis.

As the disease progresses and the joint becomes destroyed and contractures occur, deformities of the joint may develop. Frequently there is posterior subluxation of the tibia at the knee. Premature closing of the epiphyseal plate occurs. Bony ankylosis is occasionally noted.

Fig. 10.17. Severe destruction in 31-year-old adult. Knee subluxed and without normal configuration.

Fig. 10.18. Lateral view of elbow in 11-year-old child. Note irregularity of subchondral bone and radiolucency in metaphyseal region as a result of hyperemia.

584

Pathology

The pathology within the joint is a result of hemorrhage with an inflammatory reaction. This causes proliferation of the synovium. A synovial hemosiderosis may develop because of the phagocytosis of the synovial cell. Fibrin becomes adherent to the synovial surface as the disease progresses. Subsequently, intrasynovial adhensions may develop. These decrease the size of the joint cavity and joint motion. Cartilage fibrillation develops and the cartilage subsequently becomes destroyed. Hoaglund[8] was able to produce these changes in the laboratory. Stonyen described three types of tissue changes found in hemophilia. The first is a hypertrophic change which is angiomatous with vascular proliferation. Subsequently, a hypertrophic synovitis is present which is pigmented from a deposit of iron from phagocytosis. Finally, the synovium is hypertrophied and there is much fibrous material in the synovium. The synovial tissue undergoes involution with fibrosis. Ultimately, there may be pieces of cartilage and bone contained within the synovium.

The articular cartilage changes are similar to those seen in joints with degenerative arthritis except that they tend to be more diffuse. Initially there is a granular change in the cartilage surface with fibrillation and pitting. Erosion of the cartilage surface is finally noted. This is secondary to the chronic inflammatory process and enzyme destruction. Bone cysts ultimately develop which communicate with the joint and are lined by synovial tissue.

Treatment

The basic aspect of treatment is the replacement of the deficient clotting factor. Until 1965, plasma was used for this. It was noted that fresh frozen plasma was needed and that serum did not contain the deficient factor. Prolonged storage of plasma resulted in the destruction of Factors VIII and IX. In 1965, Factor VIII was isolated as a cryoprecipitate of plasma. It can be stored at -20 to $-30°C$. The remainder of the plasma may be used for other blood products. The availability of this material reduces the problem of overload of cardiovascular system which developed when plasma was used for replacement. Cryoprecipitate does not

Fig. 10.19. Ankle showing severe destructive changes as adult. Note loss of cartilage at tibiotalar joint and bony fusion at talofibular joint.

contain Factor IX. In addition, the potency is variable, which makes replacement more difficult.

More recently, other types of precipitates have been developed. These have the advantage of being stable at $-4°$ and may be stored in a dried fashion. In addition, they have a known potency for a particular dose. However, they are more expensive. Factor XI is also available as a concentrate.

The cryoprecipitate used for Factor VIII replacement normally has 125 to 140 units per bag. The concentrates have 250 units per bottle. The Konyne replacement for Factor IX has 500 units per bottle. One unit is equal to the amount of AHF or PTC in 1 ml of fresh normal plasma. This can be used to calculate the replacement. Factor VIII has a half-life of approximately 12 hr and Factor IX has a half-life of approximately 18 hr.

For an acute early hemarthrosis, a hematoma in a nonhazardous area, or external bleeding, a single dose of factor replacement sufficient to bring the level to 30% of the normal plasma volume is usually sufficient to control the hemorrhage. If more is needed, it should be given every 6 hr for the first 24 hr and then every 8 hr. Factor IX replacement may be given every 8 hr for 24 hr and then on a 12-hr program. For more severe bleeding, a hemarthrosis that has developed more than 12 hr previously, or hematuria, the level should be raised to greater than 40%. Also, a level of greater than 40% is indicated when surgery is to be performed. With severe joint bleeding, the replacement may be necessary for 2-4 days. For a fracture, it is usually advisable to give factor replacement for at least 3 days. With major surgery, 10-14 days of therapy may be indicated. With deep soft tissue operations, this may need to be extended. In addition, when a physical therapy program is being initiated following surgery or immobilization, it may be necessary to replace the factor to prevent a hemarthrosis from developing.

It should be noted that there is a risk of hepatitis at any time that blood products prepared from poor plasma are used. Therefore, a recurrent testing program for Australian antigen may be advisable.

Approximately 10% of people who have a deficiency of Factor VIII and have had replacement therapy develop an antibody to their replacement factor. This is a 7S-immunoglobulin (IgG) and acts as an inhibitor. This may be suspected when a patient fails to improve with a dose of factor replacement that is normally effective. Medical judgment must be exercised in treating a patient with this problem. Our approach has been to replace the factor with a very high dose and to treat the patient with steroids during this period. In this situation, factor replacement is used only if there is a significant threat to the patient's life or to the possible loss of a limb. More frequently, when this problem is present and a patient suffers a bleeding episode, he is treated by immobilization alone.

Pain is a frequent problem with a bleeding episode in hemophilia. It should be emphasized that aspirin is contraindicated. It impairs platelet function and may cause and prolong a bleeding episode. Any aspirin-containing product should be avoided. Other adjuncts of therapy, such as immobilization, aspiration, and steroids will be discussed under the specific problems.

Specific Problems

Acute Hemarthrosis

The clinical features of an acute hemarthrosis are swelling, pain secondary to the distention of the joint, warmth as a result of the bleeding into the joint, and loss of motion. Frequently, the patient will have observed symptoms such as an aching sensation or stiffness prior to the onset of these more familiar characteristics. The treatment program must stop the bleeding and eliminate the pain. Ultimately, the joint function must be maintained and restored and an effort should be made to eliminate chronic joint changes. As has been observed in our clinic recently, the early factor replacement is the most critical single feature in achieving these objectives. Early factor replacement maintains good joint function and minimizes the therapeutic effort. In a study of Ali,[1] 72% of 39 patients treated at the onset of their bleeding episode returned to full activity in less than 1 week, 52% of 44 patients who were not treated initially within the first 8 hr were unable to return to full activity for greater than 2 weeks. In following these patients, 1 of 39 had joint deformities if treated early, compared to 1 of 7 who did not have early factor replacement. The efficacy of early factor replacement has been demonstrated. It allows the patient to resume early activity and minimizes chronic joint deformities.

In our clinic, many of the patients are on a home program for factor replacement. The patient or parents have been instructed in the intravenous administration of the factor. At the earliest sign of bleeding into a joint, the clinic is notified and a consultation is obtained with the physician. If the physician feels that it is appropriate, the factor may be given at home. This early replacement has resulted in fewer chronic problems from an acute hemarthrosis.

Immobilization is a second essential aspect of treatment. Splinting the joint decreases the metabolic demand and allows for more rapid reabsorption of the hemarthrosis. It also decreases the amount of pain which the patient experiences. The immobilization is done initially in the position of comfort. Complete splinting is continued for approximately 24-36 hr or until the severe pain has subsided. The splinting should continue while effusion and warmth are present in the joint except for range of motion exercises which should be performed 3-4 times a day. Splinting may be discontinued when the warmth and effusion have subsided and a previous range of motion has been obtained. At that time, full activity may be allowed. If the patient had a limited range of motion at the time of onset of the acute hemarthrosis, it may be advisable to continue splinting for the weight-bearing joints and to use night splints for a few additional weeks.

Aspiration represents a controversial adjunct of therapy. In our clinic, aspiration is performed only if the joint is markedly painful. It is rarely done. If aspiration is to be attempted, the patient must be additionally treated with factor replacement. A theoretical argument for aspiration is that, by diminishing the amount of blood within the joint, there is less material to be phagocytized and therefore the breakdown products and lysosomal release with its cell destruction of the joint cartilage is minimized. In addition, the pressure within the joint which can also cause cartilage destruction is minimized. The arguments against aspiration are that bleeding will tend to occur even after the joint is aspirated and that there is increased trauma to the patient and a risk of infection.

The application of ice to the joint at the time of the acute hemarthrosis may have a beneficial effect and we use this in the first 24-36 hr.

Steroids have been suggested for use on either a local or systemic basis. The evidence that this significantly alters the course is inadequate at the present time. The local injections have a risk of infection. Systemic steroids have other potential problems, and since their efficacy has not adequately been demonstrated, these are not used at the present time in our clinic.

Hyaluronidase injected into the joints has been advocated. This is not being done at the present time.

It should be emphasized again that aspirin is contraindicated as an analgesic in hemophilia. Despite a continued warning, it is not infrequent that aspirin is used by the unweary in caring for the hemophiliac patient.

Muscle and Soft-Tissue Bleeding

After hemarthrosis, bleeding into the muscle and soft tissue is the second most common problem encountered in caring for the hemophiliac patient. With an acute bleed episode into muscle or soft tissue, the treatment is similar to that used in an acute hemarthrosis. Early factor replacement is indicated. Immobilization should also be used. This should be done in a position of comfort. Subsequently, the splinting should be corrected to prevent the development of a joint contracture. Aspiration is not indicated. Fibrosis of the muscle may occur as a result of bleeding within the muscle tissue. This may result in a muscle which has diminished excursion and power. Other problems which occur with acute bleeding in the soft tissue are nerve involvement, a compartmental syndrome, and a pseudotumor.

Nerve involvement is most likely secondary to external pressure on the nerve. This usually results in neuroproxia which takes 2-3 weeks to recover. Occasionally axonotmesis may occur which requires 6-12 months to repair. The bleeding causes a sudden increase in pressure on the nerve. It frequently starts a day or two following the onset of bleeding. The femoral nerve is most commonly involved although the median, ulnar, and tibial nerves have also been reported to be affected.

Compartmental syndromes may occur, although they are rare despite the frequency of massive soft-tissue bleeding. They most frequently occur as a Volkmann's ischemia of the forearm or in the anterior or posterior compartments of the calf. These may develop rapidly and, if they occur, can require a surgical fasciotomy to prevent muscle necrosis. This may represent a surgical emergency in the treatment of hemophilia.

A pseudotumor may develop as a result of bleeding under the periosteum or occasionally within the bone substance itself. This results in pressure on the bone and the surrounding soft tissue. The clinical picture of this may cause it to mimic a sarcoma or osteomyelitis. Progressive enlargement may occur and ultimately result in skin necrosis, ulceration, infection, and hemorrhage. The x-ray picture shows bone destruction with a surrounding soft-tissue mass. Peripheral sclerosis is seen rarely. The initial treatment of a pseudotumor is factor replacement and immobilization. If this does not respond, surgical incision and drainage are indicated.

Chronic Synovitis and Arthritis

Despite ideal therapy, many patients develop chronic synovitis and changes similar to those of degenerative arthritis. Steroids have not been shown to be helpful in this problem. Radiation therapy, which has been tried, may allow malignant degeneration. Results are accumulating which favor the use of a synovectomy for

Fig. 10.20. Progression of pseudotumor cyst of os calcis. (A) Sixteen-year-old boy. Note marked soft-tissue component; (B) 3 months later. Soft-tissue component notably decreased; (C) and (D) (opposite page) 6 months later, after onset noted in (A); (E) (p. 590) 2 years after (A).

chronic hemophiliac synovitis (Storti[14,15]). Many of these have been shown to have no recurrence on a 3-year follow-up. It should be emphasized that synovectomy in a child is a difficult procedure because it does require the patient to participate in the rehabilitation. This is often difficult for a child with a painful joint following surgery.

Joint contractures are frequently present. Serial cast correction with a Quingel or wedging

Fig. 10.20C and D

cast may be used. Precautions should be taken to restore the gliding motion of the joint. Frequently the tibia is subluxed posteriorly on the femoral condyle and may be hinged in its subluxed position. Significant contractures may require posterior capsulotomy in an effort to get the knee in a weight-bearing position. It should be emphasized that a joint in the lower extremity must be in a position to bear weight.

The degenerative arthritis changes which occur in the hemophiliac may be treated as degenerative arthritis in other areas. Most of the treatment will be performed on the adult rather than a child. It should be noted that arthrodesis

Fig. 10.20E

must be considered very carefully because of the potential problem of arthritic changes in other joints. An arthrodesis may increase markedly the stress placed on another diseased joint. With good control of the clotting mechanism, surgery may be performed in a hemophiliac as it is on a patient with degenerative joint changes. The increased risk of bleeding should not be a contraindication to surgery which can maintain or restore joint function to the patient. It should be emphasized that in the rehabilitation following surgery factor replacement may be necessary to prevent a recurrent bleeding episode.

Leg length evaluations should be performed in children who have chronic synovitis. The premature epiphyseal closure on one side may result in a leg length discrepancy which may aggrevate arthritic changes at a later date.

Preventive Treatment

With the advent of home factor replacement and the ability to treat an acute hemarthrosis earlier, the need for bracing has decreased. Bracing still is indicated in children who are subjected to repeated trauma and who lack the maturity to assist in caring for their joint function. It may also be indicated that children who have developed a chronic joint problem where it is felt that surgery is not indicated at the present time and protection is necessary. However, bracing is being used less frequently

with the availability of early factor replacement.

A good physical therapy program must be emphasized. These people have a tremendous need for maintaining good muscle function to help protect a joint. Development of a good quadriceps muscle has, without question, eliminated the frequency of acute hemarthrosis.

Since hemophilia represents a deficiency in a distinct clotting factor, the ideal treatment program would allow for replacement of this on a routine basis such as is used in managing a diabetic patient with insulin. At the present time, this is an expensive procedure. It has been tried in a number of centers. These patients are able to lead a full life with a normal physical and psychologic development. The patient is more likely to attend a regular school and participate in gainful employment. The joints remain better than those which are treated only when they have a bleeding episode. Analysis of this type of treatment has shown that it is less expensive than treatment of a hemophiliac only when he has a bleeding episode. It minimizes the requirement for hospitalization and intensive therapy. The ultimate cost to society could be reduced if this type of treatment is made available.

References

1. Ali, A. M., Gandy, R. H., Britten, M. I., and Dormandy, K. M.: Joint hemorrhage in hemophilia; is full advantage taken of plasma therapy? *Br. Med. J. 3:* 828, 1967.
2. Bennett, B., and Ratnoff, O. D.: Detection of the carrier state for classic hemophilia, *N. Engl. J. Med., 288:* 342, 1973.
3. Bennet, E., and Huehns, E. R.: Immunologic differentiation of three types of hemophilia and identification of some female carriers, *Lancet 2:* 956, 1970.
4. Boldero, J. L., and Kemp, H. S.: The early bone and joint changes in hemophilia and similar blood dyscrasias, *Br. J. Radiol., 39:* 172, 1966.
5. Dallman, P. R., and Pool, J. G.: Treatment of hemophilia with factor VIII concentrates, *N. Engl. J. Med., 278:* 199, 1968.
6. Day, A. J.: Orthopaedic management of hemophilia, *American Academy of Orthopaedic Surgeons Instructional Course Lectures,* Vol. 20, pp. 15-19, St. Louis: C. V. Mosby Co., 1971.
7. George, J. N., and Breckenridge, R. T.: The use of Factor VIII and Factor IX concentrates during surgery, *J.A.M.A., 214:* 1673, 1970.
8. Hoaglund, F. T.: Experimental hemarthrosis; the response of canine knees to injections of autologous blood, *J. Bone Joint Surg. 49A:* 285, 1967.

9. Kasper, C. K., Dietrich, S. L., and Rapaport, S. I.: Hemophilia prophylaxis with Factor VIII concentrate, *Arch. Intern. Med., 125:* 1004, 1970.

10. Kisker, C. T., Perlman, A. W., and Benton, C.: Arthritis and hemophilia, *Semin. Arthritis Rheum., 1:* 220, 1971.

11. Rabiner, S. F., Telfer, M. C., and Fajardo, R.: Home transfusions of hemophiliacs, *J.A.M.A., 221:* 885, 1972.

12. Rudowski, W. J., and Ziemski, J. M.: Extensive surgical procedures in patients with hemophilia, *Surg. Gynecol. Obstet., 135:* 571, 1972.

13. Seeler, R. A.: Hemolysis due to anti-A and anti-B and Factor VIII preparations, *Arch. Intern. Med., 130:* 101, 1972.

14. Storti, E., Traldi, A., Tosatti, E., and Davoli, P. G.: Synovectomy; new approach to hemophiliac arthropathy, *Acta Haematol., 41:* 193, 1969.

15. Storti, E., Traldi, A., Tosatti, E., and Davoli, P. G.: Synovectomy in haemophiliac arthropathy, *Schweiz. Med. Wochenschr., 100:* 2005, 1970.

16. Van Creveld, S.: Prophylaxis of joint hemorrhages in hemophilia, *Acta Haematol., 45:* 120, 1971.

RHEUMATOID ARTHRITIS IN CHILDREN

Children with severe metabolic disease due to rheumatoid arthritis become a problem in the maintenance of life. Enlargement of the liver and spleen, anemia, and severe malnutrition are overriding problems here. The functioning of their extremities often becomes a secondary problem in their care. However, good principles in the maintenance of joint function can be followed simultaneously with their general medical care so that the child who survives the onslaughts of a metabolic disturbance is not left hopelessly deformed and crippled for activity in life. In the care of the whole child, the concept that the musculoskeletal system is part of that whole child is often ignored. From the following description of rheumatoid arthritis, which is commonly seen in children without marked metabolic disturbance, the principles of maintenance of function, prevention of deformity, and rehabilitation may be employed in treating the child with metabolic disease as well.

Age and Sex Incidence

The average age at onset in our series was 5.7 years, but synovitis began in 1 child age 6 months and the oldest was 15 years. It did not matter whether the onset led to monarticular, oligoarticular arthritis, or if it was polyarticular eventually, the average age at onset was 5.9 years, 5.8 years, or 5.9 years—all very similar.

On the other hand, patients who would be classified as having Still's disease were significantly different with an average age at onset at 2.0 years, ranging from 1 to 4 years of age.

There was no female predominance of the type evident in rheumatoid arthritis in the adult. The entire series was divided into 54.7% female and 45.3% male. Only the oligoarticular group had a 2:1 female ratio.

Mode of Onset

Although 50.5% of the patients were found at onset to have involvement of a single joint, only 8.6% remained with a single joint in the course of their disease. Of those who began with two or three joints (31.6% of the total) affected, few members progressed to further involvement and remained finally at 27.4%. Only 15.4% of the total group began with four

Table 10.1. Spectrum of Disease in 117 Arthritic Patients

Table 10.2. Joints Involved within 3 Months of Onset

	No. PTS.	PERCENT OF PATIENTS
CERVICAL SPINE	30	
SHOULDER	16	
ELBOW	25	
WRIST	46	
FINGER JOINTS	50	
HIP	16	
KNEE	88	
SUBTALAR JOINT	43	
ANKLE	20	
FOOT	35	
TEMPOROMANDIBULAR	35	

Table 10.3. Erythrocyte Sedimentation Rate (Corrected)

TYPE	No. PATIENTS	NORMAL ↑20mm/h	SLIGHTLY ELEVATED 20-30mm/h	MODERATELY ELEVATED 30-40mm/h	MARKEDLY ELEVATED ↑40mm/h
MONARTICULAR ARTHRITIS	10	4 (40 %)	4 (40 %)	2 (20 %)	0
OLIGOARTICULAR ARTHRITIS	32	11 (34.4 %)	8 (25.0 %)	3 (9.4 %)	10 (31.2 %)
POLYARTICULAR ARTHRITIS	70	15 (21.4 %)	22 (31.4 %)	25 (35.7 %)	8 (11.4 %)
STILL'S DISEASE	5	0	1 (20 %)	2 (40 %)	2 (40 %)
ALL PATIENTS	117	30 (25.6 %)	35 (29.9 %)	32 (27.4 %)	20 (17.1 %)

or more joints and systemic signs. However, this group progressed to involve 59.4% of the total with polyarticular involvement.

Where the mode of onset differed from the final outcome, the change took place in the first 3 months.

Systemic Manifestations

Systemic manifestations often preceded the joint symptoms by many months. Fever, rash, fatiguability, malaise, anorexia, weight loss, iritis, lymphademopathy, and splenomegaly all represented systemic involvement. Subcutaneous nodules were found in 2 patients as compared to approximately 20% as found in adults.

Fatigue, malaise, anorexia, and weight loss tended to be closely associated with the magnitude of the fever in the children in this series. These manifestations are rarely seen in the monarticular group and only occasionally in the oligoarticular group. Lymphadenitis was found in 30 patients and only in those whose involvement was severe with multiple joints or Still's disease. One patient with polyarticular involvement and who was operated on for acute appendicitis had marked mesenteric lymphadenitis. Splenomegaly was found only in those severely ill. Fever was present in over 80% of all patients early in the disease; 47% had low grade to moderate fever (37-40°C) and 36.8% not marked febrile episodes over 40°C. The fever was intermittent. In monarticular involvement, fever was absent in 60% of the cases. Febrile episodes progressed in frequency to involve 100% of the cases of Still's disease.

Rash was present in 32.5% of all the patients in the series at onset. Good has described the rash as being characteristically a nonpruritic, erythematous, macular or slightly maculopapular eruption of the trunk, neck, or extremities. None of the monarticular patients had a rash.

Rheumatoid Arthritis without Metabolic Involvement

This type of arthritis seen in children has been designated "pauciarticular arthritis" by Green. The majority of affected children are less than 4 years of age. The involvement in the presence of generally good health varies from one to several joints. The anomaly affects females almost twice as commonly as males. The duration of joint swelling varies from several months to many years and averages approximately 3 years.

Clinical Picture

A well child notes pain and swelling of gradual onset about a major joint, most commonly the knee. Almost half of the children are affected in only one joint. In addition to the knees, the ankles, elbows, and hips are commonly involved. Two- and three-joint involvement is almost as common as single-joint involvement. In children with multiple-joint involvement, the wrists and subtalar joints also become sites of the disease.

The joint is warm and painful, and its motion is limited in all planes to varying degrees, according to the acuteness of the synovial inflammation.

Fluid is readily palpated in those joints that are easily available, such as the knee, ankle, and wrist. It is readily aspirated with a small-gauge needle, such as a No. 22 or 23, and it appears

Fig. 10.21. (A) Onset of multi-joint arthritis principally involving both hips and knees. (B) Diminished density of the bone about the major joints and extensive soft-tissue swelling 1 year later. (C) Subluxation of the hip with continued involvement 2 years later. (D) Osteoarthritis secondary to the onset of rheumatoid arthritis, 10 years later. Narrowing of the joint cartilage space and a cyst of the acetabulum are seen. (C and D are on p. 594.)

slightly cloudy. The polymorphonuclear cells are markedly increased over the normal 6% of the total cell count; they form the principal cell. The total white cell count is usually at least several thousand. The mucin is of only fair quality when it is precipitated with acetic acid. The joint fluid content of sugar is usually approximately 20 mg below the blood sugar level.

The sedimentation rate is moderately elevated. The latex fixation test is usually negative, as are tests for the febrile agglutinins. The C-reactive protein test may be positive.

Children who pass to full-fledged metabolic rheumatoid arthritis usually do so in the first 6 months after the onset of the initial joint swelling. This is a rare rather than a common occurrence.

Treatment

Once the presence of absence of metabolic disease has been determined, the problem becomes one of keeping the child a functioning individual in the home and at school and, at the same time, protecting and maintaining the function of the joint until the disease has run its course.

Rest usually brings the joint to a stable condition without tenderness, heat, or fluid in 2-4 months. Thereafter, increased activity may irritate the joint once again, and a considerable period, often of several years' duration, passes before the child can resume full normal activity. Bed rest alone takes the child out of normal contacts, and absolute fixation of the limb leads to myotatic contracture. Cortisone therapy is a two-edged sword; it quiets the joint but leads to metabolic complications. The undeformed child having full motion of the joint and attending school and home activities, yet keeping the joint at rest, appears to represent the ideal solution. In order to attain any success with the rest portion of this program, one must use a bivalved cast that the child can remove in order to exercise the limb, yet still be contained on a rest regime. Prior to establishing all phases of the child's life as fully as possible, those features of his joint disease which may limit his activity permanently must be overcome. Injection of the joint with Hydrocortone or similar substances has not

Fig. 10.21C and D

been of permanent value in our cases; usually the fluid in the joint recurs after several weeks.

Correction of Deformity

Traction is indicated to overcome deformity and restore motion. The initial traction must be applied in line with the deformity if muscle spasms are to subside. As the spasms subside, the joint is brought progressively further and further into a corrected position. As motion is regained, that portion of the joint limited by muscle spasm is overcome. The spasm that remains is due to myotatic contracture, or occasionally to actual intra-articular adhesions or deformity. A common situation complicating the correction of knee flexion contractures

Fig. 10.22 (*Left*). Rheumatoid arthritis originally with systemic symptoms. The residuals of the disease for this patient are limited motion at the major joints and foot deformities. Bilateral limitation of motion at the hip produces a particularly disabling gait.

Fig. 10.23 (*Right*). Swelling limiting the outline of the knee joint capsule in rheumatoid synovitis of the knee.

is posterior subluxation of the tibia; in this situation, although the leverage action of the lower leg allows rotation about the knee joint axis, the hamstrings prevent the gliding of the tibia forward with extension. Active contractions of the limb musculature are encouraged while the child is in traction.

In order to overcome the most rigid portion of the contracture, several possible regimes are now resorted to:

1. The child may be placed in warm water. The limb is floated, and active guided motion is used to achieve further joint range and in-

creased muscle function. In the intervals between these baths, the child remains in traction.

2. A bivalved cast is made at the point of maximal possible correction of the joint. The limb is removed from the cast several times daily for active guided motion, during which the child usually lies on his side so that the arm is supported against the pull of gravity and the insecurity and consequent muscle spasm it engenders. As correction is gradually accomplished, a new bivalved cast taking up the amount of correction achieved is made.

3. For the last few degrees of correction,

Fig. 10.24. Mucin of good quality precipitates as a soft, well formed clump of material that does not break up into shreds.

wedging type casts may be used. They are the least preferable mode of therapy since the joint is fixed during this period and pressure on cartilaginous surfaces may be great. They are sometimes necessary in resistant situations, but they should be used for no longer than several weeks. Following the correction of deformity, a bivalved cast to maintain the correction is made.

Bivalved Cast Routine

Once the joint has regained full motion and is no longer deformed, the bivalved cast ensures lack of weight bearing and is a mode of controlling the child's activity at home. It is removed at least twice daily for ½-hr periods. During this time, the child remains recumbent but carries the joint through a full range of motion and actively uses the flexor and extensor muscles without resistance.

With crutches and bivalved casts, the child may leave bed, attend school and home activities, and see his friends. Once the inflammation has completely subsided—that is, when there is no evidence of heat, tenderness, or fluid and the sedimentation rate has returned to normal—removal of the cast may be considered. It is usually well to be ultraconservative in order to avoid recurrence.

Once the child has been 1 month without the bivalved cast and with no evidence of recurrence, partial weight bearing with crutches is begun. A three-point gait is used for involvement of a single extremity and a four-point gait when both extremities are involved. If during the next interval between visits to the physician (usually 4 weeks) there is no recurrence, activity is increased partially and the crutches are discarded. During another period, the joint muscles are exercised on a progressive resistance routine in order to overcome atrophy.

Synovectomy in Childhood—Rheumatoid

The children who are brought to the point of consideration of synovectomy are principally those who have failed to respond to conservative therapy and whose general physical condition appears unaffected by the disease.

The major joint under consideration for synovectomy is the knee. In general the involvement in other joints is minor. Considerable soft-tissue thickening is evident at the knee and the soft-tissue component is major compared to the fluid distension of the joint.

Anxiety in both the child and parents is apparent, as the swelling has persisted despite non-weight bearing with repeated substance and recurrence.

When the synovectomy is performed a definite plan of action must be outlined to the parents. A gentle manipulation is often necessary at 3 weeks postoperatively, and, when done, 90° of flexion should be achieved.

The synovectomy is done anteriorly removing the suprapatellar pouch. The child is immobilized in a long leg plaster for 10 days and then placed in split Russell traction. At 3 weeks if 90° of flexion have not been achieved, a gentle manipulation under anesthesia is done. The traction is continued for 1 week, followed

Fig. 10.25. Here a manikin is used to illustrate split Russell traction in line with the deformity. Note that the foot of the bed is elevated for countertraction and that perineal straps aid in maintaining the position of the child. The knee sling is under the proximal tibia to prevent posterior subluxation as the flexion deformity is decreased. The sling is pulled at a posterior angle of about 20°. A foot board prevents the weights from catching on the bed. A rubberized bumper on the head upright prevents damage to hospital walls.

by a bivalved cast with the knee in 10° of flexion. The child is sent home with the cast removed twice daily for flexion and extension exercises. After several months this can be discontinued but partial weight bearing with crutches persists until the swelling at the knee subsides on both flexion and weight bearing. An operated joint such as this, once a good functional joint is achieved, is not the seat of a recurrence of rheumatoid arthritis.

Regimen of Therapy

A review of 117 patients has been carried out. The methods of treatment for the patients of this series could be divided into six categories. Of these 50% were seen medically only, 30% were seen chiefly by orthopaedic surgeons, and 20% had a combined approach. The more mild the disease the greater the tendency to be followed by the medical clinician, whereas the more severely affected patients tended to be followed by orthopaedic surgeons alone or with their medical colleagues.

The conservative orthopaedic approach consisted of traction, active exercises, the use of splinting and crutches. Fifty percent of all patients received either salicylates alone or salicylates with conservative orthopaedic measures. Sixteen patients received no treatment after their initial diagnosis. The other regimens of therapy were almost equally distributed between those receiving corticosteroids (13.7%), undergoing synovectomy (11.1%), or synovectomy and debridement (10.2%).

Comparison of Therapy

If all 117 patients are grouped together, the trend to more aggressive treatment of the more severely involved is evident.

No treatment was the regimen received by 16 patients. Their natural history was quite similar. Predominantly they had oligoarticular or polyarticular involvement. Many were severely ill and became well after a 1-6-month period. Fifteen of these patients were in the excellent or good category at follow-up.

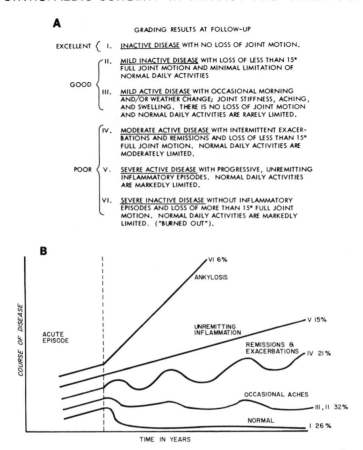

Fig. 10.26. (*A*) A follow-up study of 117 patients with juvenile rheumatoid arthritis with an average follow-up of 8.3 years used the criteria and classification listed. The study was done by Stanley Kampner, M.D. (*B*) Course of rheumatoid disease.

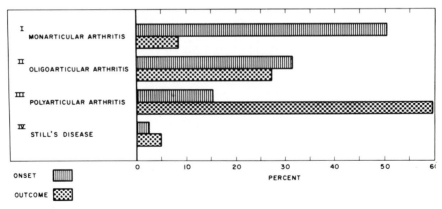

Fig. 10.27. a study of this bar graph reveals that while a large number of patients started out with monarticular arthritis, a large number soon went on to multiple joint involvement. And those who started with polyarticular arthritis were soon joined by others from the group with a minimal number of joints involved.

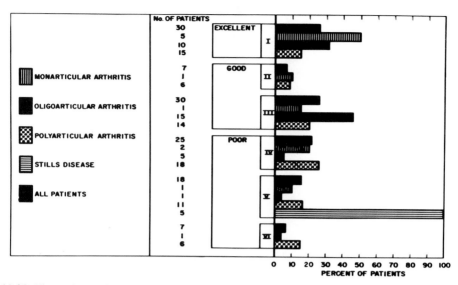

Fig. 10.28. The patients with monarticular arthritis tended to have good to excellent recovery, whereas those with polyarticular arthritis and Still's disease tended to end up in the poor category.

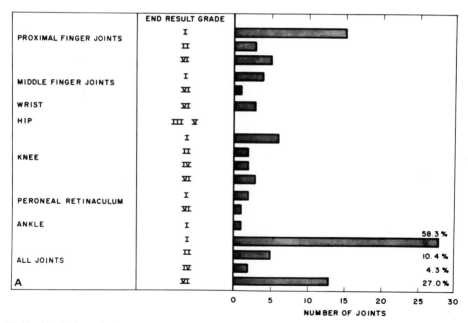

Fig. 10.29. (*A*) Patients having synovectomy alone got considerably more relief from the surgery than those patients having synovectomy and debridement (*B*) (p. 600) obviously necessitated by considerable joint destruction.

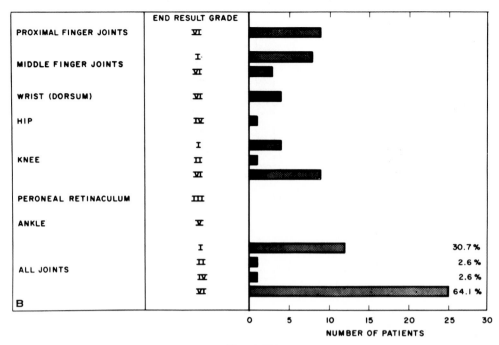

Fig. 10.29*B*

No. PATIENTS	TYPE	PATIENTS TREATED	I	II	III	IV	V	VI
			30	7	30	25	18	7
10	MONARTICULAR ARTHRITIS	0 / 0%						
32	OLIGOARTICULAR ARTHRITIS	1 / 3.1%			1			
70	POLYARTICULAR ARTHRITIS	12 / 17.1%		1	1	2	8	
5	STILL'S DISEASE	3 / 60%					3	
117	ALL PATIENTS	16 / 13.7%	0	1	2	2	11	0
			EXC.	GOOD		POOR		

Fig. 10.30. Patients treated with corticosteroids had little else in the way of therapy and ended up largely in the poor category.

Of 32 patients receiving only salicylate therapy, 19 had excellent or good results and 13 poor.

Salicylates combined with orthopaedic care, in more severe types of disease, was the therapy in 25. Fifteen were classified as having excellent or good results and 10 patients had a poor end result.

Long term corticosteroid therapy was given to the more severely involved patients and the end results showed little improvement.

Of 16 receiving corticosteroids only 3 had good results, with 13 in the poor category. Of the 13 poor results, 11 continued to have florid disease. The only death in this series was a child treated with corticosteroids for 2 years who died with an overwhelming infection.

In patients who had severe involvement with

No. PATIENTS	TYPE	PATIENTS WITH NO TREATMENT	I 30	II 7	III 30	IV 25	V 18	VI 7
10	MONARTICULAR ARTHRITIS	1 10%		1				
32	OLIGOARTICULAR ARTHRITIS	6 18.7%	4	1	1			
70	POLYARTICULAR ARTHRITIS	9 12.9%	4		5			
5	STILL'S DISEASE	0 0%						
117	ALL PATIENTS	16 13.7%	8	1	6	1	0	0
			EXC.	GOOD		POOR		

Fig. 10.31. Patients having no therapy ended up quite well and were almost exclusively in the excellent to good category. They obviously appeared to need less clinically, but some had polyarticular involvement.

frequent inflammatory episodes or progression in remitting disease, there were 13 who underwent synovectomy and 12 who had synovectomy and debridement.

Thirteen of the 15 patients in the synovectomy group had an excellent or good result, and 5 of the 12 patients in the synovectomy and debridement group who had a similar outcome spoke well for these procedures, but the only individuals with a Grade VI result were also from those surgically treated. With conservative or medical regimen of therapy, there were only Grade IV and Grade V included as a poor end result.

Surgical intervention appears to have no middle ground, being either very good or very poor as an end result.

References

1. Bywaters, E. G. L., and Ansell, B. M.: Monarticular arthritis in children, *Ann. Rheum. Dis., 24:* 116, 1965.
2. Calabro, J. J., and Marchesano, J. M.: The early natural history of juvenile rheumatoid arthritis; a 10-year followup of 100 cases; *Med. Clin. North Am., 52:* 567, 1968.
3. Cassidy, J. T., Brody, G. L., and Martel, W.: Monarticular juvenile rheumatoid arthritis, *J. Pediatr., 70:* 867, 1967.
4. Edstrom, G., and Gedda, P. L.: Clinic and prognosis of rheumatoid arthritis in children, *Acta Rheum. Scand. 3:* 129, 1957.
5. Edstrom, G.: Rheumatoid arthritis and Still's disease in children; survey of 161 cases, *Arthritis Rheum. 1:* 497, 1958.
6. Eyring, E. J.: Synovectomy in juvenile rheumatoid arthritis, *J. Bone Joint Surg., 53A:* 638, 1971.
7. Fink, C. W., Baum, J., Paradies, L. H., and Carrell, B. C.: Synovectomy in juvenile rheumatoid arthritis, *Ann. Rheum. Dis., 28:* 612, 1969.
8. Griffin, P. P., Tachdjian, M. O. and Green, W. T.: Pauciarticular arthritis in children, *J.A.M.A. 184:* 23, 1963.
9. Kampner S. L., and Ferguson A. B., Jr.: Efficacy of synovectomy in juvenile rheumatoid arthritis, *Clin. Orthop., 88:* 94, 1972.
10. Kampner, S. L., and Ferguson, A. B., Jr.: Juvenile rheumatoid arthritis; disease course and comparison of therapeutic regimens, *J. Bone Joint Surg., 53A:* 1029, 1971.
11. Laaksonen, A. L.: A prognostic study of juvenile rheumatoid arthritis. Analysis of 544 cases, *Acta Paediatr. Scand., 166* (Supp.): 1966.
12. Lindbjerg, I. F.: Juvenile rheumatoid arthritis; followup of 75 cases, *Arch. Dis. Child., 39:* 576, 1964.
13. Ragan, C.: Intermittent Hydrarthrosis, pp. 755-758, *in* Hollander, J. L. (ed.): *Arthritis and Allied Conditions,* Philadelphia: Lea & Febiger, 1966.
14. Steinbrocker, O., Traeger, C. H., and Batterman, R. C.: Therapeutic criteria in rheumatoid arthritis, *J.A.M.A., 140:* 659, 1949.
15. Still, G. F.: On a form of chronic joint disease in children. *Med.-Chir. Tr., 80:* 47, 1897.
16. Sury, N.: *Rheumatoid Arthritis in Children: A Clinical Study,* Copenhagen: Munksgaard Publisher, 1952.
17. Wissler, V. H.: Subsepsis allergica, *Helv. Paediatr. Acta, 13:* 405, 1958.

GENERALIZED AFFECTIONS

Fibrous Dysplasia

Fibrous dysplasia is a disease entity which may involve one or many bones. It may be combined with abnormal pigmentation of the skin, precocious sexual development, and early skeletal maturation. Still other endocrine-based abnormalities may be present, and there may be various combinations of effects and areas of bony involvement in any one case.

The disease appears to be a developmental defect. It is most common in childhood but may occur in adults; the adult lesion tends to be monostotic. It is a widespread anomaly of skeletal development that ranks next to multiple exostoses in incidence. It is more common in the female.

Clinical Picture

The disease may exist in various forms from the clinical point of view. It appears possible to divide it into three general types.

I. Involvement of Single Bone. The lesion is usually insidious in its onset unless a weight-bearing bone is involved, in which case it may lead to pain and limp. Rib, clavicle, maxilla, tibia, or femur have all been involved in this monostotic form which comprises approximately one-third of the reported cases. Limitation of joint motion may be present should areas such as the femoral neck be involved. Expansion of the bone and local tenderness may be evident on examination. A pathologic fracture may first bring the patient to medical attention.

II. Lesions in Several Bones. Skin pigmentation of the café au lait type may or may not be present. About 35% of the 90 cases in the literature summarized by Lichtenstein and Jaffe[1] showed a noticeable cutaneous pigmentation.

III. Multiple Lesions. Pigmentation of the skin and precocious puberty mark these cases, which represent the most severe form of the disease. Cases in which the lesions tend to

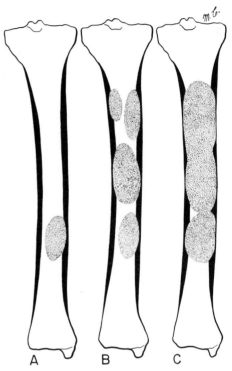

Fig. 10.32. The development of fibrous dysplasia in bone. In *A* and *B*, the single lesion is followed by multiple foci. At *C* the lesions have coalesced to give the scalloped appearance of the cortex that is characteristic of fibrous dysplasia.

Fig. 10.33. Fibrous dysplasia of femur and tibia.

Fig. 10.34. Appearance of the femur in 35-year-old woman. Femur shows multiple foci, widened medullary canal, and is scalloped; (A) anteroposterior view of proximal femur, (B) lateral view of distal femur.

Fig. 10.35. Replacement of medullary cavity contents in bone by proliferating fibrous tissue and osteoid in fibrous dysplasia.

remain unilateral may be regarded as less severe than those in which the lesions are widespread. The more severe forms are found in very young children and infants, and involvement of the skull is common. This form of disease may lead to serious deformities and crippling, and there may be repeated pathologic fractures in the past history.

Only the female appears to be subject to precocious pubert with this disease. Rarely hyperthyroidism has also been found to accompany the bone lesions. The laboratory findings have usually been within normal limits except that the serum alkaline phosphatase has occasionally been elevated beyond that expected for the age.

Roentgen Findings

Areas of decreased density appear in the bone. The involved area has a ground glass appearance which decreases the contrast with the surrounding bone and aids in distinguishing the lesion from a single bone cyst. The lesion spares the epiphyses.

With growth the cortex may become attenuated and expanded. As involvement becomes more generalized, the entire long bone reveals the thinned cortex and fine trabeculae somewhat reminiscent of osteogenesis imperfecta. There may be bone deformity secondary to previous fractures. Generalized involvement of the bone, rather than localized cystlike areas, may become the most striking feature. Rapid extension of the condition is not characteristic. Indeed many localized lesions have been observed to be dormant for years.

Sclerosis of any marked degree about the lesions is not characteristic. In the generalized disease, the base of the skull may appear sclerotic, however. There is, in addition, replacement of normal contrasting bone by areas of "ground glass" appearance in varying portions of the remainder of the skull.

Pathology

Lichtenstein and Jaffe [1] have been responsible for clarifying the pathology of this condition under the heading fibrous dysplasia. When a localized lesion is approached surgically, the cortex overlying it is frequently found to be eroded from the medullary side and more vascular than normal.

The contents of the area consist of a firm, compressible tissue that is generally whitish but has occasional red specks. The tissue is primarily connective tissue that is perhaps gritty to cut if bone formation is prevalent within

it; it occasionally contains areas of cartilage. This tissue may form virtually all of the medullary portion of the bone. Rarely some cystic softening of this tissue may be encountered.

Microscopically such tissue is composed of small, spindle-shaped cells in a loose and whorled arrangement. The cellularity varies considerably. Scattered irregularly in this tissue may be primitive osseous elements formed by metaplasia of the connective tissue. This osseous tissue is atypically calcified or frankly osteoid. The tissue tends to be avascular except in highly cellular areas. Small islands of hyaline cartilage may also be found. The presence of the cartilage foci aids the certainty of the diagnosis.

Treatment

Although the disease, particularly in severe forms, tends to begin in infancy and childhood, it is the general rule that the patient will survive into adulthood. A surgical attack of an isolated lesion with curettage and replacement of the area with bone chips is usually followed by eradication of the lesion. In the more florid and widespread form of the disease, surgery is reserved for those lesions which by location or extent are a source of clinical trouble. In widespread areas, as pointed out by Strassburger, Garber, and Hallock, the repair process may fall before the spread of the lesion, and the bone chips may be resorbed.

Isolated lesions may be attacked for diagnosis, but it should be remembered that, with cessation of growth, the lesion appears to diminish in activity and to become dormant.

Reference

1. Lichenstein, W., and Jaffe, H.: Fibrous dysplasia of bone, *Arch. Pathol., 33:* 777, 1942.

Osteopetrosis

This condition was described by Albers-Schönberg in 1904. It is characterized by a homogeneous opacity of the bones, obliteration of the marrow cavities, and a tendency toward loss of trabecular structure. The bones may be abnormally fragile. An accompanying myelophthisic anemia is the rule.

The disease is rare and has been found in both male and female. There is a strong familial tendency. It has been found in fetuses as well as in children and adults. The cause is unknown.

The disease in childhood is progressive, and anemia, hemorrhage, and infection usually lead to an early fatal outcome. Some cases run a more benign course, and with adulthood the disease tends to become stationary. According to Nussey, the condition is benign when it is inherited and malignant when there is consanguinity of the parents. The children tend to be retarded in all phases of development, and a degree of dwarfism is usually present. In

Fig. 10.36. Osteopetrosis with pathologic fracture of the femoral neck.

Fig. 10.37. Osteopetrosis in which remodeling of the metaphyseal areas of the femur and tibia is hindered.

Fig. 10.38. Involvement of the spine in osteopetrosis.

addition to the anemia, optic atrophy, deafness, and facial or ocular palsy are often found. The blood chemistry does not show any characteristic changes, although the serum calcium is occasionally raised. Analysis of the bones indicates an increased calcium and phosphorus content.

Cohen[1] reviewed the pathology of this disease and found all bones of the skeleton affected. Membranous bones showed changes analogous to the changes of cartilaginous ones. Cartilage cell columns continued to mature, but there was a disturbance of the normal sequences of resorption of the primary spongiosa. Thus there appeared to be a great quantity of unresorbed cartilage matrix upon which the usual process of deposition of bone and osteoid continued even though the matrix was not resorbed.

Fractures heal at an unusually rapid rate, but there is marked delay in the remodeling sequences associated with growth. There is no tubular marrow cavity. The cartilage and bone matrix appear well calcified, but there are large areas of osteoid formation. Cohen noted that the transverse lines in the metaphyses of osteopetrosic bone were fractures in various stages of healing.

By x-ray the bones appear to have an increased opacity and loss of structure within their outline. The metaphyses show a failure of remodeling that makes them clubbed or box-like. Transverse dense lines are frequently apparent, and they occasionally separate metaphysis from diaphysis. The skull shows an increased density that is most marked at the base.

The bones appear solid on cross section and gray-white in color. No fatty marrow is seen. The trabeculae are increased in number and thickness. Some nodules of cartilage may persist among the trabeculae. As Cohen suggests, the delay in remodeling results in the formation of chondro-osseous complexes and the absence of a marrow cavity, and it may also account for the clubbed metaphyses.

The treatment revolves around aid for the ever present anemia, which may vary in severity and be characterized by exacerbations and remissions. The child with exceptionally fragile bones is frequently seen with fractures. The duration of immobilization should be shorter than that normally used. No cure of the fundamental condition is known.

References

1. Cohen, J.: Osteopetrosis: case report, autopsy findings, and pathological interpretation; failure of treatment with vitamin A, *J. Bone Joint Surg.,* *33A:* 923, 1951.
2. Kramer, B., Yuska, H., and Steiner, M.: Marble bones. II. Chemical analysis: Albers-Schoenberg disease (marble bones), report of a case and morphologic study, *Am. J. Pathol., 23:* 755, 1947.
3. VanCreveld, S., and Heybrock, N.: On Albers-Schoenberg disease (marble bones), *Acta Paediatr., 27:* 462, 1939.

OSTEOGENESIS IMPERFECTA

The most severe form of this rare disease occurs prenatally and may cause fractures and deformities to develop in utero. A second and less severe form appears postnatally and causes mechanical weakness of the bones and blue sclerae. The disease affects both sexes but is slightly more common in females.

While the outlook for survival is poor in the hereditary prenatal case, an individual infant may survive many months even with a very severe case. Patients with milder cases may survive into adult life. A tendency to improve is frequently seen. Postnatal cases may have only an occasional fracture and a full life expectancy, although severe cases are seen in this group also. The etiology is unknown. The inheritance is a Mendelian dominant.

Bauze's Classification

Bauze summarized his findings in 42 patients and divided them into three categories. In the

Fig. 10.39. Malunion of the femur and secondary shortening of the limb in osteogenesis imperfecta.

mild category (22) there was no long bone deformity. In the moderate (3) there was mild long bone deformity. There were 17 cases in the severe category with severe long bone deformity.

Mild

The family history is prominent. The age of onset averaged 3½ years but ran from 1 to 25 years. The female was 3 times more affected then male. Fractures were relatively infrequent, averaging 8.

Ligamentous laxity was common. All had blue sclerae. Deafness was common but scolio-

Fig. 10.40. Infant with multiple fractures and deformity in osteogenesis imperfecta.

sis and dentinogenesis imperfecta were uncommon.

Fractures were few and late in appearing and disability was virtually nonexistent.

Severe

The family history is uncommon. Few had blue sclerae but most of the patients developed scoliosis. The disability was severe, deafness was uncommon, and dentinogenesis imperfecta was common.

The fractures appeared early and were frequent. Males predominated. The average age of onset was 15 months, but ran from birth to 11 years. Hyperplastic callus was seen only in this group.

Collagen Deficiency. If one continues the categorization into those with mild deformity and those with severe deformity and disability, some interesting observations could be made relative to collagen. In the mild group, the amount of collagen was depressed, accounting for the blue sclerae in this group. The stability of the structural collagen as distinct from soluble collagen was normal in the mild group. The severe group exhibited a normal amount of collagen (few blue sclerae) but with very unstable cross linkage of the structural collagen.

Clinical Picture

Another name for this disease, fragilitas ossium, gives a clue to its dominant clinical characteristic. It is the fractures of the skeleton that bring the patient to medical attention. The

Fig. 10.41. Older child with thin cortices in fragilitas ossium (osteogenesis imperfecta) and with fracture of femoral diaphysis.

relaxation of the joint capsules and the blue sclerae that frequently accompany the condition are noted secondarily. The musculature is frequently loose, elastic, and diminished in volume.

Osteosclerosis may occur in patients who survive into adult life. According to Bickel et al.,[1] it most commonly accompanies the hereditary type of the disease. Otosclerosis has also been found in adults who have blue scleritis without evidence of bone fragility.

Victims of the more severe cases exhibit diminished growth to the point of dwarfism. The skull is unusually broad and has prominent occipital and parietal bosses. The teeth in childhood are poorly calcified and translucent. Blood chemistry values have not been found of diagnostic value.

Pathology

The most striking finding on bone section is the sparse distribution and the thin, frail nature of the bone trabeculae. The cortex is poorly formed. The trabeculae are frequently osteoid. Islands of cartilage are seen, and the medulla is in part fibrous or fat-containing. The number of osteoblasts is frequently deficient.

Roentgen Findings

The mild group exhibits a minor modeling defect of the long bone. By contrast the severe group has bones that are obviously severely affected by their environment. This results in a host of patterns all part of a severe functional defect. Some bones are wide with wide medullary canals and then cortices. Others end up with needle thin wavy bones with the cortex there but the medullary canal by contrast still thinner to result occasionally in only a thin radiolucent line representing the medullary cavity. Cystic metaphyses are seen giving rise to a soap bubble appearance. In this group massive wads of hyperplastic callus are seen.

The most common type of bone seen is thinned and has a diminished trabeculation and slender cortices. Various degrees and types of

Fig. 10.42. Compression of vertebrae in osteogenesis imperfecta.

Fig. 10.43. Skull with wormian bone pattern visible in fragilitas ossium (osteogenesis imperfecta).

deformity, depending on the past history, may be seen. Many transverse lines are present in the metaphysis. The ossification of the skull is imperfect and patchy. The fibula may be a mere thin line. The vertebrae may be compressed and biconcave owing to the pressure of the intervening vertebral discs.

Fairbank [3] has differentiated a type in which the major long bones are short and widened but still have excessively thin cortices. Fractures, as well as the deformity, are frequently seen.

Healing of Fracture

The fractures in general tend to heal, although nonunion and delayed union have been seen. Some patients tend to put out a very hyperplastic callus containing a "chondroid tissue."

Treatment

The physician must tread a delicate line in treating fractures in victims of this disease. Prolonged immobilization leads to further atrophy of bone and the resultant hazard of further fracture in convalescence. Insufficient immobilization leads to bowing, which is permitted by the soft callus. Since muscle tone

is generally poor, for children who are relatively inactive and light in weight the time of immobilization can be shortened without interfering with alignment. Healing in deformity almost inevitably results in refracture.

Medical measures undertaken with a view toward providing a stronger and better calcified skeletal system have proved of little avail.

Sofield[6] reported in 1959 on 80 operations involving 22 patients with severe deformity of the long bones caused by osteogenesis imperfecta. The age of the patients, in the main, lay between 2 and 8 years. The procedure followed since 1948 appears to be a great aid in preventing recurring fractures and in procuring mobilization of the patient.

According to this technique, a subperiosteal exposure of the shaft of the long bone involved is made. An osteotomy at the proximal and distal metaphyses follows, and the shaft is removed. The shaft is then divided into the smallest number of fragments that can be threaded on a straight metal rod. It is not necessary to keep the fragments in order because they serve as a scaffolding to hold the periosteum in the shape of the new bone to be formed. The projecting end of the rod is bent to prevent migration, and the distal end approaches the distal epiphyseal line. It is often is diminished; (2) deformities are corrected; and (3) normal use, particularly of weight-bearing extremities, is achieved.

References

1. Bickel, W. H., Ghormley, R. K., and Camp, J. D.: Osteogenesis imperfecta, *Radiology, 40:* 145, 1943.
2. Fairbank, H. A. T.: Osteogenesis imperfecta, *Proc. Roy. Soc. Med., 23:* 1263, 1930.
3. Fairbank, H. A. T.: Hyperplastic callus formation with or without evidence of fracture in osteogenesis imperfecta, *Br. J. Surg., 36:* 1, 1948.
4. Fleming, B. L., Radasch, H. E., and Williams, T.: Osteogenesis imperfecta, *J. Bone Joint Surg., 19:* 725, 1937.
5. Pelner, H., and Cohen, J. N.: Osteogenesis imperfecta tarda, *Am. J. Roentgenol., 61:* 690, 1949.
6. Sofield, H. A., and Millar, E. A.: Fragmentation, realignment, and intramedullary rod fixation of deformities of the long bones in children (a 10-year appraisal), *J. Bone Joint Surg., 41A:* 1371, 1959.
7. Wright, P. B., Gernstetter, S. L., and Greenblatt, R. B.: Therapeutic acceleration of bone age in osteogenesis imperfecta, *J. Bone Joint Surg., 33A:* 939, 1951.
8. Wyatt, T. C., and McEachen, T. H.: Congenital bone dysplasia (osteogenesis imperfecta) associated with lesions of the parathyroid glands, *Am. J. Dis. Child., 43:* 403, 1932.

Fig. 10.44. Osteogenesis imperfecta in an adult. These completely disabling deformities speak for themselves. Great effort is justified to prevent a patient from arriving at such a minimal functional opportunity in life.

necessary to insert the rod in retrograde fashion, thread on the fragments, and then drive it into the distal metaphyseal fragment. The periosteum is closed over these fragments as completely as possible. The limb is then immobilized in plaster for approximately 6-8 weeks.

As the child grows, it is common for the distal epiphysis to become well removed from the end of the rod. A longer rod may have to be inserted in order to prevent refracture, which has occurred distal to the rod.

Anyone who has struggled to attain weight bearing for these children and to rehabilitate them among children of their own age group appreciates the breaking of the vicious cycle of discouraging periods of non-weight bearing, refracture, and further atrophy of the bone. Our own experience with this procedure has borne out Sofield's list of its advantages: (1) the frequency of fractures is reduced, and pain

OSTEOPATHIA STRIATA

At this writing 6 cases have been described in the literature, 3 in one family. Occasionally osteochondromas have been found accompanying this anomaly which is principally a radiographic finding.

Voorhoeve described the radiographic findings in 1924. The linear streaks appearing in the bone are not easily explained since they involve the metaphysis and diaphysis but also extend through into the epiphysis. The cortex appears normal. The striated appearance appears to be a thickening of the medullary trabeculae in long streak-like aberrations. If there is abnormality of the cortex, it is hidden from the x-ray view.

Attempts to relate this condition to other conditions such as osteopoikilosis and Engelmann's disease do not appear well founded either from a radiographic or clinical point of view.

There are no symptoms, and this condition must be classified as a skeletal anomaly not

Fig. 10.44.1. The linear streaking of thickened trabeculae although most prominent in the metaphysis at the hip (*A*) and knee (*B*). The appearance gives rise to the designation osteopathia striata.

Fig. 10.45. The surgical procedure described by Sofield and Millar is designed to maintain activity in patients with osteogenesis imperfecta who have severe deformity. The bowed bone represents an engineering structural weakness additionally predisposing to fracture. Correction of the tibia with excessive bowing is illustrated. (Redrawn from H. A. Sofield and E. A. Millar: Intramedullary fixation of deformities of the long bones, *Journal of Bone & Joint Surgery, 41A:* 1372, 1959.)

The bowed tibia is stripped of its periosteal cuff keeping it intact. The diaphysis is then divided at either end and made into segments. When the metal rod is placed through these segments it is possible to insert its projecting tip into the distal medullary canal. In order to place it proximally and still maintain length it is often necessary to make a small slot in the cortex of the proximal metaphysis. The projecting tip proximally can then be lain into the medullary canal.

Fig. 10.45

affecting either the shape, form, or function of the skeleton.

Reference

1. Hurt, R. L.: Osteopathia striata, *J. Bone Joint Surg., 35B:* 89, 1953.

MAFFUCCI'S SYNDROME (MULTIPLE CARTILAGE TUMORS ASSOCIATED WITH HEMANGIOMAS OF THE EXTREMITY)

In Maffucci's original patient, whom he described in 1881,[4] there were multiple bony hard masses of the forearm found in a 40-year-old woman. Hemangiomas overlaid these masses, but were not necessarily in direct association with them. This patient ultimately died of the consequences of a malignant transformation of a tumor of the scapula.

Patients involved with the lesions associated with this syndrome tend to be of short stature with the principle involvement occurring in the hands and feet. The bones involved become so riddled with cartilage growth that the remaining bony septa fracture easily, leading to deformity. An important secondary complication is malignant transformation to chondrosarcoma—an incidence of 14 of 75 cases (18.6%) when reviewed by Elmore and Cantrell.[2] There is no evidence of a genetic or familial control. It is well established that mothers with this involvement can give birth to normal children.

In children who will ultimately develop Maffucci's syndrome no abnormality is noted at birth. There is no six predilection. Sometime prior to adolescence nodules of bony involvement of the extremities may take place in an irregular and asymmetrical manner. A unilateral involvement is slightly more frequent than bilateral.

After the second decade the tumor growth becomes quiescent unless transformation occurs.

A complication of the clinical course is the easy fracturing of a heavily involved bone.

X-ray Examination

The roentgenogram can reveal patchy areas of calcification associated with hemangiomas in the soft-tissue masses. The bony involvement is quite different than that seen in Ollier's disease. In that disease the cartilage areas tend to be linear and progress down the metaphysis from the epiphyseal line. The long bones are shortened with widened flaring metaphyses.

In Maffucci's syndrome the areas of cartilage involvement are rounded and involve a given area of the bone completely, and break through the cortex to give rise to a tumorous growth forming a mass which is quite distinct. These areas are multiple and not related in so obvious a fashion to the epiphyseal line. The peripheral location of the most marked involvement—the small bone of the hand and feet—is striking with involvement, progressively less in frequency toward the trunk, although any one mass of cartilage may reach a large size.

Fig. 10.46. In the femur the bowing is similarly straightened by dividing into segments. The metal rod can be driven retrograde fashion into the proximal segment and then the additional segments are placed on the rod. The rod is further driven into the distal segment.

Pathology

The cartilage masses in the bone are gray-white, shiny, and discrete with occasional joining into large sheets. The cartilage is very cellular and disorganized in its arrangement of cells. The hemangiomas are cavernous in type with phlebectasia and frequent thromboses.

Treatment

Recognition of fractures with minimal trauma should be part of the education of the patient so that treatment may avoid deformity. Masses are removed that are unsightly or heavily involving a bone to the point of making its integrity precarious. Malignant transformation is common enough to warrant frequent surveillance. Occasionally masses and deformity may present when the patient is first seen sufficiently gross to warrant amputation.

References

1. Bean, W. B.: Dyschondroplasm and hemangiomata (Maffucci's syndrome), *A. M. A. Arch. Int. Med., 102:* 544, 1958.
2. Elmore, S. M., and Cantrell, W. C. Maffucci's syndrome, *J. Bone Joint Surg., 48A:* 1607, 1966.
3. Johnson, T. L., Webster, J. R., and Sippy, H. J.: Maffucci's syndrome, *Am. J. Med., 28:* 866, 1960.
4. Maffucci, A.: Di un coso di encondroma ed angioma multiple. Contribuzioni ala genesi embrionale dei tumor movimento, *Med. Chir., 25-3:* 399, 1881.

CHAPTER 11

Congenital Orthopaedic Conditions

HEMIHYPERTROPHY

Hemihypertrophy is uncommon in the pure form that it's name implies. Most of the youngsters that will be seen with this condition actually have involvement of only one limb to any marked degree. Lower extremity involvement is much more common than upper. There is no evidence of any hereditary transmission and the distribution between the sexes is equal. General involvement rather than increased length of the limb is the eventual clinical problem.

Birthmarks and evident involvement of the vascular system in terms of venous enlargement are evident early in life. Mental deficiency, an involvement in 15-20% of the cases, may be the presenting complaint. It is evident that the bone is only mirroring the general enlargement of the soft tissues rather than being the eccentric devil at the core of the syndrome. The growth centers do appear earlier than usual in the involved limb, however. There is excessive reaction of the sebaceous and sweat glands. The hair is usually thickened. Varices appear early. Many anomalies have been described in association with the abnormal enlargement of the limb such as clubfeet, congenital heart disease, polydactylism, and even Wilms' tumor. Hypertrophy of one of paired organs may occur.

Wagner originally described the condition in 1839. He was describing a case with enlargement of the lower extremities associated with lipomas and telangiectasia. There was also a tongue enlargement. Hemiatrophy is not a problem in clinical differentation since it is secondary to neurologic conditions such as lesions of the postcentral gyrus.

In Ward's classification of the varying forms of this condition, "segmented" refers to a digit or ray; "crossed" to involve one limb or side with a ray or digit involved on the other side; and hemihypertrophy includes the more common partial hypertrophy involving principally the lower extremity. So little is known of the etiology that it is hardly worthwhile to repeat the speculations.

Treatment

The syndrome of hemihypertrophy has involved following the child throughout the growth period. The initial vascular studies such as arthrograms and interosseous venograms have been disappointing in their failure to reveal an abnormality. Obviously frank arteriovenous fistulas and massive hemangiomas are treated early. Although increased blood flow is clearly evident in increased warmth of the extremity, it must occur beyond the major vessel level.

The length problem is rarely one that cannot be handled at the appropriate time by simple epiphyseal arrest. Much more troublesome are the enlarged soft tissues. This often beomes so severe that excision of subcutaneous tissue is indicated. We have not ventured beyond a third of the circumference of the extremity in doing this and have leveled the edges of our excised mass to avoid a sudden concavity in the calf. The deep fascia is exposed and the deep layer of the subcutaneous tissue is excised gradually progressing around the limb. Defatted skin laid down on the calf fails to achieve the cosmetic improvement that is the objective.

Local Gigantism

Enlargement of a digit or ray is a total enlargement of the finger or toe and may or may not include the metacarpal or metatarsal. It may accompany the syndrome of hemihypertrophy. In the finger, epiphyseal arrest of the phalanges may be indicated relatively early. In the toes, excision of the proximal phalanx is a worthwhile procedure if done early in the child's life where the size of the digit clearly indicates shoe-fitting problems. Where the whole ray is involved, amputation of the entire segment digit and metatarsus may be indicated to achieve a workable foot. In the hand, wedge resection of the soft tissue to narrow the digit or ray may have to be done early to preserve the finger and prevent enlargement to the point of interference with function. Wedge resection may also be necessary in the foot for the same reason.

Other Causes of Limb Enlargement

Arteriovenous Fistula

The congenital type is usually clearly evident at birth. The thrill or bruit associated with it is diagnostic. It is continuous but accentuated by systole. Seldom does the fistula present for the simple one connection excision; rather, extensive fistulas with multiple arteriovenous connections which prove difficult to resect are found.

The acquired arteriovenous fistula in our own experience has been iatrogenic. Knee surgery in childhood is particularly productive. The acquired type initially goes through a clinical syndrome of arterial insufficiency, and gangrene of the limb could result. Later, as collateral circulation and hypervascularity occur, venous insufficiency could result with varicose veins, edema, pigmentation, and ulcers.

Hemangiomas

The types of hemangioma most likely to occupy the orthopaedists' attention and lead to limb enlargement are those of relatively massive signs involving muscle. The capillary hemangioma involving skin, which though prominent at birth tends to regress and can occasionally be hastened in that course with judicious applications via the dermatologic route, is not ordinarily associated with a growth problem. The massive cavernous hemangioma is a resection problem of no mean magnitude on occasion. Division through the center of the hemangioma can lead to massive blood loss as if one had opened into the general circulation. It is usually readily controlled, the area being overlapped on itself and sewn. However, the real excision problem when the hemangioma has proved invasive is how much to resect without interfering with muscle function. Since this is individualized, no statement of treatment, no matter how beautifully done, could possibly encompass it all.

There are no thrills or bruit with hemangiomas. Venous dilatation as age progresses, increased skin temperature, and an occasional mass are seen. It is stated that the hemangioma is painless, but it has been found by the author to be a significant answer to unexplained limb pain with local tenderness and occasional calcification in the muscle mass by x-ray—giving the diagnosis. These phleboliths have a soft, rounded calcific density that is characteristic.

Hemangiomas may be more destructive than they would initially appear. They may result in fibrosis and contracture of muscles that markedly interfere with their function. Hemangiomas ordinarily do not enlarge after 18 to 20 years of age.

Lymphatic Aberrations

The onset of lymphatic praecox and Milroy's disease is a nebulous, poorly defined area. Certainly it is seen in children. There is no early indication of vascular involvement. The limb is enlarged by a pitting edema with a smooth skin. There is accompanying tissue hypertrophy both of the soft tissues and bone. Later varices appear, and also lymphangitis and cellulitis, in about 10% of the youngsters.

The symptoms are those of increased weight of the limb, but not pain due to the invasion of other anatomical structures.

At this writing, treatment is not efficient or curative. We have started elastic support early on recognition of edematous involvement of the limb and have reason to think that this has controlled the development of a massive elephantiasis as these children have achieved adult life.

Lymphangiosarcoma

A rare condition that has resulted in amputation of the limb in our experience.

Neurofibroma

There is no question that neurofibromatous involvement of a limb can cause massive enlargement of a limb. The only question is how does it do it? Is it merely excessive blood supply to the epiphyseal side of the epiphyseal line or is it direct neural control or lack of control? Ectodermal dysplasia leading to excessive tissue is associated with neurofibromatosis. There is often a familial history. All the secondary phenomena of excessive blood supply to the limb may result, particularly when the limb is dependent. A lesion arising in bone has still to be proven, a lesion involving bone has been reported. Excision of involved tissue leads to improvement. There comes a time when excision of tissue with peripheral nerve involvement will lead to a loss of function. Which way the decision lies, then, is a matter of the individual case and the anatomic area involved. May the surgeon choose wisely and well.

Strangely enough, there are gains to be made by excision of the tissue with nerve involvement, which may be nothing more than endoneural involvement initially. This frequently leads to arrest of the condition at least in the area attacked.

EHLERS-DANLOS SYNDROME

This syndrome is characterized by hyperextensibility of the joints and skin. Because this phenomenon may reach proportions that are intriguing from a popular point of view, it is an ancient disease in terms of recognition. Persons with the syndrome have frequently been exhibitionists. The anomaly was described in 1682 by Job van Meckeren of Amsterdam who told of a Spaniard who could easily pull the pectoral skin on the right side of his body to his left ear. Ehlers of Denmark noted the excessive mobility of the joints in 1901, and Danlos described the subcutaneous tumors which may accompany this syndrome.

Clinical Picture

Hyperelasticity of the skin is striking, and hypermobility of the joints accompanies it. Less well known is fragility of the vessels, which may be so marked that repair after trauma is jeopardized. When the skin is lacerated, sutures may not hold well, and large, gaping wounds from relatively superficial injuries are not uncommon. Ligating of the vessels has been a clinical problem.

A few people with this syndrome complain of cyanotic changes in the fingers and toes with cold weather and of a phenomenon like Raynaud's. The laxity of the ligaments and the brittleness of the skin and vessels may lead to clinical complications. Symptoms related to flat feet are not uncommon. The clavicle may be abnormally mobile, but these patients are obviously not good candidates for repair of subluxating joints.

The disease may be inherited as a simple autosomal dominant trait.

The pathologic change may be a failure of development of an intermeshing network of collagen bundles. The expected finding of a larger than normal amount of elastic fibers has not been substantiated. An increase in elastic tissue is a very relative determination, however.

Treatment

Support of the feet and measures based on the individual patient's complaints are the orthopaedic treatment. There is no available cure of the disorder.

References

1. Hass, J., and Hass, R.: Arthrochalasis multiplex congenita, *J. Bone Joint Surg., 40A:* 663, 1958.
2. McKusick, V. A.: *Heritable Disorders of Connective Tissue,* St. Louis: C. V. Mosby Co., 1960.
3. Sutro, C. J.: Hypermobility of the bones due to "overlengthened" capsular and ligamentous tissues: cause for recurrent intro-articular effusions, *Surgery, 21:* 67, 1947.
4. Tschemogobow, A.: Cutis laxa, Mhft. Prakt., *Dermatologica, 14:* 76, 1892.

PROXIMAL FEMORAL FOCAL DEFICIENCY (CONGENITAL SHORT FEMUR)

If this deformity is termed proximal femoral phocomelia there needs to be an understanding of the numerous possible variations. There may be simple shortening of the femur with or without bowing. The bowing is often accompanied by a skin dimple at the height of the bow. The short femur may be accompanied by coxa vara with a large segment of the femoral neck unossified or with full ossification, an epiphyseal line of normal width, and the deformity only. The proximal one-third to

Fig. 11.1. Congenital short femur.

one-half may be absent. The acetabulum may be absent or rudimentary.

There are many variations of congenital short femur. The disorder varies from a femur that approximates its counterpart on the opposite side of the body to a limb in which only a rudimentary portion of the femur remains and the knee approaches the inguinal fold. The calf is usually surprisingly well formed, although the tibia may be somewhat shorter on the affected than on the normal side. No bilateral case is known to the author.

Heredity appears to play no part in the development of the anomaly. Cases are not infrequent in a children's orthopaedic clinic.

In addition to the obvious shortening the deformity most obviously needing correction is the flexed, abducted, and extremely rotated

position of the thigh. The ankle is often close to the knee joint—a reflection not only of shortening, but contracture. The fibula is frequently absent on the affected side. Aitken[1] reports a 70% incidence.

Clinical Picture

The deformity is noted at birth. Examination reveals the discrepancy of leg lengths in which the lower leg plays only a minor part. The patella has a great tendency to be rudimentary, and it is often dislocated laterally.

Coxa vara deformity, which is sometimes associated with the disorder, may cause the trochanter to ride above Nélaton's line. A hip flexion deformity is frequently found. Muscular function is ordinarily sufficient to stabilize the joint at hip and knee.

The picture in females is distressing. There is a refusal to wear skirts or any form of clothing that reveals the deformity. Males can more readily cover the deformity and engage in normal activities. Unfortunately, the lesion appears to be more common in females.

A portion of the distal femur is always present. Since by age 2 1/2 the ossification of the capital femoral epiphysis will be recognizable, it should be possible to proportionate fairly accurately regarding limb length from then on. A constant growth ratio between the normal and abnormal limb occurs in 9 out of 10 cases.

Prior to 2 years of age the delay in ossification may render a clear recognition of the type of anomaly involved in the proximal femur difficult.

Classification

Amstutz and Wilson[2] have classified five distinct types of this anomaly.

Type I

The combination of bowing of the femoral diaphysis and involvement of the proximal femur with a non-progressive coxa vara. There is medial femoral cortical sclerosis. Delay in ossification of the capital femoral epiphysis leads to confusion with dislocation of the hip. The shaft is laterally displaced by the bowing.

Fig. 11.2. The short femur and relatively unaffected tibia and fibula are seen. The unossified portion of the proximal femur at the base of the neck on the involved side.

Type II

The area between the capital femoral epiphysis and the femoral shaft is occupied by a cartilaginous anlage—multiple ossification centers often appear in this area. The varus is progressive. A subtrochanteric pseudarthrosis may persist.

Type III

The acetabulum is present and ossification of the capital femoral epiphysis is naturally delayed. The proximal femoral nonossified gap between epiphysis and femoral shaft is marred with the obvious necessity of considerable varus of the rudimentary cartilaginous anlage. Ossification of this area is usually complete by 6 years. The proximal femoral shaft is bulbous.

Type IV

There is severe alteration of the proximal femur and the proximal end of the distal femoral shaft tapers sharply. The shaft is not as laterally displaced as in the first two types leading to a suspicion of a very rudimentary connection between the capital femoral epiphysis and the femoral shaft. Proximal impaction

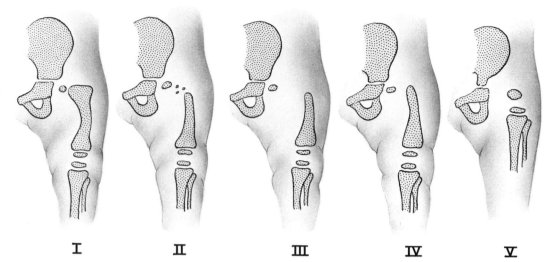

Fig. 11.3. The five distinctive types of involvement in the deformity known as proximal femoral focal deficiency according to Amstutz and Wilson. *I*, Involvement of the proximal femur in a nonprogressive coxa vara. *II*, A cartilaginous enlage between the capital femoral epiphysis and femoral shaft. *III*, A nonossified gap between epiphysis and femoral shaft with considerable lateral displacement of the femoral shaft and of necessity varus. *IV*, Severe alteration with tapering of femoral shaft and proximal impaction—a very rudimentary connection. *V*, The acetabulum and capital epiphysis are not present.

Fig. 11.4. Congenital short femur and developmental coxa vara.

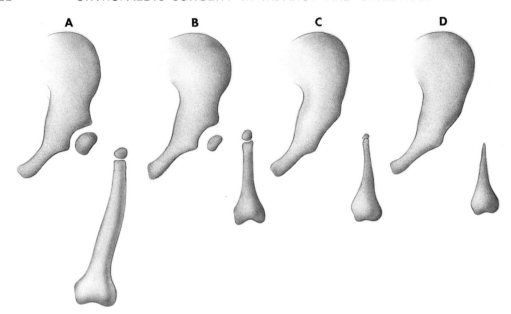

Fig. 11.5. Aitken classification of proximal femoral focal deficiency.

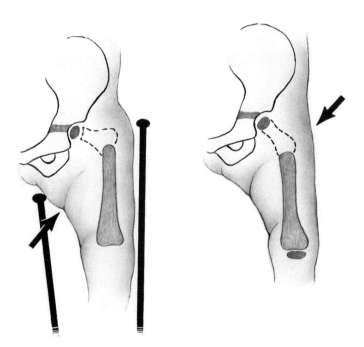

Fig. 11.6. Effect of bracing of ischial weight-bearing type in anomalies associated with congenital short femur may be to promote lateral displacement of the femur. Alignment of the leg beneath the weight-bearing line is needed.

of the femoral shaft occurs because of weakness in this area of persisting pseudarthrosis. The acetabulum becomes dysplastic as this alteration continues with lack of functional stress.

In one series the inhibition of growth averaged 64% in this group. Further migration and contractures can increase this figure with regard to functional shortening.

Type V

In this type the acetabulum and capital femoral epiphysis is not present. There is a poorly formed iliac projection just above the level of the acetabulum. The obturator foramen is spherical. Bilaterality may be present in this group.

Associated lower leg anomalies occurred in 50% of Types III and IV and to a lesser degree in Types I, II, and V. This may result in still further leg length inequality, leading to additional clinical considerations.

Treatment

The severity of the defect justifies radical measures, particularly in the female. In cases in which the ankle of the short leg is only slightly higher than that of the normal leg, an appropriate epiphyseal arrest can be performed at the proper time.

When the ankle of the short leg seems likely finally to be more nearly opposite the knee than the ankle of the normal leg, the best approach may be to secure an ankle at the level of the sound knee.

There is a fundamental approach to the anomaly. Dissatisfaction with the conservative approach arises from the fact that a prominent feature of the clinical picture is the flexed abducted and externally rotated position of the thigh. Bracing, whether a socket, ischial weight bearing, or platform with double uprights for weight bearing through the foot, encourages the continuance and growth in this position. This leaves the limb quite lateral to the trunk weight-bearing line. Progressively the deformity becomes more difficult to fit with a brace both cosmetically and functionally.

It becomes important, then, to establish the elements of the proximal femur that are available and then to get the femoral shaft aligned beneath or close to the weight-bearing line descending from the capital femoral epiphysis. Bracing them becomes cosmetically and functionally easy. Growth that exists contributes to the longitudinal axis.

As King[4] has emphasized, a simple skeletal lever must be achieved. If an acetabulum is present, a capital femoral epiphysis exists and will eventually ossify.

Each case must be individually assayed. A simple subtrochanteric osteotomy may suffice or several fragments may have to be aligned.

The first phase of treatment then consists of aligning the femoral shaft below the capital femoral epiphysis.

The second phase, once alignment, a good hip and thereafter adequate bracing have been achieved, is to ponder the problems of growth and relative alignment of ankle and knee.

No matter what will be done later, attention to the hip joint and femoral shaft alignment is the first order of business. Soft tissue release alone both at hip and knee has failed repeatedly—this is principally because bracing reconstitutes the deformity. King has demonstrated the importance of producing a single skeletal lever and the use of an intramedullary rod.

Leg lengthening is not a feasable alternative in this anomaly. The mechanical problems are too great, the knee takes too much abuse.

Knee arthrodesis is a frequently necessary procedure, depending on the shortening involved. In severe shortening, knee arthodesis is a necessary part of the rebuilding of an amputation stump that is adequate.

The aim below the hip joint appears by consensus to be to produce an amputation stump which provides improved function and cosmesis. The collective Shriner's Hospital experience summarized by Westin supports this approach. The equinus deformity of the foot does not aid the condition, being too difficult to camouflage in a prosthetic device. Rotational operations of the Van Nes[6] type have not been sufficiently successful to justify their use.

The Symes type of amputation at the level of the opposite knee when possible appears to be a very successful answer.

Where little is left of the femur, the proximal end of the tibia can be placed in the acetabulum after excising the short femoral fragment. An acetabulum must exist for the procedure to result in shaping of the proximal tibia with growth.

Valgus osteotomy of the hip is useful where sufficient ossification of the deformed proximal end of the femur is present.

The prosthesis should be designed for end bearing with a total contact socket.

References

1. Aitken, G. T.: Amputation as a treatment for certain lower extremity congenital abnormaliteis, *J. Bone Joint Surg., 41A:* 1264, 1959.
2. Amstutz, H. C., and Wilson, P. D.: Dysgenesis of

proximal femur and the surgical management, *J. Bone Joint Surg., 44A:* 1, 1962.

3. Bevan-Thomas, W. H., and Millar, E. A.: A review of proximal focal femoral deficiences, *J. Bone Joint Surg., 49A:* 1376, 1967.

4. King, R. E.: Providing a single skeletal lever in proximal focal .femoral deficiency, *Inter-Clinic Information Bull., 6:* 23, 1966.

5. Lloyd-Roberts and Stone, K. H.: Congenital hypoplasia of the upper Femur. *J. Bone Joint Surg., 45B:* 557, 1963.

6. Van Nes, C. P.: Rotation plasty for congenital defects of the femur, *J. Bone Joint Surg., 32B:* 12, 1950.

CONGENITAL ABSENCE OF FIBULA (PARAXIAL HEMIMELIA (FIBULA))

The work of Thompson, Strant, and Arnold[4] has caused a reevaluation of the treatment of this anomaly and a better understanding of it.

The disorder exhibits either complete or partial absence of the fibula. Associated with it are shortening of the extremity, various degrees of anterior bowing of the tibia, and anomalies of the foot.

Clinical Picture

The shortening of the lower extremity, which is evident at birth, is usually too great to be sufficiently corrected by either lengthening of the involved extremity or epiphyseal arrest of the opposite extremity. The discrepancy between the two legs often reaches 5 inches.

Kruger and Talbott,[3] in a study of 62 instances of absent fibula, found that a 3-inch length discrepancy occurred in the vast majority of cases, with those cases having hypoplasia of the femur being subject to still further shortening. Femoral shortening of ½–4 inches occurred in 65%. There was an inverse relationship between leg length discrepancy and absence of metatersal rays.

The average discrepancy at age 1 was 2 inches and at age 8 had increased to 5½ inches.

The anteriorly bowed tibia is often accompanied by a skin dimple anteriorly at the height of the bow. The bowing increases the length discrepancy and occurs at the junction of the middle and distal thirds.

The foot is in an equinovalgus position. One or more of the metatarsal rays are usually missing. There is a tendency for the foot to

Fig. 11.7. Absent fibula with associated shortening.

subluxate laterally as growth progresses. The condition is bilateral in 30% of the cases.

Pathology

The important element in this anomaly is the heavy fibrous band attached to the interosseous membrane and apparently representing the vestigial fibula.

Although the tibia is bowed, in most cases the medullary canal is present and of reasonable width for the bone. The talus and os calcis are often fused, and various other bones may be fused with them to the extent that there may be a single midtarsal bone mass. The appearance

Fig. 11.8. Congenital absence of the fibula with anterior angulation of the tibia.

of ossification centers is delayed, and one or more metatarsal rays may be absent.

Treatment

Preliminary assessment of the deformity is made in terms of the length of the extremity. Marked shortening leads to a guarded prognosis for the usefulness of the extremity.

Early excision of the tight fibrous lateral band has been found by Thompson et al. to give the bowed tibia a tendency to straighten spontaneously with growth. It also aids in correcting the equinus. Wedging or repeated use of corrective casts may be necessary to align the foot well under the tibia so that normal weight bearing can occur.

A shoe or a metal post elevation is usually necessary when weight bearing is begun. In addition, we have often found it necessary to add a leather gauntlet laced up the calf with lateral steel uprights in order to keep the foot

under the tibia. Osteotomy of the tibia may be necessary to correct the bow and to put the foot in a weight-bearing position. Coventry and Johnson[2] noted no difficulty in the healing of the bone in such cases.

Early ankle fusion done with injury to the distal tibial epiphyseal line may be necessary to keep the foot located correctly.

At age 5, a decision to keep the foot on some sort of patten bottom appliance in order to equalize leg length or to amputate usually has to be made. If amputation is chosen, a Syme type procedure is preferred because it permits the use of plantar heel skin for weight bearing. The stump that results is a very satisfactory one since, in this type of case with the associated shortening, it usually falls at midcalf level and thus permits cosmetically excellent prosthesis.

When a Syme amputation is done in a growing child, the problem of keeping the heel pad correctly located over the end of the tibia is a difficult one. Great care must be taken at the time of operation to fix the heel pad and to eliminate such future deformity as too tight tissues on one side. We usually keep the child in a cast that holds the tissues in a correct position for 6 weeks following such a procedure as a means of eliminating future difficulty.

References

1. Aitken, G. T., and Frantz, C. H.: The juvenile amputee, *J. Bone Joint Surg., 35:* 359, 1953.
2. Coventry, and Johnson, E. W.: Congenital absence of the fibula, *J. Bone Joint Surg., 34A:* 941, 1952.
3. Kruger, L. M., and Talbott, R. D.: Amputation and prosthesis as definitive treatment in congenital absence of the fibula, *J. Bone Joint Surg., 43A:* 625, 1961.
4. Thompson, T. C., Strant, L. R., and Arnold, W. D.: Congenital absence of the fibula, *J. Bone Joint Surg., 39A:* 1229, 1957.

ABSENT TIBIA (PARAXIAL HEMIMELIA (TIBIA))

Absence of the tibia may be partial or complete; usually some remnant remains proximally.

The lower leg is shortened not only by the absence of the tibia, but also by the fact that the fibula lies more proximal than it normally does at the knee and may be subluxated laterally at the foot. Tarsal anomalies in various combinations are the rule rather than the exception. Anterior bowing as in absence of the fibula is not a feature.

Tibial dysplasia is extremely variable in its presentation. There may be complete absence of cartilage and bone. More frequently an osteocartilagenous anlage of the proximal tibia is present (Fig. 11.10). Basing "absence" on radiographic criteria may be quite misleading. Figure 11.10 shows an allegedly absent tibia. No knee or ankle joints were present. This probably represents an early stage of the type of tibial "absence" that develops an ossification center when the child is several years old.

Tibial dysplasia results in significant shortening of the lower leg. The length inequality may be compounded by subluxation or dislocation of the fibula at knee or ankle. Bowing of the fibula is infrequent. Variable tarsal, metatarsal, and phalangeal abnormalities frequently are present. Decreased stresses at the knee joint may lessen growth of the distal femoral physis.

Treatment

Amputation with all its attendant growth problems should not be rushed into. Rather, every effort should be made to develop a leg below the knee which, if unsatisfactory in its entirety, can be used as the stump for a below-knee prosthesis and can thus increase function.

The fibula can be transplanted to the proximal portion of the remaining tibia. Hopefully, this portion will be sufficient to provide a good functional knee. Since hypertrophy of the transplanted fibula, which is desired, usually occurs to a remarkable degree, the operation should be performed as soon as sufficient bone to permit union has developed in the proximal tibial remnant. The shape of this remnant is usually such that the fibula is most directly under the femur when a long oblique cut in the fibula is opposed to the medial side of the remnant.

Fig. 11.9. Rebuilding in congenital absence of the tibia with cross union to fibula—amputation and union of os calcis to end of hypertrophied fibula. *(A)* Anterorposterior view, *(B)* lateral view.

Fig. 11.10. Absent tibia and associated anomalies of the tarsal bones. A remnant of tibia remains.

Where there is no remnant of tibia, the fibula can be moved directly under the intercondylar notch into a surgically created pocket and held there by the fibrous tissue which represents the only vestige of the tibia.

At the distal end, the fibula may be inserted into a distal tibial remnant, the astragalus, or the os calcis.

The surgery has to bring bone to bone and not fibula to cartilage portions of the remnant. Because of this requirement, the operation may have to be deferred. The treatment has to be greatly individualized to suit the variations of this anomaly.

After union is secured, exercises for the knee, including both quadriceps and hamstrings, are important. A laced leather cuff, long-leg brace with a free knee hinge is usually worn for the first several years, during which the bone is developing in order to protect it against fracture.

CONGENITAL AMPUTATIONS AND CONSTRICTING BANDS

So called "congenital amputations" exist as a single anomaly. The part involved may be a

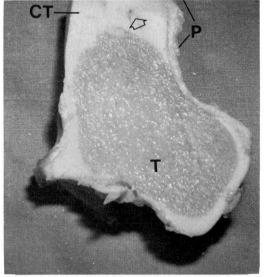

Fig. 11.11. Complete absence of tibia demonstrating distal femoral epiphyseal *(F)* and talar *(T)* ossification centers, no knee or ankle joints, and a dense cartilaginous tibial anlage *(CT)*. A perichondrium *(P)* was found only on the anterior portion. The *arrow* indicates a small focus of ossification. A relatively normal fibula, dislocated at both knee and ankle, was also present. (Courtesy of John Ogden, M.D.)

digit or the major portion of an extremity. It has been felt that these amputations may be a further extension of constricting bands, which eventually disturb the vascular system or a part. Streeter[1] believes that they are primary germ plasm defects.

Constricting bands, which have been noted most commonly in the lower leg, may exhibit varying degrees of severity. The usual clinical picture is that of a tight fibrous band about the bone through which—in an incredibly small area—pass nerves, blood vessels, and tendons. The distal part of the extremity often is enlarged and has a woody edema. After intrauterine amputations, the necrotic portion may remain attached.

Treatment

The treatment of the amputation consists in preventing deformity by active and passive exercise and by splinting. Such measures vary with the part involved. Bracing is usually accomplished with an appropriate socket and a double upright, jointed prosthesis rather than with an anatomic-appearing prosthesis, until growth is finished.

The constricting band can be very satisfactorily excised if it is not all handled at once. Approximately a third of the circumference is done at one sitting. The incision is made on the external surface, where the skin folds initially come together, rather than deep in the crevice so that the scar remains at skin level and does

not indent. Dissection must be meticulous as there is no room to spare. Some superficial adipose tissue distal to the band may also have to be excised at a later date.

Fig. 11.12. Congenital amputation (hemimelia). The necrotic tibia and fibula are still attached to the thigh stump.

Fig. 11.13. Mild degree of constricting band that needs no treatment.

Fig. 11.14. Bilateral congenital pseudarthrosis of the clavicle.

Fig. 11.15. Posterior angulation of the tibia with shortening. *(A)* Anteroposterior view, *(B)* lateral view.

Reference

1. Streeter, G. L.: Focal deficiencies in fetal tissues and their relation to intra-uterine amputations, p. 126. *Contributions to Embryology,* Publication 414, Carnegie Institute, Washington, 1930.

CLEIDOCRANIAL DYSOSTOSIS

Cleidocranial dysostosis is a hereditary defect in skeletal development that causes absence of the clavicles or aplasia of these bones to the

Fig. 11.16. Straightening of posterior angulation of the tibia with 2 years of growth. *(A)* Anteroposterior view, *(B)* lateral view. No brace is used.

degree that they are rudimentary. Associated defects include an increase in the transverse diameter of the skull due to delayed union of the sutures, delayed dentition, delayed ossification of the pubis, deformities of the metacarpals and metatarsals, and absence of bones other than the clavicles.

The clavicles may be represented by a fibrous cord. The patients may be short owing to a decrease in the longitudinal growth of long bones. Not only may the teeth be delayed in development, but loss of deciduous teeth may be delayed. Other skeletal variations, such as genu valgum, cosa vara, and scoliosis, may be noted.

Clinical Picture

The usual clinical picture is that of involvement of the clavicles and bones of the skull. The sutures are widened at birth, the fontanels gape, and the clavicles are absent. The picture may vary, and various combinations of defects may be present. The shoulders can be brought together anteriorly owing to the absence of the clavicles, and the upper portion of the thorax is narrowed and flattened.

The patient is symptomless. Motor function, for the most part, is not interfered with, and the patient is not handicapped.

Treatment

Treatment is ordinarily not indicated. Should deformity produce disability, it is corrected according to the needs of the individual.

CONGENITAL POSTERIOR ANGULATION OF TIBIA WITH TALIPES CALCANEUS

It is rather rare for children to have a posterior and medial bowing of the tibia and fibula at the junction of the middle and lower thirds. Associated with this deformity have been a severe talipes calcaneus and tightness of the anterior muscles of the lower leg and triceps surae. A dimple is frequently found over the point of maximal bow, and the limb is short.

Treatment

In infancy, bivalved plaster casts are used to hold the foot in plantar flexion once the initial tightness anteriorly has been overcome by corrective casts. When the child starts walking, a long-leg, double upright brace with an anterior strap to limit dorsiflexion is used. In the series of Heyman, Herndon, and Heiple,[2] this conservative approach was sufficient to correct the deformity.

Osteotomy for correction has been reported to result in healing of the tibia without incident. There is also a growth problem; epiphyseal arrest of the normal tibia at the appropriate time is indicated if the growth discrepancy is a clinical problem.

References

1. Badgeley, C. E., O'Connor, J. J., and Kudner, D. F.: Congenital kyphoscoliotic tibia, *J. Bone Joint Surg., 34A:* 349, 1952.
2. Heyman, C. H., Herndon, C. H., and Heiple, G. H.: Congenital posterior angulation of the tibia with talipes calcaneous; a long term report of 11 patients, *J. Bone Joint Surg., 41A:* 476, 1959.
3. Miller, B. F.: Longitudinal posterior bowing of the tibia in childhood, *J. Bone Joint Surg., 33B:* 50, 1951.

RADIOULNAR SYNOSTOSIS

This rare congenital defect is usually noted in children of 3 or 4 years, but it is seldom appreciated in infancy. Only when increasing demands for function are made is the deficit recognized. The lack of ability to pronate and supinate is masked by rotation at the shoulder and by flexion combined with radial or ulnar deviation at the wrist.

The fusion between radius and ulna involves the proximal portion of these bones and may occasionally be associated with radial head dislocation.

Treatment

Whether anything should be done or not is often debatable. The forearm is in slight to moderate pronation, and it functions quite well

Fig. 11.17. In radioulnar synostosis, some apparent pronation is developed at the wrist.

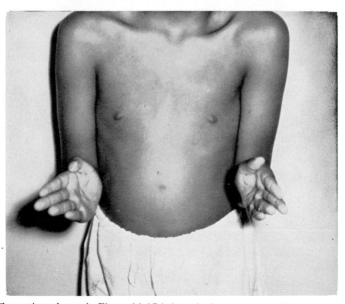

Fig. 11.18. The patient shown in Figure 11.17 brings the hands to neutral in apparent supination.

Fig. 11.19. Operation for radioulnar synostosis has exposed the entire edge of the ulna, which is seen inferiorly. The radius united to the ulna is visualized to the reader's left.

Fig. 11.20. Postoperative photograph of radioulnar synostosis after excision of proximal radius and area of union with the ulna; the interosseous membrane has also been divided at its ulnar attachment.

by adaptation. It can be improved, however, if permanent pronation-supination motion of significant degree can be obtained and actively used.

It is possible to gain a good range of motion (that is 50-60° of both pronation and supination) passively. The proximal radius is resected, and then (most important) the interosseous membrane is divided along the ulna from one end to the other. This second step is necessary because the disability includes a soft-tissue defect as well as the bony anomaly so evident by x-ray.

Gaining active motion to maintain the range obtained passively requires further procedures. The best motor for supination appears to be the extensor carpi radialis longus transplanted to the ventral side of the wrist. For pronation, the radial flexor can be transplanted dorsally.

If the disability is to be attacked at all, several operations are necessary, and as with many motions for which an eventual involuntary pattern of use is desired, they are best done in the early childhood years. The desire to begin early, however, must be tempered by judgment of the child's ability to comprehend and to train the transplant actively; most children need to be at least 6 years old.

MILROY'S DISEASE

Although often thought of as the congenital lymphedema of feet and hands noted at birth, Milroy's disease actually is more commonly first noted at puberty. It is also termed "hereditary trophedema." Just when a brawny type of edema in the extremities for which there is no evident cause is Milroy's disease and when it is merely congenital lymphedema is by no means clear; neither is it clear that there is any marked difference between the entities.

Clinical Picture

A silent onset is typical. Puberty is the usual period of occurrence. The edema often first appears about the ankle and gradually extends up the calf and down into the foot. It is often unilateral. The edema is not soft, and it pits only after prolonged firm pressure. After the edema has existed for a considerable period, fibrotic changes take place in the subcutaneous tissues and secondary skin changes appear. Episodes of lymphangitis may occur.

Fig. 11.21. Preoperative roentgenograms of congenital dislocation of the radius. The length of the radius carries it past the capitellum, and the radial head is underdeveloped.

There is no evident cause, such as a tumor or a mechanical lymphatic obstruction, for chronic edema.

The etiology is unknown.

Treatment

An elastic stocking is usually used from the time of first diagnosis onward. Later plastic reconstructive procedures, including excision of the subcutaneous areas, may be used in cases in which deformity or loss of function justifies them.

CONGENITAL DISLOCATION OF RADIAL HEAD

This is a rare anaomaly which has been reported in the past to be a familial trait. In our own series, it has occurred as an isolated anomaly in an otherwise normal child who had no familial history of the disability.

Clinical Picture

The dislocation may be either anterior or posterior. Increased length of the radius in relation to the ulna is quite apparent, as the

Fig. 11.22. A segment of the radius has been removed, and the proximal fragment has been reduced in relation to the capitellum. The proximal and distal radial fragments are aligned on a pin in a natural relation to the capitellum. The shortening of the radius allows the reduction.

radius grows past the lateral condyle either superiorly or inferiorly. Limitation of extension has always been present, and occasionally there is limitation of flexion as well. The usual age group seen is that between 5 and 9 years. The prominence of the radial head produces a deformity at the elbow.

Treatment

The anomaly may be disregarded. Function is limited but compatible with most tasks that have to be performed in life.

If parent and child are not satisfied with the appearance and function, some improvement can be gained, although absolutely normal function does not seem attainable. As a result of prolonged loss of articulation between the radial head and the capitellum, the radial head is deformed somewhat in the manner of a dislocated femoral head which has lain up against the ilium for years.

A segment of the radius sufficiently large to allow the proximal radial fragment to be reduced is removed distal to the orbicular ligament. The head is spikelike and flattened on

Fig. 11.23. Postoperative views on cast removal shows the new relation of the radial head to the capitellum.

one side. The cut surfaces of the radius are now opposed. A thin Kirschner wire or Steinmann pin is driven through the humeral condyle and down the center of the proximal and distal fragments of the radius to hold them in position. The orbicular ligament is maintained intact. The wire or pin is removed after 3 weeks, but the arm is maintained in a long arm cast with the elbow at right angle flexion until union is affected. The proximal fragment must be rotated at operation so that it will not slide by the capitellum with further growth. Great care must be taken to guard the radial nerve during this procedure.

References

1. Abbott, F. C.: Congenital dislocation of radius, *Lancet, 1:* 800, 1892.

2. McFarland, B.: Congenital dislocation of the head of the radius, *Br. J. Surg., 24:* 41, 1936.

ULNAR-DEFICIENT EXTREMITY

Ulnar deficiency (or absence) is much less frequent than radial absence. Characteristically, there are bowing of the radius, ulnar deviation at the wrist, reduction of the carpal bones (by synostosis or actual absence), and reduction in the number of metacarpal/phalangeal rays. Three significant variations may be found at the elbow: (a) normal or near normal radiohumeral joint, (b) radiohumeral synostosis (if an ossified portion of the deficient ulna is present it is usually fused to the radius and/or the humerus), and (c) dislocation of the radiohumeral joint.

Fig. 11.24. Ulnar deficient extremity. The bilateral ulnar deficiency illustrates the variable presentation. The ulna on the right was not radiologically visible for over 3 years. Note the dislocated proximal radius, curvature of the radius, and ulnar wrist deviation.

The amount of ulna present by roentgenogram may be misleading, since, unlike absence of the radius, the nonossified portion of the ulna is often present as a large fibrocartilaginous band that may insert onto the distal radius and/or carpus. This band creates a tethering effect that produced and accentuates radial curvature, abnormal development of the distal radial growth plate, deviation of the wrist, and radiohumeral joint abnormalities. In the radial clubhand, the resultant deformity is mainly determined by eccentric muscle pull. In contrast, the resultant deformity of the ulnar-deficient extremity is significantly determined by this fibrocartilaginous remnant of the distal ulna.

Initial treatment should be directed to exploration and resection of this fibrocartilaginous band. This will lessen the incidence of the aforementioned deformities. Creation of a one-bone forearm is often the treatment of choice.

NAIL-PATELLA SYNDROME (OSTEO-ONYCHODYSTROPHY)

This inherited disturbance of mesodermal and ectodermal tissue is transmitted by an autosomal dominant gene.

The patellae are hypoplastic or absent. The radial heads are dislocated, limiting elbow motion, and iliac horn formation is common. There may be a hereditary nephropathy resulting in significant renal impairment in adult life.

References

1. Beals, R. K., and Eckhardt, A. L.: Hereditary onycho-osteodysplasia (nail-platella syndrome); a report of 9 kindreds, *J. Bone Joint Surg., 51A:* 505, 1969.
2. Darlington, D., and Hawkins, C. F.: Nail-patella syndrome with iliac horns and hereditary nephropathy, *J. Bone Joint Surg., 49B:* 164, 1967.
3. Duthie, R. B., and Hecht, F.: The inheritance and development of the nail-patella syndrome, *J. Bone Joint Surg., 45B:* 259, 1963.

CHAPTER 12

Neurogenic Affections

CEREBRAL PALSY

Cerebral palsy constitutes a major classification into which fall a large number of patients who can be benefited by orthopaedic measures. Unfortunately the classification of various types is not clear. The orthopaedist tends to classify the patient according to his most predominant handicap. From this type of classification, treatment may be more readily inferred. The neurologist tends to classify according to the probable anatomic site of the deficiency. Our knowledge regarding sites of involvement in various types of cerebral palsy is still very slight.

Distraught parents seeking help for their child are driven from one physician to another until someone offers help. The disorder becomes a very difficult social and psychologic problem and demands the highest standards of judgment and character from the physician. The parent and child are not infrequently led down a path of promised recovery only to find that the child, when school or teen-age years are reached, is unable to compete; bitter disillusionment with serious consequences may be the result.

We must avoid castigating the physician as not being interested in the child because he insists on being on realistic ground. Too firm and definite a prognostication, particularly with regard to intelligence when a child is very young, is also to be avoided. Many things become evident of their own accord in a slower and kinder way with growth, which allows much time for adjustment.

Definition

This condition includes all states in which control of the motor system is interfered with by a lesion of the central nervous system. The principle characteristic is incoordination in the use of one or more of the extremities. The secondary features, which in some cases may become the principle ones, include mental deficiency, lack of balance, convulsions, and speech difficulties. The underlying etiology appears to be damage or defect of the upper motor neurone either in cord or brain.

Incidence

According to Phelps, [13,14] the incidence is 7 cases per 100,000 births. Of these 1 dies before the age of 6, usually in infancy. One-third of the 6 remaining are mentally deficient to the degree that custodial care is necessary. One is severely handicapped, 2 are moderately handicapped and capable of improvement, and 1 is so mildly handicapped that treatment is not a prominent feature. With the possible exception of polio myelitis and dependent on its epidemic incidence, cerebral palsy is the most common of the treatable neuromuscular conditions.

Classification

For years Freud's classification was used. It divides cerebral palsy into seven types:
1. Spastic hemiplegia.
2. Generalized rigidity.
3. Paraplegic rigidity.
4. Paraplegic paralysis.
5. Double hemiplegia.
6. Generalized chorea.
7. Bilateral athetosis.

This method of classifying was satisfactory from the neurologist's point of view because it included all cases and considered both the region affected and the predominant feature, which were recognizable when the patient was seen.

Phelps attacked the problem from the point of view of an "indication to treatment" and classified according to the type of involvement seen as:
1. Flaccid paralysis.
2. Spasticity.
3. Rigidity.
4. Tremor.
5. Athetosis.
6. Ataxia.

Rigidity was found clinically when excessive

Fig. 12.1. Distribution curve of intelligence rating for cerebral palsy patients as compared to the curve for the general population. (From B. Crothers and R. Paine: *History of Cerebral Palsy*, Cambridge, Mass.: Harvard University Press, 1959.)

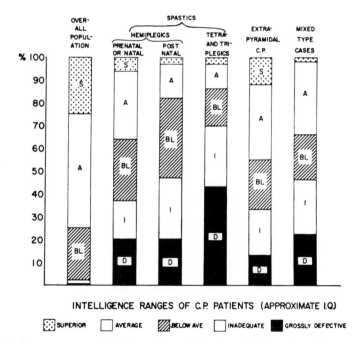

Fig. 12.2. The intelligence ranges of victims of cerebral palsy of various types is compared to that of the general population. (From B. Crothers and R. Paine: *History of Cerebral Palsy*, Cambridge, Mass.: Harvard University Press, 1959.)

Fig. 12.3. The age at which walking is achieved in the various types of cerebral palsy is shown. Note that virtually all of the spastic hemiplegics learn to walk without support. Only 70% of the spastic tetraplegics reach this level of ability. (From B. Crothers and R. Paine: *History of Cerebral Palsy*, Cambridge, Mass.: Harvard University Press, 1959.)

tone or resistance to movement was present throughout an arc of motion. Spasticity was evident when there was a stretch reflex—that is, an involuntary contraction of an antagonist muscle in response to a sudden stretch always occurring at the same point in the arc of motion. Hyperactive deep tendon reflexes are also present in children with this type of involvement.

Crothers preferred to divide his cases into two large groups:
1. Spastic cases.
2. Extrapyramidal cerebral palsies.
He also recognized that there was a combination of these two types in many cases. Only the spastic group were divided topographically into monoplegia, hemiplegia, triplegia, tetraplegia, and paraplegia. The spastic hemiplegics, representing 40% of the total, were the largest single group. Monoplegia is very rare, and, although involvement of the arm is usually first recognized, most of the cases designated as monoplegia on later examination are found to represent hemiplegia.

"Double hemiplegia" has been used by some authorities to mean as asymmetric involvement as compared to the usual spastic tetraplegia or more severe affection of the arms and legs—sometimes as an indication of causation, which is apparently not valid.

There is considerable confusion among the types of cerebral palsy when one attempts to classify too distinctly. The validity of spastic hemiplegia as a syndrome in which definite things can be expected is recognized by almost everyone. In other kinds, however, various combinations in terms of type of paralysis can be expected. There is increasing evidence that the pyramidal and extrapyramidal systems are not as clearly defined as has been accepted.

The essential features of a "spastic" type of cerebral palsy are:
1. Muscular hypertonus.
2. Hyperreflexion, including stretch reflex (constantly reduplicated).
3. Positive Babinski and Hoffmann reflexes.
4. Dimished superficial reflexes.
5. Loss of control of fine motions.
6. Interference with postural and labyrinthine reflexes.
7. Tendency to muscular contracture in

characteristic positions.

8. Clonus (a frequent but not invariable feature).

Magoun and Rhines have pointed out that spasticity probably results from a combination of interference with tracts inhibiting muscle tone and stretch reflexes (chiefly reticular in origin) and retention of sufficient facilitative tracts to augment muscle tone and responses. All cases probably involve both pyramidal and extrapyramidal connections.

In the extrapyramidal group, all possible combinations of athetosis, dystonia, tremor, rigidity, and choreiform movements may exist. The predominant feature may change with age. Crothers has pointed out that the major features of these cases are:

1. Incoordination.
2. Delayed postural development.
3. Hypotonus in infancy, which may change somewhat with growth to increased tonus in stress situations, but is never like the hypertonus of a spastic.
4. Dimished reflexes in infancy, which may become mildly hyperactive later.
5. Absence of clonus and Babinski reflex.
6. No tendency to contracture.

Etiology

This condition in one of its various forms stems from one or more of many possible etiologies.

In prenatal life the brain is subject to congenital defective development and to variations in structure that result in abnormality of function. Pathologic conditions present in the mother may affect the development of the fetus, although cases in this category are few in number.

At birth trauma may result in cerebral hemorrhage and anoxia. It is very hard to separate the effects of asphyxia from those of hemorrhage. The frequent relation to prematurity is well known and is probably to be explained on the basis is tissues not fully enough matured to withstand the sudden change in pressure relations at birth. Undue traction on the neck, forceps pressure, and birth complications such as a cord around the neck all may result in cerebral damage. Blood abnormalities may result in erythroblastosis, prolonged jaundice, and secondary cerebral palsy. Kernicterus following prolonged jaundice

after birth may result in two syndromes. One is an asymmetric mixed type of cerebral palsy involving pyramidal features but in which rigidity is most prominent, and the other is hypotonicity without evident spasticity.

After birth, causes include infections such as whooping cough occurring before the age of 6 months and encephalitis at any age. Injuries may of course result in sufficient cerebral damage to interfere with neuromuscular function. Convulsions and dehydration in early months of life may result in cerebral hemorrhage or thrombosis. Schwartz has shown that areas drained by tributaries of the great vein of Galen are affected by secondary hemorrhages from injuries to this vein.

Perlstein notes that spasticity occurs in 65% of youngsters with infantile spastic hemiplegia as the result usually of trauma and vascular damage. Twenty-five percent of these youngsters have an athetoid type of paralysis due to anoxia or other blood-borne mechanisms. Rigidity, tremor, and ataxia are divided among the remaining 10%. Almost 50% of all spastic patients are hemiplegic.

Early Diagnosis

The symptoms of neuromuscular disability are often not prominent enough in the early months of life to suggest the anomaly. By 6 months of age, however, most cases should be diagnosed. Stiffness in an extremity, failure to hold the head up or to sit, or preservation of a characteristic posture may call attention to the fault.

When a baby is presented to the physician with the question of possible disability, the signs may be elicited by careful examination. There may be excessive reaction, such as clapping the hands, to a sudden stimulus. A tendency toward hyperextension of the neck, facial grimaces, and tongue rolling may be indicative. Observation of the child's activity may reveal quick, coordinated motions of one extremity and slow, incoordinate motions on the contralateral side. It is obvious that allowance must be made for the normal variations and for the tendency of hyperactive reflexes to persist in an otherwise normal child.

Most helpful to the diagnosis is an inability to shake an extremity into floppy accompaniment to the shake in a short period, particularly when the opposite extremity is readily loosened. The lack of balance exhibited by failure to hold up the head or inability to extend the spine is additional confirmation in the 6-month age group. Such evidence alone is not sufficient, but should result in guarded observation of the child from then on.

Late Diagnosis

An athetoid state results in uncontrolled motions and habitual distorted positions. The excessive activity and purposeless motions limit the tendency to contracture, and any given joint may be passively carried through a full range of motion. In a pure athetotic state the reflexes are not increased, and the plantar response is negative. Tension develops in an attempt to control the athetosis, but muscle power throughout is good and flail muscles are not seen.

The true spastic individual exhibits increased reflexes, positive plantar responses, and stretch reflexes in the muscle. In such persons a stretch reflex is elicited by carrying the part suddenly through a range of motion. The opposing muscle contracts at the same point in the arc of motion each time and then with continued steady pressure relaxes to allow continuance through the range of motion. A readily stimulated muscle such as the gastrocnemius opposed by an inactive anterior tibial muscle may result in contractures. The true degree of contracture is elicited by first overcoming the stretch reflex—not by mistaking this response for actual contracture. Inactive, flail, or weak opposing muscles are frequently seen in spastic patients.

Rigidity, on the other hand, results in a feeling of resistance throughout the arc of motion rather than at the particular point. Such resistance is also experienced in reversing the motion and extending a previously flexed limb. It is a feeling very akin to that experienced in attempting to shift gears in a gold car in mid-winter.

Brenda[5] concludes that two-thirds of these children have impaired intelligence and that only one-third are undamaged intellectually. He divides cerebral palsy into the following categories:

1. Little's spastic rigidity (decerebrate rigidity).

2. Pyramidal type (monoplegias, hemiplegias, diplegias, paraplegias).
3. The mixed extrapyramidal-pyramidal type (paraplegias with athetosis).
4. The ataxic-atonic cerebellar type.

Little's Disease

Little[11] originally described this condition in 1853. He noted the predominance of premature birth among victims of cerebral palsy exhibiting "tetanic stiffness." Although Little covered the entire field of cerebral palsy, his syndrome is perhaps best limited to conditions involving the extremities and trunk with a decerebrate type of rigidity. This rigidity is the same in all planes of motion. The neck and back are also stiff. Such children have a short life and a progressive course. Brenda[5] noted cystic degeneration and edema of the central white matter with a relatively unaffected cortex, but cortical lesions and subdural and subarachnoid hemorrhages were also found.

Pyramidal Type

Hemiplegia in this type resembles the adult form of cerebral loss of motor function. There may be odd variations, in addition to odd limb distribution, of involvement. Thus the rotary type muscles may be involved while the flexor-extensor group is relatively unaffected. This group includes the true spastic patient with typical elbow flexion, pronation, flexed and ulnar-deviated wrist, adducted thumb, and flexed fingers in the upper extremity. In the lower extremities, the adducted leg with equinus of the forefoot and dorisiflexed first toe are typical. Where one limb only is involved or the condition is hemiplegic, the mental defect is usually slight. This group usually benefits from training and various orthopaedic measures, including reconstructive surgery.

Here also are the bilateral hemiplegic (also known as diplegic) patients in whom the legs tend to be more involved than the arms. This kind of cerebral palsy is not progressive but tends to remain stationary.

The brain lesions have been found to consist of cortical degeneration. The cortex is the site of an extensive gliosis, and the pia is thickened and attached to it. The distribution of the lesion varies from part of one lobe to an entire hemisphere. Venous or sinus thrombosis may be the cause.

Mixed Extrapyramidal-Pyramidal Type

This type is slow to become evident; only the failure to achieve a milestone in motor development may call attention to the difficulty. Convulsions may be evident in infancy. Spasticity of the lower extremities and uncoordinated flailing, flexion-extension motions of the upper extremities may call attention the athetosis which is present. The head may be noted to be small in the older child.

Venour damage, particularly to the vulnerable great vein of Galen and secondary damage through its tributaries, apparently plays a large part in this type of cerebral palsy. Areas of cortical atrophy and sclerosis beneath enlarged and sometimes thrombotic subarachnoid veins are found. The perivascular region of veins running through the white matter is demyelinated and necrotic. Subependymal cysts form and lead to degeneration of surrounding tissue.

Ataxic-Atonic Cerebellar Type

Here the pathology appears limited to the cerebellum and brain stem; the cerebrum is spared and the intelligence is relatively unaffected. Hypotonic musculature and very late walking are noted as predominant accompaniments. For a few, walking is never achieved. All motions exhibit an unsteadiness and ataxia which is characteristic. Aphonia is a prominent feature, but the child often appears to understand well.

Treatment

The cerebral palsy patient presents a multifaceted problem in treatment, which includes understanding the parents, the general condition of the patient, speech and mental defects, convulsions, and the motor disability. Although each of these features demands special understanding and skill, the parents seek stability in some one individual of the team, usually in the one who controls the major phase of the treatment. The fact that many skills are needed in the care of cerebral palsy should not cause the team to make a mass approach.

From the orthopaedic point of view, over-coming the motor defect is of particular importance.

The approach is to develop the next logical motor accomplishment. The child, in order to walk, must first learn to sit. The features of the disability that prevent him from achieving his next immediate goal must be overcome, be they deformity, contracture, ataxia, incoordination, flail or weak musculature, or inability to control motions.

Exercises

Exercises may be divided into two general types. The first is passive stretching as a means of combatting contracture, and the second is active repetition of motor acts. In active repetitive motion, the position of the limb, the confusion reflex, and rhythmic accompaniment may all be used to achieve the desired result. The conversion of exercise into a gamelike activity by whatever device increases the ease with which it is done and the duration of doing it.

Bracing in Cerebral Palsy

The brace in cerebral palsy is used as an aid to completing a coordinate movement. The problem is quite different from that of polio myelitis in which the patient has normal postural reflexes and muscular weakness is supported by blocking motion in the direction which would overstretch the weak muscle.

In cerebral palsy, generally, we want the child to complete the motion, but to do so within the limits of what we think of as a normal motor pattern. This motion in itself aids in preventing contracture if it is carried through the full range.

Background. In order to avoid some bracing mistakes, some knowledge of the relative possibilities of various roughly classified groups of patients is needed. That there is a deficit in the I.Q. level is obvious if the distribution of intelligence ratings in the normal population is compared with that in cerebral palsy patients. The intelligence of children with cerebral palsy varies somewhat, however, among the different manifestations of the disorder. Patients with extrapyramidal types come very close to the intelligence of the general population. A comparison of the ability to compete of the two

Fig. 12.4. Motor system defect in cerebral palsy increased by deformity.

groups would be a more intelligent, though less charitable, approach.

Extrapyramidal Cerebral Palsy

Well defined tonic neck reflexes accompanied by extension of the arm on the side to which the patient looks is the hallmark of extrapyramidal cerebral palsy. The rotation of the shoulders in the same direction as the head may be so involuntary that the child can be rolled over and over. These abnormalities do not mean that the patient will never walk, for they can disappear with development, but in their presence he will not. This child is a candidate for bracing when he is first seen.

Athetosis is not correlated with these reflexes, nor is an intelligence defect. Hand sensation is never affected in this group. These are the intelligent but helpless. Of those without tonic neck reflexes in this group, only 1 in 10 will be unable to walk, and intelligence will probably enter in as a factor in that one. Surgery in extrapyramidal cases is considered only in connection with contractures.

The tonic neck reflex, then, is indicative of postural immaturity. As motion patterns evolve, a neck-righting reflex takes its place, and finally a standing balance is achieved.

A chart of the walking age for the various kinds of cerebral palsy reveals that the spastic hemiplegic patient walks first. He is followed, several years later, by the extrapyramidal and spastic tetraplegic patients, although some in these groups never walk. In the extrapyramidal group classically, the children are hypotonic and have normal or slightly increased reflexes. Later, choreoathetosis may develop. In mixed types of cerebral palsy, the stiffness or rigidity may disappear when the child is emotionally secure. Contractions are not the important feature that they are in spasticity. A positive Babinski reflex is not inconsistent with extrapyramidal or mixed types. In general, with these types, the underlying principle of treatment is to encourage function by any means the patient has, even if his movements are accompanied by wild thrashing of arms. Bracing, however, renders the patient incapable of doing anything. Scoliosis, which is rare in spastic hemiplegia, can develop in this group, particularly in association with some of the substitution patterns.

In these extrapyramidal and mixed types generally, bracing does not play a part. Encouragement of substitution patterns and treatment of contractures, should they develop, by various orthopaedic measures, such as cast correction and surgical lengthening procedures, are a part of the plan.

Spastic hemiplegia

One-third of these cases are postnatal in origin. The development of a strong dominance of one arm over the other before the age of 18 months should make one suspicious, for this type of one-sided dominance is never normal before the age of 12 months. Initially, the

Fig. 12.5. Inability to extend lower extremities and assume upright posture without support in cerebral palsy.

Fig. 12.6. Foot deformity in patient with hemiplegia.

hemiplegic area is flaccid and hyporeflexive, but it progresses to hypertonus and hyper-reflexia with varying rigidity to assure the typical posture, which is characterized by pronation of the forearm, flexion of the wrist, a flexed elbow, and a clenched fist. All patients in this group walk (90% by 36 months) unless their intelligence is so low that it alone precludes walking. Athetonism can be acquired in postnatal cases.

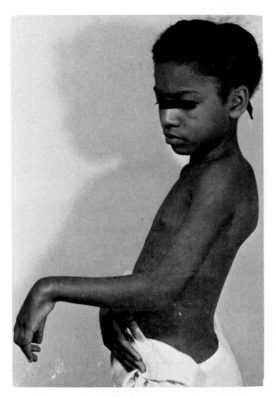

Fig. 12.7. Inability to extend wrist in hemiplegia.

Impaired sensation in the hand, which Crothers called astereognosis through ignorance, is more common in postnatal cases. Other types of sensation loss may occur as well. The entire upper extremity is frequently rather markedly underdeveloped.

Here the bracing problem is to aid the upper extremity to go through a normal motor pattern, to promote a good cosmetic result, and to prevent contracture. There is considerable controversy about the treatment of the arm, but it is generally true that emotional serenity is achieved in these children only after attempts to make them bimanual are abandoned. Impairment of the upper extremity appears to be a greater deficit than that of the lower in hemiplegia because use of the hand demands more skill than the rather gross act of walking. A brace that keeps the elbow extended and that, when the elbow is flexed, cocks up the wrist has been of help to us in achieving a normal look in use. We have never seen true skill developed to the point that the hand is on occasion used as substitute for the other extremity. Some people have described early training of the upper extremity as actually detrimental, but it appears obvious that simple motor acts, such as turning on a light switch or radio, may be taught with benefit and have a good chance of being used when the patient is involved bilaterally.

The bilateral spastic (tetraplegic paraplegic, etc.) patient is often recognized as damaged at birth. Some of these infants show only delayed motor development and lack of muscle tone or reflex change until at least the first year of life has passed. Ingram suggests that there is an orderly sequence of hypotonia, dystonic spasm, rigidity, and finally spasticity (Little's disease).

For this group, bracing, particularly for the lower extremity, can be considered. As long as balance is too poor to permit walking, some bracing may be in order. Bivalved casts with outriggers aid in limiting the development of flexion contracture at the hip, which leads later to some rather marked lumbar lordosis. To prevent overstretching of the patellar tendon by maintaining the extended knee position is important. The developing equinus is also combatted by these long-leg casts. Extensible bars can bring about abduction and, in all these planes, can work against gracilis tightness and the development of subluxation of the hip.

When balance is achieved, these patients are first seen with overstretched anterior structures at the knee, and bracing is demanded to maintain the extended position. Operation is perhaps the only means of maintaining this position permanently.

Both here and in fighting the equinus and pronated position of the foot, the braces generally should use springs rather than straps. The fundamental goal to be achieved is ability to perform the motion correctly even though the patient is still in the brace.

A preferable situation is the use not of a long-leg brace, but of a short-leg one with a dorsiflexion spring of the Klenzac type, and with an inner T-strap if there is eversion of the foot. Exercises to strengthen the quadriceps are used along with the short-leg brace. Aid in controlling the most distal joint helps the child to controll the gross motions of the hip and knee in the gait.

We have been unable to discern a rationale for encasing the child who cannot stand in rigid

Fig. 12.8A. Like other functional braces used in cerebral palsy, this brace aids in developing a motion pattern. Here spring action holds the elbow extended when the arm is at the side.

steel that includes the trunk and standing him up. We believe that he gains more by actively using his limbs in whatever way he can on a mat.

The bracing problem is quite different from that in poliomyelitis. Wherever possible, the brace should aid in accomplishing a motion, not in preventing it. In general the most distal major joint is that under poorest control and most in need of help. Particularly helpful at the ankle joint is a spring dorsiflexion brace, especially when the common problem of an overactive gastrocnemius and an anterior tibial inactive in the presence of gastrocnemius tension exists. Once an aid to dorsiflexion is incorporated in the gait, the patient can be taught to flex the knee and to exaggerate the "steppage" element in the gait, thereby improv-

ing its character. The no longer overstretched anterior tibial reenters the gait pattern, and each step the patient takes becomes a well controlled one. Repeated use of this kind of aid over the years results finally in elimination of the need for actice bracing.

In the presence of contracting tendencies, as in adducted hips, flexed thighs, equinas feet, palmar-flexed hands, and adducted thumbs, night casts or splints may be indicated. In sleep, however, the patient is usually in a relaxed position.

Stretch Reflex

The peripheral stretch reflex is activated by sensory organs in the muscle and tendon. The principle area is the muscle spindle which is oriented axially in line with the muscle fiber. Here annulospiral nerve endings are contained in a nuclear bag and stimulated as the muscle is stretched. Less important flower-spray endings are located on the myotube. The Golgi tendon organ located in the tendon requires a greater stimulus for activation. This nerve ending is responsive both to stretch and compression. Continued force will result in a sudden relaxation of the muscle as the reflex is overcome.

Connecting within the cord, these efferent nerves form part of a feedback loop stimulating efferent nerves to produce a muscle contraction.

The relationship between spindle stimulation and muscle length is an inverse one. The greater the discharge from the spindle, the shorter the muscle. Conversely, the muscle spindle excitation rises as the muscle lengthens. If diagramed, these rising and falling curves would intersect. This is the point of physiologic length at which tone is maintained. If this intersection point were moved further down the curve, a greater spindle discharge would be necessary to maintain the physiologic length.

Before this excitation point is reached there is room for greater use of the limb under voluntary control. This can be achieved by both muscle lengthening and by bone shortening relative to muscle length.

Contractures

The tendency to contracture, which is seen most often in the true spastic or pyramidal

Fig. 12.8B and C. (Top) When the elbow is extended, the wrist is allowed to come to neutral. (Bottom) With elbow flexion, the brace pulls the wrist into dorsiflexion to complete a functional pattern.

group, varies from individual to individual. It usually requires a constantly tonic muscle that is excited by minimal stimulus and a flail antagonist or one handicapped by poor mechanical function.

It is apparent in children with cerebral palsy that beneath the limitations imposed by spastic paralysis there is an ability to voluntarily contract a specific muscle. Procedures in the past, which have taken advantage of this fact,

include heel cord lengthening. This lengthening of the gastrocnemius physiologic length has diminished the triggering of the stretch reflex and has also decreased the level at which the antagonist muscle—in this case the anterior tibial—is inhibited and voluntary control is blocked by the peripheral stretch reflex.

Persistent Equinus. The measures used to combat this position include passive stretching exercises that bring the foot into dorsiflexion and inversion with the knee extended. Wedging casts are also of benefit. The anterior tibial muscle is often chronically overstretched so that, in the face of the reflex discharge from a tonic gastrocnemius, no contraction can be elicited in this muscle. Flexing the knee and thereby relaxing the gastrocnemius often elicits activity in an anterior tibial previously thought to be flail. Despite bracing with springs and the other conservative measures listed above, some radical realignment of muscle tension and power is often necessary to enable the patient to dorsiflex his foot sufficiently to achieve a heel-toe gait.

Banks[3] and Green have emphasized lengthening of the heel cord as a useful procedure in this regard. The foot should be brought into 10° of dorsiflexion with the knee extended at the time of division of the Achilles tendon and before the tendon is united surgically. The incision is made on the medial aspect of the tendon prominence posteriorly. We have not done this procedure blindly. A common method is to make a Z-shaped incision with a long central limb and short transverse cuts above and below. The proximal cut is usually lateral and the distal cut medial—just above the os calcis. After surgical repair, the limb is placed in a toe-to-groin case that holds the knee in 20° of flexion and the foot appropriately dorsiflexed.

At the end of 4 weeks, this cast should be replaced by a short-leg cast and the knee should be exercised out into full extension. If full extension is not achieved, the knee may be wedged by plaster cast to ensure actually about 10° of hyperextension. The follow-up care after healing has taken place is most important, since the anterior tibial must be actively used in the gait or the persistent equinus position of the foot will reappear. Supervision of the gait until a normal pattern has been achieved is useful, and regular follow-up studies should be made throughout the growth period.

Strayer[19] has emphasized a soudly based procedure of gastrocnemius recession which is particularly of value in those who have been unable to walk and yet have sitting balance. The aim of the procedure, in Strayer's words, is "to relieve the insertion of the biarticular gastrocnemius and plantaris from tension on the tendo Achillis until the foot is in dorsiflexion to 90° or more ... The recession of gastrocnemius allows dorsiflexion of the foot to

Fig. 12.9. Spring brace for dorsiflexion in cerebral palsy; a high shoe is necessary in younger patients.

initiate proprioceptive sensory stimuli in the soleus only until the foot reaches 90° [neutral dorsiflexion]." The value of the operation appears to lie in the removal of proprioceptive impulses originated by stretch on the gastrocnemius until that point in the arc of motion is reached at which they may be of some value in achieving progress.

The operation is done by making an incision in the proximal calf so that, first, the sural nerve can be isolated. The gastrocnemius muscle bellies are then isolated on either side and dissected from above downward to the attachment of the gastrocnemius to the soleus. The tendon is then severed, and the finger is passed underneath to make certain that all fibrous bands between the soleus and gastrocnemius have been divided. The foot is then dorsiflexed to make certain that the plantaris is also divided. Strayer uses a toe-to-groin cast for 4 weeks and then an ankle-to-groin cast that is replaced as often as necessary to achieve slight hyperextension (7-10°) at the knee.

Flexion at Hip. Here again the crux of the problem is to strengthen the glutei. Measures which attack the problem from the other side

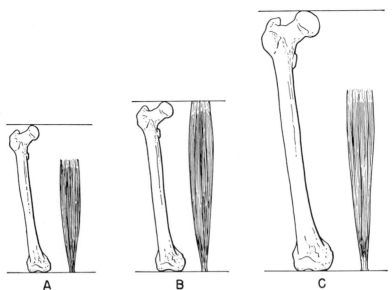

Fig. 12.10. (*A*) Relative shortness of soft tissues in relation to bone in a contracture. (*B*) Correction to normal situation. (*C*) Return of relative shortening of soft tissues with growth.

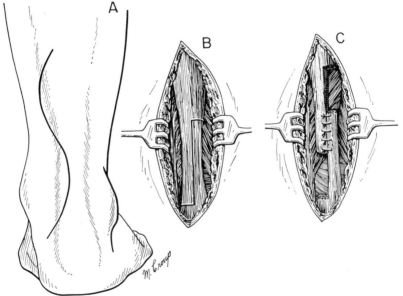

Fig. 12.11. Lengthening of the heel cord by simple Z-plasty. The incision is placed to the medial side of the Achilles tendon.

by weakening the flexors must be undertaken with caution. However, fasciotomies of the Ober type are occasionally necessary. Some patients appear improved by release of flexors, such as the rectus femoris, as advocated by Duncan.

Adduction of Hip. This is a crucial problem, particularly in spastic forms of cere-

bral palsy. The power of the hip abductors is most difficult to determine in the presence of strongly overpulling adductors and is usually rated as poor. The conservative regime includes active exercises for the glutei, adductor-stretching, and stretching of the accompanying hip flexion contracture. A bivalved hip spica that holds the legs in maximal abduction is used at night. Metal splints with adjustable bars between them may be substituted. Approximately 1 of 5 of these patients may have some degree of subluxation or frank dislocation at the hip.

Banks and Green[4] have reported on the results of adductor myotomy and anterior obturator branch neurectomy in cases of this deformity. All of the patients had undergone a considerable period of conservative therapy prior to operation. Forty-eight were not walking prior to surgery, and 27 of these were successfully ambulated. The absolute necessity for careful postoperative care until permanent lengthening of the adductor is achieved has been emphasized by these authors. This care includes the application, at the time of operation, of a cast that holds the legs in wide abduction and the use of active gluteal exercises that employ these muscles normally in the gait. The general result has been improvement in the power of the hip abductors. The use of night casts that hold the legs in wide abduction has been necessary for several years. Hips that were subluxated prior to operation have been found normal on follow-up evaluation in approximately 65% of cases. No instances of regression in motor ability attributable to the operation procedure have been noted.

When this procedure is done, a linear incision in line with the origin of the adductors is made. The deep fascia is divided and the adductor longus is isolated. The interval between the adductor longus and the adductor brevis is defined, and the branches of the anterior portion of the obturator nerve are visualized. The branches to the adductor longus, the adductor brevis, and the gracilis are divided, and 1 inch of the nerve is removed. If tightness persists after division of these muscles at their origin, then more anterior fibers of the adductor magnus are divided.

Femoral Shortening. It appears possible to gain improved voluntary control in children with severe spasticity by shortening the femur about 10% of its physiologic length. The children who could be considered for this procedure form a small group. Their involvement should be bilateral and consist of spasticity with minimal rigidity and athetosis.

The procedure could be considered in those who would require multiple surgical episodes to relieve contractures in multiple anatomic planes. It offers a multiple plane correction and

Fig. 12.12. The gastrocnemius recession described by Strayer. The incision exposes the gastrocnemius muscle. The sural nerve is identified. The gastrocnemius muscle bellies are isolated and dissected from above downward to the attachment of the gastrocnemius and soleus. The tendon is then severed to make certain that all fibrous bands between the soleus and gastrocnemius have been divided. The bellies then retract upward to their new location as the foot is dorsiflexed.

increases the range of motion possible before the stretch reflex in the antagonist muscle is called into play. As a result functional range is increased, greater steppage in the gait is possible, and adduction is no longer a prominent feature in the gait.

It does not affect the use of the lower leg and does not completely correct the gait. It is a procedure of a magnitude that should not be considered where a single plane procedure such as adduction or hamstring lengthening could accomplish. Complications are possible and holding the bone ends securely together until healing occurs requires both internal and external fixation.

Femoral shortening also decreases the level at which the stretch reflex is triggered by decreasing the bone length relative to the muscle length. A greater excursion of the joint is now necessary to achieve the same degree of stretch.

Through a lateral incision on both proximal thighs, a 1½-inch segment of femur is removed

Fig. 12.13. Lengthening of the heel cord as described by Banks and Green. (*A*) The incision is medial. (*B*) The rotation of the fibers of the tendon is studied, both cuts being made laterally. Those fibers inserting medially are divided superiorly; those inserting laterally are divided inferiorly. (*C*) The sheath is repaired after the tendon has been slid in order to avoid skin adherence. A long-leg plaster is applied. (From H. Banks and W. T. Green: Correction of equinus deformity in cerebral palsy, *Journal of Bone & Joint Surgery, 40A:* 1350, 1958.)

in an area including the lesser trochanter. This represents a 10% shortening of the femur. Later, in a relaxed state, the adductors and hamstrings will then allow a normal functional position for the limb. The adductors, on the other hand, are unaffected unless the proximal fragment goes into varus. Increased abductor power relative to the adductors should be the result. An h-beam hip nail is inserted into the proximal fragment prior to bone division. The

first division is made by a Gigli saw proximal to the lesser trochanter. The second division is made 1½ inches distal to the first. The iliopsoas muscle is thus detached from its insertion as the bone segment is removed. It is then possible to correct all contractures, extending and abducting the limb. The flexion contracture at the knee was readily overcome due to the relative laxity of the hamstrings. A bone plate is then attached to the hip nail and bone screws are used to fasten the plate to the femoral diaphysis as the fragments are held tightly opposed. The limb then remains in normal anatomic position on the operating table.

A bilateral hip spica is applied for 6 weeks, since the shortening eliminates the stability to be achieved by compression. This procedure relaxes the adductors, hamstrings, and hip flexors. The hip abductors are still at the same physiologic length. The quadriceps is slightly affected by relaxing the rectus femoris portion. No attempt is made to reinsert the iliopsoas.

Gait training and exercises are started at 6 weeks. It takes 3-4 months to regain iliopsoas, abductors, and hamstring function.

Flexed Knees. Surgery is most beneficial here. An attempt to cure the erect posture fault of standing with flexed knees by progressive resistance exercises is, in the majority of instances, doomed to failure. The quadriceps function is inhibited by the mechanical fault of an overstretched patellar tendon so that the force of the contraction is not transmitted to the tibia throughout the range of motion. Passively the full range of knee extension should be possible, and the hamstrings must be weakened until they are one grade below the quadriceps. Good quadriceps strength, as well as previous correction of deformity at the hip and knee, is necessary. A strong gastrocnemius

is also necessary. These factors, which were originally stated by Chandler, were reemphasized by Roberts and Adams.[15] Once these things have been achieved, the proximal-riding patella can be brought several centimeters distalward so that it lies in normal position. To accomplish this, the patella tendon insertion, with an accompanying block of bone, is moved distalward on the anterior tibial surface.

Eggers[7] provided for better transmission of the quadriceps force to the tibia by division of the patellar retinacula so that the patella may ascend and take up the patellar tendon slack from above rather than below.

Eggers described another procedure that has proved helpful in overcoming the flexed knee stance and greatly advantageous in improving the function of the knee in the gait. The semimembranosus, semitendinosus, and biceps femoris are removed from their tibial or fibular insertions and transplanted to the distal femur just above the origin of the gastrocnemius. We have not found it necessary to insert the tendon into the bone, but merely to sew it to the periosteum. Ability to extend the knee actively is recovered, and, with training, it can be incorporated into the gait.

Pronation of Feet. Bracing, if used, can be aided by the addition of an inner T-strap that holds the foot in inversion. The gradual

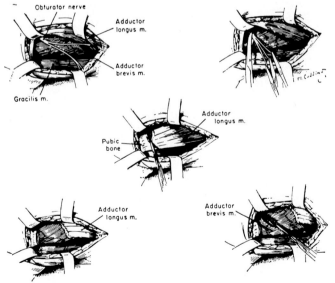

Fig. 12.14. Drawing of adductor-lengthening as done through a medial thigh incision over the adductor origins. (From H. Banks and W. T. Green: Adductor myotomy and obturator neurectomy for correction of adduction contracture of hip in cerebral palsy, *Journal of Bone & Joint Surgery, 42A:* 111, 1960.)

Fig. 12.15. An exceedingly painful situation occurs in cerebral palsy in the age group over 12 years. The persistent unbalanced muscle pull leads to acetabular deformity and femoral head deformity as subluxation occurs. The lateral third of the acetabulum is indented as the femoral head slides by. Once frankly dislocated the attempted use of the hip causes pain. This is a difficult treatment situation and mere adductor release will not relieve it. We have used an adaptation of the Colonna capsular arthroplasty to reseat and maintain the position of the femoral head. A new acetabulum is curetted in the roof of the old one. The capsule is sewn around the femoral head and the hip reseated. This has maintained position and relieved the extreme pain. (*A*) Preoperative dislocation and deformity of both femoral head and acetabulum. (*B*) Postoperative position with femoral head placed in the newly formed acetabulum.

stretching out of the tight heel cord aids in relieving this constant position. Longitudinal arch pads and inner heel wedges are usually necessary in addition. In this type of foot,

sometimes the peroneal musculature is markedly overactive and the anterior and posterior tibial musculature does not contract.

A triple arthrodesis is a very satisfactory

means of increasing foot strength, stability, and function. Such an operation can correct an equinus foot and relieve severe pronation to improve function.

Baker and Dodelin[2] reported on the use of subastragalar arthrodesis (Grice procedure) for patients in this category. Baker[1] particularly emphasized the necessity in cerebral palsy of getting rid of deformity if the child is to achieve maximal function. The rationale for the operation in these patients includes the reestablishment of balance, the correction of the deformity, and the gain in function to be expected. Baker and Dodelin reported 29 operations in 17 patients, of whom 11 had not been walking. All but 1 became ambulatory following the procedure. The possibility that the posterior tibial tendon will produce too much varus afterward must be considered; it

may be necessary to lengthen this tendon. The use of tibial bone grafts to being the os calcis into better alignment under the astragalus is described below in the section deality with poliomyelitis.

Limb Alignment. It is hard to get a maximal function in the presence of deformity. Orthopaedic principles of limb alignment hold in cerebral palsy as in other conditions. Excessive valgus at the knee, external torsion of the tibia, hyperextension of the knee, or foot deformities may result in a limb malalignment which should be corrected.

Upper Extremity. In the upper extremity the most distal joints prove to be those most difficult for the patient to control. Aid of a permanent nature to wrist, fingers, and thumb enables the patient to control the elbow and shoulder better.

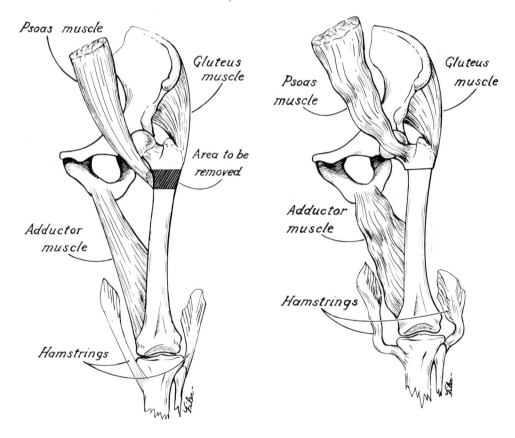

A

B

12.16. (*A*) Diagram of area for removal of bone segment from proximal femur. (*B*) Removing segment allows relative increase in length of iliopsoas (since lesser trochanter is removed) hamstrings and adductors. (From A. B. Ferguson, Jr.: The effect of femoral shortening on severe spastic paraplegia, *Archives of Surgery, 99:* 349, 1969.)

Fig. 12.17. (*A*) Preoperative roentogenogram of patient with spastic paraplegia. Valgus deformity of the femoral neck is evident. (*B*) Postoperative healing of lesser trochanter area where bone segment has been removed.

Thumb adduction that interferes with the patient's use of the palm may be treated by severance of the nerve to the thumb adductor. Fusiong of the wrist that deviates it dorsalward and ulnarward, it the fusion is indicated for other reasons as well, also gets the thumb out of the palm.

The palmar flexion and pronation of the hand presents a troublesome problem in many patients. Green[9] has suggested a transfer of the flexor carpi ulnarus tendon from its insertion to that of the extensor carpi radialis longus tendon. This procedure removes a deformity force and converts the muscle into a spinator as well as a dorsiflexor. Such a transplant works well, providing there is no loss of kinesthetic sense in the hand.

Flexor Release. For those patients with ability to fully extend the finger with the wrist a flexion it may be possible to improve function by flexor release at the elbow. The thumb is released by lengthening of the flexor pollicis longus at the same time. This latter lengthening is done just proximal to the wrist.

A curvilinear incision over the medial elbow extends distally to about mid-ulna. This length

Fig. 12.18. Transplantation of hamstring insertion from tibia to femoral condyle.

is necessary in order to divide the origin of the flexor carpi ulnaris from the ulna. As attention is paid to the origin of the flexor carpi ulnaris the ulnar nerve is isolated down to the first motor branches. By dissecting the common flexor origin from the medial condyle the median nerve is isolated. With these two nerves isolated the origin from the humerus and from the ulna can be thoroughly detached. This leaves the nerves isolated from the normal muscle packing about them down to the point of exit of motor branches. It is natural to transpose the ulna nerve forward out of its groove to the anterior surface of the humerus.

A second incision is made on the flexor surface just proximal to the wrist over the flexor pollicis longus. A simple lengthening is performed.

After incisional repair a plaster cast holds the wrist, finger, and thumb extended for 2 weeks. The finger and thumb are then released and active motion started. The entire cast is removed at 6 weeks. Intermittent wrist extension splinting may be necessary thereafter.

Drugs. Phelps, reporting on the use of prostigmine, noted that it facilitated correction of contractures, particularly in patients with rigidity, apparently lessened the stretch reflex in true spastics, and was very helpful in clearing speech difficulties in spasticity or rigidity of the tongue. No effect on pure athetosis was noted. Curare and synthetic derivatives have been used in many centers over the years with disappointing results. Anticonvulsant drugs are not the province of this text.

References

1. Baker, L. D.: Rational approach to surgical needs of cerebral palsy patients, *J. Bone Joint Surg.*, *38A:* 313, 1956.
2. Baker, L. D., and Dodelin, R. A.: Extra-articular arthrodesis of the subtalar joint (Grice procedure); results in 17 patients with cerebral palsy, *J. A. M. A., 168:* 1005, 1958.
3. Banks, H. H., and Green, W. T.: The correction of equinus deformity in cerebral palsy, *J. Bone Joint Surg., 40A:* 1359, 1958.
4. Banks, H. H., and Green, W. T.: Adductor myotomy and obturator neurectomy for the correction of adduction contracture of the hip in cerebral palsy, *J. Bone Joint Surg., 42A: 111, 1960.*
5. Brenda, C. E.: *Developmental Disorders of Mentation and Cerebral Palsies*, New York: Grune & Stratton, Inc., 1952.
6. Clifford, S. H.: The effects of asphyxia on the newborn infant, *J. Pediatr., 18:* 567, 1941.
7. Eggers, G. W. N.: Surgical division of the patella retinacula to improve extension of the knee joint in cerebral spastic paralysis, *J. Bone Joint Surg., 32A:* 80, 1950.
8. Ferguson, A. B., Jr.: The effect of femoral shortening on severe spastic paraplegia, *Arch. Surg., 99:* 349, 1969.
9. Green, W. T.: Tendon transplantation of the flexor carpi ulnaris for pronation-flexion deformity of the wrist, *Surg. Gynecol. Obstet., 75:* 337, 1942.
10. Green, W. T., and McDermott, L. T.: Operative treatment of cerebral palsy of spastic type, *J.A.M.A., 118:* 434, 1942.
11. Little, W. J.: *Disorders of the Human Frame*, London, 1853.
12. McCarroll, H. R., and Schwartzman, J. K.: Spastic paralysis and allied disorders, *J. Bone Joint Surg., 25:* 745, 1943.
13. Phelps, W. M.: Description and differentiation of types of cerebral palsy, *Nerv. Child, 8:* 1, 1949.
14. Phelps, W. M.: Recent significant trends in the care of cerebral palsy, *South. Med. J., 39:* 132, 1946.
15. Roberts, W. M., and Adams, J. P.: The patellar advancement operations in cerebral palsy, *J. Bone Joint Surg., 35A:* 958, 1953.
16. Smith, C. A.: Physiological mechanisms of fetal

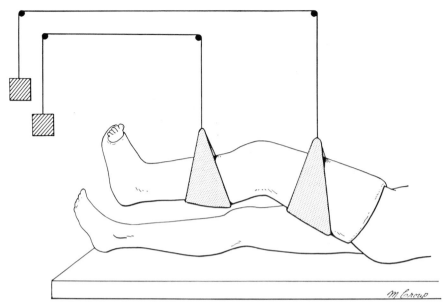

Fig. 12.19. Elevation of the limb in plaster aids to control postoperative edema.

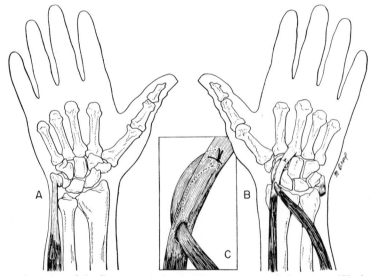

Fig. 12.20. Transplantation of the flexor carpi ulnaris (*A*) to the long radial extensor (*B*); detail of insertion of tendon into tendon (*C*).

anoxia at birth and cyanosis in the newborn *Am. J. Dis. Child., 79:* 1, 1950.

17. Strayer, L. M., Jr.: Gastrocnemius recession; a 5-year report of cases, *J. Bone Joint Surg., 40A:* 1019, 1958.

POLIOMYELITIS

Although the diagnosis of poliomyelitis frequently falls on the shoulders of the medical and pediatric practitioner, the treatment of its effects is the responsibility of orthopaedic surgery. A thorough knowledge of the disease, of the requisites for maximal recovery, of the prevention of deformity, and finally of the methods of reconstruction gives the orthopaedic surgeon tools of great use in understanding and treating other conditions in childhood.

The disease may produce an asymmetric,

flaccid, irregular paralysis without sensory involvement. Such an effect is duplicated by very few conditions.

History

Ghormley[3] states that the first monograph on poliomyelitis was published in 1840 by Jacob Heine of Connstatt. Heine put the age group affected at 6-36 months and noted that the children were enjoying unusually good health when stricken. Pain and paralysis of both lower extremities were forecast as the result.

Caverly may have been the first to describe the nonparalytic form of poliomyelitis when he reported an epidemic in Vermont in 1894. One hundred ten patients were noted to have had paralysis in some form, and at least 50 of these had fully recovered.

The first great epidemic appeared in 1905 in Norway and Sweden. Eighteen months after this epidemic broke out, 56% of the 550 patients originally reported paralyzed still had some residual paralysis, and 44% had recovered completely.

In a 1917 monograph on poliomyelitis, Rohrah and Mayer harked back to Badham, who in 1835 initiated the use of heat for comfort. They advocated wrapping the extremities in flannel and supplying heat in the form of hot water bottles.

Peabody, Draper, and Dochez in 1913 classified the forms of the disease as follows: (1) abortive cases, (2) cerebral cases (spastic paralysis evident), and (3) bulbospinal cases (flaccid paralysis). They remarked that, preceding paralysis, there is a period marked by prodromal symptoms and recommended quarantine during this stage.

Ghormley, in his article on the history of the treatment of poliomyelitis, shows that Peabody and his co-workers recommended the use of heat, passive motion, and rhythmic motion, along with activite training of muscles, to prevent contractures and hasten recovery. Placing the children in a warm bath was considered an aid to the exercising of their limbs.

Draper emphasized that resistance to anterior flexion of the spine was typical of poliomyelitis and was greater in this disease then in either the stiff neck or Kernig's sign of meningeal irritation.

Vulpian, in the same era, remarked on the muscle contracture and deformity that followed the initial stage of the disease. In total paralysis, he noted the relaxation of the joint capsule and the tendency of the limb to adapt itself more to the demands of gravity than to those of function. The shortening of active muscle groups and the development of contracture were responsible for deformity in partial paralysis. The involved muscles undergo marked atrophy and decrease in size, and the atrophied fibers become yellowish white owing to fatty degeneration. Vulpian recommended wet or dry packs (1912).

Lovett,[9] who was a keen student of poliomyelitis, laid the groundwork (1916) for much of the understanding of the disease as it occurs today. To Lovett, poliomyelitis was a generalized disease that acted on viscera as well as on the central nervous system. Spinal cord pathology could produce a fatality via the nerve cells that control respiration, or spontaneous repair of it could allow complete recovery. He described the symptoms as follows:

The symptoms are in general those of an acute infection. In many instances, however, gastrointestinal symptoms predominate; while in others, those referable to the respiratory tract, are the most marked. Stiffness of the neck to flexion of the head, sweating, marked nervous irritability and general hyperesthesia are present in many instances before the onset of paralysis, but they are not all constant.

Lovett believed that "muscle training forms the basis of the modern treatment of poliomyelitis." In theory, this training attempts to make the patient send a voluntary impulse to contract a muscle and aids the muscle to contract by means of passive movement. The limb is placed in such a position that gravity aids the movement, and further assistance is given by the hand.

There is one very important point in this connection that is often lost sight of. In an affected limb, some muscles are as a rule paralyzed, some weakened, and some comparatively normal. The muscles that we wish to exercise are those that are paralyzed or weakened. If the exercises are not carefully controlled and located, the patient is sure to use strong muscles instead of the weak ones and thus to make the muscular imbalance still worse.

Exercises loosely given by untrained persons and encouragement of the child to kick about and do anything he can are likely to do harm rather than good.

Lovett emphasized that splints to prevent deformity are an aid to treatment.

He also gave us a system of grading muscles which is in common use today for following the patient's progress.

Diagnosis

Despite widespread familarity with the cardinal signs of poliomyelitis, the disease continues to be much misdiagnosed. During the summer and fall months, virtually every child with a limp, stiff neck, or pain in the extremities is suspected of having the disease. The problem is often to separate out the cases of multiple neuritis (Guillain-Barré), meningitis, cord tumor, disease of the hip, knee, and spine from the cases of Heine-Medin's disease or poliomyelitis. The stages of poliomyelitis are:

I. The acute stage.
II. The convalescent stage.
   A. With sensitivity.
   B. Without sensitivity.
III. The chronic stage.

Acute Stage

Onset

The onset of poliomyelitis is like that of many other acute illnesses. Fever and symptoms of malaise referable to the gastrointestinal tract—i.e., vomiting, headache, and signs of a mild coryza—may all be present. The early period of mild illness may be followed by a week in which the patient feels essentially well. But the fever returns (a chart of the fever produces a double-humped curve), and it is followed rapidly by signs of meningeal irritation. When the onset is more continuous, as it quite commonly is, the fever does not subside, and the symptoms and signs gradually spread to include the central nervous system. The initial symptoms may have been overlooked because of their mildness.

In the second phase of the onset, muscle aches in the extremities are common. Stiffness of the back and neck are noted, and headaches become a frequent complaint. The irritability that is common to involvement of the central nervous system becomes prominent.

Paralysis begins usually in the second to fifth day of the febrile period. It may be maximal in 2-4 days after recognition. Subsidence of the fever has been thought by many observers to signify the end of the development of paralysis. Sensitivity may, however, cause muscles to belie this characteristic of the disease. Marked persistence of the fever may occur in cases that eventually lead to death.

As Caverly noted, there may be no paralysis at all. Sensitivity precedes paralysis. In infants, the response may be one of flaccidity such that muscle spasm and sensitivity are not appreciated by the examiner. The fever is usually of approximately 101 °F and occasionally of 103 °F, but it is rarely greater than this. An exceptionally high fever is associated ordinarily with the encephalitic type.

Clinical Picture

The patient is a very irritable child who resents attempts to handle or move the extremities. Unless the disease is encephalitic, the patient is alert and clear. Spasm of the back, neck, and hamstrings is usual. Forward flexion of the neck is painful (Brudzinski). There is a positive Kernig test. Lying on his side, the patient does not allow forward flexion of the spine. When he sits, he presents the so-called "tripod" sign of poliomyelitis. With legs extended on the table, sitting is limited, and the patient supports himself in a partial sitting posture with his arms. Straight-leg raising is limited usually in a quite symmetric fashion; the leg which will later show most involvement is not necessarily more limited than the other.

Muscles may be sensitive to pressure. Muscle sensitivity should be distinguished from nerve sensitivity by palpation of the anatomic distribution of the large nerve trunks. Spasm of the trunk muscles may be acute anteriorly as well as posteriorly and may result in confusion with intra-abdominal conditions. Even in the so-called nonparalytic type of poliomyelitis, some mild weakness may be seen on careful examination.

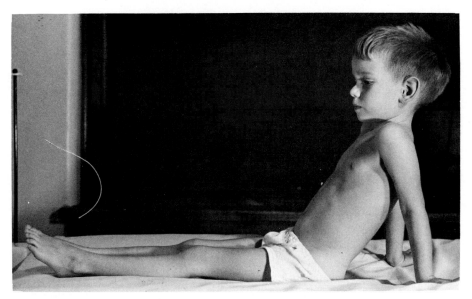

Fig. 12.21. The tripod sign in acute poliomyelitis. Spasm of the hamstrings and back muscles limits the patient's ability to sit up.

Differential Diagnosis

As Britt, Christie, and Batson have shown, the problem in diagnosis in a medical community that is alert to the disease is not that of overlooking poliomyelitis, but that of misdiagnosing other entities as poliomyelitis. Entities to be considered as the same time as nonparalytic poliomyelitis are meningitis, encephalitis, brain tumor, gastroenteritis, bacillary dysentery, meningococcemia, tick typhus, fecal impaction, and intussusception.

In patients presenting paralysis or pseudoparalysis, poliomyelitis must be differentiated from the Guillain-Barré syndrome, brain and cord tumors, osteomyelitis, pyelonephritis, scurvy, and fractures.

Treatment

In the acute phase, the patient is on bed rest and is protected against deformity by general measures, including positioning. A bed board is used so that excessive lumbar lordosis is readily seen. The bed board should not be one piece, however, since treatment of the disease includes periodic positioning of the patient in gentle spinal flexion when mobilization is begun. A knee roll that allows slight flexion of the knee

is a matter of great comfort to the patient. The foot board is separated from the end of the mattress, and the heels are allowed to drop into the interspace. A small neck roll may be comfortable. Hot packs are used to diminish sensitivity. Thdy also aid the performance of stretching type exercises when they are used just prior to the stretching. If they produce discomfort, they have little value. Hot packs in general are wrapped around an extremity and laid on the trunk. Continous use of packs can be debilitating to the patient.

There are many special therapeutic problems at this stage which cannot be covered here. They include measures to relieve difficulty in swallowing, respiration, and micturition. The respirator, rocking bed, and tracheotomy have special and definite indications.

While the patient is febrile it is important that disturbances and handling be minimized and that supportive measures be gentle and adequate. Positioning in bed to avoid deformity results in a very sensitive patient if it overstretches irritable muscles.

Convalescent Stage

The convalescent stage begins with the subsidence of fever and continues for 1½ years after the onset. It has been found that, during this period, the disease has a marked tendency to improve spontaneously in so far as paralytic involvement is concerned. With the appearance of paralysis and sensitivity, there is a marked tendency toward deformity. The paralyzed muscles, when they are opposed by muscles in spasm, become overstretched. Spastic paralysis has been seen very rarely in encephalitic types of involvement. Flaccid paralysis is the general rule.

The bulbospinal respiratory type needs special emphasis since it may be fatal. Prompt and early recognition is essential to the treatment. Facial nerves may be involved in bulbar poliomyelitis.

Examination in the stage of sensitivity must be gentle. Much can be learned merely from observing the patient's characteristic position in bed. Tendencies such as external rotation of the lower extremity, drop foot, and adduction of the upper extremity are readily appreciated. Assessment of muscle weakness at this initial stage may be general rather than specific, but it should be thorough enough to reveal what measures are necessary to block the development of deformity.

Muscle spasm in poliomyelitis is largely due to an attempt on the part of the patient to protect sensitive muscles. Spasm of this type may seem to indicate more paralysis than actually exists because the opposing muscles may be inhibited by reflex. The duration of the paralysis varies with the degree of involvement. Mild involvement may result in transient weakness only. The degree of initial paralysis is of some help in prognosticatinng the time of eventual recovery. The subsidence of sensitivity greatly aids the patient's progress. The rate of recovery is greatest in the early phases of the disease and decreases as the final stages of the convalescent period are reached. The patient at the end of this period passes to the chronic or reconstructive stage of poliomyelitis.

Pathology

Areas other than the central nervous system are involved. Lymphoid tissue generally is hyperplastic. A myocarditis has been noted at autopsy, and it occurs in approximately 25% of cases that terminate in death. The nerve cells themselves are the seat of primary injury, however. The virus is located within the neurones, and degeneration of them leads to secondary tract and nerve degeneration. There is an inflammatory and hemorrhagic reaction, the subsidence of which in the presence of undamaged ganglion cells may account for the "recovery tendency" of the disease.

The ganglion cells undergo coagulative necrosis, chromatolysis, and neuronophagia. There is no evidence that damaged ganglion cells recover. The motor cells of the cord are apparently more susceptible than cells of the cerebral cortex. The effects of the disease are not limited to the cord, however, but have been noted in medulla, pons, midbrain, cortex, and cerebellum as well. A neurogliar proliferation tends to produce a scar in 3-4 weeks.

The lesions typically tend to be distributed in the anterior horn, i.e., predominantly dorsomedially. This distribution accounts for the tendency of the clinical picture to follow certain distributions of paralysis. The anterior horn involvement is most severe, and lateral columns and posterior horns are affected.

In the late stages of the disease, the axis cylinders of the peripheral nerves degenerate. The muscles undergo the changes associated with denervation atrophy. There is a loss of striations, reduction in sarcoplasm, and alteration in electrical response. This is followed by atrophy, fibrosis, and fat replacement. Bone atrophy is a late development that follows disuse of the limb.

The development of cold legs that have a tendency to appear mildly cyanotic may be due to palsy of parasympathetic nerves from damage to the bulbar cord; the sympathetic system is spared through the lateral columns of lumbar nerves 1 and 2. Damage of anterior horn cells affects the parasympathetic system more than the sympathetic and results in failure of bladder and rectum to contract; it thereby produces the clinical problems in these areas that are occasionally seen in poliomyelitis.

Treatment

Once the patient is afebrile, the paralytic involvement is estimated. The estimate may be inaccurate owing to muscle spasm and sensitivity; it may indicate more severe involvement than actually exists. Tendencies toward deformity are noted, and the patient is positioned against them periodically during the day. The bed may be used to aid in developing spinal flexion and hamstring stretching. No positioning should be considered static, but changes in position should be frequently made.

Splints are often necessary. With young children, they are used in place of the footboard because it is sometimes difficult to keep the youngster against the board. The splint holds the foot in a neutral position so far as dorsiflexion and inversion-eversion are concerned. An outrigger attached to the splint to prevent chronic hyperextension of the knee by holding it in slight flexion is occasionally used. Splints should not be misused by being left on the patient for excessively long periods.

All of the joints should be carried through a range of motion within the limits of pain regularly during the day. Stretching is begun early and is carried to, but not beyond, the point of producing pain. Limbs are held at bony prominences, not in areas of large muscle masses, in tender patients. The period of convalescence is greatly shortened by early stretching and mobilization. The spine should be stretched in rotation as well as in flexion.

The drop foot deformity is well known in poliomyelitis. When the patient is prone, the feet should be allowed to drop into the interval between the mattress and the footboard. Less well known but quite common is the development of a flexion abduction deformity at the hip. This deformity begins with spasm of the iliopsoas, sartorius, and tensor fascia lata muscles, which tilts the pelvis forward and produces excessive lumbar lordosis. When the spasm is unilateral, a curve in the spine is produced. Full spine roentgenograms made while the patient is recumbent are often helpful in picking up early tendencies toward spinal deformities.

By the end of the first month, the patient ordinarily has full straight-leg raising and spine flexion, and an accurate estimation of the paralysis has been obtained. The following muscle-grading system is usually used:

Muscle Rating	*Definition*
Zero	No palpable contraction.
Trace	Palpable contraction but no movement of the part.
Poor	Part moves through its range but not against gravity.
Fair	Part moves through its range against gravity, but not against resistance.
Good	Part moves through its range against gravity and against resistance.
Normal	Normal.

In general, a muscle rated "zero" cannot be expected to progress beyond a "poor" rating. A muscle needs to be rated "fair" in the early stage of the disease in order to develop to "good" or "normal" in most instances. Not the extent, but the degree, of involvement is of some help in prognosis. Certain muscles have a marked tendency to be involved together, e.g., biceps femoris and gastrocnemius; and the clinical problem can often be predicted when the involvement of one is known.

The basic exercise rule is to exercise the muscle according to its rated grade. Exercising the muscle beneath its capabilities does not produce improvement except in endurance. In order to increase in power, the muscle must perform maximal work at each contraction. An increase in power is more helpful to the poliomyelitis patient at this stage of his disease than an increase in endurance. Repetitive exercises to increase endurance may be used at a late date. When the limb can be moved against gravity, progressive resistance exercises are added.

In general, bed rest is continued as long as something is to be gained from it. Residual sensitivity or tightness should be overcome before the patient is allowed up. Asymmetric tightness in the trunk should not be allowed to persist. Weakness of the trunk often calls for continued bed rest. The development of an extremely important muscle, such as the gastrocnemius, gluteus medius, or gluteus maximus, may deserve further attention before ambulation is permitted.

Except in nonparalytic cases, crutches are almost routine when ambulation is begun. Even in abortive cases, the child may have difficulty in raising the body weight with the gastrocnemius, and crutches and heel lifts help to procure the return of full function of the gastrocnemius within 2 weeks after the patient is allowed up.

Bracing is a means of preventing deformity and allowing greater activity than would otherwise be possible. Many of these children can walk without braces but with severe tendencies toward deformity in their gait. A brace aids in the prevention of overstretching a muscle, which may result in regression rather than in an increase in the power of a muscle. The gastrocnemius is so important a muscle in a child's gait that it must be protected at all costs. The young child without the gastrocnemius walks with hyperextended knees and frequently needs a long-leg brace. The older child can be taught to keep the knee flexed if sufficient muscle power is present.

A weak gastrocnemius must be prevented from allowing a calcaneus foot to develop. The particular type of brace used varies from child to child according to the individual muscle picture.

Paralytic shoulders (weak deltoid), drop feet (weak anterior tibial), knee weakness (weak quadriceps or hamstrings) are among other anomalies that must be improved by apparatus. A weak trunk must be braced according to the degree of involvement. Abdominals are particularly prone to being overstretched when the upright posture is resumed.

The pool is particularly useful in exercising patients with trunk and hip weakness, in handling large patients with extensive involvement, in stretching out resistant tightness, and in beginning ambulation in patients with minimal musculature.

So far as electrical stimulation is concerned, the present evidence indicates that in the initial phase of involvement, it temporarily slows the progress of atrophy. However, atrophy progresses nonetheless and eventually reaches the same degree in a stimulated muscle as in an unstimulated one that is similarly involved. Cessation of the stimulation causes the atrophy to progress rapidly to the level expected. There appears to be no justification for its routine use, although it may be of some help in enabling the patient to find a muscle in cases of facial paralysis or virtually flail extremities, for example.

Chronic or Residual Poliomyelitis

At the end of the convalescent period of poliomyelitis, that is, 18 months after the onset, the patient enters a period that is dominated, for the physician, by three important aims: (1) to prevent deformity, (2) to increase muscle power, and (3) to reconstruct and substitute for paralysis.

Although no further recovery can be expected, the patient may improve in the performance of practical functional tasks.

Clinical Description

These patients have usually recovered from the initial mental depression of poliomyelitis. They enter the residual stage attempting to gain as much functional ability as possible. Except in the case of a completely flail extremity, they are left with muscle imbalance, which, alone and unprotected, is sufficient to cause deformity. To this imbalance may be added the tendencies toward deformity due to use and to gravity. Atrophy of the extremity is noted within 6 weeks of the onset. A markedly diminished circulation in childhood has an effect on growth. The patient up to this point has not been allowed to substitute muscles to gain function and has become well schooled in exercise routines. The economic factor, an important consideration in adults, is not important for children.

This stage may be attended by loss of function due to progressive deformity. Flaccid paralysis is sufficient disability, but its effects may be augmented by contracture. Gravity and function may stretch ligaments and joint capsules to the point that they no longer act as adequately functioning units.

Bracing

The brace is a means of allowing increased activity without increased deformity. It is not a means of limiting activity. Bracing should be as dynamic as possible. The following outline of its uses is greatly simplified.

Lower Extremities. The foot, if completely flail, must be supported on both sides, as well as anteriorly and posteriorly, by a double upright brace with stops to limit both dorsal and plantar flexion. Such a brace ordinarily allows 10° of motion at the ankle as an aid in walking.

When the peroneal musculature alone is weak, a single upright brace placed on the

Fig. 12.22. Bracing is a means of expanding the child's horizon—not of limiting it.

medial side may be sufficient. An anterior T-strap is ordinarily added. This strap runs from the shoe to the lower tibia and upright. Lateral wedges may be used on the shoe. Stops are added when there is weakness anteroposteriorly. An anterior stop aids in preventing overstretching of the gastrocnemius. A posterior stop aids in preventing drop foot and overstretching of the anterior tibial.

Anterior or posterior tibial weakness is protected by a lateral single upright with an inner T-strap. Medial wedges on the shoe and a longitudinal arch pad are often necessary additions. Anterior or posterior stops or both may be necessary.

Different combinations of paralysis may demand double upright braces where, at first glance, a single upright may seem to be all that is necessary.

Knee. A "poor" or worse gastrocnemius may result in a tendency to hyperextend the knee despite good knee musculature. For children 6 years old and younger, a doubt in regard to the necessity for a long-leg brace should result in its use. Older children can be taught to protect their knees by walking in flexion.

Surprisingly, both strength of the quadriceps in the presence of weak hamstrings and weakness of the quadriceps may result in hyperextension at the knee. A brace to support the knee must of necessity be of double upright construction. The leather knee cap should not be so tight that it forces the knee into hyperextension. Knee braces have a number of

Fig. 12.23. Calcaneous foot produced by attempting take off in the gait without gastrocnemius power.

ingenious locks designed to allow flexion when the child is sitting. The single so-called "drop lock" works well with children.

Hip. Gluteus medius and gluteus maximus limps are largely eliminated by the use of crutches or canes. The hip weakness cannot be substituted for by a brace alone. When the hip is flail, it may be necessary to join a long-leg brace to a trunk brace by means of a hinge.

Trunk. When abdominal weakness alone is present and is relatively symmetric, a corset may suffice. The corset should be laced from the bottom upward to support the abdominal contents properly. Lateral deviations of the spine may be held well by a brace of the Barr-Buschenfeldt type whose arms are appropriately placed to eliminate the deviation. In general the lower arm supports the slump, and the upper arm corrects the curve. Check roentgenograms may be taken while the patient is held by supporting hands in the position of the arms of the brace. An x-ray film taken with the patient in the brace reveals a need for further adjustment, if there is one.

Neck. Asymmetric weakness of the sternocleido mastoids may call for holding braces of the Buchminster-Brown or collar type for a growing child. When the weakness is quite general, braces built with chin cups and occipital supports and held by a pelvic band in the fashion of Blount's brace may be needed.

Upper Extremity. The shoulder joint is subject to gravity, and weakness of the deltoid may result in a tendency toward overstretching of the capsular structures. Support for the humerus may come from the trunk or from a sling anchored at the neck. Allowing a subluxation to develop renders a later reconstruction more difficult and eliminates all possibility of improvement.

The flail elbow may be simply kept at a right angle by a sling or by a combination shoulder and elbow brace.

Hand-bracing, which varies in method with each patient, attempts to encourage the position of function; it has been more fully described in Chapter 7, Dr. Stelling's "The Upper Extremity."

The child presents a different picture from that of the adult. In children, growth in length of bone relative to soft tissue is a factor in the production of severe contractures. A child may have to be supported for many years before the skeletal maturation of a joint is sufficient to permit an arthrodesis. Children wandering from supervision may, in a short time, develop more severe deformity than adults. The problems of rehabilitation, from the points of view of both surgery and vocation, are quite different.

Progressive Resistance Exercise

Exercises during the chronic stage of poliomyelitis may be aimed at development of

Fig. 12.24. Long-leg brace for flail leg.

order to isolate function. The problem of training the muscle in the new position is then greatly simplified. The first stage in educating a transplanted muscle is to achieve use of the muscle and to suppress the use of antagonists to it. The muscle must be repeatedly "set" until a powerful sustained contraction is reduced. The proprioceptive response aids in finding the muscle when some form of resistance is used. The motion of the part involved aids in suppressing the antagonist muscles. The synergists are then suppressed one by one until the transplanted muscle alone is left. Once it has been isolated in this manner, the muscle can progressively develop greater force with increasing resistance.

Stretching Exercises

These exercises are of greatest usefulness in combatting contractures which play an active role in the development of deformity. Many of these contractures are residual from the onset of the disease—when muscle spasm resulted in habitual positioning of joints. Myostatic contractures take place only in innervated muscle and are much more likely to be seen in partially involved than in completely flail extremities.

Fixed equinus of the foot due to anterior tibial weakness in the presence of a strong gatrocnemius is most common. Flexion contractures of the hip aided by a strong iliopsoas and a weak gluteus maximus are frequently unrecognized until they are well marked. This is particularly true of a flexion-abduction contracture in which the sartorius and tensor fascia lata enter as additional factors.

Contractures of the trunk that limit the lateral bend, forward flexion, or rotation may be factors in the development of trunk deformity.

Stretching type exercises must be performed in the correct position so that the joint proximal to that being moved is immobilized. The knee is extended when the Achilles tendon is stretched, for example. Correct use of stretching exercises requires a detailed knowledge of anatomy.

Stretching exercises accomplish their purpose when they are done to the maximum each day, rather than when they are repeated many times in a single day. Muscles like the hamstrings are

hypertrophy. Progressive resistance exercises as popularized by DeLorme and Watkins are particularly valuable in this regard. The principle is that, to gain strength, the muscle must undergo a maximal contraction—that is, maximal in relation to the work load performed. Thus, if a muscle can life 5 lb against gravity, it should be exercised at this level until it can lift 6 lb. Repeated submaximal contractions may increase endurance, but not strength.

Since a heavy load increases the sensory response in a muscle, progressive resistance exercises aid also in isolating and strengthening transplanted muscle. DeLorme has advocated preoperative use of this type of exercise in

Fig. 12.25. Barr-Buschenfeldt brace used to hold early paralytic scoliosis.

particularly easy to stretch. Those about the pelvis with heavy fascia and short muscle bellies are particularly difficult.

Functional Training

The simplest example of functional training is the teaching of a patient to negotiate stairs. It is obvious that the strong leg pulls the patient upstairs and steadies him as he advances downstairs. The difficulty of such a task is appreciated when the patient confronts it, however; and the bracing and muscle power that a patient has must be converted to use in the tasks of life. The simple act of getting out of a chair can be a very complicated thing when one is handicapped. The combining of crutches and the use of them as an aid rather than a hindrance can be quickly taught. Yet if he is left to his own devices, the patient may find it impossible to leave the chair with any facility. The necessity of arms, the use of the upper extremity to extend the trunk, the locking of

braces in turn become aids under guidance.

The practical problems that the patient has to face must be met and solved. These include eating, the use of the bathroom and stairs, entering and leaving public transportation, and many others. One need not have expensive equipment to duplicate these tasks. Ingenuity and forethought bring the patient to the successful solution of these problems if they are met in some form in advance of activity.

Reconstruction of Paralytic Patient

No operation of this type is justified unless it either (1) enables the patient to use less apparatus, (2) prevents progressive deformity, or (3) increases the patient's ability to perform. It is recognized that there are many alternative procedures to the one more or less standard procedure given here.

Unstable Foot. Various types of situations have to be met under this heading, since all possible ones cannot be covered specifically. In various borderline situations individual judgment must determine treatment. Bone deformity must be corrected; the use of muscle transplant alone is of limited usefulness in the presence of deformity.

Peroneal strength, anterior and posterior tibial weakness, and good gastrocnemius—This situation results ordinarily in a valgus foot or a drop foot. Before the age of 10, the foot has been stabilized, from the skeletal point of view, by the subtalar bone block procedure of Grice.[5] A transplant alone in the presence of this deformity cannot pull the medial arch up against the body weight. In Grice's procedure, the subtalar joint is exposed. The os calcis is inverted beneath the astragalus, and a notched bed is made in the inferior surface of the astragalus and the superior surface of the os calcis, just distal to the posterior third of this joint.

The height of the bed is measured by compass. Two grafts from the proximal tibial cortex are then inserted exactly into this bed to block the ability of the os calcis to evert laterally. The grafts are wedge-shaped and are of greatest height laterally.

A transplant of the peroneus longus is then performed. The peroneus longus tendon is divided just proximal to the os peronei. The peroneus brevis is detached from the base of the fifth metatarsal and sewn to the stump of the longus. A bed is then made for the insertion of the tendon in the base of the second metatarsal. (In some feet, a still more medial insertion may be indicated.) An insertion that has worked well is accomplished in the following manner. A drill hole sufficiently large to accept the tendon is created in the superior cortex, and two small drill holes are made just distal to it. A third incision is now made on the lateral calf. The peroneus longus is identified and then retracted into the proximal wound. A long incision is made into the anterior muscle compartment. A tendon passer is introduced into this compartment and is run beneath the deep fascia to the bed prepared in the base of the second metatarsal. Silk sewn into the peroneus longus is drawn by the tendon passer down this route. If the procedure is done quickly and smoothly, the peroneus longus will lie flat without twisting.

With the use of a good tendon suture technique, the two ends of the thread (2-0) are individually passed out through the distal drill holes. The tendon is drawn down into the bone, and the thread is tied. The tendon should be taut when the foot is in maximal dorsiflexion and inversion. The patient is kept in a long-leg plaster cast in the corrected position for 6 weeks and then in a bivalved cast in which the peroneal transplant can be exercised until it is working well. When bone union is demonstrated in the grafts, the patient begins weight-bearing with crutches. When it can be estab-

Fig. 12.26. Peroneal strength and anterior and posterior tibial weakness leads to valgus deformity of the foot, as on the left.

lished that the transplant is used in the gait (about 2 months later), the crutches are discarded.

For patients past the age of 10 whose feet have a fixed valgus deformity, a triple arthrodesis is indicated. In addition, however, the muscle balance of the foot must be restored by a peroneal transplant, or the deformity will probably recur.

A triple arthrodesis corrects bony deformity by the shape of the wedges removed, and provides stability for the foot by fusing the midtarsal and subtalar joints.

A lateral incision over the sinus tarsi is made. The muscle belly of the short extensor to the toes is reflected from its origin on the os calcis. The long extensor tendons are retracted superiorly, and the peroneal tendons are retracted inferiorly. The fat filling the sinus tarsi is removed. The head of the astragalus, the astragalar surface of the navicular, and the cubocalcaneal and subtalar joints are exposed. The first osteotome cut is made in the astragalus in line with the coronal plane of the ankle joint without involving the bone further than is necessary to get in this plane. Navicular and cuboid joint surfaces are removed at right angles to the forefoot. The subtalar joint surfaces are removed, astragalar surface parallel

Fig. 12.28. Subastragalar arthrodesis described by Grice. The tibial cortex is cut on a carefully measured triangle twice the height of block needed, and the center cut is angled so that grafts can be wedged into the subastragalar joint.

Fig. 12.29. The tibial cortical grafts in place.

with the weight-bearing plane of the ankle joint, calcaneal surface with sufficient wedge to correct the hindfoot eversion. Inversion should not be produced as it will increase with weight bearing.

At the conclusion, joint surfaces should be flatly opposed. The tissues are repaired to eliminate dead space. The foot is held by the operator as a long-leg plaster cast is applied. This cast is kept on for 6 weeks. When it is removed, roentgenograms are taken, and a short-leg cast is applied if early fusion is apparent. The short-leg cast is used for 2 weeks

Fig. 12.27. Peroneus longus muscle implanted into base of second metatarsal.

Fig. 12.30. Postoperative roentgenogram of tibial cortical grafts blocking subastragalar joint into inversion.

with crutches and a walking heel, then for 2 more weeks to stimulate maturation of the fusion. The cast is then removed and partial weight bearing with crutches is begun.

When a transplant has been simultaneously done, the cast is bivalved at 6 weeks, and exercises for the transplant are done, and continued usually for a 4-6 week period until maturation of the fusion is revealed by roentgenogram as well as by the action of the transplant. Partial weight bearing with crutches is then begun.

Anterior tibial absent, peroneals strong, posterior tibial strong, toe extensors strong—

When the posterior tibial balances the everting pull of the peroneals, equinus of the forefoot may result in a cavus deformity. If it is done before fixed bony changes occur, a transplant of the extensor tendons into the metatarsal necks gives dorsiflexion.

*Weak gastrocnemius, strong peroneal, and strong anterior and posterior tibial muscle power—*Before the age of 14, the peroneal longus, posterior tibial, and long toe flexor may be moved and inserted into the posterior inferior angle of the os calcis. When there is no gastrocnemius power, such a transplant, although it does not give sufficient power to substitute for a brace, may prevent progression of a calcaneous deformity.

When there is some gastrocnemius power, such additions may be sufficient to substitute for a brace and to give a normal gait.

After the age of 14, an ankle fusion is preferable in the presence of a laterally stable foot.

An incision is made anteromedially and is carried down to the ankle joint between the long extensors of the toes and the anterior tibial tendons. A Hatt type of procedure is followed. The cartilage surfaces of the ankle joint are denuded and fitted together. A graft of tibial cortex is elevated from the anteromedial surface of the distal tibia. The most distal inch of tibial cortex is left intact as a bridge. A Hatt osteotome is inserted into the medullary cavity of the tibia and driven across the ankle joint and well into the astragalus. The bone graft is then driven down the track made by the osteotome. The foot is very carefully positioned as this is done so that the position determined as optimal preoperatively can be achieved and held by the graft. Ten degrees of equinus are usually necessary, but there may be some variety dependent on sex, type of heel worn, and other factors.

Knee. *Hyperextension deformity of knee—*This deformity quite frequently needs to be corrected. It results from the gait habit of locking the unstable knee by placing it in hyperextension. The procedure for correcting it is not done until growth is completed. A Steinmann pin or Kirschner wire is driven into the most proximal tibia. Force is applied to the pin as the tibia is divided distal to it. The proximal fragment is thus held in hyperextension as the distal fragment is lined up with the femur. This position is held as a plaster cast is applied.

Absent quadriceps; strong semimembranosus, semitendinosus, and biceps femoris—Not every patient who lacks a quadriceps needs muscle power anteriorly at the knee. Where a fundamental gain is possible, one or more of the hamstrings may be transplanted forward to the patella.

Hip. The most troublesome situation here is that of weak or absent gluteals with a strong hip flexor. The result is a tendency toward hip flexion contracture, which unleashes a series of events that may result in a paralytic dislocation of the hip.

Barr found that anterior fasciotomy at the hip with reenforcement posteriorly did not prevent a recurrence of deformity. Such reenforcement is available in the erector spinae transplant of Ober.[9a] It is insufficient to substitute for a gluteus maximus, but it can be used as a check to the development of a hip flexion contracture.

In this procedure, after preliminary fasciotomy anteriorly, a second incision is made to detach the fascia lata at its insertion into the fibula. It is withdrawn and run from the insertion of the tensor fascia lata into it through a subperiosteal tunnel below the greater trochanter, posteriorly over the pelvis, through the substance of the gluteus maximus, to the erector spinae. The lower end of the erector spinae is fashioned into a cone in its

Figs. 12.31 and 12.32. Inverted foot with poor gastrocnemius and good peroneal and anterior and posterior tibial power.

Fig. 12.33. Functional hand and elbow with flail deltoid but good scapular muscles—a candidate for fusion.

lower segments, and the fascia lata is sewn around it while the hip is in an extended position.

Shoulder. Paralysis of the deltoid can be very well substituted for by fusion. There are fundamental conditions to be met, however, before fusion can be considered. The muscles controlling the scapula must be rated "good" or better, and the hand and elbow must be functional. The situation of the other arm must be considered. The patient should be past age 12. The joint is usually denuded of cartilage, the surfaces are opposed, and the acromion is osteotomized and bent down to notch into the humerus.

The usual position is such that the hand reaches the mouth when the elbow is flexed. This usually means about 45° of abduction, 15° of forward flexion, and 15° of internal rotation.

The postoperative shoulder spica is made preoperatively so that the position is accurate. The spica is removed and replaced after operation. The usual period of necessary immobilization is 4 months.

Elbow. Lack of elbow flexion must be overcome to restore useful function to the upper extremity. It is fairly common to have good forearm flexors with weak or absent biceps. If the hand has function, a Steindler transplant may be performed.

Here the common flexor tendon is isolated at its origin from the medial epicondyle and transplanted approximately 1 1/2 inches proximally up the shaft of the humerus. This improves the lever action across the elbow joint so that the hand can be elevated against gravity

Fig. 12.34. Muscle transplant—in this case, the fourth sublimus tendon to the metacarpal and first phalanx of the thumb.

Fig. 12.35. Muscle transplant provides motor power.

Fig. 12.36. Muscle transplant increases function.

and against some resistance.

References

1. Bouman, H. D., and Schwartz, R. P.: The degree, the extent and the mechanism of muscle spasm in infantile paralysis, *New York J. Med., 44:* 147, 1944.
2. Colonna, P.: Hamstring transplantation for quadriceps paralysis, *J. Bone Joint Surg., 5:* 472, 1923.
3. Ghormley, R. K.: History of the treatment of poliomyelitis, *J. Iowa Med. Soc., 37:* 343, 1947.
4. Green, W. T.: Diagnostic and therapeutic considerations in anterior poliomyelitis, *Rhode Island Med. J., 28:* 89, 1945.
5. Grice, D. S.: Further experience with extra-articular arthrodesis of the subtalar joint, *J. Bone Joint Surg., 37A:* 246, 1955.
6. Johnson, R. W.: Results of modern methods of treatment of poliomyelitis, *J. Bone Joint Surg., 27:* 223, 1945.
7. Jones, R.: On arthrodesis and tendon transplantation, *Br. Med. J.,* March 28, 1908.
8. Legg, A. T., and Merrill, J. B.: *Physical Therapy in Infantile Paralysis,* Hagerstown, Md.: W. F. Prior, Inc., 1932.
9. Lovett, R. W.: *The Treatment of Infantile Paralysis,* Philadelphia: Blakiston Co., 1916.
9a. Ober, F. R.: Tendon transplantation in the lower extremity, *N. Engl. J. Med., 209:* 52, 1933.
10. Peabody, C. W.: Tendon transplantation—an end-result study, *J. Bone Joint Surg., 20:* 193, 1938.
11. Sabin, A. B.: Pathology and pathogenesis in human poliomyelitis, *J. A. M. A., 120:* 506, 1942.
12. Steindler, A.: *The Rehabilitation of the Paralyzed Patient,* New York: Appleton-Century-Crofts, Inc., 1925.
13. Yount, C. C.: The role of the tensor fascia femoris in certain deformities of the lower extremities, *J. Bone Joint Surg., 8:* 171, 1926.

PROGRESSIVE MUSCULAR ATROPHY OF THE PERONEAL TYPE (PERONEAL ATROPHY, CHARCOT-MARIE-TOOTH DISEASE)

Progressive muscular atrophy of the peroneal type is a familial disorder. It virtually always begins in the lower extremity progressing thereafter to the upper. Although the peroneal muscles are usually the first involved, the anterior and posterior tibial, extensors of the toes, and the gastrocnemius-soleus group exhibit weakness shortly thereafter. It is a disease with symmetrical involvement of the distal extremities with a flaccid paralysis without sensory involvement.

It is most commonly inherited as a dominant trait, but may be inherited either as a recessive or a sex-linked recessive. In general, when inherited as a dominant trait the progress of the disease is relatively mild and consistent with survival into the 6th and 7th decades of life. The disease is rarely seen in infancy and is usually recognized in the 2nd and 3rd decade. When involvement is extensive the disease usually begins around the age of 8 or 9.

Clinical Picture

The disease first presents in children late in the 1st decade or in the teens with symmetrical weakness in the lower extremities. A cavus foot deformity may be a presenting complaint and is usually the case with late onset. The upper extremity weakness begins distally with involvement of the ulnar nerve and the development of clawhand.

The reflexes are diminished to absent without the development of hyperactivity first, such as may be seen in diseases involving the long tracts of the cord, e.g., syringomyelia and Friedreich's ataxia. The symmetrical involvement distally aids in distinguishing it from the residuals of poliomyelitis.

The gait may become quite disabling with the development of a drop foot and calcaneus element.

Electromyographic Findings

The conduction velocity of the peroneal, median, and ulnar nerves may be measured as a means of confirming the diagnosis. The distal latency of response is obtained by measuring the time interval from the moment of stimulation of the nerve to the appearance of action potentials recorded over the hypothenar, thenar, and extensor digitorum brevis muscle groups. Over the age of 5, conduction velocities less than 47 m per second in the medial nerve and 40 m per second in the peroneal nerve are considered abnormal.

Dyck, Lambert, and Mulder[3] have shown that all patients who have a definite clinical picture of Charcot-Marie-Tooth disease had slow conduction velocity in these peripheral nerves. Relatives of patients with the disease may show slow conduction velocities even without clinical involvement, but this is not frequent.

Conduction velocities are lower in infants and very young children.

Pathology

The peripheral nerves show atrophy with empty sheath; occasional regenerating fibers may be found. The pathology in the spinal cord has not been well delineated but it is believed to be simply an involvement of the anterior horn cells without tract degeneration. The muscle fibers show the results of neural atrophy with some fatty replacement.

Treatment

Jacobs and Carr[4] have emphasized the prognosis for a long life and usual function. As a result such procedures as bracing to prevent deformity and stabilizations are indicated.

The triple arthrodesis frequently is of great aid to the patient. Ankle fusion may be necessary with drop foot and gastrocnemius weakness. Tendon transplantations are not ordinarily indicated due to the progressive involvement.

Bracing may support a drop foot, stabilize lateral instability of the foot, and prevent the development of further deformity in the growing child.

References

1. Allan, W.: Relation of hereditary pattern to clinical severity as illustrated by peroneal atrophy, *Arch. Int. Med., 63:* 1123, 1939.
2. Duncan, S. A.: Orthopedic treatment of the muscular dystrophies and muscular atrophies, *Va. Med. Mon., 64:* 40, 1937.
3. Dyck, P. J., Lambert, E. H., and Mulder, D.: Charcot-Marie-Tooth disease; nerve conduction and clinical studies of a large kinship, *Neurology, 8:* 1, 1963.
4. Jacobs, J. E., and Carr, C. R.: Progressive muscular atrophy of the peroneal type, *J. Bone Joint Surg., 32A:* 27, 1950.

SPINA BIFIDA SYNDROME (MYELOMENINGOCELE AND HYDROCEPHALUS)

General Discussion

An intensive therapeutic attack on children born with myelomeningocele was spawned in the late 1950s and continued through the decade of the 1960s. As a result, the 4-year survival rate rose from 46% to 61%. The severe disability present in most of these surviving children caused a careful statistical reevaluation of what had been accomplished.

The problems of these children present in varying combinations including hydrocephalus treated with a mechanical shunt and necessitating repeated revisions, paraplegia and the necessity to use braces and/or wheel chair, kyphosis, scoliosis, extreme dwarfing, repeated fractures, low intelligence quotient, and occasionally blindness and fits. The severity of many of these disabilities was sufficient to prevent the child from having any future, other than as a ward of the state. The cost of care was beyond the reasonable allocation of its benefit to society, the load impossible to carry, and the services required from physicians and surgeons spread them thin and diluted their efforts for those who could benefit most from their attention.

John Lorber was able to put together the experience at Sheffield, England, where a center for the care of these children was established. Physicians were encouraged to refer the infants at birth. He reported that, of 848 admissions to the center, 424 who were alive revealed only 6 or 0.7% with no handicaps, 73 or 8.6% had a moderate handicap, that is, they were incontinent but had not developed pyelonephritis, had a limp, used crutches, had segmental analgesia, and hydrocephalus without need for a shunt or well controlled with a shunt.

Beyond these were the severely affected with two or more systems and functional disabilities affected to the point of inability to compete in life.

The intelligence quotient in this group ranged as follows:

Intelligence Quotient	Number	Percentage
Over 80	201	23.72
60–79	93	11.09
Below 60	51	6.09

The loss of sensation in the lower extremities led to problems with trophic ulcers, the kyphosis and scoliosis to severe disfigurement, the paralysis to inability to achieve ambulation, the osteoporosis to fractures and dwarfism, and the bladder neurology to pyelonephritis and death.

So far as locomotion was concerned, in 134 patients 13% were normal, 20% had a limp, 18% used crutches, 18% used a wheelchair most of the time, and 37% were confined to a wheelchair.

There was good evidence that the hydrocephalus that occurred existed prior to the closure of the myelomeningocele, rather than being caused by the surgery. It occurred in 80% of the myelomeningocele cases and was made clinically apparent sooner by the closure. Blindness, relatively rare, occurred when the patient was unmanaged for sufficient periods of time. Twenty percent of the patients receiving a shunt procedure died as a direct result of the operation within 7 years.

In severe hydrocephalus there were no survivors without severe sequelae.

It became apparent that society could not support the maintenance of survivors without function and prevent their suffering one complication after another without an expense and service effort that it was unable to mount.

Lorber was able to post some adverse criteria leading to the selection of those needing treatment and prognosticating accurately the inability of medicine, surgery, the patient, and the parent to rise in any functional way above the severe malformation that existed at birth. Normal function, if anything, decreased (it did not increase) with removal of the myelomeningocele.

A policy of selection was based on adverse criteria. The criteria of bad import included any two of the following:

1. A thoracolumbar lesion.
2. A paraplegia with level above the third lumbar.
3. A head circumference 2 cm above the 90th percentile related to body weight.
4. Associated gross congenital anomalies.

Other criteria included severe prematurity and a heavily infected and ruptured spina bifida sac.

Selection was possible either at birth during the first day, during the first hospital admission, after closure, or anytime later such as for a life threatening situation, i.e., revision of the shunt.

Of children with adverse criteria, none survived to the 9th month, most died within the first 3 months.

The child with myelomeningocele represents a complex problem in treatment because his future as a human being is involved and can be thwarted by deficiencies in the neural, genitourinary, and motor areas.

A team approach involving the neurosurgeon, genitourinary surgeon, and the orthopaedic surgeon is necessary from birth to full growth in order to achieve the maximum function for these children.

It has been found by the neurosurgeon that virtually emergency resection of the myelomengocele at birth gives the most promise for maximal neural function. A wait of over 48 hr allows secondary infection to begin to develop, and resection at 9 or 10 days is fraught with hazards. If the early resection period is missed it is better to delay resection until further epitheliazation and stabilization of the hydrodynamics of the spinal fluid has occurred, a period of many months. The hydrocephalus is controlled by appropriate types of shunting procedures developed by neurosurgery.

Kidney function must be preserved. Price has delineated the rapid development of hydronephrosis when these children are bedridden either electively while undergoing hospital treatment or by necessity. He has also shown the importance of a Credé maneuver in emptying the bladder and relieving back pressure on the kidney. A well taught regime can markedly effect the hydronephrosis and improve kidney function. In addition, much of the odor and consequent social stigmas associated with constant or involuntary dribbling can be controlled. In an occasional case, the problem of urinary incontinence may be alleviated by a surgical procedure.

Detailed examination of the genitourinary system should be made at regular intervals. The construction of an ileal bladder to avoid reflux into the kidneys must be considered.

These children tend to become constipated despite a patulous anus. A program of regulated bowel control including bulk-producing medication is important. Enemas and manual assistance in emptying may be necessary. Laxatives that initiate the bowel are in general to be avoided.

Fig. 12.37. Typical myelomeningocele involving the lumbar region.

When hydrocephalus and myelomeningocele are associated, the child has an Arnold-Chiari syndrome. Secondary to this malformation, with herniation of the brain stem, paralysis of the vocal chords may occur and should be watched for.

Anatomy

Confusion about the pathology of myelomeningocele relates to the variability of the neurologic and osseous abnormalities. Despite their complexity, however, a basic pattern becomes evident. The infants have dysplasia of both spinal cord and meninges that causes irreversible neurologic disability. However, the neurologic loss is not static and may worsen with growth if a coexistant deformity such as diastematomyelia is present. Figure 12.38 shows a representative defect. The skin usually extends only partially over the defect and is confluent with the arachnoid, which covers the remainder of the defect. The dura mater is present ventrally, but usually fuses with the lateral skin edges. The dysplastic cord or attenuated nerve elements generally are fused to the arachnoid. Any cord elements that may exist beyond the gross defect are invariably

Fig. 12.38. (*Top*) Schematic transverse and longitudinal views of myelomeningocele. (*A*) Arachnoid,, (*B*) dysplastic cord, (*C*) dura, (*D*) skin, (*E*) peripheral roots, (*F*) vertebral body. (*Bottom*) Gross appearance of lumbosacral myelomeningocele in 2-month-old infant.

abnormal, causing a complete lower motor neuron type of flaccidity (no spinal reflex arc) below the highest level of the myelomeningocele defect. Often the cord above the dysplastic area, even though surrounded by normal vertebrae, may be abnormal, causing neurologic levels seemingly higher than the gross defect. Peripheral nerve roots develop relatively normally, but have abnormal connections with the spinal cord elements. The main osseous defect is arrested development of the laminae, with abnormal lateral deviation of the pedicles.

Fundamental Objectives

Every effort should be made to get these children ambulant as soon as possible. This aids in preventing the development of secondary urinary tract complications and increases the opportunity for learning experiences for the child. Although many of these children have a mental deficit, the mere presence of hydrocephalus does not rule out adequate cerebral function.

Arm exercises should be started as a game as soon as the child's attention can be held. Because most of these children have virtually flail lower extremities, the upper extremities must substitute for the lower. Wheelbarrow games in which the parent holds the child's legs and the child progresses by means of his arms are helpful. A chinning bar should be available. Push-ups and progression by means of the arms are to be encouraged.

Care is enormously complicated by sensory loss or anesthesia, which usually involves only the foot. It is obvious that foot deformity and lack of a well distributed weight-bearing surface lead to ulceration.

Feet

The child may be born with a foot deformity such as equinovarus, or deformity may develop with growth owing to unbalanced musculature. Most often, the anterior tibial musculature is present, but the other musculature, including the gastrocnemius, is virtually flail. A fixed equinus may easily develop, when virtually no muscle power is present, owing to a persistent recumbent position. Wherever such tendencies or an unbalanced musculature is noted, the feet should be supported in well padded bivalved casts that hold them in a neutral position. Because of associated knee and hip flexion problems, the casts are usually long-leg ones and are often joined by an outrigger or a bar to prevent the development of rotational deformities at the knee and hip.

The deformities present at birth should be corrected as rapidly as possible by repeated cast changes followed by the use of bivalved casts.

Hips

The associated skeletal anomalies of the lumbar spine and pelvis may be such that there is a fixed pelvic obliquity and no possibility of changing the bony anomaly. With care, the child will develop despite this anomaly. The hip should be stretched to secure good axial alignment and to overcome adduction and abduction contractures; it should then be held in neutral position by a bivalved spica.

When a child is first seen, the hips very commonly slide into the acetabulum on abduction or internal rotation but subluxate laterally when the child is brought to a weight-bearing position. In these children, valgus of the femoral neck is extreme. The hip musculature is flail or very weak, and sensation of the skin about the hip area has been partially lost. It is well to remember that although the glutei are innervated principally by the sacral roots, the hip joint itself is innervated principally by the lumbar roots (femoral and obturator nerves, for the most part).

Achieving a stable hip, with the aid to ambulation that sensation in this area provides, is important and should not be ignored. A varus osteotomy done in the intertrochanteric area seats the femoral head in the milder cases.

The innominate osteotomy of Salter (described in Chapter 4, under "Treatment of Dislocated Hip at Age Two to Four") brings the acetabulum over the head in others. Transplant of the iliopsoas to the greater trochanter may improve the hip situation, although it does not

Fig. 12.39. (*Left*) Sitting posture with extensive myelomeningocele and fixed pelvic obliquity secondary to lumbar spine anomalies. (*Right*) Lateral view of patient with myleomeningocele, extensive lumbar spine anomalies, and hip flexion contractures. Loss of trunk height and maldevelopment of lumbar spine are evident.

Fig. 12.40. Thermal injury to foot with diminished sensation secondary to myelomeningocele.

provide normal abductor power. The procedure has been described by Mustard and by Sharrard.[59] Movement of the hip flexor aids in preventing persistent hip flexion contracture. The added power in abduction keeps the femoral head seated in the acetabulum. These procedures or various combinations of them are used according to the requirements of the individual case.

Bracing

Long-leg braces are usually used with children from 1 to 4 years old because of the tendency to hyperextend the knee despite the presence of some power in the quadriceps or the hamstrings, or in both. The gastrocnemius paralysis that is common in these children aids the development of this deformity and further indicates long-leg braces. Rather than use pelvic bands, we prefer to stabilize the hips (surgically, if necessary) and to teach the child to substitute with his arms for his hip instability by using crutches. The greater ease of living without the pelvic band is worth the slower period of ambulation. Parallel bars in the home are helpful in developing arm power and in learning to use the arms as a substitute. The

child later progresses to saw horses, to crutches, and finally to crutch walking.

Development with Growth

To be prepared for school, the child must make contact with other children. Ambulation aids this. A bladder- and bowel-emptying routine must be established if the child is to go to school, as he may if his intellect is adequate. The tendency of this disease to cause the parents to reject the child is great. The child smells and is often unsightly, and his demands for care are enormous. The parent must be educated along with the child, and he must be brought to realize what possibilities the child has if an early start is made and a persistent followup is carried out.

Neurotrophic Joints

Myelodysplasia is the most frequent cause of the development of neurotrophic joints in childhood. When sensory loss in the lower extremity is profound, great care must be taken to make the braces fit accurately so that weight-bearing pressure is adequately distributed. Deformity must be corrected since localized persistent trauma will almost assuredly lead to difficulty. The only good treatment of neurotrophic joints is prevention.

Muscle Transplant

It is frequently found that the anterior tibial is a relatively strong muscle in an otherwise flail lower leg. The foot assumes a calcaneous position as the weak gastrocnemius becomes overstretched. It is frequently advantageous to transplant the anterior tibial muscle through the interosseous membrane and into the os calcis. The foot is held in equinus for several months thereafter and is then braced against dorsiflexion as weight bearing is begun.

Treatment

BY H. ANDREW WISSINGER, M.D.

Philosophy

The orthopaedic problems of the myelomeningocele are rather clear-cut. They are due to

Fig. 12.41. (*A*) The unstable hip in a patient with myelomengocele. (*B*) The same hip after a varus osteotomy to gain stability in the acetabulum.

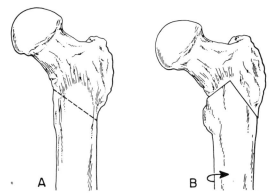

Fig. 12.42. The varus osteotomy done in the intertrochanteric region with the hip internally rotated as in *A*. In *B*, as the distal fragment is rotated externally, the head and neck slide into varus.

the abnormal innervation caused by a defect in the spinal elements. The level of the defect determines the level of the denervation. This level of denervation remains constant throughout life unless there is further insult locally. Abnormal innervation causes muscle imbalance.

Neurogenic deformity is caused by muscle imbalance acting across a moveable joint.[60] The magnitude of the deformity is proportional to the magnitude of the imbalance and the length of time this imbalance existed. Great imbalances need only a short time to cause significant deformity. A little imbalance needs a long time to cause significant deformity.

Deformities have a predictable sequence of development which is time related. Early, they are passively correctable (Fig. 12.45); later, they become rigid but there is still no skeletal adaptation to the deformity (Fig. 12.46); and, finally, the deformities become fixed with bony change (Fig. 12.47).

In the patient with a myelomeningocele, the level of denervation can be determined by clinical examination early in life.[57] Because this level remains constant, it is possible to anticipate the problems the patient will have in the future. The ability to anticipate deformities before they occur permits the orthopaedist to act while the deformities are passively correctable and without skeletal adaptation. The advantage of early intervention is tremendous. Not only are the procedures themselves technically less difficult, but the results are better. *The only treatment for neurogenic deformity is to correct the muscle imbalance in this normally balanced system.* Muscle imbalance can be corrected only in two ways: one must either strengthen the weak muscles or weaken the strong muscles acting across the joint. It is possible to strengthen a muscle with a program of progressive active-resistive exercises if the muscle rates fair or better and is under voluntary control. Unfortunately, this situation is rarely present in the deforming joint of a

Fig. 12.43. The iliopsoas transplant devised by Mustard to aid abduction. The iliopsoas is mobilized with the lesser trochanter, passed laterally through the ilium, and sutured to the femur by means of a trap door type of fixation. (From W. T. Mustard: A follow-up study of ilio-psoas transfer for hip instability, *Journal of Bone & Joint Surgery*, 41B: 289, 1959.)

patient with a myelomeningocele. Muscle transfer is the most reliable method to strengthen the weak muscles in the deforming joint in this disease.

Weakening the strong muscles in the face of imbalance to prevent neurogenic deformity is also applicable in the patient with a myelomeningocele. This may be accomplished by lengthening the muscles, shortening the skeleton, or transferring the muscles.

Any treatment program designed to treat neurogenic deformity which cannot in some way strengthen the week muscles or weaken the

strong muscles in an unbalanced system is not useful because it will be unsuccessful.

Passive stretching, positioning, and bracing have no place in the treatment of the neurogenic deformity caused by an unbalanced system acting across a limber joint for none of these modalities have the ability to either strengthen or weaken muscles.

Positioning and bracing are, in effect, external supporting measures which do have a place in the treatment program designed for the patient with a myelomeningocele. External support is a valuable and necessary part of the program which must be designed to offer the patient maximum function. but external supports will not prevent or correct deformity in a joint acting in an unbalanced system. External supporting devices are used to increase function and are applied only to balanced systems. One may brace a joint that is flail or that has been balanced surgically. To brace a joint that is

Fig. 12.44. Patient with myelomeningocele removed and osteotomies of the femur performed for hip stability. Short-leg braces and crutches are used to aid ambulation and to prevent deformity. Early ambulation is a goal for these patients.

Fig. 12.45. Anteroposterior roentgenogram of the pelvis showing location reduction of neurogenic dislocated hips in abduction and internal rotation.

Fig. 12.46. Anteroposterior roentgenogram of the pelvis showing irreducible neurogenic dislocated hips without skeletal adaptation. Note normal appearing acetabuli.

unbalanced will result in the "crooked child-straight brace syndrome" manifested by a patient with pressure sores, a weeping mother, an angry orthotist, and a frustrated doctor.

The child with neurologic deficit secondary to a myelomeningocele should be prepared to achieve major motor milestones on time if at all possible. This means the patient should be prepared to sit at about 6 months and stand at approximately 1 year.

Optimum care for the child with neurologic deficit due to myelomeningocele demands that the orthopaedist:

1. Establish the level of motor loss in the

Fig. 12.47. Anteroposterior roentgenogram of the pelvis showing neurogenic dislocated hips with skeletal adaptation. Note shallow acetabuli and formation of false acetabuli superiorly.

newborn;

2. Anticipate deformity on the basis of the imbalance dictated by the level of the loss;
3. Correct all imbalance in systems that are deforming; and
4. Provide external support to increase function so that the child's motor development might progress in an orderly manner.

If these steps are realized and acted upon, the child with the myelomeningocele will attain his maximum motor function.

Application

To establish the level of motor loss, one must identify the functioning muscles with the lowest root innervation. This is best accomplished by examination of the feet. Deformities are often present at birth, and they are reflections of deforming forces. The root levels of the extrinsics of the feet have been identified (Fig. 12.48).

Because the musculature of the hips and the extrinsics of the feet are innervated by common roots, foot and hip muscle imbalance must be related. It follows that foot deformities reflect deformities in the hip. To understand the hip in the patient with a myelomeningocele, *it pays to watch the feet.*[61]

ANTERIOR TIBIALIS	L4
POSTERIOR TIBIALIS	L5
PERONEUS LONGUS	SI
INTRINSICS	S2 S3

Fig. 12.48. Innervation of foot musculature.

The hip surrounded by normally innervated muscles (Fig. 12.49) does not deform because the system is balanced.

The hip that is surrounded by denervated muscles (Fig. 12.50) does not deform because the system is balanced.

Patients with innervation levels of T12 and above have flail hips and feet which are balanced and rarely deform unless subjected to abnormal external forces. Therefore, in this group of patients, proper positioning and bracing are essential but present no technical difficulties. Our plan would be to provide the patient with appropriate external supports (Fig. 12.51) so that major motor milestones might be achieved on time.

This group of patients present only one problem that requires major surgical intervention. The kyphosis which is present in 12% of patients with a myelomeningocele rarely is seen in patients with levels of denervation below T12. It is our feeling that the kyphosis is best resected at the time of closure of the meningocele.[63]

Failure to resect the kyphosis in the past has established the natural history of the deformity, it always is progressive. In our hands, bracing difficulties and pressure ulcers over the kyphosis prevented this group of patients from attaining their maximum functional level. These children should be able to ambulate with a "swing to" gait utilizing crutches and long-leg braces with a double pelvic band.

Patients with denervation below L1 or L2 (Fig. 12.52) are also noted to have flail feet. The presence of the iliopsoas which is a potential deforming force may be missed upon initial examination. Serial examination of the hips will show progressive flexion contractures if the iliopsoas is a deforming force. Progressive flexion contracture in the patient with a flail foot is the harbinger of neurogenic dislocation of the hips. If the progression of the deformity is slow, iliopsoas release will weaken the deforming force and possibly balance the sys-

Fig. 12.50. At level of T12, the hip is flail.

PACK BOARD	WHEN SKIN IS COVERED
CASTOR CART	HEAD CONTROL
STANDING SPLINTS	SITTING WITH SUPPORT
PARAPODIUM	INDEPENDENT SITTING
RECIPROCAL GATE BRACE	ABILITY TO FLEX HIPS 45° AGAINST GRAVITY

Fig. 12.51. Objective criteria for external support.

Fig. 12.49. Innervation of muscles about the normal hip.

tem, preventing eventual dislocation of the hips. If the progression of the flexion contracture is rapid, iliopsoas transfer to the greater

L1 L2

Fig. 12.52. Innervation of muscles about the hip in the patient denervated below L1 or L2.

trochanter would be appropriate treatment.[59]

It is our practice to stage the hip surgery. On the first admission, the left iliopsoas transfer is accomplished. The patient is discharged in a double hip spica. Standing in the hip spica is encouraged, the feeling being that dependency may decrease the incidence of urinary tract infections and weight bearing makes osteoporosis less of a problem.

At the time of the second admission, 6 weeks following the first operation, measurements are taken for bracing. Fabrication of the braces takes place during the time that the patient is in plaster following the second hip operation. The feet need no surgical correction for they are flail and do not deform.

These children are capable of ambulation. A "swing-through" gait with crutches and bracing consisting of a double pelvic band attached to long-leg braces with hip and knee locks should be expected. It is desirable to have surgical correction of the hips completed by 12 to 18 months.

If the lowest functioning motor is innervated by L4 motor roots, the flexion adduction movers of the hip will be unopposed (Fig. 12.53) and the foot will show a calcaneovarus deformity. The magnitude of the imbalance across the hip is great. The dislocation is inevitable. Our plan would be to balance the foot so as to prevent calcaneus by transferring the anterior tibial muscle to triceps surae.[46] Prevention of dislocation of the hips in this gorup can be achieved by iliopsoas transfer to the greater trochanter.[59] Because of the magnitude of the imbalance across the hip, deformities are far advanced even in the infant and usually exhibit coxa valga which is a skeletal adaptation to muscle imbalance. In the presence of coxa valga, iliopsoas transfer alone has been disappointing in our hands. For this reason, for patients affected at L3-L4 with established coxa valga, we add iliopsoas transfer to varus derotation osteotomies (Fig. 12.54). The osteotomy is accomplished at the subtrochanteric level at the same time of the iliopsoas

L3 L4

Fig. 12.53. Innervation of muscles about the hip in the patient denervated below L3 or L4.

Fig. 12.54. Postoperative roentgenogram of patient who has undergone iliopsoas transfer and varus derotation osteotomy of the proximal femur.

transfer. Combining transfer with osteotomy in these patients has improved our results.

Our operative plan is to accomplish the entire surgical reconstructive program before the time that the baby would ordinarily attempt to stand at approximately 1 year. This involves three hospital admissions staged 3 weeks apart. On the first admission the left hip is done, 6 weeks later the right hip, and, 12 weeks after the initial admission, both feet are operated. The patient is measured for braces consisting of a double pelvic band, hip and knee locks, a 90° ankle stop, and surgical shoes just prior to the foot surgery. At this time accurate measurements can be obtained and fabrication can be accomplished while the child recovers from the foot surgery. These children are able to ambulate with crutches and braces utilizing a "four-point" gait.

The patient with an L5 level innervation has minimal imbalance across the hip joint (Fig. 12.55). Neurogenic dislocation will be slow and preceded by the development of hip adduction contractures. Serial examination of the hip with accurate recording of hip adduction in flexion is necessary so that neurogenic dislocation of the hip may be anticipated and iliopsoas transfer can be accomplished while the deformity is minimal. Those patients have neurogenic clubfeet. Medial release combined with posterior tibial tendon transfer through the interosseous membrane to the dorsum of the foot will correct the deformity and prevent

Fig. 12.55. Innervation of muscles about the hip in the patient denervated below L5.

recurrence.[20] On occasion, troublesome valgus has been a late sequel of this procedure. If valgus is a problem, subtalar bone blocks[23] have been useful and have provided a plantargrade foot.

These patients are excellent ambulators but often need external support because of inadequate rotary control of the hips. If rotary control of the hips is missing, the pelvic band is still necessary.

In patients with S1 level innervation, the muscles about the hips are balanced (Fig. 12.56) and dislocation is not apt to occur. If the S1 contributtion to the hip abductors is weak, then a rather marked gluteus lurch may be a problem to the patient. The peroneus musculature are the lowest functioning extrinsic motors to the foot. The feet exhibit calaneovalgus deformities. Transfer of the peroneous longus in continuity has been the best balancing operation in our hands.[39] Surgical balancing of the foot is all that is needed to make this group of patients independent ambulators without external supports. However, their gait is grotesque and disappointing to the patients. They ambulate with hips and kees flexed. A gluteal lurch plus calcaneus further mars the gait. Our attempts to imporve the situation have been disappointing in that improvement requires a large amount of surgery to reap an unimpressive correction in the gait. Nonetheless, we have used iliopsoas transfers to decrease the lurch[59] and transfer of the biceps femoris to the patella[8] to decrease the knee flexion observed in the stance phase of gait.

These patients have very little difficulty from an orthopaedic standpoint. Their hips are normally intervated (Fig. 12.57). The extrinsics of the feet are normal, but there is appreciable weakness of the intrinsic musculature of the feet. The foot exhibits a cavus deformity. It is our practice to balance the foot musculature prior to the time the cavus deformity becomes fixed. Tendon transfers are useful only in the passively correctable deformities.

Passively correctable clawtoes are corrected by transferring flexors into extensors. If the clawtoes are accompanied by an equinus forefoot, extensor tenton recessions are done. If the deformities are fixed, the therapeutic approach must be changed for tendon transfers are not

Fig. 12.56. Innervation of muscles about the hip in the patient denervated below S1.

Fig. 12.57. Innervation of muscles about the hip in the patient denervated below S2 or S3.

applicable in the presence of fixed deformity. Interphalangeal fusion in the toes, dorsal tarsal wedges in the forefoot, and valgus osteotomies of the os calcis are applicable either separately or in combination, depending upon the nature of the presenting fixed deformity.[61] This group should ambulate with a normal gait. Their foot problems, if handled promptly, should never amount to more than a nuisance. If ignored, major problems leading to amputation are not unusual.

Normal lower extremity musculature allowing prolonged ambulation, decreased sensation on the plantar surface of the foot, and the uneven contour of a neglected cavus foot provide perfect circumstances for neurogenic ulcers. Neurogenic ulcers in the feet then secondarily involve the bone causing osteomyelitis that leads to amputation.[29] To avoid this horrible complication, foot deformities in this active group must be cared for promptly.

Surgical reconstruction to obtain maximum function and geared to the time table of normal motor development requires that multiple stage procedures be accomplished in a relatively short period of time. These procedures require postoperative immobilization. Repeated periods of immobilization, though necessary, have the disadvantage of predisposing the patient to disuse osteoporosis and pathologic fracture.[25] In the past the vicious circle of immobilization, fracture, more immobilization and more fracture deprived a significant number of children from attaining maximum function commensurate with their level of neurologic loss. For this reason, we have adopted a rigid attitude toward pathologic fracture in the patient with neurologic deficit.

All stable, undisplaced fractures are treated by immobilization in braces. The braces are worn 24 hr per day, with the joints locked until local swelling at the fracture site disappears. The patient's normal program is then resumed.

All unstable fractures are reduced and immobilized in plaster for 6 weeks.

In the event that a child suffers two fractures in the extremity in 1 calendar year, the patient is admitted at the time of the second fracture and all long bones of the lower extremities are treated by prophylactic intramedullary rodding. The rods are introduced through the knee (Fig. 12.58). Since the institution of this program,

Fig. 12.58. Anteroposterior roentgenogram of lower extremities treated by prophylactic rodding for multiple pathologic fractures.

lost time due to pathologic fracture has ceased to be a serious problem in our myelomeningocele population.

In summary, early evaluation of the level of neurologic deficit, a timely surgical reconstruction program, and an awareness of the problems peculiar to the patient with neurologic deficit should enable one to help this group of patients to attain maximum capability in keeping with their loss.

Nothing has been said about patchy loss and skip levels. It is the author's contention that a clear understanding of the pure lesion is necessary. This information can be easily adapted to variants seen in the clinical situation.

In the last decade, varied approaches to paralytic deformity have been recorded in the orthopaedic literature (entire bibliography). It has been our plan to provide the reader with a time-tested, single approach to the problems of the child with paralytic deformity secondary to myelomeningocele. It is not our intention to suggest to the reader that this is the only suitable solution to the problem.

References

1. Allen, J. H.: Challenge of spina bifida cystica, *J. Bone Joint Surg., 46A:* 462, 1964.
2. Amuso, S. J., and Mankin, H. J.: Hereditary spondylolisthesis and spina bifida, *J. Bone Joint Surg., 49A:* 507, 1967.
3. Baker, G. C. W., and Stark, G.: Patterns of spinal cord lesion in myelomeningocele, *J. Bone Joint Surg. 49B:* 187, 1967.
4. Bobechko, W. P.: Management of spinal deformity in spina bifida, *J. Bone Joint Surg., 54A:* 772, 1971.
5. Brown, J. C., Bonnett, C. S., Perry, J., and Sherman, J. M. The surgical treatment of spine deformity in the childhood and adolescent myelodysplastic, *J. Bone Joint Surg., 54A:* 198, 1972.
6. Buisson, J. S., and Hamblen, D. L.: Electromyographic assessment of the transplanted iliopsoas muscle in spina bifida cystica, *J. Bone Joint Surg. 54B:* 752, 1972.
7. Buisson, J. S., and Hamblen, D. L.: Electromyographic assessment of the transplanted iliopsoas muscle in spina bifida. *J. Bone Joint Surg., 54B:* 752, 1972.
8. Caldwell, G. D.: Transplantation of the biceps femoris to the patella by the medial route in poliomyelitis quadriceps paralysis, *J. Bone Joint Surg., 37A:* 347, 1955.
9. Carroll, N. C., and Sharrard, W. J. W.: Long-term follow-up of posterior iliopsoas transplantation for paralytic dislocation of the hip, *J. Bone Joint Surg., 54A:* 551, 1972.
10. Cruess, R. L., and Turner, N. S.: Paralysis of hip abductor muscles in spina bifida, *J. Bone Joint Surg., 52A:* 1364, 1970.
11. Curtis, B. H., and Brightman, E.: Spina bifida; a follow-up of 90 cases. *J. Bone Joint Surg., 41A:* 1342, 1959.
12. Diamond, L. S.: An evaluation of the Sharrard posterior iliopsoas transfer, *J. Bone Joint Surg., 51A:* 1044, 1969.
13. Drennan, J. C., and Sharrad, W. J. W.: The pathological anatomy of convex pes valgus, *J. Bone Joint Surg., 53B:* 455, 1971.
14. Dunlap, J. P.: Sciatic-nerve section in the paraplegic spina bifida patients, *J. Bone Joint Surg., 49A:* 977, 1958.
15. Eckstein, H. B., and Vors, R. M.: Spinal osteotomy for severe kyphosis in children with myelomeningocele, *J. Bone Joint Surg., 54B:* 328, 1972.
16. Exner, G.: Observations of an extensive periosteal change as a result of trans-section paralysis with myelodysplasia, *J. Bone Joint Surg., 43A:* 302, 1961.
17. Eyring, E. J., and Wanken, J. J.: Spinal osteotomy for kyphosis in myelomeningocele, *J. Bone Joint Surg., 53A:* 1032, 1971.
18. Forrester-Browne, M.: Spina bifida with meningocele, *J. Bone Joint Surg., 31B:* 485, 1949.
19. Freehafer, A. A., Vessely, J. C., and Mack, R. P.: Iliopsoas muscle transfer in the treatment of myelomeningocele patients with paralytic hip, *J. Bone Joint Surg., 54A:* 1715, 1972.
20. Fried, A.: Recurrent congenital club foot; the role of m. tibialis posterior in etiology and treatment, *J. Bone Joint Surg., 41A:* 243, 1959.
21. Gordon, L. H., and Raichle, M. E.: The morphology of myelodysplasia produced in rats by trypan blue, *J. Bone Joint Surg., 47A:* 1098, 1965.
22. Gordon, L. H., Shurtleff, D. B., and Fortz, E. L.: Meningomyelocele, *J. Bone Joint Surg., 47B:* 381, 1965.
23. Grice, D. S.: An extra-articular arthrodesis of the subastragular joint for the correction of paralytic feet in children, *J. Bone Joint Surg., 37A:* 246, 1952.
24. Griffin, G. D., and Stark, G.: Correlation of neurological deficit and limb deformity in myelomeningocele, *J. Bone Joint Surg., 53A:* 386, 1971.
25. Handelsman, J. E.: Spontaneous fractures in spina bifida, *J. Bone Joint Surg., 54B:* 381, 1972.
26. Hayes, J. T., and Gross, H. P.: The orthopedic implications of myelodysplasia, *J. Bone Joint Surg., 44A:* 1488, 1962.
27. Hayes, J. T., Gross, H. P., and Dow, S.: surgery for paralytic defects secondary to myelomeningocele and myelodysplasia, *J. Bone Joint Surg., 46A:* 1577, 1964.
28. Heyman, C. H.: Long-term results following a bone-shelf operation for congenital and some other dislocations of the hip in children, *J. Bone Joint Surg., 45A:* 1113, 1963.
29. Hogshead, H. P.: Management of the anesthetic, paralytic foot in patients with myelodysplasia, *J. Bone Joint Surg., 48A:* 1016, 1966.
30. Hogshead, H. P., and Ponseti, I. V.: Vascia lata transfer to the erector spinae for the treatment of flexion-abduction contractures of the hip in patients with poliomyelitis and meningomyelocele, *J. Bone Joint Surg., 46A:* 1389, 1964.
31. Hoppenfeld, S.: Congenital kyphosis in myelomeningocele, *J. Bone Joint Surg., 49A:* 276, 1967.
32. James, C. C. M., and Lassman, L. P.: Spinal dysraphism, the diagnosis and treatment of progressive lesions in spina bifida occulta, *J. Bone Joint Surg., 44B:* 828, 1962.
33. Jones, G. B.: Paralytic dislocation of the hip, *J. Bone Joint Surg., 44B:* 573, 1962.
34. Kilfoyle, R. M., Foley, J. J., and Norton, P. L.: Spine and pelvic deformity in childhood and adolescent paraplegia, *J. Bone Joint Surg., 47A:* 659, 1965.
35. Kilfoyle, R. M., and Foley, J. J.: The hip in myelomeningocele, *J. Bone Joint Surg., 52A:* 827, 1970.
36. Kummel, B. M., Lasoff, M. E. L., and Stockman, J. C.: Management of spina bifida in a community hospital, *J. Bone Joint Surg., 54A:* 1568, 1972.
37. Lane, G. H.: The posterior iliopsoas transfer in myelodysplasia, report of 62 cases, *J. Bone Joint Surg. 51A:* 1036, 1969.

38. McKibbin, B.: Conservative management of paralytic dislocation of the hip in meningomyelocele, *J. Bone Joint Surg., 53B:* 758, 1971.

39. Makin, M., and Yossipovitch, Z.: Translocation of the peroneus longus in the treatment of paralytic pes calcaneus, *J. Bone Joint Surg., 48A:* 1541, 1966.

40. Martin, R. F.: An orthopedic review of spina bifida in children, *J. Bone Joint Surg., 51B:* 194, 1969.

41. Menelaus, M. B.: Dislocation and deformity of the hip in children with spina bifida cystica, *J. Bone Joint Surg. 51B:* 238, 1969.

42. Menelaus, M. B.: Posterior iliopsoas transfer, *J. Bone Joint Surg., 48B:* 592, 1966.

43. Menelaus, M. B.: Talectomy for equinovarus deformity in arthrogryposis and spina bifida, *J. Bone Joint Surg. 53B:* 468, 1971.

44. Menelaus, M. B.: The management of orthopedic disabilities in spina bifida, *J. Bone Joint Surg., 50B:* 681, 1968.

45. Merril, R. E.: One hundred cases of hydrocephalus and myelomeningocele or both, *J. Bone Joint Surg., 44A:* 808, 1962.

46. Peabody, C. W.: Tendon transposition; an end result study, *J. Bone Joint Surg., 20:* 193, 1938.

47. Piggot, J.: Leg movements after closure of myelomeningocele, *J. Bone Joint Surg., 53B:* 758, 1971.

48. Piggot, J.: Meningomyelocele, *J. Bone Joint Surg., 50B:* 885, 1968.

49. Pollock, J. H., and Carrell, B.: Subtalar extra-articular arthrodesis in the treatment of paralytic valgus deformities, *J. Bone Joint Surg., 46:* 533, 1964.

50. Raycroft, J. F.: Spinal curvature in myelomeningocele; natural history and etiology, *J. Bone Joint Surg., 54A:* 1335, 1972.

51. Regan, B. G.: Myelomeningocele, *J. Bone Joint Surg., 51B:* 775, 1969.

52. Rueda, J., and Carroll, N. C.: Hip instability in patients with myelomeningocele, *J. Bone Joint Surg., 54B:* 422, 1972.

53. Seymour, N., and Evans, D. K.: A modification of the Grice subtalar arthrodesis, *J. Bone Joint Surg., 50B:* 372, 1968.

54. Sharrard, W. J. W.: Congenital paralytic dislocation of the hip in children with myelomeningocele, *J. Bone Joint Surg., 41B:* 622, 1959.

55. Sharrard, W. J. W.: Congenital paralytic dislocation of the hip, *J. Bone Joint Surg., 41B:* 427, 1959.

56. Sharrard, W. J. W.: Immediate closure of myelomeningocele and management of paralytic deformities in myelomeningocele, *J. Bone Joint Surg., 45B:* 434, 1963.

57. Sharrard, W. J. W.: Mortality, Paralysis and Deformity in Spina Bifida Cystica, Ch.M. Thesis, University of Sheffield, 1966.

58. Sharrard, W. J. W.: Paralytic deformity in meningomyelocele, *J. Bone Joint Surg., 45B:* 616, 1963.

59. Sharrard, W. J. W.: Posterior iliopsoas transplantation in the treatment of paralytic dislocation of the hip, *J. Bone Joint Surg., 46B:* 426, 1964.

60. Sharrard, W. J. W.: Paralytic deformity in the lower limb, *J. Bone Joint Surg., 49B:* 731, 1967.

61. Sharrard, W. J. W.: The management of deformity and paralysis of the foot in myelomeningocele, *J. Bone Joint Surg. 50B:* 456, 1968.

62. Sharrard, W. J. W.: Osteotomy-excision of the spine for lumbar kyphosis in older children with myelomeningocele, *J. Bone Joint Surg., 54B:* 50, 1972.

63. Sharrard, W. J. W.: Spinal osteotomy for congenital kyphosis in myelomeningocele, *J. Bone Joint Surg., 50B:* 466, 1968.

64. Sharrard, W. J. W.: Spinal osteotomy for congenital kyphosis in myelomeningocele, *J. Bone Joint Surg., 51B:* 181, 1969.

65. Sriram, K., Bobechko, W. P., and Hall, J. E.: Surgical management of spine deformities in myelomeningocele, *J. Bone Joint Surg., 53A:* 198, 1971.

66. Sriram, K., Bobechko, W. P., and Hall, J. E.: Surgical management of spinal deformities in spina bifida, *J. Bone Joint Surg., 54B:* 666, 1972.

67. Stoyle, T. F.: Prognosis for paralysis in meningomyelocele, *J. Bone Joint Surg., 48B:* 195, 1966.

68. Till, K.: Spinal dysraphism, *J. Bone Joint Surg., 51B:* 415, 1969.

69. Tzimas, N. A., Thompson, W. A. L., Swinyard, C. A., and Greenspan, L.: The child with spina bifida, *J. Bone Joint Surg. 50A:* 1274, 1968.

70. Walker, G.: The early management of varus feet in myelomeningocele children, *J. Bone Joint Surg., 52B:* 178, 1970.

71. Walker, G.: The early management of varus feet in myelomeningocele, *J. Bone Joint Surg., 53B:* 462, 1971.

72. Williams, P. F.: Surgery for spina bifida, *J. Bone Joint Surg., 49A:* 805, 1967.

73. Winckworth, R. F., Jowett, A. E., and Hubbard, M.: Talipes equinovarus with spina bifida and meningocele, *J. Bone Joint Surg., 40B:* 824, 1958.

PARAPLEGIA IN CHILDHOOD

The most frequent causes of paraplegia in childhood are congenital. But whether the paraplegia is congenital or acquired, severe deforming forces are at work and may be expected to cause progression until growth ceases. Excessive lumbar lordosis, kyphoscoliosis, and fixed pelvic obliquity all act to affect the deformities present in the lower extremities. Kilfoyle, Foley, and Norton[1] have studied the natural history of these spine and pelvic deformities. Patients with acquired paraplegia have their lesion principally at L1 level and above into the dorsal spine, usually with complete paralysis. In congenital lesions the

Fig. 12.59. Diagrammatic representation of the various crutch gaits. The swing through gait is a rapid means of ambulation fondly used by children once the arms are built up to their use. The legs progress ahead of the crutches. The swing-to gait brings them even with the crutches. The non-weight bearing three point gait requires a flexed knee of the involved leg and is difficult over the distances. If the foot can touch down the involved leg can go through the usual gait motions and requires less energy. In the alternate two-point gait the crutch on the same side is brought forward with the leg and repeated on the alternate side. The four point gait is a good stable gait, easier, but slower, and requiring a rhythmic cadence. On going upstairs with crutches the good leg leads to pull the patient upstairs; on going down the good leg remains on the step behind to let the patient down.

Fig. 12.60. (*A*) Strong iliopsoas and weak glutei result in increasing forward tilt of the pelvis and secondary lordosis. (*B*) Balance must be achieved by getting head and shoulders over the pelvis. In order to enable the patient to get the pelvis tilted back up to this position surgery may be necessary. (*C*) Increasing kyphosis in the lumbar spine may result in "jack-knifing" of the spine and the necessity to support the sitting posture with the upper extremity. (From R. M. Kilfoyle, J. J. Foley, and P. L. Morton: *Journal of Bone & Joint Surgery, 47A:* 659, 1965.)

principal site of involvement is the lumbar spine with patchy loss of sensation and motor power.

The spinal deformities may be divided into the following:

Lordosis. The development of increased lordosis occurs in almost all of these children. It may be low, ending at the third lumbar vertebra, or high, extending through the lumbar spine into the lower dorsal segments.

The development of lordosis is favored by the frequent finding of innervation of the iliopsoas and loss of the gluteus maximus due to its sacral innervation—a more distal level more likely to be involved is with congenital etiologies. In addition, the natural tendency of the child with paraplegia to stand with a forward inclination of the trunk when using crutches in order to maintain balance favors lordosis development. In order to become erect the lordosis must be increased, and, if the child is going to be balanced as defined by Kilfoyle et al.,[1] the kyphosis above it must bring the center of gravity of the trunk over the feet. Crutches are needed if off balance, and the deformity of one area of the spine may be so great when not compensated by an anteroposterior curve either above or below it that standing even with crutches is impossible.

Lateral curvature of the spine may be added to the lordosis or kypkosis; and, again, if unbalanced, may progress to the point of inability to sit without external support.

Balance would mean level shoulder and pelvis with occiput centered over the first sacral body.

Lordosis primarily affects walking, and scoliosis, the ability to sit.

Pelvic Obliquity. The accurate determination of pelvic obliquity in terms of the area causing it to be fixed is an exercise in physical diagnosis. A fixed abduction deformity at the hip can be appreciated by performing a Thomas test—stabilizing the opposite side by full flexion. Full abduction of the involved hip is then necessary to eliminate the tendency of the limb to go into flexion if an abduction contracture is present. The abduction or adduction component at the hip can be further evaluated by bringing both hips into a position in which the pelvis is at right angles to the spine; this may result in considerable displacement of the limbs to either side. Inability to get the pelvis to neutral by this maneuver speaks for a contracture above the pelvis. Further evaluation can be made by pulling the limb downward against the quadratus lumborum and erector spinae musculature above.

With poliomyelitis infrequent fixed pelvic obliquity is principally caused by paralysis and chronic posture associated with spina bifida syndromes.

Collapsing Spine. The collapsing flaccid spine is principally seen in high thoracic levels of paralysis and has been designated as a "rope spine" by Kilfoyle et al.[1] It is a clear-cut indication for spine fixation before deformity that is fixed develops.

Kyphosis. Increasing kyphosis can involve the lumbar spine and culminate in a jack-knifed position of the spine, making it impossible for the patient to stand without support. The sitting posture tends to be supported by the upper extremities as the center of gravity is thrown forward. In dorsal hemivertebra the vertebrae above and below may converge in front of the hemivertebra to form an extreme deformity for which there appears to be no treatment.

Treatment

Treatment is based on a careful assessment of the forces producing the deformity and a recognition of the inevitable further progression if active forces in a growing child cannot be held by bracing, training, and careful attention to sitting and crutch-walking posture. The child's whole day must be laid out with attention to the posture used in performing all functions.

The attention is to the spine before the hips, since hip position cannot be maintained if the spine cannot be controlled. Spine fusion is used early in preventing excessive kyphosis, lordosis, and scoliosis.

Sectioning of adductors, transplant of the iliopsoas, and adductor tendon division are all necessary in controlling the pelvis if deforming contracture exists. When correcting hip flexion contractures the opposite hip must be held in a flexed position in plaster to stablize the pelvis while the correction is being obtained or the result will be disappointing.

The usual orthopaedic procedures are used as indicated to stabilize the lower extremity at the ankle, foot, and knee. Harrington instrumentation appears to have a place in the treatment of some of the severe lordotic deformities, but it is not fully established as yet. Spine fusion accompanying the correction frequently must include the sacrum.

References

1. Kilfoyle, R. M., Foley, J. J., and Norton, P. L.: Spine and pelvic deformity in childhood and adolescent paraplegia, *J. Bone Joint Surg., 47A:* 659, 1965.

NEUROFIBROMATOSIS

Manifestations of neurofibromatosis are seen in childhood as the cause of some difficult and bizarre orthopaedic problems. Café au lait spots and skeletal and joint changes are an entity in a variety of conditions.

Von Recklinghausen in 1882 originally described the relationship between peripheral nerves and the subcutaneous nodules which are typical of the disease in the adult. The advanced form of the disease he described has been supplemented by childhood manifestations in which tumors of the skin and subcutaneous tissue are seldom evident visually, but may be palpable. The incidence has been variously calculated at between 1 in 2,500 and 1 in 3,300 of the general population.

Clinical Picture

The pigmentation and skin nodules of the adult are a serious cosmetic problem. In childhood the cutaneous manifestation consists of café au lait pigmentation and occurs in 80% of the cases. Still more threatening manifestations of the disease include a rapidly progressive scoliosis. Tumors extending from the spinal canal into the major body cavities may undergo sarcomatous change with a grave prognosis.

Soft tissue involvement of an extremity is a cause of massive enlargement through lymphatic and vascular proliferation. It tends to be unilateral.

The skeletal changes include the scoliosis, a nonunion of very stubborn type in the tibia but also occurring in other bones such as the clavicle and radius.

Recognition

The macules of neurofibromatosis are tan in color with smooth margins (coast of California) as compared to the irregular (coast of Maine) configuration seen in Albright's disease. Although an occasional spot seen in normal persons (20% of 100 student nurses) their presence in any number and their grouping in skeletally involved areas is significant. The café au lait spot immediately raises clinical suspicion. The development of tumors and pigmentation increases with puberty.

Tumors with central nervous system involve-

Fig. 12.61. Patient with neurofibromatosis involving spine. There are a mild structural scoliosis of the dorsal spine and café au lait spots of skin pigmentation.

ment tend to occur in 20% of the persons without the café au lait spots. Cranial nerves with optic glioma and widening of the optic formamen are found. Acoustic neuromas involving the eight nerve occur. According to the study of Gardner and Frazier, 84% of bilateral nerve neuromas occurred in patients with neurofibromatosis.

The neurofibromas occur both centrally and peripherally and show malignant degeneration in 5-15% of recorded series.

There is an element of mental retardation. In Borberg's series of 71 patients, 85% had low normal or moron intelligence levels.

Peripherally the tumors are of three types: (1) those resulting in a "fibroma molluscum" subcutaneous lesion, (2) discrete lesions along the course of peripheral nerves, and (3) the plexiform neuroma associated with hamartomatous overgrowth resulting in local giantism. The plexiform neuroma may result in a large pedunculated mass, a "pachydermatocele."

Skeletal Lesions

About 50% of patients with this disease have at least some x-ray evidence of skeletal involvement. Erosions or scalloping along the ribs are the most common. When the neurofibroma is adjacent to the cortex of a long bone, a saucer-like depression will occur in the cortex. The thinning of the cortex in this area will give a cystlike impression when the x-ray is taken at right angles to it. Periosteal new bone may form about the lesion. The edges are smooth— metaphysis or diaphysis could be involved. When the lesion occurs at the point of exit of spinal or cranial nerves, the opening is smoothly eroded. The spinal nerve lesion thins the pedicles and enlarges the neural foramen.

Scoliosis

The incidence of scoliosis has been reported in from 5 to 17%.

Scott[10] (1965) studied the scoliosis of neurofibromatosis and found no uniform length or direction of curves, no association with number of café au lait spots, or tumors. Of 33 patients with scoliosis, 9 had gradual "C"-shaped curves, i.e., ≤30° the other 24 had curves ≥30° mostly thoracic and thoracolumbar. He noted the similarity of these acute curves with those of "progressive infantile idiopathhic scoliosis."

The point to be made is that while the severe angular curve with twisted ribbon ribs and erosions is pathognomonic of neurofibromatosis, often these findings are not present. Often the curve is indistinguishable from idiopathic scoliosis.

The x-rays of 18 patients seen here at Children's Hospital since 1957 confirms the findings of Scott. A third of these scoliosis lesions are not the "characteristic" type with short, sharp angular curves.

Nonunion

The nonunion of the tibia associated with neurofibromatosis is associated with bowing of the tibia and a thin, waving fibula. Congenital nonunion of the tibia can occur for several reasons, including fibrous dysplasia. The occurrence of nonunion in patients with neurofibromatosis is a real clinical fact although actual demonstration of the neurofibroma has been rare. Green and Rudo[3] reported a case and we have seen one adult with nonunion of the radius and gross clinical neurofibromatosis. The entity was described by Cucroquet in 1937. The nonunion is characteristic in that there is progressive narrowing and sclerosis of the tibia (pencilling) toward the nonunion site with obliteration of the marrow cavity. In Meszaros' 11 cases of pseudarthrosis, 9 had neurofibromatosis. The clavicle is a fairly common site in addition to the tibia.

Skeletal overgrowth occurs with gigantism and with marked involvement of the soft tissues of a limb.

Orbital Defects

Orbital defects were first reported as part of the syndrome by LeWald in 1933. Hunt and Pugh found the defect in 7% of a series of 192 patients.

The defect involves the posterior wall of the orbit. It may be due to erosion but more often no neurofibroma is found and dysplasia must be evoked. Usually the greater and lesser wings of the sphenoid and the orbital part of the frontal bone are absent. Pulsating exophthalmos results because of the direct contact of the temporal lobe with the orbital soft tissues.

Overgrowth

Asymmetric disorders of bone growth can be due to neurofibromatosis. Brooks and Lehman reported shortening of bones of the lower extremity secondary to invasion of the epiphyseal plate by neurofibroma. Several investigators including Holt[4] (1948) found only increased bone length presumably secondary to increased blood supply. According to Meszaros, the altered bone growth is found most often in association with plexiform neuroma and local gigantism.

In localized areas of hypertrophy, café au lait spots, palpable nodules, enlargement of the part, and erythema are all seen. If such a process involves an entire leg, it gives rise to a picture very much like that of elephantiasis. In a growing child it produces great inequality of leg length and overgrowth of the affected side.

Sarcoma

Sarcomas associated with the disease are often found contiguous with other neurofibromatous tissue. Such sarcomas are difficult to excise as they ramify through and around major nerve plexuses and appear usually as a neurofibrosarcoma under the microscope. Bone cysts in localized subperiosteal areas have been described. The treatment of these various lesions is highly individualized, and the general principles have been described elsewhere.

A large mass occurring in the chest or abdominal cavity identified as neurofibromasarcoma carries with it a dire prognosis in our experience. A fatal outcome may be expected due to the inability to excise the lesion.

References

1. Aegarter, E. E.: Possible relationship of neurofibromatosis, congenital psyeudarthrosis, and fibrous dysplasia, *J. Bone Joint Surg., 32A:* 618, 1950.
2. Benedict, M.: Melanotic macules in Albrights and Von Recklinghausen, *J. A. M. A., 205:* 618, 1968.
3. Green, W. T., and Rudo, N.: Pseudarthrosis and neurofibromatosis, *Arch. Surg., 46:* 639, 1943.
4. Holt, R.: Radiologic features of neurofibromatosis, *Radiology, 51:* 647, 1948.
5. Hunt, E., and Pugh, D.: Skeletal lesions in neurofibromatosis, *Radiology, 76:* 1, 1961.
6. Laws, S.: Spinal deformities in neurofibromatosis, *J. Bone Joint Surg., 45B:* 675, 1963.
7. Levin, M.: Neurofibromatosis-clinical and x-ray manifestation, *Radiology, 71:* 48, 1963.
8. McCarroll, H. R.: Clinical manifestations of congenital neurofibromatosis, *J. Bone Joint Surg., 32A:* 601, 1950.
9. Moore, B. H.: Some orthopaedic relationships of neurofibromatosis, *J. Bone Joint Surg., 23:* 109, 1941.
10. Scott, J.: Scoliosis and neurofibromatosis, *J. Bone Joint Surg., 47B:* 240, 1965.

RADIAL NERVE PARALYSIS ASSOCIATED WITH FRACTURES OF HUMERUS

Approximately 20% of the radial nerve paralysis following fractures of the humerus occur in children. In virtually all cases the trauma has been severe. Virtually all fractures are located in the middle or lower third of the humerus, and the severe injury with marked displacement and angulation or comminution appears more important than whether it is spiral, oblique, or transverse. However, the medial angulation of the proximal portion of the distal fragment is significant. The outlook can be very optimistic when the paralysis is partial, and it is the usual rule for the full recovery to occur in those patients whose paralysis occurred when the humerus was fractured. The onset of spontaneous recovery usually occurs by 2 weeks. The time required for full recovery varies from 3 days to 8 months, the average being 4 months. Two-thirds of the patients with complete paralysis will regain full nerve function spontaneously.

In all the patients with partial paralysis, recovery begins within 2 months so that lack of spontaneous recovery or evidence of beginning spontaneous recovery at 2 months justifies exploration.

The findings at exploration may include divided nerves, large neuromas in continuity with partial involvement of the nerve, small neuromas, and contusions of the nerve. Neurolysis alone of the nerve is not associated with a good prognosis; and although approximately 25-30% will evince some recovery, many will not. If the nerve is really crushed at the time of exploration and recovery not evident 7-8 weeks after operation, a resection of the neuroma and resuture should be performed. If the paralysis follows open reduction of the humeral fracture, prognosis is also excellent, the average time for full recovery being approximately 3 months for partial paralysis and 8 months for complete paralysis. In this instance, should recovery be delayed, neurolysis would be of some help.

CONGENITAL INDIFFERENCE TO PAIN

Children are seen in pediatric clinics who early on develop swelling about the epiphyses due to repeated trauma, but who are not subject to abuse. Underlying the problem is a neurologic deficit centering about a congenital indifference to pain. The condition is rare and may be confused with rickets as bowing of unrecognized fractures may take place along with the epiphyseal swelling evidence on clinical examination. The children are otherwise normal.

The complicating features that might be expected are burns and bruises, trauma to the eye, and biting of the fingers, tongue, or lips as the teeth appear. The joints when subject to repeated trauma develop synovial thickening and laxity of the ligaments secondary to chronic hemarthroses. As in hemophilia, aseptic necrosis of the femoral head can occur.

As the age of the patient progresses the trauma to weight-bearing joints, particularly the ankle, may lead to dissolution and a picture of a Charcot neuropathic joint. The appearance of such a joint in a child without obvious neurologic deficit such as that due to myelodysplasia should arouse suspicion of congenital pain indifference.

The peripheral and central nervous system is otherwise intact except for the failure to respond to pain. The peripheral nerves should be demonstrated as being intact by electromyographic and nerve conduction studies.

There are other syndromes (all very rare) which may be thought of in connection with this syndrome, including the Riley-Day syndrome (familial dysautonomia). These children are of Jewish ancestry and tend to be mentally and emotionally operating at a below normal level. There is no lacrimation at birth. There is excessive sweating and temperature control abnormalities.

There is a lack of fungiform papillae on the tongue and the normal reflex to histamines of the cornea and axion is absent.

In congenital sensory neuropathy all modalities of reaction to light touch, pain, and temperature change are affected. Conduction is absent over sensory cutaneous nerves although the motor nerve conduction is normal. It may be inherited as a dominant trait.

Obviously recognition of the underlying defect in these children is of prime importance in saving them from marked disability secondary to unrecognized trauma. With recognition and maturity the incidence of repeated difficulty diminishes. Bracing of the neuropathic joints is necessary.

References

1. Abell, J. M., Jr. and Hayes, J. T.: Charcot knee due to congenital insensitivity to pain, *J. Bone Joint Surg., 46A:* 1287, 1964.
2. Denny-Brown, D.: Hereditary sensory radicular

neuropathy, *J. Neurol. Neurosurg. Psychiatry, 14:* 237, 1951.

3. Dimon, J. H., Funk, F. J., Jr., and Wells, R. E.: Congenital indifference to pain with associated orthopaedic abnormalities, *South. Med. J., 58:* 524, 1965.

4. Johnson, J. T. H.: Neuropathic fractures and joint injuries, *J. Bone Joint Surg., 49A:* 1, 1967.

5. Mooney, V., and Mankin, H.: A case of congenital insensitivity to pain with neuropathic arthropathy, *Arthritis Rheum., 9:* 820, 1966.

6. Riley, C. M., Day, R. L., Greely, D. M., and Lanceford, W. S.: Central autonomic dysfunction with defective lacrimation, *Pediatrics, 3:* 468, 1949.

CHAPTER 13

Affections of Muscle

PSEUDOHYPERTROPHIC MUSCULAR DYSTROPHY

Pseudohypertrophic muscular dystrophy, a progressive condition of loss of muscle function, is seen quite commonly in orthopaedic clinics. It is a primary myopathy. The cases are often hidden among patients reporting because of flat feet.

The disease is often familial, and its frequent incidence in male siblings is familiar. The onset usually takes place before the age of 6. The weakness is symmetric and progressive, and it is featured by enlargement of muscle groups, most strikingly those of the calf. At the same time, or slightly later, atrophy about the shoulder girdle may be noted.

Its incidence was reported as 4 per 100,000 for North Carolina.

The Duchenne type occurs almost entirely in males and the onset is usually in the first 4 years of life—coming into clinical notice at about that time. The transmission is sex-linked recessive, and the mutation rate is high. Landouzy and Déjérine[6] described muscular dystrophy of the facial, pectoral, and shoulder-girdle muscles. Erb[5] reported a condition with limb-girdle dystrophy and little or no facial involvement. The latter two types occur in both sexes.

The onset of the facioscapulohumeral type may arise symptomatically from early childhood to late adult life. Transmission is by an autosomal dominant gene. Involvement may be very mild. The limb-girdle type occurs in both sexes with an onset of symptoms usually in the first 3 decades of life.

Pseudohypertrophic muscular dystrophy is often familial and has a frequent incidence in male siblings. The weakness is symmetric and progressive and is featured by enlargement of muscle groups, most strikingly those of the calf. Mild cases may be found first presenting because of flat feet.

Etiology

The theory that there is an underlying involvement of the central nervous system has not been substantiated. A familial history can usually be obtained. The muscle defect causing the atrophy is unknown, but it is conceded to be hereditary.

Progressive muscular dystrophy is an inherited disease with various modes of transmission, but spontaneous occurrence accounts for approximately one-third of the cases. There are various disturbances of the enzymes systems concerned with muscle metabolism but it is not clear that they are primary.

Clinical Picture

The onset is insidious, and the symptoms are first noted in the 3-7 age group. That the patient is weak is usually not appreciated by the family. Difficulty in climbing stairs, easy fatigue, or flattening of the arch of the foot may be a complaint.

The pseudohypertrophic type is more common in males. The feet are pronated, and contracture of the gastrocnemius is noted early in the development of the disease. Difficulty in the gait, such as stumbling and frequent falls, is noted. The calves are enlarged and have a doughy feel on palpation, not the hard feel of normal muscle. The child placed on the floor arises by aiding extension of the knee by the quadriceps with the hand. He then extends the hips by pushing further on the thigh.

Atrophy of the shoulder girdle, particularly the pectorals, may be noted on palpation. Muscle test reveals diminished muscle power, particularly in the quadriceps and proximal limb muscles, until late in the disease.

The facioscapulohumeral type of Landouzy-Déjérine is marked by early involvement of the muscles of the face, which gives a masklike, dull expression. Expression remains about the eyes longer than elsewhere in the face, although difficulty is experienced in closing the eyes. The lower lip hangs down and out. Atrophy of the shoulder girdle and arms is marked. Later there is involvement of the pelvic girdle.

In the juvenile scapulohumeral form of Erb,[5] atrophy of the shoulder girdle is the first form of involvement. The onset is later than that of the early childhood type; the disease begins in pseudohypertrophic muscular dystrophy and usually occurs in the teen-age group. The reflexes are absent in muscle that are severely involved.

Late forms of muscular dystrophy with pelvic girdle atrophy shows a gluteus maximus and medius limp. Scoliosis and trunk weakness are found and are progressive, even in those patients confined to a wheelchair.

There is also an increase in the amount of creatine secreted in the urine. The electromyogram is of considerable value in diagnosis. The pattern of voluntary effort recorded by means of concentric needle electrodes is characterized by a disintegration of motor unit potentials, many of which become polyphasic and of short duration. No fibrillation potentials are seen. Nerve conduction velocities are normal.

On palpation the hypertrophic muscles feel firm and rubbery. The atrophic muscles are often difficult to feel on account of the overlying fat. The involvement of the muscles is symmetrical. Abnormal movements are not present and fibrillary twitchings of the muscles occur only rarely. Pseudohypertrophy may

Fig. 13.2. Scapulohumeral form of muscular dystrophy.

precede atrophy, or atrophy may develop in muscles never hypertrophied.

The sensory examination is normal and there are no sphincter disturbances. The deep reflexes may be lost early in the course of the disease or they may persist in atrophied muscle. Cutaneous reflexes are preserved and the plantar responses are usually flexor.

Serum Enzymes in Muscular Dystrophy

The diagnosis of muscular dystrophy has been helped recently by serum enzyme studies, notably creatine kinase and aldolase. Of these the most striking is creatine kinase and this is particularly true in the Duchenne type of muscular dystrophy.

Creatine kinase is present primarily in skeletal muscle, and reversibility transfers a phosphate group from creatine phosphate to adeno-

Fig. 13.1. Roentgenogram of the calf enlargement with streaks of fat density. Enlargement is limited initially to the area of the calf.

sine diphosphate. The average normal level is 2 units (per mole of creatine formed per hour per milliliter of serum). Values have ranged up to several hundred units in muscular dystrophy. The evidence points to an abnormality of metabolism as the cause of the leakage of this enzyme according to Ebashi, Toyokura, Momoi, and Sugita[4] in 1959.

Female carriers of the Duchenne type of dystrophy have also been found to have elevated levels. The proportion showing an elevated serum aldolase has been smaller.

The enzyme aldolase is present in most tissues and is a catalytic agent in one of the steps of glucose breakdown, namely, the splitting of fructose 1,6-diphosphate. Although normally found at levels less than 10 Bruns units, figures over 100 have been found. Principal values are found early in the disease, with lesser values found as the disease progresses. Less marked values have been found in adult dystrophy. A rise has been reported in polymyositis and dermatomyositis, but only rarely and low in neuromuscular disease.

Both these enzymes offer a nice distinction between neural atrophy and primary myopathy.

Pearson[8] found a rise before clinical signs of weakness were evident. He also found evidence of widespread histologic changes before the clinical disease was evident.

Increased serum levels of aldolase, creatine phosphokinase (CPK), lactic dehydrogenase, phosphohexoisomerase, and transaminase have been reported. Serum enzyme levels, especially CPK, are most consistently elevated in the early stages of the Duchenne variety of muscular dystrophy. Detection of the disease in the preclinical stage of Duchenne's dystrophy can be made by determination of the serum enzymes, and detection of the carrier state in unaffected females is manifested by an increase in the serum CPK and aldolase.

Pathology

The essential muscle changes are similar in all types of dystrophy. The gastrocnemius in a marked case of hypertrophy looks fatty. The muscle color varies from pale grayish to yellowish.

There is considerable variation in fiber size, fatty replacement, and connective tissue invasion of the muscle. Swelling of the fiber is apparently the first change.

Sarcolemmic nuclei are increased in number and may be increased in size. In some forms of dystrophy, the nuclei may occupy a central position in the fiber. Denny-Brown[3] has noted that the biopsy site, if rebiopsied 10-14 days later, exhibits such degenerative changes as loss of myofibrils without evidence of regeneration of muscle buds. In later cases vascular and granular degeneration of the fibers is found. Changes in sensory and motor nerve fibers are not seen. Changes late in the disease are relatively minor and do not point toward a neural atrophy.

Differential Diagnosis

Progressive muscular dystrophy must be distinguished from the diseases of infancy and childhood which are accompanied by muscular wasting. The atypical adult-onset cases must be distinguished from diseases of adult life accompanied by muscular wasting.

Infantile muscular atrophy is recognized by its onset in infancy, the presence of fibrillations, and the rapidly fatal course.

Myotonic muscular dystrophy is distinguished from the cases of muscular dystrophy of relatively late onset by the absence of pseudohypertrophy and by the presence of myotona, cataracts, testicular atrophy, and early baldness.

Peroneal muscular atrophy may be confused with the rare cases of progressive muscular atrophy with an unusual degree of atrophy in the distal portion of the extremities, especially the legs. The presence of cutaneous sensory loss or impairment of the proprioceptive senses should establish the diagnosis of peroneal muscular atrophy.

Amyotrophic lateral sclerosis is distinguished by the extensive degree of atrophy in the distal parts of the extremities, the fibrillary twitchings, hyperactive reflexes, and by the absence of hypertrophy.

In infectious polyneuritis the muscular weakness may occasionally be greatest in the girdle muscles. The acute onset of the symptoms, the increased cerebrospinal fluid protein and the subsequent regression of symptoms establish the diagnosis.

Pseudohypertrophy of the muscles may

Table 13.1. Progressive Muscular Dystrophies

Diagnostic Criteria	Duchenne	Facioscapulohumeral	Limb-Girdle
Age at onset	Childhood	Adolescence	Early or late
Sex	Male	Either	Either
Pseudohypertrophy	Common	Rare	Uncommon
Initial distribution	Pelvic girdle	Shoulder girdle	Either
Involvement of Face	Rare	Always	Possibly never
Rate of progression	Relatively rapid	Slow (abortive)	Intermediate
Contractures and deformity	Common	Rare	Occasional
Inheritance	Sex-linked recessive	Dominant	Either

Fig. 13.3. Enlargement of the calves in pseudo-hypertrophic muscular dystrophy.

occasionally be seen with syringomyelia, but other features should leave no doubt about the diagnosis.

The differential diagnosis between myositis or dermatomyositis and progressive muscular dystrophy can be made by biopsy of the affected muscles.

Treatment

A specific treatment to stop the progress of the disease has not been found. Various medications have been thought helpful, at least for periods in the patient's course. These include glycine taken by mouth and subcutaneous injections of epinephrine and pilocarpine. a-Tocopherol (vitamin E) has been found to inhibit the creatinuria in some of these patients. A program of resistive exercises for key muscles, such as the gastrocnemius, quadriceps, and gluteus maximus, has been helpful, providing the course is periodically interrupted to allow the patient's interest to freshen.

There is no treatment which has been known to be effective in arresting the course of the disease. Obesity, of course, should be prevented by dietary measures.

In the absence of curative medical therapy management by the orthopaedist should include:

1. Strengthening muscles where possible.
2. Preventing or correcting contractures to ensure *full* use of available *strength* and *function.*
3. Bracing (after correction of deformities) to extend the length of the ambulatory period.
4. Surgery to correct contractures and deformities as well as to remove deforming forces.

With regard to contractures, it is best to prevent rather than to treat contractures. Spencer[1,12] advocates a program of stretching and night splinting. The contractures that occur first and are usually most severe are those of the heel-cord and iliotibial band followed later by equinovarus deformity secondary to the strong pull of the frequently normal or near-normal posterior tibial muscle.

Gucker has found that frequently light plaster shells with prevent contractures of the knees and heel cords if they are used for prolonged periods when the deformities are first diagnosed.

A combination of surgery followed by

bracing shortly before or after a patient ceases to walk can preserve amublation, on the average, for 4 or more years. Crutches have not been useful in prolonging ambulation because of weakness of the shoulder depressor muscles.

Spencer[11,12] has found a typical pattern of muscle weakness when the patient is about to stop ambulation. The quadriceps have dropped to fair minus on manual muscle testing. However, the plantar flexors continue to be good for exceedingly long time. The evertors are fair minus, and the dorsiflexors and anterior tibials remain fair.

Stretching exercises are particularly necessary for the gastrocnemius. The tendency toward contracture is marked and provides an additional handicap to the already overburdened patient. Tenotomy of the tendo Achillis is rarely necessary to release such a contracture. Bivalved night casts that hold the limb in the corrected position may be an aid to prevention.

Prolonged periods of bed rest must be avoided because they weaken the patient further. Muscle biopsy of the gastrocnemius, when done to confirm the diagnosis, should be followed by use of a protective splint and by early weight bearing to prevent contracture.

The iliotibial bands are corrected by a low Yount fasciotomy in which a large rectangular section of the iliotibial tract is excised, including a section of the lateral intermuscular septum down to the linea aspera of the femur.

The equinus contractures are corrected by a closed Achilles tenotomy. Open tenotomy contributed to prolonged postoperative disability of the patient with increasing disuse atrophy. After a transverse tenotomy the correction is held by applying the cast with as much dorsiflexion and eversion of the ankle as can be obtained.

To prevent recurrence of the equinus deformity and to correct varus deformity, the posterior tibial tendon is transferred to the third cuneiform through the interosseous membrane.

The principal factor in loss of independent ambulation is progressive muscle weakness. However, loss of independent ambulation often occurs prematurely due to contractures. Another major factor leading to premature loss of amubulation is obesity which, with diet, can be controlled.

Eventually, even surgery and braces cannot maintain ambulation. The wheelchair becomes a necessity. Eventually, seat belts, folding desks, and an electric-powered chair may be necessary. For patients confined to a wheelchair, Spencer believes that measures that might help to prevent or lessen scoliosis include: (1) light plaster jackets, (2) corsets, (3) standing tables, and (4) Rodpri braces.

Respiratory function always deteriorates as the disease advances until vital capacity measures little more than tidal volume. Acute respiratory arrest is the common course. Even a common cold may cause the patient to succumb.

The dystrophic process inevitably involves the myocardium with enlargement of the heart and electrocardiographic abnormalities. Practically, there is no indication for treatment until symptoms occur. Chronic cardiac failure with either pulmonary or peripheral edema is the case. Friedberg reports that in 12 muscular dystrophy patients at rest cardiac catheterization was essentially normal, but during exercise revealed the typical findings associated with congestive heart failure.

References

1. Adams, R. D., Denny-Brown, D., and Pearson, C. M.: *Diseases of Muscles*, New York: Paul B. Hoeber, Inc., 1953.
2. Danowski, T. S., and Fetterman, G.: Muscular dystrophy history, clinical status, muscle strength and biopsy findings, *J. Dis. Child., 91:* 326, 1956.
3. Denny-Brown, D.: The nature of muscular diseases. *Can. Med. Assoc. J., 67:* 1, 1952.
4. Ebashi, S., Toyokura, Y., Momoi, H., and Sugita, H.: High creative phospokinase activity of sera of progressive muscular dystrophy patients, *J. Biochem. (Tokyo), 46:* 413, 1959.
5. Erb, W. H.: Uber die "juvenile form" der progressiven Muskelatrophie; ihre Beziehungen zur sogenannten Pseudohypertrophie der Muskeln, *Dtsch. Arch. Klin. Med., 34:* 464, 1884.
6. Landouzy, L., and Déjérine, J.: De la myopathie atrophique progressive; Myopathie sans neuropathie, débutant d'ordinaire dans l'enface, par la face, *Rev. Méd., 5:* 81, 253, 1885.
7. Miller, W.: Management of muscular dystrophy, *J. Bone Joint Surg., 49A:* 1205, 1967.
8. Pearson, C. M.: Serum enzymes in muscular dystrophy and certain other muscular and neuromuscular diseases. I. Serum, glutamic, oxalacetic transaminase, *N. Engl. J. Med., 256:* 1069, 1957.
9. Pearson, C. M.: Histopathological features of muscle in the preclinical stages of muscular dystrophy, *Brain, 85:* 109, 1962.
10. Siegel, et. al.: Subcutaneous lower limb tenotomy in the treatment of pseudohypertrophic muscular

dystrophy, *J. Bone Joint Surg., 50A:* 1437, 1968.

11. Spencer, G.: Orthopedic care of progressive muscular dystrophy, *J. Bone Joint Surg., 49A:* 1201, 1967.

12. Spencer, G.: Bracing for ambulation in childhood progressive muscular dystrophy, *J. Bone Joint Surg., 44A:* 234, 1962.

13. Vignos, J.: Maintenance of ambulation in childhood muscular dystrophy, *J. Chronic Dis., August:* 273, 1960.

DERMATOMYOSITIS

This is a rare, highly disabling disease whose activity leads to marked contractures. When it involves muscles of respiration and deglutition, it may lead to a fatal outcome. The activity of the disease is marked by a nonsuppurative inflammation of striated muscles that is usually accompanied by skin lesions.

Etiology

Attempts have been made to implicate parasitic, viral, and bacterial agents, but they have not been substantiated. No definite nutritional disturbance has been found. The disease has been grouped with so-called "collagen diseases," such as scleroderma.

Clinical Picture

The onset is usually insidious and marked by weakness and chronic fatigue. The development of limb stiffness and muscle pain follows these initial symptoms. Dermatomyocitis may eventually cause considerable weakness, which is usually irreversible if extensive. The muscle soreness leads to flexion contractures of the joints.

A low grade fever is present at some time in the course of the disease. The skin of the face may be involved early in the disease. The extremities tend to become wasted and to feel brawny and inelastic. Shiny or scaly skin tends to be drawn tightly over bones and atrophied muscles. The atrophy is extensive.

A fatal termination, if the disease follows that course, usually takes place in the first 2 years, the disease thereafter tending to become quiescent.

Pathology

A biopsy of skin, subcutaneous tissue, and muscle taken in continuity from one area may be helpful in establishing the diagnosis. Early changes show edema of subepithelial tissues and collections of polymorphonuclear leukocytes in both skin and muscles. The leukocytes are mainly eosinophils. Later, foci of lymphocytes and monocytes are seen, particularly at the junction of fascia and muscle. Muscle necrosis may be seen. In the late stages, atrophy with disappearance of muscle fibers without inflammation is usual.

Treatment

The measures to combat the disease are centered upon prevention of deformity and compensation for muscle weakness. Periods of rest in the corrective position and bivalved casts, if the tendency to deformity is great, are essential. Use of casts must be balanced by periods of exercise out of casts during the day. To correct an existing deformity, traction, splints, corrective operations, and stretching by active and passive manipulation may all be necessary.

Improvement is characterized by increase in muscle strength, decrease in fever, if present, subsidence of skin lesions and muscle soreness, and gain in body weight. Active exercises of a resistive type may be given when the muscles are no longer sore.

Medication has ranged from hormones, including adrenocorticotropic hormone, to vitamin E. Results have not been encouraging, but occasionally there is a suggestive improvement which is difficult to evaluate because of the tendency toward spontaneous remission.

ARTHROGRYPOSIS MULTIPLEX CONGENITA

This disease of uncertain etiology was first described by Otto in 1841. The unfortunate youngster frequently has multiple deformities of the extremities, although the trunk is relatively unaffected. Rosenkranz named the disease "arthrogryposis" because of the curved joints it causes but "amyoplasia congenita" is a more popular term among the pathologists. The condition is best thought of as involving principally the muscles, which may be represented by only a few undeveloped fibers. It is not progressive. Meade, Lithgow, and Sweeney have delineated the features of its clinical course very well in their series, which included 12 patients followed into adulthood. Mental retardation is not a feature. Clubfeet, club-hands, and dislocated hips are common forms of involvement. The joints are fixed, and their motion is extremely limited.

Etiology

Various forms of intrauterine compression have been thought to be the primary cause of the thin, atrophic limbs. The joint limitation has sometimes, however, been attributed to intrauterine arthritis, but there is no evidence for this etiology in the clinical cases seen. The skeletal muscles have not developed in the involved area, and Middleton[4] has suggested that the primitive myoblast failed to mature. That the muscle picture is secondary to disease of the central nervous system has seemed plausible to other authors, who noted degenera-tion of anterior horn cells, and intrauterine poliomyelitis has been postulated as the under-lying factor. The cause of what is often a very severe clinical picture is not clearly known, however.

Clinical Picture

The outline of the involved extremity is often cylindrical and lacking muscle promi-nences and normal skin creases. Any extremity or any joint area, or any combination of extremities and joint areas, may be involved. Most often all four extremities are affected. Even though the joints are contracted, some motion is usually possible, although it may be small in degree. This motion is painless, free, and often greater in the passive range than in the active.

The extremities feel softer than normal and are conical in shape. The picture of the entire body reveals equinovarus feet, clubhands, dis-located hips, and knee and elbow contractures. The disease is suspected, however, in cases of more discrete lesions, such as the equinovarus foot with a thin calf at birth or a congential contracture of the knee or elbow.

Roentgen Picture

Roentgen studies reveal the contracture or an associated deformity. The muscle shadows are nothing more than thin strands of water density that run through the extremity, which appears to consist largely of fat. The joint space is unaffected, except when a condition such as a dislocated hip is associated with the disorder.

Pathology

Adams, Denny-Brown, and Pearson,[1a] in their text, point out that, in one of their cases of hip flexion contracture due to this disease, the flexors of the hip were well developed, but the extensors were atrophied. Their finding lends some credence to a neurologic etiology. Some muscles cannot be found at all in the masses of fatty tissue; others are represented by occasional, rudimentary, pale pink fibers. The smallness of the muscle fibers seen is note-worthy. Degeneration of muscle fibers is not a

Fig. 13.4. Contractures of the hands, feet, and knees in amyoplasia congenita.

Fig. 13.5. Roentgenogram revealing thin strands that represent muscular tissue running through shadows of fat density in the leg in a case of arthrogryposis.

marked finding. The joints themselves are unaffected; their cartilaginous surfaces appear normal. It is apparent that the cause of the limited motion and contractures lies in the soft tissues. In the cord, the anterior horn cells are markedly reduced in number, and in some areas they may be completely absent. Mead et al. have been impressed by the increased fibrosis about the joints and the lack of loose areolar tissue under the skin.

Treatment

Correcting the contracture and increasing the range of motion are exceedingly difficult. Some gain can be achieved by slow, patient application of plaster casts that hold the limb in a correcting position. The gain is important because it is frequently great enough to enable ambulation in a reasonable position. Surgical correction is not as rewarding as the surgeon might hope since the inelastic skin, vessels, and nerves prove to be limiting factors. It is sometimes indicated and necessary, however. The range of passive motion achieved is greater than the patient can handle actively, but, as in clubfoot, it is a nonetheless necessary achievement for satisfactory ambulation. Bracing is usually necessary to hold the correction, in view of the lack of active muscle power. The foot must be brought to a weight-bearing position, or a rocker bottom deformity may result.

When the hip is dislocated, the soft tissues frequently hold it rather rigidly in abduction and flexion. In some cases the deformity must be accepted; however, a conservative attempt at reduction is always justified, and, when this fails, an open reduction should often be attempted. Traction, which is helpful in patients with a congenital dislocation but good soft tissues, is of little avail against the rigid structures present in this disease.

The knees may be fixed in a range of flexion deformity or occasionally in hyperextension. Quadriceps action often appears to be absent, and bracing is frequently necessary.

At the elbow, a rather rigid extension deformity is frequently a problem, and flexion of one elbow is often desirable. Passive flexion can be achieved by capsulotomy, but active flexion is usually absent.

At the wrist, there is usually a flexion deformity which does not respond to conservative attempts at correction. Absence of dorsiflexion power is a common finding. Surgical correction in the older age group frequently includes fusion to hold the wrist for better function, but each patient must be individually evaluated in terms of what function is present.

Little can be done for the rather rigid tapering fingers, except the thumb, in which the adductor web can frequently be lengthened to gain function. Since the patients have had to confront the problem since birth, there is frequently more function in the hands than the extent of the contractures would lead one to anticipate.

References

1a. Adams, R. D., Denny-Brown, D., and Pearson, C.: *Diseases of Muscle*, Ed. 2. New York: Paul B. Hoeber, Inc., 1962.
1. Brandt, S.: A case of arthrogryposis multiplex congenita, *Acta Paediatr., 34:* 365, 1947.
2. Ealing, M. I.: Amyoplasia congenita causing malpresentation of the fetus, *J. Obstet. Gynaecol. Br. Emp., 51:* 144, 1944.
3. Gilmour, J. R.: Amyoplasia congenita, *J. Pathol. Bacteriol., 58:* 675, 1946.

4. Middleton, D. S.: Studies on prenatal lesions of striated muscle as a cause of congenital deformity, *Edinburgh Med. J., 41:* 401, 1934.

MYOSITIS OSSIFICANS (CIRCUMSCRIPTA)

The formation of bone in heterotypic fashion in muscle occurs most commonly in the quadriceps and brachialis muscle groups and exhibits two distinguishing clinical features: (1) an association with the age group of 16 and 17 years and (2) trauma or repeated trauma.

Myositis ossificans circumscripta must be distinguished from myositis ossificans progressiva a familial disease which progresses to "turn the man to stone" as motion is lost at joints and in the chest wall to the point of inhibiting respiratory function and threatening life. The involvement here is related to tendons and ligaments. In the isolated form, the lesion is solitary and related to muscle, including the collagenous supportive tissue of the involved muscle.

It is also necessary to distinguish an ossifying hematoma from myositis ossificans. This is not developed in irregular extending fashion into the body of the muscle, but has a smooth exterior wall. It is closely related to the bone and does not continue to proliferate in a tumorous fashion as does myositis in its early phases. This type of ossification is not limited by age group as is myositis. There are also various forms of heterotype bone formation occurring in paraplegia, following burns, and after massive trauma around joints involving the capsule in an ossifying repair reaction.

Clinical Picture

The patient is usually male and in the 16-17

Fig. 13.6. Lengthening the tendo-calcaneus by the method of Kuhlmann and Bell. There is a short transverse incision made above the insertion of the tendon into the os calcis. The foot is plantar flexed and a medial transverse incision is made. As the foot is dorsiflexed the long limb of the Z is made in an oblique fashion through the center of the tendon. The fibers are separated rather than divided. The length of the cut is 1/2 to 1 inch as needed. With dorsiflexion the posteriolateral portion of the tendon is divided by retracting the superior margin of the skin incision. The tendon is not sutured, the skin incision is closed.

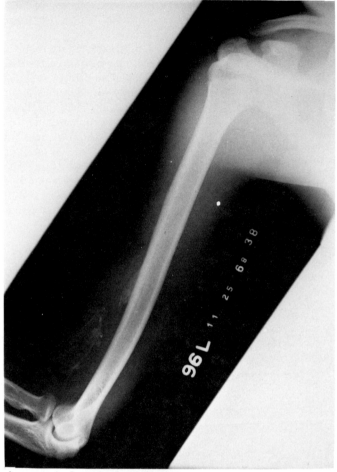

Fig. 13.7. Blocker's exostosis. Irregular bone formation within the brachialis muscle with swelling of the muscle and soft tissues about.

year-old group. The athletic activity of the individual is prominent in the history and a major contusion is often remembered at the onset. Thereafter, repeated blows seem to be suffered in the same area as tenderness and swelling become apparent. The biceps-brachialis area gives rise to a progressively more tender swelling known as a "blocker's exostosis." The quadriceps in mid-thigh progressively enlarges, is markedly tender, and ability to flex the knee is progressively restricted. The early stages may be complicated by vigorous stretching therapy to get the joint motion back, which only results in increasing swelling and progressive limitation.

Pathology

In the early stages there is definite inflammation about the lesion which appears to be a

hematoma and necrosis secondary to muscle tear and contusion, but such an initial inflammatory response will he resorbed and the inflammation subside normally. In myositis ossificans (circumscripta) there is a definite cellular proliferative response. There is metaplasia of the collagen into osteoblasts and chondroblasts. The formed bone is normal in appearance. There may be viable muscle cells persisting in the areas of osteoblastic proliferation. At the periphery the cellular activity is more a reaction than neoplastic. There are three definite zones of maturity in the area of myositis rather than the uniform cellular proliferation of an osteosarcoma. The cells are more regular.

Treatment

Initially the inflammation should be allowed

Fig. 13.8. The irregular formation of bone in the quadriceps muscle in a 17-year-old boy after a football injury. The bone is separate from the underlying femur. There are irregular projections into the muscle belly itself. (*A*) At end of football season, (*B*) 6 weeks later. An ossifying hematoma would have a smooth outline and be closely adherent to the underlying femur. A tumor would present a rounded mass rather than a poorly defined inflammatory swelling and would not have the irregular extension through the muscle.

to subside. Physical therapy at this juncture in any form—electrical, manual, or stretching— can keep the activity of the lesion alive. The motion of the limb should be carried out by the patient alone within the range which is pain free. As the swelling and tenderness subside, the active range of motion may be gradually increased. If treatment has been vigorous initially there may be a large bony mass form. This begins with indistinct outline next to the bone but not attached to it and extending through the muscle belly and along septal planes. Over a 3-4-month period it gains a regular, distinct outline and appears as mature bone.

At this juncture one does not palpate heavily swollen tissues about the bony lesion.

Where the limitation of motion is apprently permanent, surgical excision of the bony mass may be considered. Where operated on at the correct stage the muscle separates readily from it and a space between the bony mass and the adjacent bone may be found. Hematoma formation is minimized by clean surgery and keeping the limb at rest for 10 days before guarded active motion is started by the patient. Full motion will be regained unless bone formation again takes place.

Reference

1. Aegerter, E., and Kirkpatrick, J. A.: *Orthopaedic Diseases,* Ed. 2, pp. 345-346, Philadelphia: W. B. Saunders Co., 1963.

CHAPTER 14

Infections of the Bones and Joints

SEPTIC ARTHRITIS

BY HAROLD SWENSON, M.D.

Thomas Smith's classic review in 1874[13] discussed 21 cases of septic arthritis in infants, 13 of whom died. Treatment through the years was restricted to surgery, which reduced both the death rate and complication rate. Sulfa drugs, introduced in the late 1930s changed the course very little, but the antibiotic era beginning in the 1940s resulted in significant changes. The greatest effect was a dramatic drop in mortality in bone and joint infections uncomplicated by major systemic illness. Death is not longer so possible and prevention of permanent joint destruction and growth alteration are the goals. Anything less than a normal joint falls short of that goal.

Etiology

Joint infection is usually the result of hematogenous spread from a primary focus. In the majority of cases the site of entrance into the body is not of clinical importance. The most common portal of entry is the upper respiratory tree. Furunculosis, otitis media, pneumonia, meningitis, and urinary tract infections are all known to precede joint invasion. Direct penetration, either by trauma or iatrogenically is also a cause.

Enough experience has now been amassed so that the etiologic agent is predictable in a high percentage of cases. This accomplishes two things. First, treatment can be initiated prior to complete bacteriologic identification, and second, treatment can be successfully accomplished when bacteriologic diagnosis cannot be made. An uncomfortably large number of cases occur in which no etiologic agent is isolated (see Table 14.1).

The most common organism producing septic arthritis from birth to age 16 is still *Staphylococcus aureus.* In all series reviewed this proved to be the case.

However, different organisms tend to predominate at different ages. In the first 6 months staphylococcal and streptococcal infections are encountered most frequently. Most of these tend to occur in the first 3 months. Recent reports seem to demonstrate a reduction in incidence of streptococcal bone and joint infections over what it was in pre- and early antibiotic years.

Infections by pathogens of the colon-bacillus family of bacteria are also seen occasionally in infancy, but rarely later. These are aerobic, gram-negative nonsporogenous rods found typically in the excreta of man and animals. Relative immunity against these pathogens develops within 6 months in an otherwise healthy child.

The past 20 years has seen a significant increase in septic arthritis secondary to *Haemophilus influenzae.* This gram-negative pleomorphic bacillus generally strikes the child in the 6-36-month age range producing bronchitis, pneumonitis, otitis media, and meningitis, as well as arthritis.

After age 3 the most common infecting organism is the staphylococcus, with no particular age group evidencing a predilection. However, with the increased incidence of gonorrhea, there also has been an increase in gonococcal arthritis in children, most particularly in the teen-age years.

Clinical Picture

The onset of septic arthritis may be preceded by a variety of infections, but in most cases the focus is the upper respiratory tract. In the newborn the umbilical stump is a potential invasive site. A history of trauma may be given in the cases involving active, otherwise healthy children. Systemic diseases such as blood dyscrasias, dysgammaglobulinemia, and rheumatoid arthritis are also on occasion complicated by pyogenic arthritis.

Fever, anorexia, and irritability usually herald the onset of septic arthritis anywhere from hours to several days prior to specific joint involvement. In the infant the initial symptoms may be subtle, with the baby failing to feed well and displaying a greater than usual amount of fussiness. Pseudoparalysis of the affected limb may also occur.

The child with septic arthritis usually appears acutely ill or "toxic." The temperature may be 39.5° C or higher. Tachycardia and tachypnea are present. Those children on steroid therapy may have significant masking of symptoms.

Pain, loss of motion, and a local increase in heat then involve the joint. Refusal to walk or an antalgic gait are early signs when the lower extremities are involved. Erythema and articular swelling are evident in the more superficial joints. Swelling may even be seen around the hip and shoulder if the process is more advanced. The hip is typically held in a position of abduction, flexion, and external rotation to accomodate the effusion and an increased intra-articular pressure. Most other joints are rigidly splinted in flexion and any attempt at passive motion produces pain.

Pathology

Bacterial invasion of the joint occurs by the hematogenous route with involvement of the synovium as the initial stage. Less frequently, infection results secondary to direct extension from an osteomyelitic focus. This is particularly true in the hip where the proximal femoral metaphysis is within the articular capsule.

Edema and hyperemia of the synovial tissue occur first. An effusion develops which if aspirated early may appear turbid or cloudy and, within 24 to 48 hr, frankly purulent. Polymorphonuclear leukocytes predominate. The protein content of the fluid is high and fibrin pannus may be evident as early as 3 days after invasion. If opened at this point, the joint appears to contain much debris, usually fibrinous, as well as pus.

Destruction of articular cartilage seems to result from loss of nutrition because of the local environment and more actively by proteolytic enzymes. Studies by Curtiss and Klein[4] demonstrated release of hexosamines from cartilage in the presence of lysosomes and streptococcal and leukocytic proteinases. They felt that the matirx was initially lost, and the subsequent breakdown of collagen might be secondary to pressure and use. This process of

Table 14.1. Reported Proved Etiology of Septic Arthritis

Series	Cases	Positive Cultures	
		no.	%
Nelson and Koontz[8] ...	117	57	48.7
Borella et al.[3]	52	17	32.7
Almquist[2]	50	16	32.0
Children's Hospital of Pittsburgh	92	24	26.1

cartilage breakdown and loss seems to occur most rapidly in staphylococcal and streptococcal infections, although it is seen with all.

Extension of the infection from the joint may occur with the further passage of time. In the untreated case extension to the adjacent osseous structures generally does not occur in less than 5 days. Spread is probably along vascular channels since direct penetration through the articular cartilage and growth plate is rarely seen.

The hip, which is the most commonly infected joint, may also develop septic necrosis of the capitular femoral epiphysis. Increased pressure and/or thrombosis of the intra-articular vessels resulting in ischemia appears to be the cause. In addition, since the growth plate and metaphysis are within the capsule, bony destruction and growth arrest are more likely to occur. Growth arrest and avascular necrosis are rare in any other joint.

X-Ray Appearance

Initially there is evidence of deep soft-tissue swelling with displacement or obliteration of fat pads particularly at the elbow and knee. Later, not much earlier than 1 week, there may be evidence of osteoporosis about the joint. Subluxation or dislocation of the hip joint can occur and may be evident within several days after onset of the septic process.

Evidence of bone destruction or new bone formation can be seen later, most particularly in the region of the hip. Actual loss of cartilage space is not usually seen radiologically at least not until after there has been resumption of some degree of activity.

Diagnosis

Critical in the handling of any case of septic

Fig. 14.1. (A) Three-week-old infant. Two-day history of fever and swelling of right knee and distal thigh. Note lytic area in distal femoral metaphysis. Pneumococcus was isolated from the knee. (B) Three weeks after incision, drainage, and immobilization. Note irregularity of epiphyseal line; the right knee is still swollen. (C) Four years later. No evidence of growth disturbance and right knee appears intact.

arthritis is the bacteriologic diagnosis. No child with an inflammed joint should receive antibiotics prior to aspiration of that joint and culture of the fluid obtained. In addition, nose and throat and at least two blood cultures should be gotten. If the initial urinalysis demonstrates a pyuria, the urine should also be cultured.

Of all inflammatory conditions of joints, pyogenic arthritis is the most rapidly destructive and potentially one of the most treatable. If the suspicion of sepsis is present, aspiration should be done. Anaerobic and some gram-negative infections produce a lesser effusion and consequently it may be necessary to irrigate the joint with saline to obtain sufficient quantities for study. The aspirate may appear creamy yellow in the case of staphylococcal sepsis, gray and possibly bloody with streptococcal sepsis, and dirty, watery, gray-yellow in the presence of haemophilus infections.

Culture and Gram stain should be done immediately after arthrocentesis. Thioglycolate broth is inoculated and may be most productive

Fig. 14.1C

in the isolation of microaerophilic and an-aerobic organisms. Plating should be done on blood agar and chocolate agar specifically to culture haemophilus organisms. There are a number of commercially available enriched media which will satisfactorily accomplish specific bacterial growth.

Bacterial morphology and staining character-istics are then determined on the Gram stain. *Haemophilus influenzae* is pleomorphic and classed as a gram-negative coccobacillus. It is important that an expert review slides when *H. influenzae* is suspected because identification is sometimes difficult other than by a bacteriol-ogist. White cell type and predominance can also be observed on the Gram stain. Granulo-cytes will be present in greatest percentage, often with many immature forms in evidence.

Fluid should also be placed in a tube with heparin to determine the cell count. This should be diluted to the proper concentration with saline. In septic arthritis the count may be as low as 10,000 or as high as 100,000, but generally it is about 30,000-50,000 cells per cubic millimeter.

If a sufficient amount of fluid remains, a joint fluid glucose content is determined. Simultaneously a blood glucose level is done. In the presence of joint sepsis the synovial fluid glucose level may be one-half or less than that of blood. If sufficient fluid remains it may be checked for mucin content. In the presence of infection the mucin clot may not form or it may be very friable. Peripheral blood will usually reveal an elevation in the white blood count with the predominance of polymorphonuclear leukocytes and a shift to the left. This count may be as high as 35,000 but, particularly in the case of infants, not notably elevated. Often the hemoglobin and hematocrit are lower than expected, an indication of the preinfection status of the child or as the result of hemolysis. Almost invariably the sedimentation rate is elevated (see Table 14.2).

Treatment

Antibiotic therapy is initiated after all culture samples are obtained. The smallest needle used in aspiration of the joint should be 18 guage. Note should be made of the amount of particulate matter aspirated, and whether or not the needle clogs. Irrigation with saline can be accomplished after samples are obtained, if there is a free flow of fluid. A smaller syringe such as a 5 or 10 cubic milliliter, facilitates aspiration because less suction is applied and synovium is not drawn into the needle tip. The synovial fluid is often under enough pressure so that one may not have to apply any force.

Enough is now known about septic arthritis so that different treatment modalities can be applied rationally without being excessively dogmatic. The goal is to restore a normal joint with no loss of growth potential. Our predeces-sors have given us the tools to prevent death so that it is rarely, if ever, of great concern unless the septic joint is but one of multiple body sites infected by microorganisms. Early recognition followed by adequate therapy invariably ends

Fig. 14.2. (*A*) Two-year-old girl, treated at home for 10 days for fever and hot, swollen left ankle. Had received penicillin and tetracycline. Culture of joint fluid was sterile. (*B* and *C*) Two and a half years later; now age 4 1/2. Film demonstrates loss of articular cartilage and flattening and irregularity of talus. (*D*) Four years after onset and advanced degenerative changes.

in the desired results. Therefore, education of colleagues in general medical and pediatrics will result in referral for early definitive treatment. If partially treated or untreated cases are being seen at pediatric treatment centers 1 week or longer after onset, those involved in definitive care have not been fulfilling their proper role in education of their colleagues. Cases seen 12 hr after onset may not present the so-called classical or full-blown picture, but they do allow some latitude in treatment in terms of time.

If seen early, satisfactory drainage can be accomplished by means of arthrocentesis. This means within 48-72 hr of onset. Beyond that period it becomes difficult or impossible to satisfactorily remove pus and debris from most septic joints by repeat aspiration. An arthrotomy must then be done.

Decompression of hips is obviously a treatment necessity and this is accomplished only temporarily and partially by needle drainage. Therefore, arthrotomy by the posterior Ober muscle splitting approach should be done as soon as it is possible for the child to receive an anesthetic safely. Retrospectively, it seems evident that open drainage of the hip has reduced necrosis of the femoral head and damage to the femoral growth plate.

Numerous studies have demonstrated that antibiotics readily cross the synovial membrane barrier in sufficient concentrations to destroy sensitive bacteria. It consequently is unnecessary to directly instill antibiotics into the

Fig. 14.2*C* and *D*

involved joint in acute cases. There is also evidence that high antibiotic concentrations injected directly into a joint may produce additional synovial irritation, an undesirable side effect of an unnecessary mode of therapy.

The antibiotic of choice prior to identification of the infecting organism is determined primarily by two factors. One is the result of the Gram stain where morphology and stain characteristics are decided, and the second is the patient's age. As mentioned before, gram-positive cocci are found most often in the septic joints of infants. Therefore, penicillin and penicillinase-resistant synthetic penicillins are used in this young age group until cultures and sensitivities are obtained. In the age group from 6 to 36 months, *Staphylococcus aureus* or *Haemophilus influenzae* are generally isolated. In this age group ampicillin is the therapy of choice when the organism cannot be differentiated on Gram stain. In a child beyond 3 years of age the staphylococcus is far and away the most commonly isolated bacteria, and therefore, penicillin and the penicillinase-resistant penicillins are the drugs of choice.

Repeat joint aspiration after initiation of antibiotic therapy will usually produce fluid in which no organism can be seen by staining or isolated by culture. In those cases where no organism can be retrieved because of prior antibiotic therapy, the safest choice seems to be to treat on the basis of the child's age and the usual infecting agent of that age group.

Intravenous administration provides the surest route by which satisfactory levels of antibiotic concentrations can be reached. Intramuscular injections also seem to give high enough serum levels, although this method of therapy may prove to be difficult, particularly in the infant where the subcutaneous tissue and muscle mass is not so great. Unpredictable levels are achieved by the oral pathway since

Fig. 14.3. (*A*) Six-month-old boy treated with antibiotics at home for 3 weeks for fever, irritability, and failure to move the left lower extremity. Left hip is subluxed. (*B*) Two months after incision and drainage and spica immobilization. *Haemophilus influenzae* was isolated. Note dense left capital femoral epiphysis (*C*) One year later there is absence of the osseous growth center and widening of the proximal femoral metaphysis. (*D*) Age five. Coxa magna and plana. (*E*) Age eleven. Femur is 1/2 inch shorter on left. Coxa magna and plana.

absorption varies in different individuals and is also affected by the time relationship to feedings.

The satisfactory duration of antibiotic therapy is difficult to assess objectively. If therapy has been started early after the onset of joint involvement it logically follows that eradication of the organism will occur early if that particular bacteria is sensitive to the antibiotic being given. Successful reversal of the infectious process also occurs more rapidly in the infant and the younger child. Experience seems to indicate that the intravenous and intramuscular method must be used for at least 1 week in these cases. In those instances where prior antibiotics have been given and successful isolation has not occurred despite the persistence of signs and symptoms of joint infections, therapy must necessarily be continued by parenteral means for a longer period, usually for 2 weeks or more. On those occasions where septic arthritis is complicated by the presence or apparent presence of osteomyelitis, parenteral therapy should be continued for 3 weeks or more.

When arthrocentesis has been chosen as the means of joint drainage, repeat aspirations are necessary. How often this is done is dependant upon the reaccumulation of the effusion, the continued presence of bacteria in the synovial

Fig. 14.3*C–E*

Fig. 14.4. (*A*) Septic dislocation of left hip in 21-month-old boy. Had been treated with penicillin. *Staphylococcus aureus* was isolated from blood culture. (*B*) Three and a half months after incision, drainage, and cast immobilization. (*C*) Eleven months after onset. (*D*) Now age 3 1/2. Full range of motion and no limp. New bone formation at proximal femoral metaphysis.

fluid, a persistently high white blood count, and a failure to improve systemically. As noted before, if local and systemic signs and symptoms persist for longer than 72 hr from the time of onset, arthrotomy should be performed. There does not seem to be any necessity for insertion of drains in acute cases.

In all cases the joint should be put at rest. This may satisfactorily be done in the case of the shoulder, hip, and knee by the use of cast immobilization or suspension. All other joints seem to respond best to splinting or whole cast immobilization.

Successful therapy transfers the joint to a sterile state very rapidly. An aseptic synovitis will usually persist to some degree for a number of days or even weeks. Immobilization or splinting should continue until all evidence of joint inflammation has cleared, even though antibiotic therapy may have been stopped (see Table 14.3).

References

1. Almquist, E. E.: The changing epidemiology of septic arthritis in children, *Clin. Orthop., 68:* 96, 1970.

Fig. 14.4 *C* and *D*

2. Badgely, C. E.: Study of the end-results in 113 cases of septic hips, *J. Bone Joint Surg., 18:* 1047, 1936.
3. Borella, L., Goobar, J. E., Summitt, R. L., and Clark, G. M.: Septic arthritis in childhood, *J. Pediatr., 62:* 742, 1963,
4. Curtiss, P. H., and Klein, L.: Destruction of articular carilage in septic arthritis, *J. Bone Joint Surg., 47A:* 1595, 1965.
5. Eyre-Brook, A. L.: Septic arthritis of the hip and osteomyelitis of the upper end of the femur in infants, *J. Bone Joint Surg., 42B:* 11, 1960.
6. Lloyd-Roberts, G. C.: Suppurative arthritis of infancy; some observations upon progress and management, *J. Bone Joint Surg., 42B:* 706, 1960.
7. Nelson, J. D.: Antibiotic concentrations in septic joint effusions, *N. Engl. J. Med., 284:* 349, 1971.
8. Nelson, J. D., and Koontz, W. C.: Septic arthritis in infants and children, *Pediatrics, 38:* 966, 1966.
9. Ober, R.: Posterior arthrotomy of the hip joint, *J. A. M. A., 82:* 1500, 1924.
10. Samilson, R. C., Bersani, F. A., and Watkins, M. B.: Acute suppurative arthritis in infants and children, *Pediatrics, 21:* 798, 1958.
11. Schmid, F. R., and Parker, R. H.: Treatment of infection forms of arthritis, *Mod. Treat. 6:* 1969.
12. Schmid, F. R., and Parker, R. H.: Ongoing assessment of therapy in septic arthritis, *Arthritis Rheum., 11:* 529, 1969.
13. mith, T.: On the acute arthritis of infants, *St. Bartholomew Hospital, Rep. 10,* p. 189, 1874.
14. Weissman, G., and Spilberg, I.: Breakdown of cartilage protein polysaccharide by lysosomes, *Arthritis Rheum., 11:* 162, 1968.

Gonococcal Arthritis

The incidence of gonorrheal infections has climbed steadily since 1960. Along with the increase in genitourinary infections, there has been a concomitant rise in gonococcal arthritis. However, joint involvement has been reported to occur in less than 1% of cases of gonorrhea.

Fig. 14.5. (*A*) Four-day-old infant with fever and irritability for 1 day. Subluxation of both hips. Bilateral incision and drainage was done on the same day. *Staphylococcus aureus* was isolated from blood and hips. (*B*) One month later. Treatment by cast immobilization and methicillin for penicillin-resistant staphylococcus. Note proximal femoral new bone formation. (*C*) Two years later. Clinically normal.

Systemic manifestations in addition to arthritis include tenosynovitis, meningitis, endocarditis, maculopapular skin lesions, and septicemia. Arthritis and tenosynovitis are the most common complications in disseminated gonorrhea. Females are afflicted with joint sepsis 3 or 4 times as often as males, a reversal of statistics from the pre- and early antibiotic era. This is most likely because genitourinary symptoms in men are more apparent, and consequently successful treatment is received earlier. Symptoms of disseminated infection occur disproportionately more often during menses and pregnancies.

Gonorrheal arthritis, other than neonatal, has occurred as early as age 3. However, most cases are seen in the late teens and 20s. In the majority of instances involvement is polyarticular. Wrists, knees, ankles, and the small joints of the hands and feet are the most frequent sites of involvement.

Two phases of gonococcal arthritis have been described. The first is the bacteremic characterized by fever, chills, skin lesions, and tenosynovitis or polyarthritis. Little or no fluid is evident in the joints in this phase. The second or septic joint phase occurs later and is characterized by single joint infection with a large effusion. The gonococcus recovery rate is generally much higher from the joint aspirate in this phase.

Diagnosis requires, first, a high index of

Fig. 14.5*B* and *C*

suspicion. Blood and cervical or urethral cultures should be obtained as well as those from joints. In addition, to the usual plating, inoculation should be done on a Thayer-Martin medium. Gram staining will frequently reveal the gram-negative intracellular diplococci. The peripheral white blood count is usually elevated. Synovial fluid cell count may exceed 50,000. The synovial fluid glucose level will be less than one-half that of the serum. A poor mucin clot is formed.

Most cases respond within several days to parenteral penicillin G therapy. This should be in a range of 10 million units per day in a mature patient. In the face of penicillin allergy, tetracycline is the alternative drug of choice. Arthrotomy and joint debridement is usually not necessary, but splinting or cast immobilization should be done to protect the inflamed joint.

The response to parenteral penicillin therapy is usually rapid and reversal of the process occurs in several days. It is now relatively unusual to see a gonococcal arthritis which has

Table 14.2. Synovial Fluid Analysis*

	Appearance	Viscosity	Mucin Clot	Cell Count	Cell Type	Glucose	Bacteria
Normal	Clear	Normal	Good	<200	Mononuclear	>80% of serum	None
Post-traumatic	Clear, bloody, or xantho-chromatic	Normal	Good	Few to many <peripheral blood	Mononuclear to many RBCs	>80% of serum	None
Rheumatic fever	Cloudy, yellow turbid	Decreased	Good to fair	18,000	50% polys, RBCs	>80% of serum	None
Rheumatoid arthritis	Cloudy, yellow turbid	Decreased	Fair to poor	15,000	60% polys	80% of serum	None
Septic arthritis	White, yellow gray, turbid	Decreased	Poor	20,000 to 100,000	90% polys	50% of serum	Present

* From Ropes and Bauer: *Synovial Fluid Changes in Joint Disease,* Cambridge, Mass.: Harvard University Press, 1953.

Table 14.3. Remission of Septic Arthritis

	No. of Cases	Time for Complete Remission in Days	
Etiology		Range	Average
Staphylococcus ...	13	10-70	28
Streptococcus	9	10-30	21
Haemophilus influenzae	4	10-50	
Diplococcus pneumoniae	2	8-38	
Escherichia coli	2	37-45	
Pseudomonas	2	40-45	
Proteus	2	65-80	
Salmonella	1	27	

produced any significant degree of damage in a joint, when treatment has been begun within 5 days of onset.

TUBERCULOSIS OF HIP

The onset of this disease is seen as a rule in young children. It accounts for 20% of the cases of bone and joint tuberculosis. The hip is more frequently involved with tuberculosis than any other single joint.

The infection is hematogenous and due to Koch's bacilli. The initial lesion may be synovial in the superior acetabulum or in the inferior neck adjacent to the epiphyseal line. Since it is impossible to excise the local site of involvement with hope of success, it is best to think of the disease as generally involving the joint.

Clinical Picture

The onset is insidious, and there is a history of chronic limp and hip or knee pain, usually encompassing many months, when the patient is first seen. Cries and sudden awakening in the night may mark the illness. There are systemic complaints that often include anorexia, loss of weight, and afternoon fever. The child limps, drops out of activities with his fellows, and avoids weight bearing.

On physical examination, the atrophy of the limb is often striking. The hip motion is limited, and a hip flexion contracture is evident when the uninvolved hip is flexed so that the lumbar spine is flattened. The patient may guard against pain on attempted motion in all planes, but early in the disease, most particularly in internal rotation and abduction as well as in extension.

The rate of progression of the disease may vary from individual to individual.

The limp is antalgic, and there is a short stance phase on the involved leg. Hip flexion contracture may result in marked lumbar lordosis on standing. Local tenderness of the joint may be evident over the femoral head, located beneath the femoral artery one finger's breadth below the inguinal ligament. Posterior joint tenderness may be present as well.

It is not common in these times to see a tuberculous hip accompanied by abscess formation when it is first diagnosed. Shortening of the limb from bone destruction is also a late finding. Relative shortening due to an adducted position may, however, be present in the early stages. Some cases late in the disease show extensive shortening—as much as 10 inches. Gill has shown that such shortening may be due in part to premature central closure of the distal femoral or proximal tibial epiphysis.

Pathology

The disease can begin in the synovia, in the metaphysis adjacent to the proximal femoral epiphysis as in the acetabulum. The place of origin is not important.

Even if synovial, the tuberculous granulation tissue begins to invade the subchondral area very quickly. Metaphyseal foci spread to the same area, but usually not by going through the epiphyseal line. A primary epiphyseal foci is uncommon. The trabeculae of the articular cortex are absorbed, and there are granulations both over and under the joint cartilage. This cartilage may be free of its attachment to the parent bone. Areas of contact of joint cartilage

Fig. 14.6. (A) Early tuberculosis of the hip—note destruction of subchondral bone of the acetabulum with narrowing of the joint. (B) Later development of the disease reveals extensive bone atrophy on the affected side. In addition, destruction of bone on both sides of the joint has become marked.

Fig. 14.7. Early tuberculosis of the hip with atrophy and bone envolvement.

constitute a barrier to the extension of the disease and cause destruction to take place first at the joint margins.

With the advancement of the disease, complete destruction of cartilage and subchondral bone occurs. Lymphocytes and plasma cells infiltrate the granulomatous tissue lying intermixed with fibroblasts and vascular tissues. The typically tuberculous arrangement of epipeloid and giant cells about a central area of caseation may be found. In children, healing may occur spontaneously, but when it does, a fibrous ankylosis usually results.

Roentgen Picture

Despite the relative resistance of cartilage to the infection, the most noticeable roentgen finding may be narrowing of the joint space. Apparently no proteolytic enzyme that will digest cartilage, as in pyogenesis, is associated with tuberculous infection. Nonetheless, progression of the disease is so slow and chronic that narrowing of the joint space actually stands out.

There is active destruction of bone, which proceeds irregularly rather than in a rounded distribution as in a tumor; both sides of the joint are often affected. Later, marked bone atrophy occurs in the involved area. There is distention of the capsular shadow and a hazy loss of distinctness of the trabeculae over a wide area. The disease may progress to gross destruction.

Treatment

The first objective is to make a diagnosis of this destructive lesion that is without doubt. While studies are proceeding, the child should be confined to bed, and traction should be applied at the line of his flexion deformity with the object of reducing the degree of contracture, eliminating muscle guarding, and securing comfort for the patient.

There is a positive tuberculin test virtually without exception. A negative test in a patient suspected of having tuberculosis should cause the antigen to be checked and another source to be used. The laboratory work usually reveals an elevated sedimentation rate and may reveal a leukocytosis. The lymphocyte-monocyte ratio may be altered. Secondary anemia may be present.

The joint should be inspected, and a biopsy should be done. The degree of cartilage involvement in both sides is noted at the time of biopsy. With confirmation of the diagnosis, one proceeds with treatment

An attempt should be made to save a joint that still has intact surfaces. This usually means immobilization in a hip spica which also covers the unaffected leg to the knee. The spica is bivalved, and the patient is allowed to carry the joint briefly through a range of motion twice daily. The spica is not applied until the joint flexion and adduction contracture has been corrected in traction.

The patient's systemic response should subside rapidly if the treatment is to be successful.

Chemotherapy with streptomycin, isoniazid, and p-aminosalicylic acid is used as outlined in the treatment of the knee with this disease.

Failure of the systemic symptoms to subside rapidly and progression of destruction is seen by roentgenogram indicate a need for complete immobilization with the hip in neutral position in relation to the pelvis.

Such treatment is also indicated if the patient first presents with a destroyed joint which cannot be functional. Abscesses of the hip are drained and closed primarily.

When the case is destined for fusion, the systemic symptoms are first brought under control. The younger the patient, the more difficult the fusion is to secure and, therefore, the longer the delay in attempting it. For patients younger than 10, fusion is frequently inadvisable.

Attempts at fusion directly through the area involved by disease do not do well and subject the grafts to the ravages of the tuberculous granulation tissue. Operations for hip fusion try

in general to by-pass the diseased area by proceeding either above or below the hip joint.

In Wilson's technique, a rectangular section of ilium is turned down into the trochanter. In Hibb's technique, the greater trochanter and a portion of the shaft are cut out and reversed, and the shaft end is sunk into a hole in the ilium, the cortex of which has been levered out. The cut surface of the graft faces the neck, which can be denuded where healthy. All fusions superiorly have one defect in common: the muscles guarding the hip tend to pull it into adduction, and thus to separate the graft from bony contact. Thus some force tends to compress into the graft when it is inferior. Brittain's method runs the graft from the femoral to the ischial region. A tibial graft is run through a subtrochanteric osteotomy of the femur into an ischial bed. In the Trumbell operation the tibial graft runs from femoral shaft to ischium, but without a subtrochanteric osteotomy.

In all hip fusion operations the task is easier if hip motion is limited and the joint quite firmly fixed; if the joint is unstable, difficulty in fusion may be encountered. The simultaneous use of a subtrochanteric osteotomy in order to obtain fusion has been found of great value by the author.

All of these operations require immobilization in a bilateral hip spica for at least 6

Fig. 14.8. Hip flexion contracture with infection of the hip.

months. Thereafter, release from immobilization depends on the state of bone fusion. Bony union takes place last through the diseased area. The bypass graft acts as a stabilizing start to eliminate motion and to permit healing of the diseased area.

References

1. Bosworth, D. M.: Treatment of bone and joint tuberculosis in children, *J. Bone Joint Surg., 41A:* 1255, 1959.
2. Cleveland, M.: Surgical treatment of joint tuberculosis, *J. Bone Joint Surg., 21:* 607, 1939.
3. Girdlestone, G. R., and Somerville, E. W.: *Tuberculosis of Bone and Joint,* New York: Oxford University Press, 1952.
4. Key, J. A.: Pathology of tuberculosis of spine, *J. Bone Joint Surg., 22:* 799, 1940.
5. Luck, V.: *Bone and Joint Diseases,* Springfield, Ill.: Charles C Thomas, 1950.
6. Phemister, D. B.: Changes in articular surfaces in tuberculous arthritis, *J. Bone Joint Surg., 7:* 835, 1925.
7. Phemister, D. B., and Hatcher, C. H.: Correlation of pathological and roentgenological findings in the diagnosis of tuberculous arthritis, *Am. J. Roentgenol., 29:* 736, 1933.
8. Pimm, L. H., and Waugh, W.: Tuberculous tenosynovitis, *J. Bone Joint Surg., 39B:* 91, 1957.
9. Pomeranz, M. M.: Roentgen diagnosis of bone and joint tuberculosis, *Am. J. Roentgenol., 29:* 753, 1933.

RETROPERITONEAL ABSCESS

In septic arthritis of the hip the muscle spasm is marked and resistance occurs when rotation is attempted either way from a usual fixed externally rotated and abducted position. The internal rotation mode may be limited in retroperitoneal abscess, but further external rotation may be possible. Both septic hip and retroperitoneal abscess, of course, have a flexion contracture held so by the patient to maintain comfort. March et al. brought out the possibility of the physical signs of septic hip being duplicated in children by retroperitoneal abscess and that rectal examination is very helpful in differentiating the two as a tender mass may be palpated by this route.

Any condition that could cause a hip flexion contracture can cause diagnostic confusion. Uncorrected inguinal hernia and the multitudinous causes giving rise to psoas and retroperitoneal abscess must be considered. This includes appendicitis with abscess formation. It includes spinal abscess descending via this route anteriorly.

PYOGENIC INFECTION OF HIP

The septic hip problem is still very much with us. The long term trend since the advent of antibiotics is an increased incidence, and in the early 1970s specifically an increased incidence due to *Haemophilus influenzae.*

Not only is the incidence increased but the disease is often masked by early antibiotic therapy for undiagnosed illness. This leads to softening of the diagnostic signs, delay in arrival of the concept that a serious destructive process is going on in an infant's hip, and consequent important tissue destruction—never to be replaced.

A contrast of the picture of septic hip, prior to the advent of antibiotics and since, reveals that the mortality has virtually been eliminated by antibiotic therapy. The masking of symptoms and signs and the delay in diagnosis exhibit increased incidence and severity since antibiotics have arrived on the scene. The epiphyseal line is destroyed and the femoral head isolated from its blood supply and possibly destroyed as well during this delay.

Over age 2 *Staphylococcus aureus* becomes increasingly the etiologic agent arriving fairly obviously via the blood stream from a skin lesion. In the early months of infancy the *Staphylococcus* and *H. influenzae* are the common organisms.

Infected hip joints are seen most frequently in infancy and may easily be overlooked in the early stages; yet early diagnosis is necessary to save the hip joint. Pyogenic infection occurs most often as a complication of a general septicemia. The initial lesion may be respiratory, dermal, or enteric, or it may be an umbilical vein infection. It is not unknown as a complication of femoral vein puncture in a septicemic infant.

The disease may begin as an osteomyelitis of the femoral neck metaphysis rather than as a primary synovial infection. The femoral neck, because it is contained within the joint, allows the infection to progress rather easily directly into the joint. Destruction of cartilage is particularly possible with staphylococcic infection owing to its proteolytic enzyme.

Clinical Picture

The patients fall into two groups: those who are acutely ill and appear so, and those who are acutely ill and do not appear so. In infants, fever and a high leukocyte count help to determine the diagnosis but are not necessary to it. The child's failure to move the limb may be the first clinical observation. Swelling in the hip and trochanteric area may be another. Some possible portal of entry for the organism is usually known. The most common agents are the streptococcus, staphylococcus, pneumococcus, or *Escherichia coli.*

Examination reveals limited motion of the hip. Neither internal nor external rotation is evident. Swelling obscures bony prominences and makes palpation of the femoral head beneath the femoral artery difficult or impossible. Tenderness is present both anteriorly and posteriorly over the hip joint.

Roentgen Picture

The early signs are those of distension of the capsular shadows of the hip joint and widening of the joint space. Later, areas of destruction in the metaphysis of the femoral neck may be seen. If the infecting agent is the staphylococcus, bony proliferation may also be noted relatively early. In infants, because much of the femoral epiphysis and neck consists of cartilage, the amount of destruction may not be evident.

In the untreated case, further distension of the joint with purulent material, plus the associated muscle spasm, leads to dislocation. Subperiosteal new bone may be present well down the diaphysis in late cases.

Treatment

The disease is an emergency since drainage and removal of purulent material in contact with the cartilage of the femoral epiphysis may be the only means of saving the epiphysis from destruction. The general condition of the patient may, if necessary, be reinforced by blood transfusion before proceeding.

On clinical suspicion, the joint is aspirated anteriorly with a No. 18 spinal needle. When the needle enters the distended hip joint, purulent material wells up into and out of it. Smears and cultures of this material are made.

If pus is obtained, the patient is turned over and the buttock area is reprepared and redraped. Drainage of the hip is done through a linear Ober type incision. This incision is made in line with the femoral neck and over it. The landmarks are a point one-third of the distance along the iliac crest from the posterior superior spine and the trochanter of the femur. In infants, care should be taken to keep the incision well lateralward to avoid the sciatic nerve. The incision splits the fibers of the gluteus maximus, separates the quadratus femoris from the gemellus, and then incises the hip joint capsule. The joint is thoroughly irrigated so that all fibrin clots are removed. A suitable chemotherapeutic agent is instilled. The edges of the capsule are sewn open with a few catgut sutures. A catheter is led down to this opening, but not into the joint itself, and held in place by a skin silk. The would falls together and the skin is loosely approximated.

Postoperatively the patient is treated on a Bradford frame. The posterior incision allows for gravity drainage and does not interfere with nursing care. The catheter is gradually removed whenever, during the next 5 days, the patient's clinical course suggests that it may be.

During therapy and from the time of recognition, the patient has both legs in traction in order to prevent dislocation and allow for the resumption of early motion. Immobilization in a hip spica during this period is contraindicated because it is too likely to lead to a limited hip motion.

Reconstruction of Old Septic Hip

The indications for the reconstruction are: (1) the loss of the normal anatomy with the head and neck frequently destroyed by the original septic process, (2) the unilaterality of the disease with the need for preventing a secondary deformity due to unequal growth of the limb, and (3) the need for stability to correct an unsightly limp.

When the deformity is recognized in infancy the femur is kept pulled down opposite the acetabulum and abducted until the age of 2. Weightbearing or other activity that will cause the femur to slide up the face of the ilium is not allowed on the basis that it complicates the eventual reconstruction.

The reconstruction procedure is borrowed in part from Colonna's arthroplasty. There are, however, no loose capsular tissues to enclose

Fig. 14.9. Fifteen-month-old infant with widened hip joint space and lateral displacement of the femur with extensive soft-tissue swelling.

Fig. 14.10. Abscess of the thigh secondary to infection of the hip in a 3-week-old infant. Progression of the disease unrecognized to this point means virtually certain destruction of the femoral head and neck.

the trochanter. The object is to seat the trochanter in the newly carved acetabulum and have the trochanter convert to a femoral head substitute. To do this all tendinous portions of muscles attaching to the greater trochanteric area such as gluteus medius, gluteus minimus, the gemelli, piriformis, and so forth, are left on the trochanter in as great an abundance as possible. The procedure is done at a relatively young age in the hope of getting greater adaptation and conversion of these tissues. The trochanter is placed against the bare bone of the newly reamed acetabulum and the trochanteric musculature allowed to lie against the bare femoral shaft by widely abducting it. The youngster is kept in position in a spica for 6 weeks. Motion from the bivalved spica is then allowed for the next several months.

References

1. Dunham, E. C.: Septicemia in the newborn, *Am. J. Dis. Child., 45:* 229, 1933.

Fig. 14.11. Soft-tissue inflammatory swelling, widening of the joint space, and displacement of the femoral shaft at the hip in acute pyogenic infection of the hip.

Fig. 14.12. Actual dislocation resulting from hip joint infection.

2. Ferguson, A. B., Anderson, R. L., and Braude, A. I.: Bacteriostatic effect of tetracycline in bone, *Antibiot. Chemother., 9:* 2, 1959.

3. Obletz, B. E.: Acute suppurative arthritis of the hip in the neonatal period, *J. Bone Joint Surg., 42A:* 23, 1960.

4. Sieber, W. K., and Ferguson, A. B., Jr.: Surgical and orthopedic aspects of infections in newly born

Fig. 14.13 (*left*). Preoperative roentgenogram reveals destruction of head and neck due to sepsis of the hip joint. If the femur is left in this position, the gait is poor, and shortening of the limb with lack of normal stress becomes excessive.

Fig. 14.14 (*right*). Postoperative follow-up roentgenogram of reconstructed hip joint. The trochanteric epiphysis and shaft have been transplanted into a reconstructed acetabulum.

and young infants, *Pediatrics, 24:* 145, 1961.
5. Watkins, M. B., Samilson, R. L., and Winters, D. M.: Acute suppurative arthritis, *J. Bone Joint Surg., 38A:* 1313, 1956.

OSTEOMYELITIS

Although osteomyelitis occurs directly—for example, after compound fractures—we are considering here principally the blood-borne, hematogenous infection of bone. This disease once occupied a most prominent position in texts as a difficult and dangerous entity requiring great skill in treatment. The incidence of bone infection has been greatly reduced, but unfortunate situations in which the disease has been underestimated or not recognized are still regularly seen, particularly in the first 3 years of life. It is primarily a disease of early childhood, and it is 4 times as frequent in boys as in girls.

Osteomyelitis is most commonly caused by one of the pyogenic organisms. Green and Shannon have noted the high incidence of streptococcal infections apparently secondary to respiratory involvement in the first 2 years of life. The *Staphylococcus aureus* rises in incidence, as skin lesions liable to cause a bacteremia begin to occur in the ensuing decade.

Etiology

The disease is most frequently secondary to a blood-borne organism which tends to localize in the metaphysis of bones, owing apparently to a peculiarity of the vessels, and which, with its anatomic loops, tends to produce a relatively stagnant situation.

The tendency to localize in the metaphysis is so strong that it frequently is helpful in differential diagnosis. Although the staphylococcus and streptococcus lead the list, infections with gram-negative organisms occur and

Fig. 14.15. A Bradford frame for the care of infants in a hip spica. The pelvis is higher than the head on this frame and plastic inserted into the plaster spica leads to the bed pan. The patient's cast is strapped to the frame to prevent accident. The frame, made of pipe with canvas laced tightly around it for support, is sent home with the patient along with instructions for its use in order to prevent soiling of the cast. The frame on top of the crib is used for those youngsters who are standing and inquisitive to the point of leaving the crib, but it is not necessary with a Bradford frame patient who is strapped to the frame and in a plaster spica. Although there are youngsters who could surmount this handicap, they are rare.

fever, lassitude, and usually pain in an extremity. The primary infection may not have required medical attention, however, and the child in this case is first seen because of the secondary infection.

In an infant, the tendency of the involved extremity to lie flaccidly may lead to confusion with diseases such as poliomyelitis. If a lower extremity is involved, a limp may lead to similar confusion.

The most helpful diagnostic sign is the anatomic position of the tenderness, which early in the disease is maximal in the metaphyseal area. Late in the disease, a spread of an abscess to the midshaft may result in more diffuse tenderness. There is often local heat and swelling, depending on the area involved. The child frequently experiences such agony upon motion of the limb that any attempt to move it is resisted. It is possible, if one is careful not to press on a tender area, to gain enough cooperation from the patient to carry the joints of the area through a range of motion and thus to rule out pathology in the joint itself.

The child may be seriously ill with a

must be considered as diagnostic possibilities early in the disease when the organism may not yet be known. The pneumococcus, *E. coli*, and typhoid bacillus are occasional offending agents.

Clinical Picture

The most usual history in these times of antibiotic agents is a primary respiratory infection, skin abscess, abscess of the teeth, or intestinal infection which was treated apparently in adequate fashion. However, 1 or 2 weeks later, the child may have a recurrence of

Fig. 14.16. Hip flexion and adduction with fixed deformity following previous sepsis of the hip joint.

Fig. 14.17. Swelling of the ankle joint in a 5-year-old child with evidence of metaphyseal destruction, pointing to origin of disease mistaken for rheumatoid arthritis (8-week duration).

Fig. 14.18. Six weeks after incision and drainage, the metaphyseal involvement extending into the epiphysis and then anteriorly to the ankle joint is clear as the ankle joint swelling subsides.

septicemia in addition to his local disease. The blood picture indicates an inflammatory response with a rise in polymorphonuclear leukocytes and an increase in young forms. Rarely the osteomyelitis in infants may be part of an overwhelming infection that does not elicit the usual systemic response.

The antibiotic regime which the child has previously been subjected to may make diagnosis quite difficult. The bone may be carrying an abscess with a low grade inflammatory response, development of physical signs may be slow, and only a stubborn failure of the fever to subside from a low grade elevation to normal

Fig. 14.19. Osteomyelitis of proximal femoral metaphysis with involvement of the diaphysis, sequestration of the shaft, and wrapping of the diaphysis in reactive subperiosteal ossification (involucrum).

following treatment may arouse suspicion.

In infants osteomyelitis is still occasionally seen late in its development. Such infections, if in the region of the shoulder or hip, may have broken through into the joint, and the proteolytic enzymes of the purulent material may have done irreparable damage to the cartilage of the epiphysis. Phemister is responsible for calling our attention to the existence of these enzymes and to the rapidity of their digestion of cartilage.

Advent of Antibiotics

Gilmour[3], analyzing the Perth Children's Hospital figures, noted that penicillin treatment beginning in 1944 constituted a massive experiment. *Staphylococcus aureus,* always the predominant organism, was virtually wiped out. There was progressively a tendency to regard the disease as completely curable by administration of penicillin alone. The staphylococcus reacted by developing a resistant strain. This was evident by 1951. The disease began to increase in frequency. Sequestra reappeared. The disease appeared at a lower age and neonates became prominently involved. The mortality went from 25-30% prior to antibiotics to 1% or less depending on the incidence of neglected cases. Papers appeared bent more on promoting a medical stance than the child's welfare. One proved that osteomyelitis was no longer a surgical disease by showing that 7 cases involving the distal femur failed to drain and subsided without recurrence. Four of these 7 children had their epiphyseal lines destroyed in the process. What was becoming evident was that the mortality due to septicemia was markedly improved. On the other hand, the disease could not be inadequately treated, the symptoms masked, and the morbidity due to tissue destruction increased.

A review of the statistics at Pittsburgh Children's Hospital revealed that the essential truths were there with the advent of penicillin. The mortality went down, but masking the disease with antibiotic therapy led to a rise in aseptic necrosis and total destruction of the infant's hip with late diagnosis of the condition.

Dennison, dividing the patients into preantibiotic, those treated with sulfathiazole, and those treated with penicillin, noted the progressive decrease in mortality. The incidence of complications did not subside, however. Twenty-seven of 75 patients died before any antibiotics. Even sulfathiazole reduced this to 12.7%. Pathologic fracture and limb overgrowth as well as arthritis by direct extension remained common problems. He found that aspiration was not enough.

As the staphylococcus learned to live with penicillin the battle between new chemicals and the ability of the staphylococcus to adapt was joined. A review of the history of this battle reveals that, in moments of enthusiasm when surgical drainage has been neglected, later review has left us with destroyed tissue and complications for full function in the life of a growing child.

Paterson[1] in Adelaide, Australia, adopted an immediate arthrotomy program with installation of penicillin for septic hips in 1960. The improvement in results thereafter was dramatic. Fifty joints were clinically and radiographically normal on follow-up. Of 33 other joints treated

Fig. 14.20 (*Top*). Deep metaphyseal swelling in early osteomyelitis as compared to superficial cellulitis. On the left, the swelling involves superficial subcutaneous as well as deep tissues. On the right, the swelling involves the deep soft tissues only.

Fig. 14.21 (*Bottom*). On the left, the cellulitis area is seen 1 week later. On the right, subperiosteal reaction can be seen 11 days later.

by a variety of other methods, 15 were destroyed.

Pathology

Osteomyelitis tends to begin in the metaphysis because the circulation slows, the arteries and endarteries, and cells to combat the infection become less evident as these sinusoids abut against the epiphyseal line. Inflammation and exudate follows the initial lesion. The pressure forces the purulent material out beneath the periosteum raising it up—it runs into the epiphyseal line and often through it and into the epiphysis and, in the case of the hip and shoulder, where the metaphysis is intracapsular, frequently into the joint.

The metaphyseal abscess may follow any one of many possible courses. It may subside with treatment and not extend. If a condensation of bone forms around it, the abscess may become chronic. This kind of abscess was more frequently seen before the introduction of antibiotics and was known as Brodie's abscess. The infection may spread through the cortex, elevate the periosteum, and form a subperiosteal abscess. A more massive development of the same trend causes the purulent material to extend up and down the diaphysis and circumferentially around the bone. The entire shaft, or a portion of it, may be cut off from its blood supply, and a sequestrum may form. Such an avascular segment of bone complicates treatment. New bone of a coarse type may wall off the abscess by forming what is called an

Fig. 14.22. (A) Chronic osteomyelitis can occur in children as in this 15-month-old patient. There is sclerosis and proliferation of bone about a metaphyseal focus. (B) Lateral view of the femur with bone proliferation and deformity.

Fig. 14.23. Osteomyelitis of proximal tibial metaphysis with bone abscess, destruction of adjacent cortex, and periosteal reaction.

involucrum. Pathologic specimens have been obtained in which the original bone is encased in an involucrum of similar form.

A less common course for the metaphyseal abscess is that of rupturing into the joint and forming a pyogenic arthritis. Such a development is more common at the shoulder or the hip where, depending on the location of the infection, little or no periosteum or fibrous septa may separate it from the joint space.

Although the disease is most commonly localized in the metaphyseal areas of long bones such as the femur and the tibia, it should be remembered that other metaphyseal areas, such as that of the os calcis, have the same arterial configuration and are suprisingly common sites of involvement.

Roentgen Picture

The x-ray is very helpful and indeed most helpful early in the disease (during the first 11 days), when it is commonly thought to be valueless.

In order to be able to diagnose osteomyelitis at this stage, when it is most helpful to do so, the examiner must be able to distinguish deep from superficial swelling. Deep swelling in-

volves the area spoken of as of muscle density and having the anatomic configuration of muscle. The area of the subcutaneous tissue is not involved. A superficial skin abscess, on the

Fig. 14.24. In this infant, the osteomyelitis that was originally centered in the metaphysis (where an area of destruction can be seen) has extended through the epiphyseal line into the epiphysis. New bone is laid by the periosteum, and deep soft-tissue swelling is apparent.

Fig. 14.25. Chronic osteomyelitis in childhood. This 15-year-old boy had a 2-year history of pain, limp, and inability to use the extremity actively. Previous treatment included 1 year's use of antibiotics of various types without amelioration of symptoms. In this anteroposterior view of the distal femoral metaphysis, destruction and new bone proliferation about it can be seen.

other hand, involved the subcutaneous tissue with increased vascular markings and the hazy loss of definition associated with inflammation. The deep shadows in superficial cellulitis are not thickened or swollen. It is also necessary to remember that, in the early stages, osteomyelitis is metaphyseal in location. Thus a deep swelling of the inflammatory type localized to the metaphysis is most helpful in recognizing osteomyelitis before changes of bone destruction have appeared.

Later bone destruction, inflammatory swelling, periosteal new bone (involucrum), and new bone distant from the lesion associated

with stasis of the circulation make an obvious picture.

The radiolucent areas that appear track irregularly through the metaphysis. The destroyed areas may break out through the cortex. The destruction may progress into the epiphysis. Soft-tissue swelling appears down into the diaphyseal region. The original metaphyseal location can usually be seen, however.

In late disease solitary radiolucent areas with hazy outline may appear. These are often filled with granulomatous tissue. Periosteal ossification is often evident.

Certain specifics in the x-ray pictures enable the physician to gain an impression of the probably causative organism. The staphylococcus is rapid, acutely destructive, and early

Fig. 14.26. The lateral view of patient shown in Figure 14.26 shows the original nidus and a dimly seen tract toward the cortex proximally.

Fig. 14.27. The postoperative view of patient shown in Figures 14.25 and 14.26 shows excision of the infected granuloma and primary closure of the wound. Full healing resulted and activity was regained without further antibiotic therapy. The body tends to isolate the infected lesion from the systemic circulation and thus renders antibiotics useless.

on provokes an ossifying reaction about the areas of involvement. Salmonella involving children with sickle cell anemia tends to run up and down the shaft in a chronic way, providing minimal reaction but extensive mottling of the bone over most of its length.

Tuberculosis does everything the staphylococcus does in the x-ray but takes months to do it. This evidence of chronicity becomes prominent, such as atrophy of the bone and musculature. This evidence for chronicity is prominent, relative to the amount of active destruction and walling off by ossific reaction that may appear. Streptococcus excites little ossific reaction but much cellulitis as evidenced by soft-tissue swelling.

Treatment

If the disease involves only a metaphyseal focus, it may be treated and cured with the correct antibiotic, given a sufficiently long period of time to prevent recurrence and provided that the limb is immobilized during that time.

Some of the cases in which there is a small subperiosteal abscess in addition may get by with antibiotics alone. Most, however, need aspiration or drainage to avoid unnecessary complication, such as interference with growth, the development of a sequestrum, or a prolonged course.

Cases which have already developed beyond this point may need surgical intervention to save the child, the limb, an epiphyseal line, or a joint or to secure a sequestrum and prevent the development of chronic osteomyelitis.

The judgment as to what procedure will secure the maximal benefit for the child must be based on bedside findings, not on a textbook; but, in general, unnecessary guttering and removal of bone are to be avoided. The healing powers of childhood are equal to restoring even a sequestration of the entire shaft. Cartilage of the epiphysis and epiphyseal line, if damaged, is damaged permanently, however.

The general antibiotic approach is through wide spectrum drugs, which are used until the organism is known and the most useful drug can be prescribed (Tables 14.4-14.7). Dosage is high; it is continued for a minimum of 3 weeks and at least 2 weeks beyond the subsidence of fever and preferably also of the sedimentation rate. A slight elevation of the sedimentation rate may persist for several months, however, if there has been extensive tissue destruction.

Rest is still good treatment for infection, and, in the presence of resistant organisms, it gives the natural antibody processes the greatest help in overcoming the disease. Bed rest alone, however, has many times been found insufficient rest for the part. A comfortable splint or bivalved cast ensures real rest for the extremity involved.

A general principle and safe working rule is to incise and drain the subperiosteal abscess when it is clearly evident and fluctuation is apparent, or when there is any possibility of

Fig. 14.28. Extensive osteomyelitis due to salmonella infestation. This low grade, widespread process is seen in blood dyscrasias (in this case, sickle cell anemia) in children.

Table 14.4. Antibacterial Spectrum of Antimicrobial Agents

Mode of Action	Gram-Positives	Broad-Spectrum	Gram-Negatives
Bactericidal	Penicillins Bacitracin	Kanamycin-Neomycin Cephalothin Ampicillin (Penicillin)*	Streptomycin Polymyxin B-Colistin Gentamycin
Bacteriostatic	Erythromycin Oleandomycin Lincomycin	Tetracyclines Methacycline Sulfonamides Chloramphenicol	Nalidixic acid

* In very large doses, penicillin may be bactericidal against a number of gram-negative organisms.

involvement of the epiphyseal line. Cellulitis alone is not drained in infants. To drain the bone, an incision is made and holes are drilled through the cortex without elevating the periosteum. It is important to maintain the blood supply to the bone and yet secure adequate decompression of the medullary cavity. In infants, this cavity has a tendency to decompress spontaneously due to the spongy nature of very young bones.

In older children with an established bone abscess, the abscess must be reached and emptied completely. It will often contain granulation tissue requiring curettement. The abscess is left unroofed, and the soft tissues are closed primarily with catgut rather than with silk or cotton. The periosteum is not stripped to accomplish this surgery.

References

1. Altermeier, W. A. and Helmsworth, J. A.: Penicillin treatment in acute osteomyelitis, *Surg. Gynecol. Obstet., 81:* 138, 1945.
2. Altermeier, W. A., and Helmsworth, J. A.: An evaluation of penicillin therapy in acute osteomyelitis, *J. Bone Joint Surg., 30A:* 657, 1948.
3. Gilmour, W. N.: Acute hematogenous osteomyelitis, *J. Bone Joint Surg., 44B:* 840, 1962.
4. Harris, N. H., and Kirkaldy-Willis, W. H.: Primary subacute pyogenic osteomyelitis, *J. Bone Joint*

Table 14.5. Choice of Anti-Infective Agents

Organism (and Gram Reaction)	Drugs	
	First choice	Second choice
Actinomyces (+)	Penicillin + tetracycline	Sulfonamide
Aerobacter aerogenes (−)*	Kanamycin, neomycin, cephalothin	Streptomycin + tetracycline, polymyxin, colistin, gentamycin
Bacillus anthracis (+)	Penicillin	Tetracycline, erythromycin
Bacteroides (−)*	Tetracyclines	Penicillin
Brucella (−)	Tetracycline + streptomycin	Kanamycin
Clostridium (+)	(Antitoxin) penicillin	Erythromycin, kanamycin
Corynebacterium diphtheriae (+)	(Antitoxin)penicillin	Erythromycin, lincomycin
Diplococcus pneumoniae (+)	Penicillin	Erythromycin, cephalothin, tetracyclines, lincomycin
Erysipelothrix (+)	Penicillin	Tetracyclines, erythromycin
Escherichia coli (−)*	Ampicillin	Kanamycin, streptomycin, tetracyclines, colistin, cephalothin, sulfonamides
Haemophilus influenzae (−), H. pertussis	Ampicillin	Chloramphenicol + streptomycin
Klebsiella pneumoniae (−)	Kanamycin, neomycin, cephalothin	Streptomycin + tetracyclines, polymyxin, colistin, gentamycin
Leptospira icterohaemorrhagiae	Tetracyclines	Penicillin
Listeria monocytogenes	Tetracyclines	Penicillin, bacitracin
Lymphogranuloma venereum, psittacosis, and trachoma agents	Tetracyclines	Chloramphenicol, sulfonamide
Mycobacterium leprae (+)	Sulfones	Sulphetrone, diphenylthiourea, sulfoxone
M. tuberculosis (+)	Isoniazid + streptomycin + p-aminosalicylic acid	Viomycin, cycloserine, ethionamide, pyrazinamide
Moniliasis (*Candida albicans*)	Amphotericin B	Nystatin
Mycoplasma (Eaton agent)	Tetracyclines	
Neisseria gonorrhoeae (−)	Penicillin	Ampicillin, tetracyclines Erythromycin, chloramphenicol
N. meningitidis (−)	Penicillin + sulfonamides	Ampicillin, cephalothin, erythromycin, tetracyclines
Nocardia (+)*	Sulfonamides + tetracyclines	Sulfonamides + agent chosen by sensitivity tests
Pasteurella pestis, P. tularensis (−)	Streptomycin + tetracyclines	
Proteus mirabilis (−)*	Ampicillin, penicillin	Cephalothin, neomycin
P. vulgaris, P. morganii, P. rettgeri (−)*	Kanamycin, streptomycin	Cephalothin, chloramphenicol, gentamycin
Pseudomonas aeruginosa (−)*	Polymyxin B, colistin	Gentamycin, tetracyclines, kanamycin, neomycin
Rickettsia (−)	Chloramphenicol	Tetracyclines
Salmonella (−)	Ampicillin	Chloramphenicol, cephalothin, tetracyclines, kanamycin
S. typhosa (−)	Chloramphenicol	Ampicillin
Shigella (−)	Sulfonamides	Ampicillin, tetracyclines, cephalothin, chloramphenicol
Spirillum minus (−)	Penicillin	Tetracyclines
Staphylococcus (+)*, if sensitive	Penicillin	Erythromycin, lincomycin, oleandomycin
Staphylococcus (+), if resistant	Methicillin, oxacillin, nafcillin, cloxacillin	(See above)
Streptococcus (+)	Penicillin	(See above)
S. faecalis (+)*	Penicillin + streptomycin	Ampicillin
Treponema pallidum	Penicillin	Cephalothin, erythromycin, tetracycline

* Sensitivity tests usually indicated.

Table 14.6. Sensitivity of Common Pathogens to Major Antibacterial Agents: Minimal Inhibitory Concentration, μg/ml

Boxed values (indicated below with [ ]) = preferred antimicrobial(s) in clinical use.

Pathogen	Sulfonamide (0.029)	Penicillin G (0.02–2)	Ampicillin (0.02–5)	Methicillin (0.15–2.6)	Cephalosporin (0.15–8)	Erythromycin (0.03–1)	Vancomycin (0.5–1)	Tetracycline (0.25–2)	Chloramphenicol (0.5–16)	Streptomycin (0.1–32)	Kanamycin (1–8)	Polymyxin (0.1–1)
Staphylococcus aureus (a)	PS	[0.03]	0.06	2	0.25	0.12	1	0.12	4–8	2	0.5	R
S. aureus (b)*	V	R	R	[2]	0.25	0.12	1	0.12	4–8	V	0.5	R
Streptomyces pyogenes	S	[0.015]	0.03	0.12	0.12	0.03	0.5	0.25	2	32	R	64–128
Streptococcus faecalis	R	[2]	2.0	32	>8	0.5	1	0.5	2	[64]	64–128	R
Pneumococcus	S	[0.015]	0.06	0.25	0.12	0.03	0.5	0.25	2	64	R	R
Mycobacterium tuberculosis	R	R	—	—	—	5–20	—	10	10	[0.1]	0.5	R
Gonococcus	[S]	[0.015]	0.12	0.06	0.12	0.06	R	1	1	4	8	R
Meningococcus	[S*]	[0.03]	0.06	0.25	—	—	R	1	1	—	—	R
Haemophilus influenzae	PS	0.25–2	[0.25]	2	8	1.0	R	1	[0.5]	2–4	2	0.1–1
Haemophilus pertussis	PS	0.5–2	—	—	—	0.2	—	0.2–2	0.2–2	2–64	—	0.2–1
Escherichia coli*	[S]	16–R	[8]	R	16	R	R	1	2–8	4	[1–4]	0.25
Klebsiella-Aerobacter*	PS	R	16–R	R	8–R	R	R	2–R	2–R	2–R	4–R	0.25
Proteus mirabilis (a)*	V	[16–32]	[4]	R	16	R	R	32–64	4–16	4–8	4–8	R
P. mirabilis (b)*	V	R	R	R	[16]	R	R	32–64	[4–16]	4–R	[4–8]	R
Proteus vulgaris*	V	R	64	R	128–R	R	R	4–32	[4–8]	2–8	[1–4]	R
Proteus morgagni*	V	R	128	R	R	R	R	4–64	[4–64]	4–R	[2–4]	R
Salmonella sp.	PS	[2–16]	[2]	R	4–8	—	R	1	2	8	2–4	0.12
Shigella sp.	[PS]	16	[4]	R	8–16	—	R	[0.5–2]	1–8	8	4	0.12
Pseudomonas*	R	R	R	R	R	R	R	20–R	R	16–64	64–128	[0.12]

*Variable sensitivities—should always be tested. (a) = non-penicillinase producers, (b) = penicillinase producers, □ = preferred antimicrobial(s) in clinical use.

R = all resistant; S = all sensitive; PS = probably sensitive; V = variable.

Table 14.7. Incompatibilities of Commonly Used Drugs for Intravenous Administration

Agent	Incompatible agents
Amphotericin B	Potassium penicillin G, tetracyclines
Cephalothin	Calcium chloride or gluconate, erythromycin, polymyxin B, tetracyclines
Chloramphenicol	B-Complex vitamin preparations, hydrocortisone, polymyxin B, tetracyclines, vancomycin
Methicillin	Tetracyclines
Nafcillin	B-Complex vitamin preparations
Potassium penicillin G	Amphotericin B, metaraminol, phenylephrine, tetracyclines, vancomycin, ascorbic acid
Polymyxin B	Cephalothin, chloramphenicol, heparin, tetracyclines
Tetracyclines	Amphotericin B, cephalothin, chloramphenicol, heparin, hydrocortisone, methicillin, potassium penicillin G, polymyxin B
Vancomycin	Chloramphenicol, heparin, hydrocortisone, potassium penicillin G

Surg., 47B: 526, 1965.
5. Hook, E. W., Campbell, C. G., Weens, H. S., and Cooper, G. R.: Salmonella Osteomyelitis in patients with sickle-cell anemia, *N. Engl. J. Med., 257:* 403, 1957.
6. Morse, T. S., and Pryles, C. V.: Infections of the bones and joints in children, *N. Engl. J. Med., 262:* 846, 1960.
7. Paterson, D. C.: Acute suppurative arthritis of infancy and childhood, *J. Bone Joint Surg., 52B:* 474, 1960.
8. Trueta, J.: The three types of osteomyelitis, *J. Bone Joint Surg., 41B:* 671, 1959.
9. White M. and Dennison, W. M.: Acute hematogenous osteitis in childhood, *J. Bone Joint Surg., 34B:* 608, 1952.

INFLAMMATION OF INTERVERTEBRAL DISC SPACE IN CHILDREN

Particularly in the child age 2-6, the clinical syndrome accompanying inflammation of the intervertebral disc can be a puzzling diagnostic problem. The child frequently refuses to walk.

The child will characteristically splint the entire spinal column rigidly. This results in a stiff gait with minimal flexion of the hips and difficulty with a sitting posture. On the floor the child tends to sit with the trunk thrown back and rising on the outstretched arms behind the body. (The old tripod sign of poliomyelitis and occasionally meningitis.) The child in imitable.

Palpation of the spine with the child prone when done carefully will elicit highly localized tenderness. The straight leg raising may reveal marked hamstring spasm. The lumbar lordosis is straightened.

The average age of the child is 4 years but cases have been reported from 15 months to 15 years. The vast majority are under 6 years of age.

In addition to refusal to walk (the commonest complaint) back pain and thigh pain are common complaints. Loss of appetite and vomiting may occur.

The most common disc spaces involved are at the thoracolumbar junction or at L4-L5 or L5-S1 interspaces.

Laboratory Findings

The sedimentation rate usually shows a mild elevation but may be slow in developing. The white blood cell count tends to run in the high normal range only occasionally getting over 10,000 per cubic millimeter.

Tuberculin, brucellergin, and febrile agglutinin tests are ordinarily negative, but we have had one patient with a very high brucellosis titer.

Blood cultures and cerebrospinal fluid determinations are ordinarily negative.

Cultures obtained by needle biopsy have generally been negative with an occasional coagulase-positive *Staphylococcus aureus* entering the picture.

Roentgen Findings

Narrowing of the disc height is the earliest finding, usually present by the 2nd to 3rd week of symptoms. There follows invasion of the adjacent cortical bone of the vertebrae on either side of the disc space. This is clearly

Fig. 14.29. Narrowing of the intervertebral disc space with destruction of subchondral bone on either side of the disc space.

defined active destruction. Smith and Taylor[3] point out that this destruction may progress to well defined cavities in the vertebrae, the vertebrae do not lose height, and there may be some reactive sclerosis, but it is minimal.

Treatment

The usual treatment is immobilization in a double hip spica for 3 months. Antibiotics are used for a period of 3 weeks at onset of treatment. This usually consists of methicillin, oxacillin, or penicillin in combination with broad-spectrum agents. Even though positive cultures are not frequent and the value of the spica immobilization well established, there is still sufficient evidence of delayed response

without antibiotics that their use continues to be justified.

Course

The clinical course is ordinarily benign and the patient is left without residual symptoms or vertebral deformity. The patient never appears to be in critical conditions. Spontaneous interbody fusion is rare. Six months following onset, the child is usually back on full activity, with roentgen signs stable or possibly with some irregularity of the cortical surface of the vertebrae remaining, but no loss of height.

References

1. Bremmer, A. E., and Neligan, G. A.: Benign forms of acute osteitis of the spine in young children, *Br.*

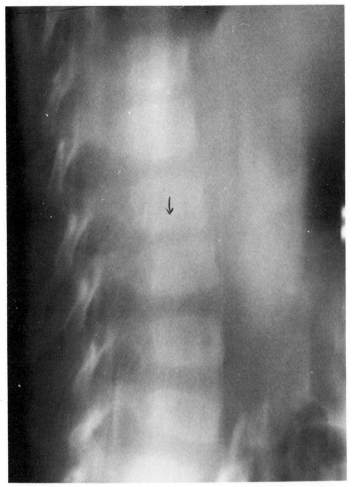

Fig. 14.30. The tomogram further accentuates the irregular destruction of the subchondral bone on either side of the intervertebral disc space.

    Med. J., 1: 856, 1953.

2. Menelaus, M. B.: Discitis; An inflammation affecting the intervertebral discs in children, *J. Bone Joint Surg., 46B:* 16, 1964.

3. Smith, R. F., and Taylor, T.: Inflammatory lesions of intervertebral discs in children, *J. Bone Joint*

Surg., 49A: 508, 1967.

4. Wiley, A. M., and Trueta, J.: The vascular anatomy of the spine and its relationship to pyogenic vertebral osteomyelitis, *J. Bone Joint Surg., 41B:* 796, 1959.

CHAPTER 15

Benign and Malignant Tumors of Bone

BENIGN TUMORS IN CHILDHOOD *

Benign tumors involving bone tend to have a cystic appearance. The area involved is generally totally lytic and the juncture of tumor with bone is smooth rather than having the irregular, finely spiculated edge of active destruction seen in malignancy. A discussion of simple bone cyst and osteoid osteoma is included here solely to aid in their differentiation, since they are not true tumors.

Giant cell tumor is included here, but it is neither truly benign nor characteristically a childhood lesion. Its presence at the far end of the scale as a cystic, invasive, locally recurrent, and occasionally frankly malignant tumor which can occur in the late teen-age group makes it necessary to include it.

The difficulty in deciding when a lesion is an osteogenic fibroma and when an osteoid osteoma as the less characteristic forms of the two merge illustrates some of the difficulties with this group of conditions.

Osteogenic Fibroma and Osteoid Osteoma

Attempts have been made to identify a lesion as ossifying fibroma or benign osteoblastoma. The cases fade imperceptibly into the osteoid osteomas and appear to be one edge of the spectrum of this condition. As in osteoid osteomas there is no evidence that the lesion has the power of autonomous growth, and it has many of the elements of repair. The use of the terms, "fibroma" and "osteoma" is unfortunate.

The age group and location of ossifying fibroma is identical with that of osteoid osteoma. They occur roughly from age 6 to age 26. It is true that they may rarely be found beyond this span. The principal incidence is in

the late teens. As one might expect in a process which may represent prolonged repair under difficulty, the males are heir to the condition twice as often as females.

Pain, worse at night and relieved by salicylates, is a characteristic feature. Clinically, the low grade, insidious nature of the lesion results in a history of many months' duration before being seen, and atrophy of the involved limb is usually marked and common. It is very wise clinically to suspect osteoid osteoma or osteogenic fibroma when atrophy is present and a history of prolonged pain exists with little else in the way of a clinical finding to guide the orthopaedist to the lesion. A careful search of the roentgenogram, making sure the suspected bone is entirely covered, is then indicated. Local tenderness exists over the lesion if it can be found.

In osteoid osteoma there may be very little evidence on the film of the lesion when it is early in it course. In those cases likely to be interpreted as osteogenic fibroma the lesion is more fluid and large, giving rise to still a third term, giant osteoid osteoma. Some of the cases of giant osteoid osteoma coming into our experience have eventually turned out to be osteosarcoma.

As in so many lesions in bone the diagnosis is based on the clinical course, roentgen findings, and view of the microscopic section rather than on the microscopic pathology alone.

Roentgen Findings

The lesion occurs principally in the diaphysis and is eccentric or cortical. Once this is said it is appropriate to add that they have been found in the small bones of the hand, foot, vertebra— in the posterior elements, sacrum, ilium, and, rarely, in the epiphysis. For osteoid osteoma the nidus is radiolucent and small, occasionally

---

* Reprinted in part from A. B. Ferguson, Jr.: Benign tumors of bone in childhood, *Pediatric Clinics of North America*, 14: 683, 1967.

Fig. 15.1. (*A*) Osteoid osteoma of the acetabulum in a 6-year-old girl. In the inferior acetabulum a rounded radiolucent area with central dense nidus is visible to the reader's right. The cartilage joint space of the affected hip is widened. (*B*) The tomogram brings out the details of the lesion. There is a shell of sclerosis about the nidus and the central density is irregular.

Fig. 15.2. Specimens of cortex involved with lesion diagnosed as osteoid ostemoa. Note that there are two separate and distinct nidi. This example helps to support contention that this is not a true tumor.

with some flecks of calcific density within it. Around it, as the lesion develops, new bone may form from both the endosteum and periosteum. This eventually gives rise to considerable sclerosis and localized, axial thickenings of the diaphysis on one side. The ossifying fibroma could be described as having a more central location and less sclerotic reaction.

Pathology

The area occupied by the essential process is sharply delineated from the surrounding bone. It is rather dark reddish brown and cuts with a gritty feel. The bone around it is dense when the location is cortical; where it lies in antomic areas that are principally cancellous the bony reaction is thinner and less noticeable.

On microscopic section, there are areas of osteoid in the center of the lesion. The cells are principally fibroblasts lying in a loose vascular matrix. Denser osteoblasts line the spicules of osteoid and are about bony spicules at the edge. There is not fat and no hematopoietic marrow.

The ossifying fibroma or osteoblastoma varies only in size and, being larger, has less sclerotic reaction. The basic elements are the same with giant cells being perhaps more evident in the large lesion. These are consistent with the giant cells of repair rather than turnover. The lesion may be quite cellular with large numbers of fibroblasts and osteoblasts in some areas. Osteoid formation is still a prominent feature although mineralization of this material may be quite sparse.

Treatment

The treatment consists of an en bloc excision

Fig. 15.3. Osteoid osteoma of the lumbar spine. The enlargement of the pedicle and transverse process at the third lumbar vertebra is easily seen. The scoliosis is secondary to protective muscle spasm guarding this painful lesion.

of the nidus. Because of the difficulty of identifying the nidus beneath the bony reaction about it, an intelligent approach is to perform the surgery using x-ray marker films while the bone is exposed so that the involved area is removed with certainty.

When a fair sized block of bone has been removed the surgeon must support the skeleton in plaster while repair fills in the area. This process is ordinarily rapid and complete without evidence of disturbing tumorous bone formation. Should this occur, it is well to review the entire case, including the pathologic section, to make certain the diagnosis is correct and that the lesion has not been underinterpreted.

Although some of these lesions have eventually proved to be osteosarcoma, it is usually apparent on final review that the features of tumor were there from the onset.

There is little to suggest that osteoid osteoma or ossifying fibroma (benign osteoblastoma) are tumors and a great deal to suggest that they represent repair which has been interfered with in some way. Some of the lesions have been reported as eventually healing themselves after a prolonged course.

References

1. Dahlin, D. C., and Johnson, E. W., Jr.: Giant osteoid osteoma, *J. Bone Joint Surg., 36A:* 559, 1954.
2. Jaffe, H. L., and Lichtenstein, L: Osteoid-osteoma; further experience with this benign tumor of bone, with special reference to cases showing lesion in relation to shaft cortices and commonly misclassified as instances of sclerosing non-suppurative osteomyelitis or cortical-bone, *J. Bone Joint Surg., 22:* 645, 1940.
3. Lichtenstein, L.: Benign osteoblastoma; category of osteoid- and bone-forming tumors other than classical osteoid osteoma, which may be mistaken for giant-cell tumor or osteogenic sarcoma, *Cancer, 9:* 1044, 1956.

Nonosteogenic Fibroma (Benign Cortical Defect)

There is little real evidence that nonosteogenic fibroma differs materially from so-called benign cortical defects. The more extensive involvement of the cortex leads to the use of the term "fibroma," particularly where no osteoid is seen on microscopic section. In neither of these lesions is there any evidence that the process is neoplastic. A conversion defect appears to be the nature of the pathology with the tissue laid down by the epiphyseal line failing to be converted to bone. The metaphyseal area is the only area involved—or at least only that area of the bone derived from the epiphyseal line as compared to the original fetal bone segment.

In order to understand the development of this process, which is usually seen as an incidental roentgen finding, it is important to remember a fundamental of x-ray interpretation. In order for the pathologic process to be seen on the x-ray film at all the cortex must be involved, otherwise the x-ray density of the cortex hides the abnormalities within it. The bone is analogous to a metal pipe, the wall of which must be thinned or a hole drilled through it in order to appreciate on a roetgen film that something has occurred within it.

Thus this lesion could occur in the medullary cavity and be unnoted. Consequently it is thought of as primarily a cortical lesion since this involvement results in its being seen.

Large lesions obviously do involve the medullary canal as well as the cortex. These are relatively rare and may come to clinical attention because of pathologic fracture. A benign cortical defect is generally regarded as asymptomatic.

Following the lesion in time sequence as the child grows one finds that it goes through a fairly characteristic sequence. It is first seen as the metaphysis under-goes tubulation. As age progresses more and more of the lesion appears. The epiphyseal line by this time has laid down additional bone and the lesion consequently is still further exposed as it occupies a position closer to the diaphysis.

The lesion is linear. The long axis is parallel to the long axis of the bone and has a thin cortical wall at its edge. Either the anteroposterior or lateral view confirms its eccentric cortical position. It is important to remember that more of the lesion may exist than is seen by x-ray. As growth progresses the lesion may disappear roentgenographically at the diaphyseal end, and more of the cortical defect appears at the epiphyseal end. The lesion itself may have existed throughout in its original form. The roentgenographic visibility of the lesion varies with its position in the metaphysis.

The age span when the lesion is seen is roughly from 4 to 14 years. Time from first being noted roentgenographically to disappearance varies from 2 to 5 years. It disappears entirely or leaves a small area of sclerosis at its site as it reaches a portion of the metaphysis where remodeling of the involved bone is complete.

The commonest bone involved is the femur, particularly the medial posterior distal metaphysis. The medial proximal third is also common. Any area that is formed of bone laid down by an epiphyseal line can be a site.

It is obvious that the epiphyseal line is these patients over a large or small portion of its surface lays down tissue which, rather than being converted to bone, becomes fibrous tissue. It then, as a result of the bone's undergoing tubulation, appears to the roentgen film viewer. There is no evidence of expansion—the lesion is never wider than the epiphyseal line.

Pathology

A thin layer of cortical bone is often seen about the lesion, although, when biopsied, portions of the lesion are usually exposed without bone covering. It is yellow white in color, soft, and fibrous. There is no osteoid, but occasionally some of the collagen areas appear hyalinized. The lesion cuts without a gritty sensation. The cells are spindle-shaped fibroblasts with fairly minimal collagen production. Occasionally there are some large pale cells which give rise to the thought (when these are plentiful) that this is a xanthoma. Occasional giant cells are seen among the fibroblasts; their nuclei are small. Hemosiderin deposits have been noted.

Fig. 15.4. The typical medial femoral cortical defect of non-osteogenic fibroma.

Treatment

Since the lesion is largely asymptomatic, the most important treatment is to recognize it. Peculiar anatomic locations can occasionally cause the lesion to be implicated as a cause of pain with muscle pull, etc., but there does not appear to be much justification for this thought. The lesion may be biopsied if it is necessary to make the diagnosis in children who are complaining of pain in the area without other evident cause. Where it is large enough to cause a pathologic fracture, removal of the tissue and bone grafting are ordinarily successful.

References

1. Caffe, J.: *Advances Pediat., 7:* 13, 1955.
2. Ponseti, I. V., and Friedman, B. J.: Evolution of metaphyseal fibrous defects, *J. Bone Joint Surg., 31A:* 582, 1949.

Osteochondroma

The relationship between nonosteogenic fibroma and osteochondroma can be recognized if one dwells on one essential feature, i.e., the process which gives birth to each. At first we had fibrous tissue as the product of the metabolism and degradation of the epiphyseal line, visible when its location was cortical. Now we have cartilage left as the product of the maturation of the epiphyseal line and left, due to some fault as yet unknown, to live as cartilage rather than being converted to bone. Again, if its location is cortical, many changes will be obvious; but, if its location is central, it may exist unrecognized by our prime detector, the x-ray film. It may be true that cartilage with the ability to grow following its isolation from the epiphyseal line exists only as a product of the cells at the periphery, where, for a moment, epiphyseal, metaphysis, and epiphyseal line join. These cells indeed are peculiarly reproductive. Cartilage which has been found centrally in bone has been particularly acellular and consists principally of matrix.

A peculiarity of products of the epiphyseal line—be they fibrous tissue, cartilage, or abnormal bone or any percentage mixture of these

Fig. 15.5. Non-osteogenic fibroma involving a sufficient amount of the bone to allow fracture. The lesion is linear, convoluted, metaphyseal, and smooth-walled and does involve the cortex of the distal tibia (*A*). Distal tibia at the time of fracture, (*B*) 3 months later after healing of the fracture and bone grafting.

ingredients—is their failure to respond to the remodeling so characteristic of the normal metaphysis as it narrows into the diaphysis. This abnormal degeneration of material other than normal bone by the epiphyseal line can be designated chondrodysplasia. An osteochondroma with peripheral cartilage based on bone which is not subject to remodeling and with ability of the cartilage to resume growth is a form of chondrodysplasia.

Experimental Osteochondroma

True osteochondromas were produced in the laboratory by D'Ambrosia and Ferguson.[1] Articular cartilage transplants and transplants in which the polarity of the epiphyseal line was reversed did not give rise to true osteochondroma formation. A true osteochondroma occurred almost uniformly when all elements of an epiphyseal line were transplanted in a definite polarity. There was a direct communication of the medullary cavity of the rabbit's tibia into the medullary cavity of the osteochondroma and modeling of the metaphysis occurred in characteristic fashion about the lesion.

There have been many theories about the origin of these cartilage-capped bony lesions. Virchow suggested in 1891 that a portion of the epiphyseal line for reasons unknown became separated from the parent tissue. Muller (1913) suggested that the cartilage cap formed from the "cambium layer" of the periosteum. Keith (1920) felt that the osteochondroma was made possible by a defect in the periosteal ring surrounding the growth zone (aclasis). Geschickter and Copeland (1949) emphasized tendon attachments pulling on local accumulations of embryonic connective tissue as a starting point for these tumors. The laboratory creation of the tumors and the importance of polarity of the epiphyseal line in the successful creation support the thought that their origin is an offshoot of the epiphyseal line separated traumatically in the isolated osteochondroma or by genetic code in multiple exostoses.

Clinical Picture

The osteochondroma is the commonest bone tumor of childhood. Although any one tumor in a patient with multiple lesions may be similar to a tumor occurring as an isolated instance, it is quite evident that more than just the development of the tumor is involved in the patient with multiple lesions. In hereditary multiple exostoses there is a strong tendency for a familial involvement (80%). Males are heirs to the condition 3 times as often as females and appear to be the chief carriers of the syndrome.

The effect on growth is profound in the patient with multiple cartilaginous exostoses, and it is exceedingly typical for the ulna and fibula to be short in relation to the radius and tibia. This results in curving of the radius, producing a wrist deformity similar to Madelung's and occasional dislocation of the radial head. The extremities are short, the patient is short, and the long bone involvement very evident in both the upper and lower extremities. Involvement is fairly symmetrical.

There is little reason to call this disease diaphyseal aclasis since it is primarily a disease of the metaphysis and epiphyseal line. A portion of the cartilage of the epiphyseal line is not converted to bone. The area of bone beneath this periphearl anomaly is not subject to remodeling. Thus as the epiphyseal line grows away from the cartilage cap left behind, the normal remodeling of the metaphyseal bone takes place, leaving the osteochondroma jutting out as the metaphysis falls away. On top of the unremodeled bone lies a cartilage cap which has many of the characteristics of the epiphyseal line from which it came. Although initially the osteochondroma is not wider than the epiphyseal line, if further growth remains to the child, the cartilage cap may also grow, resulting in an increase in size of the bony mass as the cartilage in converted to apparently normal bone. This eccentric growth may result in pressure defects in an adjoining bone, bursae over the prominence, bowing deformity of a paired bone, snapping tendons as the muscle course must fall over the prominence and be displaced as motion occurs, or, finally, limited motion due to bony abutment.

The cartilage cap appears to be subject to the same influences as the epiphyseal line. As the end of growth nears, the adventitious cartilage becomes less cellular and cell columns begin to disappear. Growth in an osteochondroma is not to be expected after general body growth has ceased.

Fig. 15.6. (A) Normal human epiphyseal line at the junction of blood vessels and the cartilage cell columns as bone formation begins. (B) Cartilage cap of osteochondroma. The slight disorganization and irregular lineup of the cartilage cells is evident but so, too, is the basic similarity to the epiphyseal line.

Fig. 15.7. The laboratory creation of an osteochondroma in the rabbit by epiphyseal line transplant to the proximal metaphysis of the tibia. (*A*) The gross specimen reveals cartilage cap and widened metaphysis behind the osteochondroma. (*B*) The effect on the width of the medullary cavity and of the cortex proximal to the lesion is related to failure of modeling, a characteristic of chondrodysplasia. Remodeling is evident in those areas not affected by the growth of the cartilage cap (*C*) Detail of the cartilage cap and demonstration of continuity of the medullary cavity into the lesion (8 weeks post transplant).

		GROWTH PRODUCED				REMODELING
		TOTAL RABBITS	NO GROWTH	OSTEOCHONDROMA	CARTILAGE ISLAND	
TOWARD TIBIA		13	3	10	0	10
AWAY FROM TIBIA		13	4	0	9	0
CONTROL		8	8	0	0	0

ZONE OF ENCHONDRAL OSSIFICATION

Fig. 15.8. Polarization of the transplant so that the metaphyseal side of the cartilage is toward the cortex is very important in achieving experimental osteochomdroma formation. When polarity was reversed, only a cartilage island remained. The controls had a periosteal defect made but not carried to the point of inserting a cartilage transplant from the epiphyseal line.

Fig. 15.9. Proximal fibula from a 4-year-old girl with multiple osteochondromas. The osteochondromas are separated from each other and from the normal growth plate by fibrous bridges. The cell columns appear vacuolated, disarrayed, and are lightly stained. These osteochondromas were juxtaposed to a similar osteochondroma of the lateral proximal tibia. (*A*) Gross specimen with separation of osteochondromatous growth plates from the epiphyseal line. (*B*) Diagram of the photograph of the gross specimen (cut surface). The areas are labeled for easy identification in the photograph. (Courtesy, of John Ogden, M.D.)

Malignant change is heralded from the x-ray point of view by the development of increasing density in the tumor or by continued growth after the normal epiphyseal lines have closed. Malignant change as a possibility is rated from 17% down to 8% of the cases seen, but the real incidence is not really known since most series have been preselected by referral of the more

Fig. 15.10. (*Left*) Osteochondroma of the distal femoral metaphysis. Note that the area supporting the cartilage cap is not subject to normal metaphyseal remodeling.

Fig. 15.11. (*Right*) Multiple osteochondromas are frequently involved with growth abnormalities at the epiphyseal line. This is not so true of the solitary exostosis. Here deficient ulna growth has resulted in bowing of the radius and a resultant Madelung's deformity.

unusual cases to an authority.Malignant change is more likely in the case with multiple exostoses.

Solitary exostoses, although identical on microscopic examination, are not ordinarily accompanied by the profound disturbances of growth from the involved epiphyseal line. In the instance of single lesions, a case can readily be made out to support the contention that they represent the end result of a traumatic peripheral detachment of a portion of an epiphyseal line which is otherwise normal.

Treatment

Excision of the osteochondroma may be done because it is producing deformity, interfering with growth or joint motion, or is cosmetically unappealing. Rarely, pain due to overlying bursitis or tendinitis may occur.

It is possible to produce disability if the exostosis is not correctly removed. The base should be well beyond the cartilage cap area and should depress into the parent bone. It is very easy to take out to little

The overlying soft tissue should be repaired across the defect of bare bone that is left. This

is particularly important where a broad flat surface of muscle will lie against the defect and could adhere to it. The end result of this occurrence would be limited motion of the involved joint.

Cast immobilization aids postoperative comfort, prevents excessive hematoma formation, and allows healing of the repaired tissues without tearing apart and subsequent adherence. The cast should be on for at least 3 weeks.

Reference

1. D'Ambrosia, R., and Ferguson, A. B., Jr.: The formation of osteochondroma by epiphyseal cartilage transplantation, *Clin. Orthop. Res., 61:* 103, 1968.

Simple Bone Cyst

If we carry on the concept of origin from the epiphyseal line by failure of conversion to normal bone we find that the simple bone cyst fits readily into this picture. Very definite is the feature of these lesions which is evident roentgenographically—namely, that in the case of simple bone cysts the entire epiphyseal line is involved. The lesion, once fully formed, extends from cortex to cortex. It always is limited to the metaphysis. It never extends beyond the width of the epiphyseal line and accordingly has no evidence for the existence within it of autonomous growth.

As a form of chondrodysplasia the area involved by the cyst responds to the fundamental rule of areas so involved—that is, it does not respond to remodeling. Consequently the normal bone distal to it remodels to meet the diaphysis, and, proximally, once normal bone has again been laid down by the epiphyseal line, it too begins to remodel. This leaves the area

Fig. 15.12. (*A*) Epiphyseal osteochondroma of talus and navicular. T.. approach is from the medial side of the foot the talus exhibits a cartilage capped irregular protuberance (*left*) followed next in line by a similar lesion projecting from the navicular. (*B*) The excised osteochondromas. This left the parent bones of normal size and shape. The astragalar lesion is on top.

Fig. 15.13. The simple bone cyst involves the entire width of the metaphysis at its widest point. This should not be wider than the epiphyseal line. The cystic tissue narrows as the epiphyseal line begins once again to lay down normal bone, leading to a false appearance of expansion. The cyst area is not subject to remodeling—the bone proximal and distal to it is.

occupied by the cyst apparently expansile—an optical illusion, for it never progresses beyond the maximum width of the metaphysis or the epiphyseal line. The area of radiolucency extending the width of the bone has no evidence of independent density within it.

It is occupied by fluid and a thin membrane tending to be pale rather than reddish or brown, which would be its characteristic color with the hemosiderin deposits of recent trauma and fracture. It is one large cavity occasionally ridged but not divided by bone septa. The septa contains fibroblast macrophages with hemosiderin and occasional clusters of giant cells. The predominence of any cell is not such that one would consider the diagnosis of tumor.

It is so often said that it is a lesion of the growing years—roughly from 3 to 16. One wonders why it is so rarely seen in adult life. The explanation is fairly obvious when one remembers that in older children bone usually begins to be laid down once again by the epiphyseal line. The cyst comes to lie more distally in the metaphysis. The bone continues to enlarge and new cortex is formed over the cyst area, obliterating it from x-ray view, as the cortex resumes normal thickness.

Treatment

Most series agree that the later in life that a cyst is operated upon the greater the chances of success. Some feel this is due to the removal of the cyst from direct contact with the epiphyseal line. It is also apparent that the further down the metaphysis toward the diaphysis the cyst occurs the easier it is for strong cortex to form in a bone now enlarging beyond the character of the cyst.

Some cysts in the proximal metaphysis have been extraordinarily troublesome to obliterate and Fahey has replaced most of the cyst with bone graft, on occasion, leaving only a thin strut of bone to maintain the normal anatomic outline.

The thoroughness with which bone grafts are packed into the defect obliterating unfilled space has played a part in healing the lesion.

Fracture through the cyst exerts a healing influence of callous formation for about 1/8 inch on either side of the frature line and exerts a neglible effect on large cysts.

Aneurysmal Bone Cyst

The name derives from the fact that this lesion breaks through the cortex of the parent bone and new bone is laid down about it. This gives rise to the appearance of "blow out" or "soap bubble," both of which terms have been used to characterize the lesion. Because of its vascular nature, the term "aneurysmal bone cyst" has stuck.

On occasion, the location, combined with the expansile characteristic, has given rise to secondary complications. In vertebra, where the

Fig. 15.14. Bone cysts involving the femoral neck lead to varus deformity with repeated fractures and must be attacked early by grafting to prevent deformity.

lesion occurs in the posterior elements and progresses forward, pressure on the spinal cord has given rise to paraplegia.

The lesion produces pain, low grade usually, but the patient has noted its painful nature when pressure has been accidentally applied. If superficial, a mass or swelling about it had been noted. It is a lesion of late childhood extending into early adult life. The youngest case reported, however, was 2 years and 3 months of age.

Roentgen Appearance

It is a cyst of bone, totally lucent in the area it occupies. It is distinguished in long bones from simple cysts by several characteristics. It is eccentric in its location in the metaphysis rather than extending completely across it. The fact that is has broken through the cortex rather than being enclosed by it is usually evident. A thin layer of new bone encloses it, but this layer extends beyond the original

width of the epiphyseal line. The long axis parallels the long axis of the bone. It may extend well beyond a line dropped from the edge of the epiphyseal line parallel to the parent bone. This feature is never seen in simple bone cyst.

In vertebra its appearance is very characteristic. The spinous process is enlarged and a lacelike new bone envelops it. As the lesion extends through the posterior elements it may invade the body, but only from its posterior aspect, giving rise to a very diagnostic appearance. Only the posterior one-third or one-quarter of the vertebral body is involved.

Pathology

On cutting into the lesion blood wells up, tending to obscure sight of the lesion. It is not filled with dense tissue, but the abundant vascular spaces make the tissue appear fragmentary. It may be gritty to cut as calcification of the tissue is occasionally present. Extraperi-

Fig. 15.15. The aneurysmal bone cyst destroys the old cortex and lays down a thin shell of new bone about the lesion. In this fifth metatarsal, it occupies the entire width of the bone but in long bones it is more usual for it to be eccentric.

Fig. 15.16. Aneurysmal bone cyst occupying the medial portion of the distal femoral metaphysis. Note the eccentric position, the destruction of the old cortex, and the laying down of a thin layer of new bone about the lesion which extends beyond the confines of the old bony outline.

osteal dissection is simple as the lesion easily separates from surrounding tissue. Dissection from the bome is difficult as it invades the intraosseous area. There are fibrous septa. Spaced in these septa are small giant cells of the foreign body type. The vascular spaces do not have well marked endothelial lining. The septa have a collagenous matrix with occasional areas of osteoid formation, some of which may be calcified.

Treatment

The lesion responds well to simple curettage. Apparently the surgical trauma and division of blood supply is sufficient to ablate most lesions. The bone then goes on to repair itself with normal bond. There have been recurrences after simple curettage, however, and it must be thoroughly ablative. The lesion also responds to x-ray therapy, and, once the diagnosis is made, this form of therapy may be indicated in inaccessible locations.

References

1. Donaldson, W. F.: Aneurysmal bone cyst, *J. Bone Joint Surg., 44A:* 25, 1962.

Chondromyxoid Fibroma

Chondromyxoid fibroma is a painful and rapidly progressive tumor of bone, a considerable number of which have occurred in children. This statement characterizes the lesion. It is true that the peak of incidence is in the 3rd decade. It is rather definitely a metaphyseal lesion giving rise to the suspicion that the parent cells may represent offshoots from the epiphyseal line which have failed to heed their genetic code.

Fig. 15.17. Septa from aneurysmal bone cyst, primarily fibrous with some giant cell formation. Osteoid formation is not uncommon.

Roentgen Appearance

The area of bone involvement is totally lucent—it appears to arise at the cortical edge perhaps in the subperiosteal region with a multipronged involvement of the metaphysis. There is considerable periosteal reaction. Nothing, however, suggests malignancy, the edge remaining smooth despite considerable sclerotic reaction. The lesion appears to have bone septa, as the bone extends into areas between lobular extensions; it definitely is eccentric rather than extending across the total width of the bone.

Pathology

There is a greyish yellow cast to the tissue. A lobulated appearance is confirmed as the whole lesion is viewed in cross section. The mass is stiffened by fibrous tissue septa, not bone. The cells lying in a homogenous ground substance are scarce and stellate or triangular in shape. The ground substance is abundant and enclosed by the fibrous tissue septa, giving form to the lesion. Metachromasia of the ground substance has been noted by Scaglietti and Stringa.[2]

Treatment

Definite, complete local excision beyond the edges of the tumor is indicated. There have been recurrences after simple curettage. Because of the normal bone still remaining due to the eccentric location it is usually possible to easily graft the area of removal with reasonable expectations of filling in as the grafts are replaced by normal bone.

References

1. Dahlin, D. C., Wells, A. H., and Henderson, E.:

Fig. 15.18. (*A*) The eccentric position of a recurrent aneurysmal bone cyst is a distractive feature when contrasted with a simple bone cyst which occupies the entire width of the metaphysis. Note the junction of the lesion with the distal cortex of the tibia. The old metaphyseal cortex has been destroyed and the new bone laid down about the lesion abuts onto the exterior surface of the old cortex. It is not a direct continuation of the cortex as in a simple bone cyst. (*B*) After excision and grafting, the lesion is ablated, but growth of the lateral portion of the epiphyseal line appears deficient as some valgus of the tibia is apparent.

Chondromixyoid fibroma of bone, *J Bone Joint Surg., 33A:* 831, 1953.
2. Scaglietti, O., and Stringa, G.: Myxoma of bone in childhood, *J. Bone Joint Surg., 43A:* 67, 1961.
3. Stout, A. P.: Myxoma, the tumor of primitive mesenchyme, *Ann. Surg., 176:* 706, 1948.

Desmoplastic Fibroma

This lesion looks so much like a simple bone cyst that it could escape recognition on first encounter. There is one important difference: it can occupy the diaphysis as well as the metaphysis of the bone. This is a very important difference as it establishes the fact that it does not arise from the epiphyseal line but is a tumor arising from fibroblasts in a local area, and as experience with it grows one might expect that many bizarre locations would eventually be reported. Two cases have been reported that extended into the epiphysis.

It occurs principally in children although cases have been reported at age 40. Series of cases have run an age span from 8 to 21 years in one and 8 to 40 years in the other. The humerus, radius, femur, and tibia carry by far the majority of the cases, although scapula,

ilium, calcaneus, and lumbar vertebrae have been reported as involved. There is no sex predilection.

The clinical complaint that calls attention to the lesion is the presence of pain or pathologic fracture

Roentgen Appearance

Like a simple bone cyst the lesion is totally lucent and tends to extend across the full width of the bone without exciting a marked bony reaction or periosteal proliferation. As one grows more sophisticated it is possible to appreciate that as in giant cell tumor there is a density to the lucent area all its own giving a homogeneous appearance to the lucent area occupied by the tumor. The edge is smooth as it meets bone, not invasive.

Pathology

The defect in the bone is totally filled by the lesion. It does not consist of a few scrapings from the wall of a cyst. The material is greyish white and collagenous. The characteristic cell is

Fig. 15.19. (*Left*) Desmoplatin fibroma giving a very similar appearance to simple bone cyst. There is a hazy density to the lesion as the result of being filled with fibrous tissue very difficult to differentiate on occasion from fibrosarcoma. (From P. Cohen and R. R. Goldenberg: Desmoplastic fibroma of bone, *Journal of Bone & Joint Surgery, 47A:* 1620, 1965.)

Fig. 15.20. (*Right*) Chondroblastoma occupying an epiphyseal location of the humerus. Small flecks of calcification are occasionally seen.

the fibroblast and careful study of the cells is necessary to differentiate the lesion from fibrosarcoma. The cells are small by comparison with those associated with fibrosarcoma, approximately half the size of those seen in the malignant lesion. The cells are sparse, spindle-shaped, and with uniformly small, oval nuclei. Mitotic figures are not seen.

Treatment

Complete local extirpation of the lesion is indicated. This is better done by so-called segmental resection than by curetting, leaving the periosteum and hopefully a stub or two of uninvolved bone. Bone grafts are then used to maintain its skeletal outline. The results of surgical attack to date have been good

References

1. Cohen, P., and Goldenberg, R. R.: Desmoplastic fibroma of bone, *J. Bone Joint Surg., 47A:* 1620, 1625, 1965.
2. Sheer, G. R., and Kuhlman, R. E.: Vertebral involvement by desmoplastic fibroma, *J.A.M.A.,* *185:* 669, 1963.
3. Whitesides, T. E., and Acherman, L. V.: Desmoplastic fibroma, *J. Bone Joint Surg., 42A:* 1143, 1960.

Chondroblastoma

Ewing in 1928 referred to atypical giant cell tumors producing areas of punctate calcification in the humeral head as essentially benign. Codman[2] referred to these tumors as epiphyseal chondroblastomas, Their chondroblastic nature was still further delineated by Jaffe and Lichtenstein as they sharpened their delineation from giant cell tumors of bone.

A chondroblastoma is a lesion that occurs in adolescents and young adults. As the chondroblast fades as a type cell with the closure of the epiphyseal line, one would expect that the origin of these tumors must have taken place prior to epiphyseal line closure.

Recognition of the tumor may occur in adolescents and young adults, but it is often possible to trace the origin to an earlier date.

Pain occurs as the presenting symptom in some, for others existence has been prolonged

Fig. 15.21. Eosinphilic granuloma of the tibia—considerable sclerosis about the lesion may occasionally be seen. This particular lesion has had roentgen therapy, resulting in considerable bony density. A thin area of sclerosis is more typical. The lesion is totally lytic.

sufficiently and pain so low grade that a mass is the presenting symptom.

Roentgen Appearance

An epiphyseal location is characteristic, but extension from the original site may occur into the metaphysis. The tumor produces a radiolucent defect with a benign smooth edge often accompanied by a thin scalloping of bone. There is very little reaction in the adjacent bone, although, as the tumor progresses into lower reaches of the metaphysis, some periosteal reaction may occur. The presence of flecks of calcification within the tumor is very characteristic.

Pathology

Since there is often considerable cartilage produced by the tumor it tends to a pale grey or reddish grey color. The presence of calcified cartilage areas gives a gritty sensation as it is cut.

The lesion appears to be derived from proliferation of the chondroblast, a cell that disappears from the area the epiphyseal line closes. This accounts for its characteristic age group onset in adolescence. The rounded chondroblast may produce little cartilage, giving rise to highly cellular areas. There is considerable variation from section to section with myxomatous and collagenized fibrous tissue also present. The presence of giant cells accounts for its earlier inclusion in th giant cell variant group of tumors.

Treatment

The tumor is highly responsive to local excision, including incomplete removal, and one suspects the cartilaginous material produced within the lesion could be induced to convert to bone with the trauma of surgery. Radiation appears contraindicated and has been implicated in one case where this ordinarily benign tumor later developed into a chondrosarcoma.

References

1. Aegerter, E., and Kirkpatrick, J. A.: *Orthopaedic Diseases,* Ed. 2, pp. 574-580, Philadelphia: W. B. Saunders Co., 1963.
2. Codman, E. A.: Chondroblastoma, *Surg. Gynecol. Obstet., 52:* 543, 1931.

Eosinophilic Granuloma

This disease produces an area of radiolucency within bone without any particular habit so far as location is concerned. It is inserted here under the category of "mentioned in passing." It does not conform well to the habits of true tumors and its cause is unknown. However it does produce a cyst-lesion in bone which may lead to confusion.

The picture is still further complicated by the fact that Hand-Schüller-Christian disease produces lesions in bone which are indistinguishable from the standpoint of pathology. The clinical picture is vastly different, however, with one child (Hand-Schüller-Christian disease) subject to a severe illness which involves liver and spleen enlargement and leading to anemia and a fatal termination. The child with eosinophilic granuloma as a solitary lesion exhibits no systemic manifestations whatever and is in exceedingly good general health. Despite this obvious difference many authors have attempted to link the two conditions together. It leads one to think that eosinophilic granuloma may be one of the ways that bone can react as visualized pathologically and there easily may be no relation between the two conditions.

Most of the cases in our series have occurred about the pelvis and proximal femur.

Eosinophilic granuloma does represent an important consideration in the differential diagnosis of radiolucent lesions of bone in childhood. There is usually some bone reaction consisting of a very thin walling off of the lesion which does not extend for any distance into the general bone structure.

On the microscopic slide the appearance is exceedingly characteristic. Histiocytes, rather pale and large, reticulate with one another in a

Fig. 15.22. (*A*) Chondroblastoma involving the proximal humeral epiphysis. There are irregular flecks of calcification in the lesion. (*B*) After excision.

characteristic background. Over them flows a mass of eosinophilic leukocytes, occasionally exceedingly dense in concentration, varying to relative thinly populated areas. Charcot-Leyden crystals have been reported in the cytoplasm, leading to a suspicion that the lesion represents an allergic reaction. Occasionally giant cells occur. Lipid-filled cells are not obvious except in very long standing lesions.

It should be mentioned that this lesion has been implicated as the cause of vertebral collapse which occurs in Calvé's disease or vertebral plana, a condition which runs a benign course.

The only real connection between patients with solitary eosinophilic granuloma and Hand-Schüller-Christian disease lies in the fact that initially the picture might momentarily be very similar if one considered only the microscopic findings. The differentiation into a systemic disease soon occurs in the latter, however, leading to a very sick child.

Treatment

Many lesions have been cured by the curettage which accompanied biopsy. It is very sensitive to low doses of x-ray therapy as well. It is important to biopsy the initial lesion if possible—one or two others may occur. If this occurs, the possibility of dealing with Hand-Schüller-Christian disease must be kept in mind.

References

1. Compere, E. L., Johnson, W. E., and Coventry, M. B.: Vertebra plana (Calvé's disease) due to eosinophilic granuloma, *J. Bone Joint Surg., 36A:* 969, 1954.
2. Green, W., Farber, S., and McDermott, L.: Eosinophilic granuloma, *J. Bone Joint Surg., 24:* 499, 1942.

Giant Cell Tumor

It is difficult to consider the giant cell tumor as anything but a malignant tumor which is locally invasive but rarely metastisizes. It characteristically occurs after closure of the epiphyseal line but most series report a considerable percentage in the group from 10 to 20 years of age. This is partially explained by the high incidence in females in this younger age group. In one series, 8 of 11 patients under 20 were girls, but only 2 of these were under 15 years of age. The female sex predominates over all, almost 2 to 1. The highest age group incidence occurs between the ages of 20 and 30.

It was orginally described in 1818 by Cooper and Travers, but clearly recognized as an entity distinct from other tumors containing giant cells by the delineation of Jaffe, Lichtenstein, and Portis[1] in 1940.

The area about the knee, either distal femur or proximal tibia, accounts for most cases, but two other sites deserve particular mention. The distal end of the radius is thought of as highly characteristic but surprisingly high is the occurrence in the sacrum. This is true in most series. Other sites include the proximal humerus, distal ulna, and proximal fibula. It can occur in vertebra and in small bones but is rare there.

Pain is a prominent presenting feature, although it may be sufficiently low grade that a number of months elapse before the patient comes to clinical attention. A mass may be the presenting complaint or pathologic fracture.

Roentgen Appearance

A giant cell tumor in a long bone has features that give it sufficient personality that the diagnosis should be readily made.

The epiphyseal origin is obvious although the lesion readily extends into the metaphysis. It destroys bone, but leaves in its place the x-ray density of the soft-tissue mass which is homogenous and recognizable. No bone is formed except that which walls off the tumor at its periphery and appears definitely as a host reaction rather than tumor bone. Such bone as appears in the lesion has been left behind by the enveloping tumor. At the junction of the tumor with normal cortex of metaphysis, the lesion has clearly broken through, and new periosteal bone has been laid down over the cortex, which extends often as a thin layer of bone about the expanded tumor. This layer may not be complete but ceases shortly after it leaves the tumor-cortex junction.

In the vertebra or sacrum the lesion may start in the posterior element and has considerable tendency to fill the outline of the vertebrae before breaking out through the cortex.

Fig. 15.23. Giant cell tumor of the distal ulna. The bone has been totally destroyed and the tumor is now walled off by a thin layer of new bone. Note the typical junction of this new bone with the remaining old cortex. It is seen on the radial side most characteristically.

Reaction of the host bone to the tumor is not marked.

Pathology

The tumor fills the area of destruction with a reddish gray mass with occasional hemorrhagic areas. The edge may cut with the gritty feel of a thin layer of bone. It is not unusual to find the tumor invading into the surrounding soft tissues. Some cyst formation may occur within the tumor secondary to necrosis.

The tumor is cellular with the stromal cells fairly uniform in size. The supportive collagen framework is moderately abundant. Mitoses are extremely variable, a factor that led to grading the lesion, although there is little correlation with grading and subsequent course. Various parts of the lesion may exhibit variable giant

cell concentration as well. These cells contain abundant nuclei.

Treatment

The results of treatment with irradiation, currettage, and partial excision are extremely poor with recurrence the rule. In one series of 9 patients treated by irradiation, 8 recurred. The course following the other two forms of treatment is similar and leads to clear definition of the most advantageous treatment.

The lesion should be thought of as invasive, locally recurrent, and malignant. Neither the term "benign giant cell tumor" or grading the tumor help the clinical approach.

En bloc excision is the treatment of choice, leaving the defect to be filled by surgical reconstructive measures. This en bloc excision

Fig. 15.24. The active stroma of giant cell tumor with tumor rather than foreign body giant cells.

usually means partial removal of a long bone or even amputation. Grafts and prostheses may be used to fill the area of excision and maintain function.

Sacral tumors have a poor prognosis because of the difficulty of applying en bloc excision. There appears to be little justification for the use of the phrase "malignant transformation." Good results are obtained in anatomic locations where en bloc excision is easy. Poor results are obtained where it is difficult or impossible.

References

1. Jaffe, H., Lichtenstein, L., and Portis, R. B.: Giant cell tumor of bone, its pathological appearance, grading supposed variants and treatment, *Arch. Pathol., 30:* 993, 1940.
2. Johnson, E. W., Jr., and Dahlin, D. C.: Treatment of giant cell tumor of bone, *J. Bone Joint Surg., 41A:* 895, 1959.
3. Mhaymneh, W. A., Dudley, H. R., and Mhaymneh, L. G.: Giant cell tumor of bone, *J. Bone Joint Surg., 46A:* 63, 1964.
4. Schajowicz, F.: Giant cell tumor of bone (osteoclastoma); a pathological and histological study, *J. Bone Joint Surg., 43A:* 1, 1961.

Congenital Generalized Fibromatosis

A rare condition has been noted at birth. It is characterized by multiple fibrous tumors available for clinical inspection in the subcutaneous tissues, but also found in other tissues such as the muscles, viscera, and bone.

Of the 16 cases found in the literature by Schaffzin et al.,[3] bone involvement occurred in only 4. Death in infancy is common but regression can occur. The fatal cases have all had visceral involvement. No cases of development of the lesion after the first few months of life have been described.

The lesions consist of fibroblastic tissue, with

elongated spindle cells. The mass is not encapsulated and there is a striking lack of atypical nuclei or mitoses. The histologic pattern of neurofibromatous tissue is absent. The fibrous tissue invades bone. Heiple et al.[1] described a case apparently limited to the skeleton with regression of the lesion in 9 months.

The cases may be confused with congenital fibrosarcoma or neurofibromatosis. The other possibilities are reticuloendotheliosis, neuroblastoma, fibrous dysplasia, hemangioma, lymphangioma, and lipomatosis.

The microscopic examination differentiates this condition from the others.

References

1. Heiple, K. G., Perrin, E., and Aikawa, M.: Congenital generalized fibromatosis, *J. Bone Joint Surg., 54A:* 663, 1972.
2. Kauffman, S. L., and Stout, A. P.: Congenital mesenchymal tumors, *Cancer, 18:* 460, 1965.
3. Schaffzin, E. A., Chung, S. M. K, and Kaye, R.: Congenital generalized fibromatosis with complete spontaneous regression, *J. Bone Joint Surg., 54:* 657, 1972.

MALIGNANT TUMORS

BY JAMES H. McMASTER, M.D.

Osteogenic Sarcoma

Osteogenic sarcoma is the most common primary malignancy of bone and is characterized by rapid growth, early metastasis, and a grave prognosis. Typically arising in the metaphysis of a long bone, its distribution pattern in the body is directly related to the rate of bone growth. Thus, the distal femur, proximal tibia, and proximal humerus are the most frequently involved sites. Osteosarcoma in children is seen from ages 3 through 20 with most cases concentrated in the pubertal years. A 2 to 1 male to female ratio has been reported by many authors. The etiology of childhood and adolescent osteosarcoma is unknown.

In adults this tumor is seen in association with Paget's disease, previous enchondromas, and bone infarcts. There are many differences between osteosarcoma in the adult and osteosarcoma in children. In children, the site predilection is for the lower extremity, distal to midfemur. In adults preexisting disease such as Paget's disease of bone or previous irradiation is a common antecedent. Also, it has been induced through the use of localized radiation therapy in excess of 1,500 R, radium implants, strontium-90 ingestion, beryllium ingestion, and the use of Thoratrast. No convincing epidemiologic, virologic or immunologic evidence exists implicating a virus as the etiologic agent. Although a history of trauma is frequently obtained from patients presenting with osteosarcoma, its role as an etiologic factor has not been demonstrated.

Symptoms

The insidious onset of extremity pain which becomes unrelenting, associated with a palpable mass in an adolescent is characteristic of osteosarcoma. The tumor is usually metaphyseal in location and produces minimal to severe functional impairment.

Physical Examination

The patient presenting with osteosarcoma usually appears to be in good health although one occasionally is first seen with anorexia and distant metastasis. The tumor mass is palpable in the metaphysis of the long bone with variable tenderness on direct palpation. Highly vascular lesions are usually warm with distention of the overlying veins. Metastases are typically blood borne, although regional lymph node involvement has been reported. Since osteogenic sarcoma arises from intramedullary elements, x-ray examination reveals an alteration in the normal bony structure of the metaphysis. A portion of the cortex is usually destroyed, and adjacent to it is subperiosteal new bone formed in response to periosteal elevation. The amount of extraosseous bone

Fig. 15.25. Clinical appearance of patient with osteogenic sarcoma. There is swelling of the metaphyseal area of the distal right femur.

proliferation. The tumor is usually contained by the adjacent epiphyseal line, but there is no barrier to its diaphyseal extension. X-ray examination usually fails to reveal the true extent of the diaphyseal spread. Radioscopic scanning is of value, helping to determine the appropriate level of amputation.

Laboratory Data

The usual clinical laboratory studies on patients suffering from osteogenic sarcoma add little to the diagnosis. In some cases, the serum alkaline phosphatase and erythrocyte sedimentation rate may be elevated but these findings are variable and nonspecific. In order to make a definite diagnosis of osteogenic sarcoma, biopsy material must be obtained. It should be taken under tourniquet so that the best possible selection of gross material can be made. The biopsy should be adequate in size and taken from the radiolucent portion of the tumor, avoiding areas of necrotic or liquefied material. Accuracy of diagnosis is of overriding importance in evaluating the biopsy material obtained, with care taken to avoid hasty, inaccurate interpretation. Permenent sections should be made and evaluated thoroughly by special, competent bone pathologists before definitive therapy is instituted.

Pathology

Osteogenic sarcoma most often arises from within the intramedullary canal of the metaphysis of the long bone. The tumor fills the intramedullary canal and perforates the cortex, forming a nodular, asymmetric mass about the shaft. Longitudinal sections of such a specimen usually demonstrate containment of the tumor by the epiphyseal line with variable diaphyseal extension through the intramedullary canal. The peripheral, actively growing portion of the tumor is usually fibrous or cartilaginous in nature and not as densely sclerotic and calcified as the more central regions. Most tumors remain metaphyseal in location; occasionally one is seen that extends throughout the length of the involved bone. Failure to amputate above the level of diaphyseal involvement is the cause of local recurrence of tumors when midshaft amputation is performed. For this

formation varies from tumor to tumor. The sclerosing osteosarcomas may form a large extraosseous mass. Other tumors are more nodular and the lytic variety forms virtually no new bone at all. The intraosseous reaction beneath the cortical destruction causes areas of radiolucency due to dissolution of the trabeculae of cancelous bone by the tumor. Other areas demonstrate endosteal or tumor bone

Fir. 15.26. Multiple fibromas of the hand in a child.

Fig. 15.27. Roentgen features of osteogenic sarcoma: metaphyseal location, bone formation, globular shape, early destruction of the cortex, Codman's triangle of subperiosteal bone at the periphery, active destruction, sunburst appearance, and radial deposition of bone.

reason some surgeons advocate routine disarticulation at the joint proximal to the long bone involved. The microscopic examination of an osteogenic sarcoma shows great variation from tumor to tumor and even within different areas of the same tumor. One constant feature is tumor bone or osteoid formation. This new osseous tissue may arise from a stroma pre-dominantly of cartilaginous tissue. Other areas of sclerotic bone are so dense that the cellular details are obliterated. A supposedly typical field is that of very active pleomorphic osteoblasts forming irregular tumor bone with a vascular marrow and occasional malignant giant cells.

Classification

A great amount of energy has been expended on classifications of osteogenic sarcoma. In general, such classifications are based on the amount of bone produced by the tumor and on the type of stroma producing it. Thus, the tumor which destroys bone and produces little of its own would be called an "osteolytic osteogenic sarcoma." Other sarcomas cause much bone production and are called "sclerosing osteogenic sarcomas." There are other classifications based on the predominate stroma of the tumor, and thus terms such as "telangiectatic," "chondroblastic," and "fibrous" osteogenic sarcoma may be used. There seems to be some correlation between certain types of osteogenic sarcoma and prognosis. In general, osteolytic tumors and those that have a stroma that is principally cartilaginous (chondroblastic osteogenic sarcomas) give practically no survival rate. The sclerosing osteogenic sarcomas seem to metastasize late, and some give long survival periods even with metastases. The classification

Fig. 15.28. Roentgenogram of the scapula of a 13-year-old girl. It demonstrates an osteogenic sarcoma probably radiation-induced. At age 2 years, this child had a hemangioma that was removed by x-radiation, and two randon seeds were implanted. The sarcoma quickly metastasized and caused her demise.

of osteogenic sarcomas seems to have helped to identify a rather succinct type of tumor known as "parosteal osteosarcoma." It is important to recognize this tumor because of the much better prognosis it affords. It usually occurs in an older age group than osteogenic sarcoma. The earliest age is about 10 years, and 40 years is the upper limit. Parosteal osteogenic sarcoma typically occurs as an extraosseous lesion adjacent to the planum popliteum of the femur. Here it appears as one to three islands of dense new bone with a surrounding mass and causes a proliferation of the posterior cortex of the femur. As the tumor ages, the extraosseous new bone becomes confluent with the posterior cortical reaction, and then the tumor surrounds

Fig. 15.29. Osteogenic sarcoma of the femoral metaphysis with osteoplastic metastases to the lungs.

Fig. 15.30. Bone formation in osteogenic sarcoma.

the entire shaft of the femur and may assume a remarkable size with little systemic effect on the patient.

Parosteal osteogenic sarcoma can be successfully treated by local excision, if this is technically feasible. If the tumor is so large that it demands amputation, this can be done with a good chance of long survival in the majority of cases.

Grossly, the parosteal osteogenic sarcoma

Fig. 15.31. Distribution of sclerosing (*left*) and osteolytic (*right*) osteogenic sarcoma. The greatest incidence is in the metaphyseal areas above and below the knee (*shaded black*). (From C. T. Geschickter and M. M. Copeland: *Tumors of Bone,* Ed. 3, Philadelphia: J. B. Lippincott Co., 1949.)

does not invade the intramedullary canal of the bone to any great extent. The tumor seems to arise from the periosteal region and to mushroom out into the soft tissue. The tumor is sclerotic toward the center and becomes less so peripherally.

Finally, it must be noted that the position of origin of osteogenic sarcoma influences the survival rate. Osteogenic sarcomas arising in the proximal metaphysis of the humerus or femur give practically no survival. Those tumors arising in the distal femoral metaphysis give a small percentage of 5-year survival. Those arising in the proximal tibial metaphysis give a still better prognosis.

Recent studies may provide a clue as to why this neoplasia is so well tolerated by its host. The host-immune response has long been implicated as a vital component in the body's defense against neoplasia. Extensive investigation into the role of the immune response in patients with osteosarcoma have been performed. These studies clearly indicate that

osteosarcoma patients are immunologically competent but their tumor is nonantigenic. This lack of antigenicity permits tumor growth to occur, unimpeded by the suppressive effect of the host-immune system.

Recent in vitro experiments have demonstrated estrogen suppression of DNA-synthesis in osteosarcoma cells. The biochemical pathways responsible for producing this effect have already been elucidated and clinical investigation is now in progress.

Treatment

Eight-five percent of patients with histologically proven osteosarcomas succumb to their disease within 24 months of diagnosis. Radical amputation has proven to be the only treatment modality consistently associated with survival. No case of spontaneous regression has been recorded, nor has cure attributable to the use of radiation therapy and/or chemotherapy without amputation been seen. These results support amputation as the best treatment available at this time and clearly indicate the need for basic investigation into the biology of this tumor.

Radical amputation has long been considered the only proper treatment for osteogenic sarcoma. Some reports still state strongly that any surgeon who treats this sarcoma otherwise is negligent. As series of cases are accumulated, however, the instances of 5-year survival are about 5-10%. The Tumor Registry of the Hospital for Sick Children in Toronto revealed 18 children with osteosarcoma diagnosed from 1924 to 1958 with no 5-year survivors regardless of treaatment, according to Jenkil et al.[6]

It is difficult to continue to support a method that fails almost 90-95% of the time, and one wonders if the inevitable variability which is biology would not allow 5% of the patients to survive were no treatment given. With such poor results, it seems wise that at least some surgeons explore other methods.

The statistics regarding osteogenic sarcoma reveal that patients with late amputation (that is, amputation after a period of months in which the tumor was known to exist) have a higher survival rate than those with immediate amputation (Ferguson[4]). Whether this finding reflects only a lower degree of malignancy among the former group of patients or is a valid indication of correct treatment may still be argued. However, patients who have had a delayed amputation and preliminary x-ray treatment have had a better than expected course in our direct observation. These tumors are thought to be insensitive to x-ray therapy. There is, however, a maturing influence since the tumor tends to become more osteoplastic, denser by roentgenogram, and less painful after x-radiation.

The patient gains weight; fever, if it is present, subsides; and the sedimentation rate, if it has been elevated, declines. When the tumor is quiescent and has no new radiolucent areas, the limb is amputated. The level of amputation is not necessarily that of disarticulation, but is as far removed from the tumor as possible. Recurrence in the stump is rare.

References

1. Badgley, C. E., and Batts, M., Jr.: Osteogenic sarcoma, *Arch. Surg., 43:* 541, 1941.
2. Colby, B. L.: *Neoplasms of Bone and Related Conditions,* New York: Paul B. Hoeber, Inc., 1949.
3. Coventry, M. B., and Dahlin, D. C.: Osteogenic sarcoma, *J. Bone Joint Surg., 39A:* 741, 1957.
4. Ferguson, A. B.: Treatment of osteogenic sarcoma, *J. Bone Joint Surg., 22:* 916, 1940.
5. Hatcher, C. H.: The development of sarcoma in bone subjected to roentgen or radium irradiation, *J. Bone Joint Surg., 27:* 179, 1945.
6. Jenkil, R. D. T., Allt, W. E. C., and Fitzpatrick, P. J.: Osteosarcoma, *Cancer, 30:* 393, 1972.
7. Marcove, R. C., Mike, V., Jajek, J. V., Levin, A. G., and Hutter, R. V. P.: Osteogenic sarcoma under the age of 21; a review of 145 operative cases, *J. Bone Joint Surg., 52A:* 411, 1970.
8. McMaster, J. A., Ferguson, R. J., and Weinert, C.: The host-immune response in osteosarcoma, *Clin. Orthop.,* in press.
9. Sweetnam, R., Knoweldon, J., and Seddon, H.: Bone sarcoma; treatment by irradiation, amputation, or a combination of the two, *Br. Med. J., 2:* 363, 1971.

Ewing's Sarcoma

Original Description

In 1921 Ewing[5] described a lesion he called diffuse endothelioma of bone. He reported a total of 7 cases and characterized the disease as a primarily lytic lesion of bone that is extremely radiosensitive and readily metastasizes to the lungs and to other bones. All of his cases apparently died of the disease. Histologically, the tumor was stated to be "composed of broad sheets of small polyhedral cells with pale cytoplasm, small hyperchromatic nuclei, well defined cell borders, and complete absence of extracellular material." He postulated the probable endothelial origin of this tumor. No postmortem examination was performed on any of these patients. The course was that of rather rapid development of metastases to the lung and skull and of exophthalmos.

Since this original report, the literature has contained an interesting running debate as to whether such a disease entity actually exists, and if it does, what its clinical and histologic picture really presents.

Clinical Picture

The most common period of onset of Ewing's sarcoma is the 2nd decade of life. The average age is about 15 years, but the extremes are 3 and 40 years of age. Most reports suggest it is twice as common in boys as in girls.

Symptoms. The first complaint is pain in the

Fig. 15.32. Roentgenogram of Ewing's sarma exhibiting infiltrative type of destruction, tendency to run axially along the shaft, and multiple layers of subperiosteal ossification. A disphyseal location is more typical.

Fig. 15.33. Ewing's sarcoma with sheets of endothelial cells separated by fibrous tissue septa.

region of a bone. The pain may be intermittent for several weeks or months, but it then becomes constant. It is unrelated to activity, and it usually interferes with sleep. If the lesion is in the region of a rather superficial osseous structure, it may present a tender mass, but otherwise it causes a diffuse swelling of an extremity. The symptoms quickly become totally disabling. Fever may be noted soon after the onset of pain, and it is usually intermittent.

Signs. Physical examination early in the disease reveals tender enlargement of the shaft of a long bone. Should the lesion be near the metaphysis of a long bone, it causes some limitation of motion of a major joint. If the patient is seen when two or more bones are involved, he appears cachectic and may have fever.

Fig. 15.34. Distribution of Ewing's sarcoma. (From C. T. Geschickter and M. M. Copeland: *Tumors of Bone,* Ed. 3, Philadelphia: J. B. Lippincott Co., 1949.)

X-ray Examination

Much has been written of the characteristic roentgenographic appearance of Ewing's sarcoma. It should be a lytic diaphyseal lesion of subperiosteal new bone that has an onion skin appearance. Such a typical lesion was seen in 65% of cases in a review of a series by Sherman. Coley[4] found the typical roentgenographic picture in less than half of his cases.

Ewing's sarcoma causes rapid lysis in whatever bone it affects. It appears locally multifocal, as if arising from myeloid elements. Its rapid growth results in sudden elevation of the periosteum, and the roentgenogram reflects this by evidence of periosteal new bone beyond the limits of the lesion. Directly over the area of destruction, the tumor cells may be growing so rapidly that subperiosteal new bone may not be seen. Within the medullary canal, the tumor grows so quickly that the host bone rarely responds by sclerosis. Only 10% of the lesions in Sherman's series showed sclerosis.

Laboratory Data

The most consistent change in the hemogram is a hypochromic, normocytic anemia. The erythrocyte sedimentation rate is elevated. In patients with fever, there may be a moderate leukocytosis.

Pathology

Grossly, Ewing's sarcoma causes a much more extensive involvement than the roentgenogram suggests. Nodules of tumor are found in the intramedullary canal beyond the areas of obvious bone destruction. These tumors appear as grayish white, glistening nodules.

Microscopically, the characteristic lesion differs from that which Ewing originally described. The tumor appears as sheets of closely packed, dark-staining, rather uniform cells. There is very little cytoplasm and no clearly defined cell boundaries. The typical cell nucleus contains finely divided chromatin and is about twice the size of the nucelus of a lymphocyte. Vascularity is not the predominant picture. True rosettes are not seen in this lesion.

Differential Diagnosis

From the foregoing description, it is evident that the clinical picture may be confused with those of other more common diseases. Not infrequently, a patient with pain in an extremity, fever, leukocytosis, and a roentgenogram showing a destructive mottled lesion of bone may be considered to have osteomyelitis. Grossly at surgery, fluid-simulating pus may be seen surrounding a sequestrated portion of diaphysis. Microscopic examination may show tissue that suggests an abscess lining. Further research on the tissue may reveal the sheets of cells that are considered to characterize a

Fig. 15.35. Metastases to the lung from Ewing's sarcoma of the femur.

Ewing's sarcoma. The prognosis in these cases that resemble osteomyelitis seems universally poor.

Eosinophilic granuloma may present with the same clinical and roentgenographic changes as Ewing's sarcoma and must be included in the differential diagnosis.

Treatment

One of the characteristics of this tumor that was originally noted by Ewing is its very gratifying disappearance after roentgen therapy. He also noted that the lesion soon reappeared, if not in its original site, as a "metastasis" to another bone or in the lungs. Some report long term survivals following roentgen treatment of a single lesion, but these are exceptions. Surgical ablation, locally or by amputation, has not given any more satisfactory results. The combination of surgery and x-ray therapy has failed to increase the survival rate. At present the most universal treatment is roentgen therapy to the destructive lesion of the bone and to as much of the adjacent normal-appearing bone as possible.

Past experience amply documents the futility of radical amputation in this disease. Recently, the combination of supervoltage radiation in combination with *Vincristin* and cyclophosphamide has greatly improved the patient's chances of surviving this tumor. The role of the orthopaedic surgeon should be strictly limited to obtaining adequate biopsy material to permit accurate histologic diagnosis. Radical surgical procedures are no longer indicated in patients suffering from Ewing's sarcoma.

Course

The patient presenting originally with a single lesion receives dramatic relief from 3,000 to 4,000 R of x-radiation. Usually, the symptoms of persistent pain return within 6-12 months, and a second course of treatment gives much less relief, or none at all. It is not uncommon for the presenting lesion to remain quiescent, yet for the patient to expire from pulmonary metastases. Regardless of treatment, 95% of all patients with this disease succumb to it within 5 years.

References

1. Bardin, R. P.: Similarity of clinical and roentgen findings in children with Ewing's sarcoma and neuroblastoma, *Am. J. Roentgenol., 50:* 575, 1943.
2. Boyer, C. W., Jr., Barkner, T. J., and Perry, R. H.: Ewing's sarcoma; case against surgery, *Cancer, 20:* 1602, 1972.
3. Charpure, V. V.: Endothelial myeloma, *Am. J. Pathol., 17:* 503, 1941.
4. Coley, B. L., Higenbotham, N. L., and Bowden, L.: Endothelioma of bone, *Ann. Surg., 128:* 533, 1948.
5. Ewing, J.: Diffuse endothelioma of bone, *Proc. New York Pathol. Soc., 21:* 17, 1921.
6. Foote, F. W., Jr., and Anderson, H. R.: Histogenesis of Ewing's tumor, *Am. J. Pathol., 17:* 497, 1941.
7. Histo, H. O., Pinkel, D., and Prah, C. B.: Treatment of clinically localized Ewing's sarcoma with radiotherapy and combination chemotherapy, *Cancer, 30:* 1522, 1972.
8. Stout, A. P.: A discussion of the pathogenesis and histogenesis of Ewing's tumor, *Am. J. Roentgenol., 50:* 334, 1943.
9. Wang, C. C., and Schultz, M. D.: Ewing's sarcoma, *N. Engl. J. Med., 248:* 571, 1953.
10. Willis, R. A.: Metastatic neuroblastoma in bone presenting the Ewing syndrome, *Am. J. Pathol., 16:* 317, 1940.

Neuroblastoma

This tumor is derived from sympathetic formative cells. The primary tumor is, therefore, located wherever the sympathetic ganglia are found or in the suprarenal medulla. Neuroblastoma should be considered as an embryonal tumor in spite of the fact that it is seen in patients in the 2nd decade of life. In children less than 2 years old, it is usually confined to the thorax or abdomen. Such tumors are usually amenable to surgical ablation and x-ray therapy, and they give an appreciable survival rate. Neuroblastoma of this clinical type does not frequently metastasize to bone.

The orthopaedist is concerned with those cases of neuroblastoma in which the initial complaint is due to an osseous metastasis. Such cases are unusual before the age of 2 years and are most commonly seen between 5 and 15 years of age. Because of the retroperitoneal origin of neuroblastoma, it may give rather unusual complaints and findings. Ten cases in the literature simulated appendicitis closely enough to force an abdominal exploration, which revealed a large retroperitoneal tumor in the right iliac fossa. Neuroblastoma arising anterior to the sacroiliac joint may cause pain in the femoral nerve distribution or femoral nerve paralysis. The most common complaint, however, is the spontaneous onset of constant deep pain in the extremity, which is usually accompanied by swelling and is ultimately disabling.

The patient not infrequently presents with weight loss and fever, as if he were suffering from an infectious process. Laboratory data may support this impression by showing anemia, leukocytosis, and an elevated sedimentation rate. Gaffney[5] reported finding characteristic tumor cells in the bone marrow smears from 15 patients with neuroblastoma. In 13 of these 15 positive cases, the marrow smears contained tumor cells when the patients were first observed.

Roentgenographic examination of the osseous lesion reveals bone destruction and usually no bone reaction. The periosteum is soon elevated, and there is an adjacent soft-tissue mass. Some suggest that femoral lesions tend to be symmetric.

Microscopic examination of biopsy material shows a tumor composed of sheets of deep-staining cells of uniform size. These cells possess very little cytoplasm and no extracellular material. There are usually large areas of necrosis within the tumor. A supposedly characteristic microscopic finding is the presence of rosettes. These are circular collections

Fig. 15.36. Marrow smear from a child with metastatic neuroblastoma. Illustration shows neuroblastoma cells assuming a rosette-like arrangement. (From P. C. Gaffney, C. F. Hansman, and G. H. Fetterman: Experience with smears of aspirates from bone marrow in diagnosis of neuroblastoma, *American Journal of Clinical Pathology, 31:* 213, 1959.)

of tumor cells around a central collection of fibrils. They may not, however, be present in a metastasis of neuroblastoma or even in all of the primary lesion.

Treatment

Neuroblastoma of bone is a metastatic lesion that is usually sensitive to x-radiation. Because the osseous lesion is a metastasis, surgical ablation is not rewarding. After the administration of large doses of x-radiation (2,500-3,500 R) to the neuroblastoma, the tumor usually recedes only to recur locally or as another metastasis.

This tumor tends to metastasize to the skull, orbit, and maxilla, as well as to the lungs. The course is usually very rapid and ends fatally 6 months to 1 year after diagnosis.

Neuroblastoma is unique in its high rate of spontaneous regression, particularly in young infants. This phenonemon is seen more frequently in neuroblastoma than any other human cancer. Considerable investigative effort has been extended in attempting to define the role of the host-immune system in this disease. The concept of host suppression of tumor through the immune mechanism is supported by the positive correlation of lymphocyte infiltration of tumor with enhanced survival. Also important in the prognosis is the age of the patient (younger patients having the more favorable prognosis) and the presence of the primary lesion in the chest. Bone marrow involvement does not preclude survival but lytic bone disease usually has a fatal outcome. Although chemotherapy and radiation therapy are widely used in treatment of this disease, their role remains poorly defined.

Bodian[1] was enthusiastic about the arresting effect of vitamin B_{12} on the tumor. His enthusiasm has not been shared by others, for the most responsive cases occurred in the younger age group, in which the tumor has a good prognosis under surgical and radiation therapy also. A combination therapy of α-methopterin, actinomycin D, and Cytoxan is being used, and a new agent, Leuropristin, shows some promise. The nitrogen mustards have not been effective.

It should be evident from the foregoing description of Ewing's sarcoma and neuroblastoma—the onset, clinical and roentgenographic findings, pathologic description, and course—that these lesions are quite similar. Not infrequently it is impossible to distinguish between the two entities unless an autopsy is performed. The literature records that frequently a postmortem examination of a patient who dies of what seemed to be Ewing's sarcoma reveals a large retroperitoneal tumor that proves to be a neuroblastoma, and the original diagnosis is changed. At the Children's Hospital of Pittsburgh, there have been 45 diagnoses of neuroblastoma in the past 10 years. Twelve of these have been confirmed by autopsy. Ewing's sarcoma has been diagnosed in 15 patients, but none of these have been autopsied. For the arguments in favor of the opinion that these lesions differ, one should read Foote, Charpure, Lichtenstein, and Jaffe. Other authors believe that these two lesions are most frequently identical. The evidence in favor of this opinion is presented by Willis, Bardin, and Stout.

References

1. Bodian, M.: Neuroblastoma, *Pediatr. Clin. North Am., 6:* 449, 1959.
2. Charoche, H.: Neuroblastoma, *Am. J. Surg., 87:* 545, 1954.
3. Evans, A. E.: Treatment of neuroblastoma, *Cancer, 30:* 1695, 1972.
4. Farber, S.: Neuroblastoma, *Am. J. Dis. Child., 66:* 749, 1940.
5. Gaffney, P. C., Hansman, C. F., and Fetterman, G. H.: Experience with smears of aspirates from bone marrow in the diagnosis of neuroblastoma, *Am. J. Clin. Pathol., 31:* 213, 1959.
6. Hendren, W. H.: Pediatric surgery, *N. Engl. J. Med., 289:* 562, 1973.

Reticulum Cell Sarcoma

Reticulum cell sarcoma was distinguished as an entity by Parker and Jackson[2] in 1939. It is believed to be derived from the reticulum cells of the bone marrow and offers a more hopeful outlook than Ewing's sarcoma. Typically, the general condition of the patient is unaffected. The tumor has a tendency to remain localized to a single bone for a considerable time before it metatasizes to regional lymph nodes or distantly via the blood stream. The tumor ordinarily affects adults, but some cases have been seen in children.

The roentgenographic picture resembles that of Ewing's sarcoma somewhat, except that the reticulum cell sarcoma involves the metaphyseal area. It is osteolytic and tends to break out through the cortex on one side. There is little or no cortical or periosteal reaction. The tumor readily involves the epiphyseal region.

The tumor cell has a round or oval nucleus, approximately twice the size of a lymphocyte. It may be elongated or lobulated. There may

Fig. 15.37. Reticulum cell sarcoma.

be a fair amount of cytoplasm. Giant cells are not seen, but mitoses are present. A reticulum stain brings out strands running around areas of tumor cells.

The prognosis, if appropriate treatment is given, is apparently much better than in cases of Ewing's tumor. Treatment includes amputation or radical resection followed by roentgen therapy.

References

1. Francis, K. C., Higenbotham, N. L., and Caley, B. L.: Primary reticulum cell sarcoma of bone, *Surg. Gynecol. Obstet., 99:* 142: 1954.
2. Parker, F. Jr., and Jackson, H., Jr.: Primary reticulum cell sarcoma of bone *Surg. Gynecol. Obstet, 68:* 45, 1939.
3. Valls, J., Muscolo, D., and Schajowicz, F.: Reticulum cell sarcoma of bone, *J. Bone Joint Surg., 34B:* 588, 1952.

INDEX